DISEASES OF THE PANCREAS

Levan Maglakelidze

ALLIED
HEALTH
PRESS

Diseases of the Pancreas

Author: **Levan Maglakelidze**

Allied Health Press
4164 Lakeshore Road
Burlington ON L7L 1A4
Canada
www.alliedhealthpress.com
Email: orders@arclereducation.com

ISBN: 978-1-77956-802-1

ABOUT THE AUTHOR

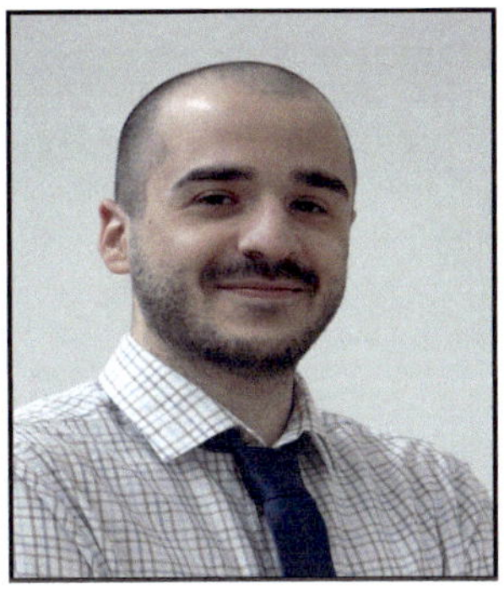

Levan Maglakelidze holds an M.D. from David Tvildiani Medical University, Tbilisi, with a clinical background in intensive care, cardiac and neurosurgical assistance, and psychiatry. He is currently working as a Research Study Coordinator at Evexi Clinic, Tbilisi, contributing to international clinical trials with organizations including ICON, Merck, and PPD. He also serves as an invited lecturer in American medical programs at the University of Georgia. His research interests include psychiatry, precision medicine, and medical data analysis. He holds a Good Clinical Practice (GCP) certificate obtained through his research work, and has previous experience as an ICU junior doctor, surgical assistant, and junior psychiatrist.

Brief Table of Contents

Detailed Table of Contents

CHAPTER 12

Pancreatic Neuroendocrine Tumors (PNETs) 375

CHAPTER 13

Metastatic and Rare Tumors of the Pancreas 411

CHAPTER 14

Trauma to the Pancreas 447

CHAPTER 15

Surgical Interventions in Pancreatic Diseases 481

Index 515

LIST OF FIGURES

PREFACE

The pancreas performs both digestive and endocrine functions, and thus its pathologies are difficult to manage. Its exocrine function is the release of enzymes required for the digestion of nutrients, whereas its endocrine function controls blood sugar levels by releasing insulin and glucagon. Inflammation, as seen in acute pancreatitis, intraglandular enzyme activation can result in tissue damage, systemic inflammatory responses, and, in extreme cases, distant organ failure. Chronic inflammation, as seen in chronic pancreatitis, usually leads to chronic pain, progressive exocrine tissue loss, malabsorption, and secondary diabetes, all of which have the potential to critically diminish the quality of life in the patient.

Pancreatic tumors have a wide range of behavioral and prognostic implications. Cystic neoplasms can be categorized as benign or with a high potential for malignant transformation, and accordingly, careful assessment of imaging features and cytologic analysis of the fluid is required. Pancreatic ductal adenocarcinoma is among the most aggressive malignancies seen in clinical practice, with early intrapancreatic spread and a tendency for metastasis. Neuroendocrine tumors, however, have a characteristic pattern, at times presenting with hormonal syndromes and characteristically following a slow growth behavior. Therapeutic success depends on precise diagnosis, proper staging, and individualized planning of treatment that can include endoscopic, surgical, or pharmacologic therapy.

Providers are asked to make subtle distinctions on cross-sectional images, navigate changing definitions of cystic lesions, and incorporate genetic information into individualized treatment regimens. Treatment strategies go well beyond pharmacotherapy to encompass endoscopic drainage, minimal-access surgery, and palliative care pathways. As investigations continue to advance, clinicians need an accurate integration of available evidence, best-practice guidelines, and emerging modalities to be able to maximize the outcomes for their patients.

This volume, *Diseases of the Pancreas*, has been constructed as an all-embracing reference for every professional engaged in the management, study, and treatment of pancreatic disease. It brings together contributions from gastroenterologists, surgeons, radiologists, pathologists, and oncologists to guarantee that each topic is considered from a number of professional viewpoints. The intention is to present the most up-to-date information in an understandable, ordered way to support both clinical and academic applications.

Chapter 1 provides a comprehensive description of the anatomy and physiology of the pancreas, including its embryonic development, vascular supply, ductal anatomy, and association between exocrine acini and islet cells. It is a prerequisite to the comprehension of the pathophysiologic processes of different disease states and proper interpretation of the diagnostic findings.

Chapter 2 covers diagnostic modalities, compiling the indications, sensitivities, and limitations of ultrasound, CT, MRI, endoscopic ultrasound, and new functional imaging modalities. Particular attention is given proper ordering of tests and standard reporting guidelines to maximize diagnostic accuracy.

Chapter 3 addresses the acute state of pancreatitis, starting with the etiologic etiology of gallstones and alcohol and then outlining autodigestion, systemic inflammatory response, and risk stratification measures. The management options—fluid resuscitation, nutrition, and indications for endoscopic or surgical procedures, are outlined in the context of recent clinical trials.

Chapter 4 is a discussion of chronic pancreatitis, including the spectrum of inflammatory alterations, pain management, the impact of pancreatic exocrine insufficiency, and alternatives to endocrine replacement. Both chapters also have case studies to demonstrate the practical use of guidelines developed.

Chapter 5 addresses pancreatic cystic neoplasms on imaging, separating serous, mucinous, and intraductal papillary lesions by imaging characteristics and potential for malignancy. Chapter 5 addresses the surveillance imaging protocols, guidelines for fine-needle aspiration, and the cyst fluid analysis role.

Chapter 6 concludes with histopathologic classification and molecular bases of these cystic tumors, correlating microscopic features to clinical behavior and therapeutic modalities, including indications for surgery and recommendations for prolonged follow-up.

Chapter 7 concludes autoimmune pancreatitis with diagnostic criteria, typical imaging features, serologic features, and corticosteroid response. Differentiation from pancreatic carcinoma is emphasized because there is a risk of misdiagnosis and unwarranted surgery.

Chapter 8 deals with pancreatic infection and abscess, describing patterns of microbial invasion, common pathogens, and suggestions for antibiotic choice, percutaneous drainage, or surgical debridement. New data on antimicrobial stewardship and resistance patterns are added.

Chapter 9 discusses pancreas pseudocysts, from their onset as acute fluid collections, indications for drainage, and endoscopic versus surgical drainage procedures. Follow-up methods to identify recurrence and complications are discussed.

Chapter 10 addresses congenital pancreatic abnormalities like annular pancreas, pancreatic divisum, and other developmental abnormalities by outlining their clinical presentation, diagnostic problems, and treatment modalities.

Chapter 11 covers pancreatic ductal adenocarcinoma, including tumor biology, staging systems, and multidisciplinary treatment approaches from neoadjuvant chemotherapy to advanced surgical resections. Quality-of-life issues and palliative care options are added.

Chapter 12 covers pancreatic neuroendocrine tumors (PNETs), functional versus nonfunctional, hormonal syndromes, and the newest in targeted therapies and peptide receptor radionuclide therapy.

Chapter 13 outlines metastatic and unusual pancreas tumors, such as metastatic renal cell carcinoma lesions and rare stromal tumors. Diagnostic methods and tailored treatment protocols are discussed.

Chapter 14 addresses trauma to the pancreas, penetrating and blunt, addressing diagnostic approaches, indications for operative versus nonoperative care, and late results.

In general, Chapter 15 addresses surgical management of pancreatic disease and offers a thorough review of classical operations such as the Whipple procedure, distal pancreatectomy, and newer minimally invasive surgery, as well as postoperative management and management of complications.

This book is intended for gastroenterologists and surgeons, who will appreciate practical tips on evidence-based practice. Radiologists and pathologists will appreciate the careful correlations between imaging and histology. Oncologists and internists will learn about the evolution of systemic treatments. Residents in all specialties will appreciate the use of clear descriptions, teaching case studies, and up-to-date references allowing for continued learning and clinical competence.

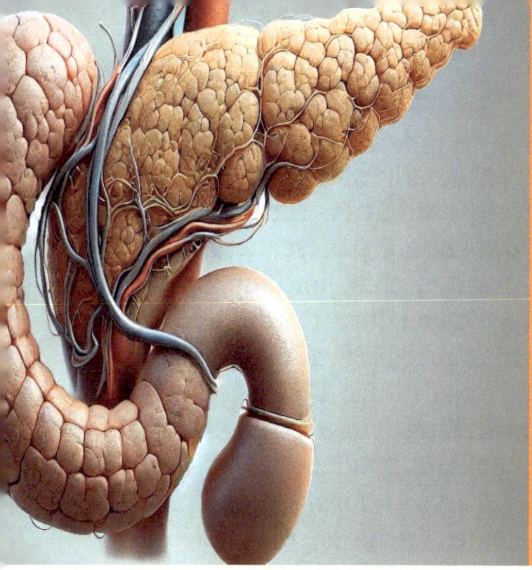

Chapter 1

ANATOMY AND PHYSIOLOGY OF THE PANCREAS

Contents

Introduction

Knowledge of the pancreas's anatomy and physiology is necessary for understanding its multi-faceted role in the human body. This organ plays not only a vital role in the digestive system but also a key role in the regulation of metabolism through hormone secretion. The pancreas is both an exocrine and an endocrine gland, a feature that enables it to secrete digestive enzymes into the small intestine and also release hormones like insulin and glucagon into the bloodstream. The dual role points to the sophistication of relationships between digestive processes and metabolic homeostasis, hence making the pancreas the central point of study for various disorders, such as diabetes and pancreatitis. Further examination of the physiological mechanisms of the pancreas uncovers complex regulatory pathways that ensure the maintenance of glucose levels within a very narrow range, vital for overall health. Insulin, secreted by beta cells in the islets of Langerhans, promotes the uptake of glucose into cells, hence reducing blood sugar levels. On the other hand, glucagon, secreted by alpha cells, increases blood glucose when levels become too low. This interaction between insulin and glucagon is the quintessential example of the dynamic process of metabolic regulation. In addition, recent research has identified the role that various signaling molecules play in influencing pancreatic function, indicating that the regulation of metabolism is much more complicated than initially thought. The coordination of these hormonal functions provides vital information into the homeostatic mechanisms the body uses to adjust to metabolic demands. In current research, the pancreas has been of great interest due to its role in various pathophysiological conditions. Diseases such as diabetes mellitus illustrate the consequence of pancreatic failure, making it crucial to study its anatomical and physiological features. Successful management and control of such diseases hinge on a thorough understanding of pancreatic secretions and the consequences of hormonal imbalance. Scientific investigations also continue to reveal new therapeutic strategies, including pharmacologic and regenerative therapies, to maintain normal pancreatic function. As new research uncovers previously underemphasized features of pancreatic biology, it enables the development of new strategies that potentially benefit patients. The urgent need for such developments underscores the importance of a thorough study of the anatomy and physiology of the pancreas, serving as a bridge between fundamental science and clinical medicine (Figure 1.1).

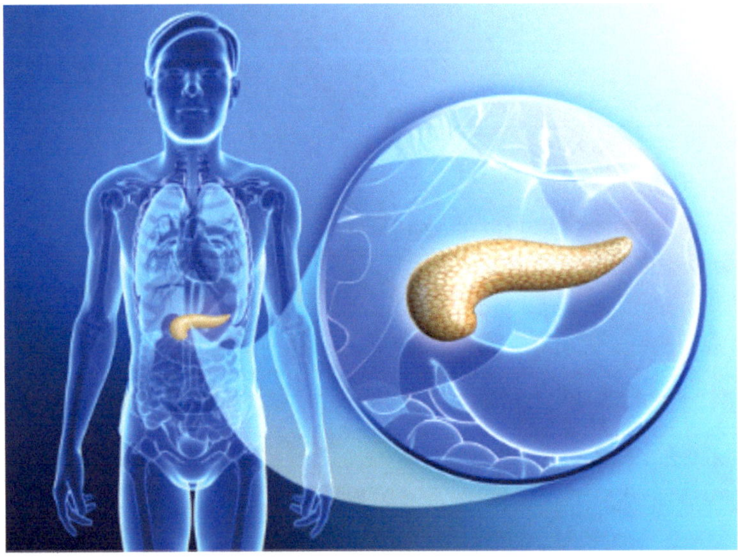

Figure 1.1. Pancreas.

Source: https://external-content.duckduckgo.com/iu/?u=https%3A%2F%2Fi0.wp.com%2Fcdn-prod.medicalnewstoday.com%2Fcontent%2Fimages%2Farticles%2F010%2F10011%2Fpancreas.jpg%3Fw%3D1155%26h%3D1692&f=1&nofb=1&ipt=4ee45104fac73eaa7947ac847a2c777dd4d9f18518b716811ab0c6e09d796a58.

Definition of the Pancreas

The pancreas is a vital organ that lies within the abdominal cavity, serving a dual purpose in the digestive and endocrine systems. Anatomically, it is shaped like a flattened pear, measuring about 6–10 inches long and lying horizontally along the posterior wall of the abdomen. This unique morphology allows it to be nestled comfortably between the stomach and duodenum, where it secretes digestive enzymes via the pancreatic duct. Functionally, the pancreas is divided into two main components: the exocrine and endocrine tissues. The exocrine portion is responsible for the production of digestive enzymes, which aid in the disintegration of proteins, carbohydrates, and fats in the small intestine. On the other hand, the endocrine portion secretes hormones like insulin and glucagon, which play a central role in the regulation of blood glucose levels. Therefore, the pancreas is a complex organ that plays a vital role in metabolic processes and digestion, and its importance in ensuring homeostasis within the organism is underscored. Aside from its anatomical and functional complexity, the pancreas is central to various physiological processes that are crucial for health. The exocrine activity of the organ involves the secretion of enzymes like amylase, lipase, and proteases, which are vital for the breakdown of macronutrients. By maximizing the digestive process, the pancreas ensures that nutrients are absorbed maximally in the intestine, thus fulfilling the body's energy requirements. At the same time, the hormonal secretion of the endocrine system, including insulin and glucagon, plays a central role in glucose metabolism. A delicate balance between these hormones is essential to prevent conditions like diabetes mellitus and hypoglycemia. Examining the complex interaction between the exocrine and endocrine functions demonstrates the pancreas's wide-ranging influence on physiological health and disease, underlining its obligatory role in both digestion and metabolic control. In addition, insulin metabolism regulation, a central part of pancreatic endocrine function, emphasizes the importance of this organ in systemic physiology. The selective secretion of insulin is triggered by an increase in blood glucose levels after a meal, thus promoting cellular glucose uptake and energetic homeostasis. Conversely, glucagon's function is to increase blood glucose levels under fasting conditions, which demonstrates the pancreas's involvement in energy balance and metabolic signaling. The complexity of this system is further enhanced by the integration of an object-oriented knowledge base related to insulin metabolism. This allows systematic comprehension of the different states and events of insulin secretion and its metabolic effects, ultimately leading to a comprehensive model that could facilitate future research and clinical interventions in diabetes management (Ensing et al., 1994). All in all, the pancreas is not just a digestive organ; it is an integral part of the intricate regulation of metabolism, influencing a wide range of physiological processes across the organism.

Importance of the Pancreas in the Human Body

The pancreas has a bifunctional role in the human body, acting as both an exocrine and endocrine gland at the same time. As an exocrine gland, it secretes digestive enzymes like amylase, lipase, and proteases, which are critical for carbohydrate, fat, and protein hydrolysis in the small intestine. Enzymatic activity is critical for nutrient absorption, thus enabling the body to efficiently utilize energy-rich substrates. The interaction between the anatomical structuring of the pancreas and its diversified functions is a testament to a refined design that underlies digestive physiology. The acinar cells, where enzymes are secreted, and the ductal cells, for the conveyance of pancreatic juice, are harmoniously interdependent to enable digestion to occur. The understanding of this functional role is at the core of understanding how defects in pancreatic function cause malabsorption disorders and nutritional deficiencies, thus placing the role of the organ at the master level of human health. In addition to its exocrine role, the pancreas plays a critical role in modulating blood glucose levels through the release of hormones, such as insulin and glucagon, from the islets of Langerhans. Insulin lowers blood glucose levels through cellular glucose uptake, whereas glucagon is involved in increasing blood sugar levels as a corrective response. This delicate balance is critical in ensuring homeostasis within the body, thus implicating the pancreas in metabolic processes critical to overall health. Aberrations in these hormonal processes can lead to severe conditions, such as diabetes mellitus, thus placing the role of the pancreas in endocrine regulation. The interplay between its hormonal and digestive function not only captures the complexity of pancreatic physiology but also the consequences when such systems break down. Therefore, it is indispensable to have a full understanding of these mechanisms for the treatment of metabolic disorders that could be induced by pancreatic malfunction. The anatomical structure of the pancreas also enhances its functional properties and clinical significance.

This gland is particularly noteworthy for being clearly composed of a diverse set of cell types that are involved in both its exocrine and endocrine functions, as indicated in research that investigates its embryonic and ontogenetic development. A scientific investigation of the pancreas confirms that its complex vascular supply and neuronal innervation are significant for the regulation of the secretion process and the preservation of overall well-being. As researchers delve deeper into pancreas physiology, they explain how normal and pathological processes are influenced by these structural features. This foundational knowledge is necessary for the formulation of medical knowledge and the creation of successful interventions for pancreatic illnesses such as pancreatitis and pancreatic cancer. The remarkable relationship between anatomy and function in the pancreas underscores its relevance in attaining human health and in the treatment of many diseases that could be triggered by its malfunction, as emphasized by recent studies on this subject (Dolenšek et al., 2017; Tonetti et al., 2017) (Figure 1.2).

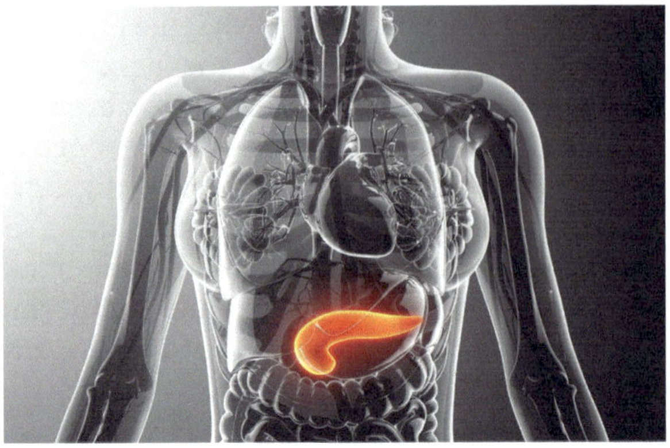

Figure 1.2. Pancreas in the human body.

Source: https://d33ljpvc0tflz5.cloudfront.net/dims3/MMH/1380ba5/2147483647/strip/true/crop/4564x2971+0+429/resize/1536x1000!/quality/75/?url=https:%2F%2Fd26ua9paks4zq.cloudfront.net%2Fda%2Fb9%2Fbaeabc3b4ad6b6678883c9e29b2e%2Fimage-getty-478189511.jpg.

1.1. Anatomy of the Pancreas

The pancreas, an important organ housed in the abdominal cavity, is responsible for numerous functions in the endocrine and exocrine systems. The pancreas is located dorsal to the stomach and is roughly six inches in length, with a flattened, pear-shaped morphology. The pancreas is anatomically divided into three regions: head, body, and tail, with the head housed in the duodenal curve. The organ is made up of acini, clusters of cells secreting digestive enzymes, and the islets of Langerhans, responsible for hormone production, such as insulin and glucagon. This arrangement is what enables the pancreas to efficiently carry out its dual role in digestion and metabolism regulation, making it an integral component of homeostasis maintenance in the body. An understanding of the pancreas's anatomy is imperative since it forms the basis of understanding its physiological processes and health-related implications. The endocrine roles of the pancreas are performed by the islets of Langerhans, responsible for only 1%–2% of the mass of the organ. These clusters of cells play a vital role in the regulation of glucose metabolism, secreting hormones regulating blood sugar levels. Of these hormones, insulin increases the uptake of glucose by cells for energy use or storage, and glucagon stimulates the release of glucose from the liver during fasting. The balance provided by these hormones is not only significant for energy regulation but also for overall metabolic wellness. Interruptions in this regulatory function, such as in diabetes mellitus, can have devastating health effects, thus making the thorough understanding of islet physiology and the anatomical basis that enables their function all the more significant. In addition, the pancreas is in close association with the lymphatic and blood vascular systems, which play an essential role in its development as well as physiological functions. Early reports suggested that lymphatic vessel formation and blood vessel formation take place at key periods of pancreatic organogenesis, determining their role in the provision of nutrients and regulation of immune response. As studied, the blood vessels along the peri-pancreatic mesenchyme are visible as early as gestation W9, supporting early pancreatic development, whereas lymphatic vessels start developing relatively late, indicating a coordinated growth process among the two vascular systems. Such detailed association not only preserves the these exocrine and endocrine functions but also lays the foundation for the development of therapeutic interventions for diabetes and other pancreatic diseases, since their successful management depends heavily on an intensive understanding of both vascular systems (Roost et al., 2014; Tonetti et al., 2017) (Figure 1.3).

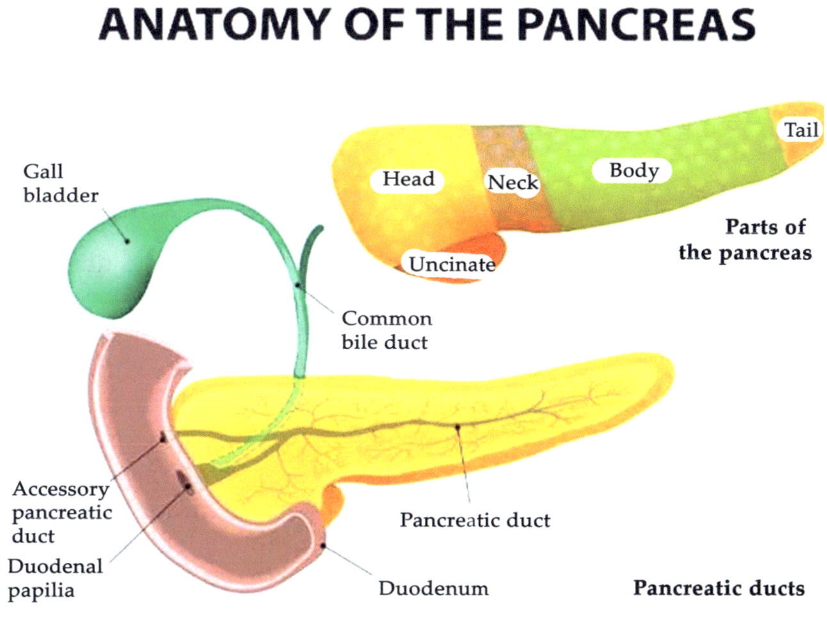

Figure 1.3. Anatomy of the pancreas.

Source: https://www.omicsonline.org/journal-highlight-images/pancreas-anatomy.jpg.

1.1.1. Location and Size of the Pancreas

The pancreas, an essential organ of the human body, is located in the posterior cavity of the abdomen in the retroperitoneal space, lying horizontally in its location. Located behind the stomach, it lies between the duodenum to the right and the spleen to the left. This posterior location allows the pancreas to efficiently perform its two functions in digestion and the regulation of the endocrine system. In terms of size, the typical pancreas is approximately 15–20 centimeters in length with an estimated weight of 70–100 grams. The pancreas anatomically is divided into four main parts: the head, neck, body, and tail. Each section has a corresponding function to the function of the organ, specifically the role of secreting digestive enzymes and hormones, in support of its function in the digestive and endocrine systems. The head of the pancreas is the widest part and is directly associated with the duodenum, from which it secretes into the pancreatic juices via the major duodenal papilla. Located next to the head is the thin neck, which is a transition to the body, the largest part of the pancreas. The body tapers towards the tail, which is located next to the spleen and may be hard to visualize using typical imaging modalities. The anatomical location of these sections allows for efficient secretory mechanisms and is a conduit for both exocrine and endocrine secretions. The close location of the pancreas to the major blood vessels, such as the splenic artery and vein, and its location with the biliary system further support the organ's integral function to the overall digestive system. Knowledge of the size and location of the pancreas is not merely significant for its physiological role but also for diagnosis and surgery. With its posterior position behind other organs in the abdomen, the pancreas may be inaccessible during surgery, making accurate anatomical information all the more necessary. Its size may also vary with disease processes like pancreatitis or pancreatic cancer, which may reflect underlying pathology. As emphasized in other anatomical references, including large laboratory manuals, the function of the pancreas in the human body is well established, demonstrating its complexity and central role in metabolic and digestive homeostasis (Horst et al., 1984; Beebe et al., 2019). The anatomical information forms the foundation for exploring the complex physiological processes of the pancreas in the latter sections of this essay.

1.1.2. Structure of the Pancreatic Tissue

The pancreas is an interesting organ, specially designed to carry out its dual role in exocrine and endocrine functions. Composed of discrete areas, pancreatic tissue is organized into the head, body, and tail, each of which contains clusters of specialized cells in their functions. The exocrine tissue constituting approximately 90% of the pancreas is organized into acini—small sac-like structures secreting digestive enzymes. The enzymes are transported along a complex network of ducts, flowing into the main pancreatic duct, which opens into the small intestine. Contrary to this, the endocrine component is concentrated in the islets of Langerhans. These islets, composed of mixed cell types such as alpha and beta cells, are dispersed throughout the pancreatic tissue, enabling efficient secretion of hormones into the blood supply, highlighting the organ's complex architecture and functional specialization. The vascular organization of the pancreatic tissue plays a crucial part in augmenting its physiological processes and regulation mechanisms. The blood vessels supply the necessary nutrients and oxygen, as well as enable the transportation of islet-secreted hormones. As early as gestation in nine weeks, research indicates that peri-pancreatic mesenchyme is composed of blood vessels and lymphatic vessels, indicating the complexity of vascular development in pancreatic organogenesis. Blood supply to the islets increases from approximately W14.5, indicating their increasing metabolic requirements. Interestingly, lymphatic vessels, which play a major role in immune response and fluid regulation, are restricted to the peri-pancreatic region until later developmental stages. The complex interaction between these vascular components illustrates their importance in the structural integrity as well as functional efficiency of the pancreatic tissue (Roost et al., 2014). Besides, the organization of pancreatic tissue closely resembles its developmental process, as highlighted in recent literature on angiogenesis and lymphangiogenesis. The formation of the blood and the lymphatic vessels during early development is paramount to the preservation of endocrine functions, as seen from weeks 17 to 22. This is not just the maturation of the islets but also their extensive vascularization to support effective release of the hormones. The sequential formation of lymphatic vessels, although initially limited to the peri-pancreatic mesenchyme, is a later expansion and maturation to support the pancreas structural requirements. These interrelations are at the core of developing regenerative therapies for diabetes and other pancreatic pathologies, as it informs the reader on how structural elements of the pancreas enable its functionality (Huang et al., 2016) (Figure 1.4).

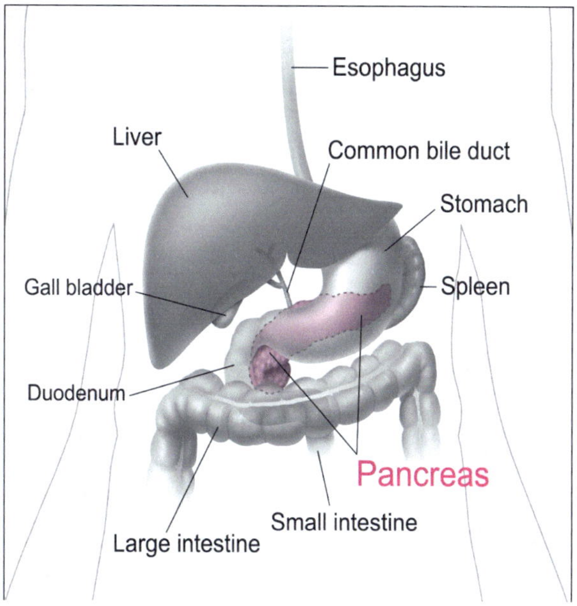

Figure 1.4. Structure of the pancreas. Pancreas tissue consists of both exocrine and endocrine glands.

Source: By Don Bliss (Illustrator) - This image was released by the National Cancer Institute, an agency part of the National Institutes of Health, with the ID 4363 (image) (next)., Public Domain, https://commons.wikimedia.org/w/index.php?curid=24052171

1.1.3. Major Anatomical Features (Head, Body, and Tail)

The pancreas is an essential organ with a unique anatomical structure comprising three major components: head, body, and tail. The head, which lies alongside the duodenum, is the widest part of the pancreas, lined with a protective layer of connective tissue. This part is important in the sense that it harbors major structures, such as the ampulla of Vater, where the pancreatic duct and bile duct join. The anatomy of the heads is beneficial for the maximum release of digestive enzymes into the small intestine, emphasizing its functional significance in the digestive system. Furthermore, the existence of pancreatic duct glands (PDGs) in this part of the pancreas is evidence of the complexity of the pancreatic structure, as the PDGs serve as progenitor niches and are involved in the organ's regenerative power, and most importantly, likely influences the anatomy and function of the head of the pancreas (Carpino et al., 2015). Transcending from the head to the body, the pancreas narrows and traverses obliquely across the posterior wall of the abdomen. This region is a mid-structure for enzymatic secretion and hormones, a smaller duct compared to the head. The body harbors acinar clusters responsible for secreting digestive enzymes such as lipase and amylase necessary for digestion in the small intestine. The body also harbors islet cells, which are central to endocrine function, regulating blood glucose levels through the secretion of insulin and glucagon. The anatomical structure within this part emphasizes the pancreas's dual role in exocrine and endocrine function, exhibiting an elevated level of integration of form and function necessary for homeostasis (Beebe et al., 2019). Lastly, the tail of the pancreas becomes narrower and tapers into the spleen, which is the end of the organs. Though the smallest portion, the tail is notable since it has an abundance of vascular structures and a more dense supply of islet cells than the rest of the parts. Being close to the spleen facilitates the exchange of blood and improves endocrine functions needed for the regulation of metabolism. Moreover, the anatomical characteristics of the tail enable it to help the overall health of the pathways involved in insulin secretion. Such associations demonstrate the intricacy of pancreatic anatomy since the unique features of the head, body, and tail are related to one another and play a part in the organ's important role in digestion and metabolism, thus proving the importance of appreciating these anatomical structures in the study of pancreatic physiology (Carpino et al., 2015).

1.2. Histology of the Pancreas

In histology studies of the pancreas, it is important to note the organ's dual nature, endocrine and exocrine. The pancreas is made up of acinar cells and islets of Langerhans, with acinar cells encompassing the exocrine component that secretes digestive enzymes and islets carrying the endocrine cells that secrete hormones, such as insulin and glucagon. Pancreatic acini histologically appear as pyramidal-shaped acinar cells covered by a basement membrane. The cells, which are packed with zymogen granules, engage in synthesizing and secreting digestive enzymes into the duodenum. The structural organization reflects the functional specialization of the pancreas and the pivotal role of histology in appreciating its physiological function. Investigation of the histological changes in the pancreas under pathological conditions further elucidates its functional capability. For instance, investigations on combined extracts of *Vernonia amygdalina* and *Gongronema latifolium* in diabetic models demonstrate the regenerative capability of the pancreas. With treatment in diabetic Wistar rats, there were hallmark histological changes observed in pancreatic β-cells, reflecting a regenerative action opposing the distortion and degeneration that is typical of diabetes (Akpaso et al., 2011). A significant increase in the proliferation of islet cells and a normalization of the surrounding exocrine tissue reflects the sensitivity of pancreatic histology to treatment. Such findings alert us to potential treatment of diabetes, contributing to our knowledge of pancreatic histopathology. Further, the development of the pancreatic vasculature is integral to its histological architecture and overall function. The formation of both blood and lymphatic vessels in the pancreas is pivotal to its endocrine function, particularly in supporting islet vascularization. During human development, blood vessels filled the peri-pancreatic mesenchyme by week 9, and lymphatic vessels began to appear a short while later (Roost et al., 2014). The complex relationship between the vascular networks is essential to the delivery of nutrients and removal of waste, and thus the significance of the comprehension of histological development within the context of pancreatic health and regenerative medicine. A deep understanding of these subtleties of pancreatic histology not only makes its physiology easier but also guides potential interventions for pancreatic disease (Figure 1.5).

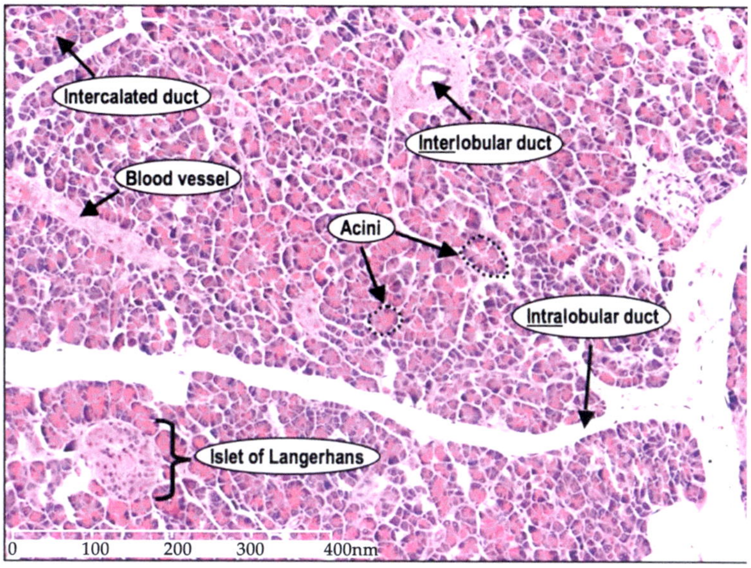

Figure 1.5. Histological structure of pancreas.

Source: https://image.slidesharecdn.com/histologicalstructureofpancreas-141010043222-conversion-gate01/95/histological-structure-of-pancreas-6-1024.jpg?cb=1412916677.

1.2.1. Types of Cells in the Pancreas

The pancreas is a vital organ with both exocrine as well as endocrine cells, each performing unique but related processes. The exocrine component is made up of acinar cells, which secrete pancreatic digestive enzymes critical to small intestine carbohydrate, protein, and fat digestion. The enzymes, including amylase, lipase, and proteases, are secreted into the pancreatic duct and ultimately into the gastrointestinal tract to enable digestion. The exocrine cells also secrete bicarbonate to neutralize gastric acid and provide an ideal environment for enzyme activity. This understanding of cell types and specialization highlights the role of the pancreas in digestion and underscores the organ's dual role in digestion and metabolism. In addition to the exocrine cells, the pancreas also contains the endocrine islets of Langerhans, which play a crucial role in regulating glucose homeostasis. The islets contain many distinct cell types, i.e., α-cells, β-cells, and δ-cells, each secreting different hormones. α-cells secrete glucagon, a hormone that raises blood glucose, and β-cells secrete insulin, which lowers blood glucose by stimulating cellular uptake. δ-cells secrete somatostatin, a regulatory hormone that suppresses the release of insulin and glucagon, thus fine-tuning the hormonal response to changing blood glucose. The delicate balance of these cell types is critical to metabolic health; malfunction, especially of insulin-secreting β-cells, can result in diseases such as diabetes mellitus, highlighting the significance of these specialized cells in the pancreas (Zhou et al., 2019). More recent research into pancreatic regenerative potential has also uncovered the role of pancreatic stellate cells (PSCs), which have been shown to possess the potential to differentiate into a range of different cell types, including insulin-secreting cells. Such versatility in cell type switching provides valuable insights into the potential for treating diabetes, as in observations that induction of other cells of the pancreas to adopt β-cell-like characteristics is a process by which functional insulin production can be restored. Significantly, the presence and role of PSCs in regeneration sheds light on their contribution to the expanded model of the role of the pancreatic cell. Furthermore, the physiological functions of the pancreas are necessarily linked to the vascular system, as shown by studies that illustrate the organ's endocrine functions are maintained by the blood and lymphatic vessels during development (Roost et al., 2014). This interaction is intended to illustrate the complexity of the pancreas and its cellular components with respect to the maintenance of metabolic homeostasis and pancreatic disease therapy (Figure 1.6).

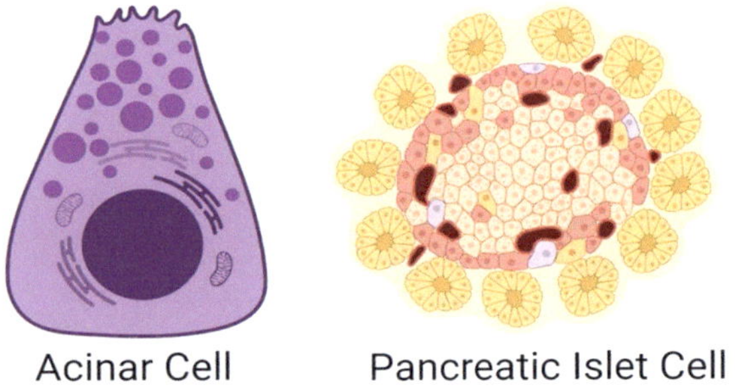

Figure 1.6. Pancreatic cells.

Source: https://external-content.duckduckgo.com/iu/?u=https%3A%2F%2Fmicrobenotes.com%2Fwp-content%2Fuploads%2F2024%2F04%2FTypes-of-Pancreatic-Cells-1024x536.jpeg&f=1&nofb=1&ipt=b03a44fa96e636fa2b53c5ddfaa0e49cbb248e1fae83c4c447a1c8f415afc16c.

1.2.2. Exocrine Versus Endocrine Functions

The pancreas possesses a singular dual role, an exocrine and endocrine organ, vital for global body homeostasis. The exocrine role of the pancreas is primarily the secretion of digestive enzymes, such as amylase, lipase, and proteases, which facilitate carbohydrate, lipid, and protein digestion in the small intestine. Acinar cells secrete these enzymes and release them into the pancreatic duct, which combines to form pancreatic juice and empties into the duodenum. Regulation of the process is tightly coordinated with a multitude of hormonal stimuli and neural inputs, amplifying acinar cell function during feeding. Moreover, the physiological regulation of this exocrine process is the foundation of understanding digestive health and the potential ramifications of pancreatic dysfunction, highlighting the pancreas's role in nutrient metabolism and absorption, as discussed in some physiological texts (Dolenšek et al., 2017). Alternatively, the endocrine role of the pancreas is primarily mediated by the islets of Langerhans, clusters of cells that secrete hormones into the circulation. The two primary hormones secreted by these cells, insulin and glucagon, play a critical role in the regulation of glucose homeostasis. Secretion of insulin from beta cells stimulates the uptake of glucose by tissues, thereby lowering blood sugar levels; secretion of glucagon from alpha cells stimulates glycogenolysis and gluconeogenesis by the liver, raising blood sugar levels as required. This homeostatic equilibrium between insulin and glucagon secretion illustrates the pancreas's critical role in metabolic control and energy balance. Disruption of this endocrine process leads to metabolic disease, and diabetes mellitus, illustrating the need for a comprehensive understanding of these hormone interactions in the overall context of pancreatic physiology (Norland et al., 2022). Additionally, interaction between the endocrine and exocrine components of the pancreas is required for the adaptability of the organs under varying physiological demands. For instance, the overproduction of insulin during states of excess nutrients for absorption and energy storage can be consistent with the excess secretion of digestive enzymes during such states. Moreover, during fasting or low-energy conditions, the exocrine secretion can be diminished as hormonal signals induce glucagon-induced processes for energy conservation. This symbiotic relationship illustrates the pancreas's integrated function in digestion and metabolic regulation. Understanding the anatomical and physiological complexities of these pancreatic functions is required for clinical relevance, particularly in the diagnosis and treatment of pancreatic diseases. Disease in one component may significantly affect the other, illustrating the complex nature of pancreas (Dolenšek et al., 2017) (Figure 1.7).

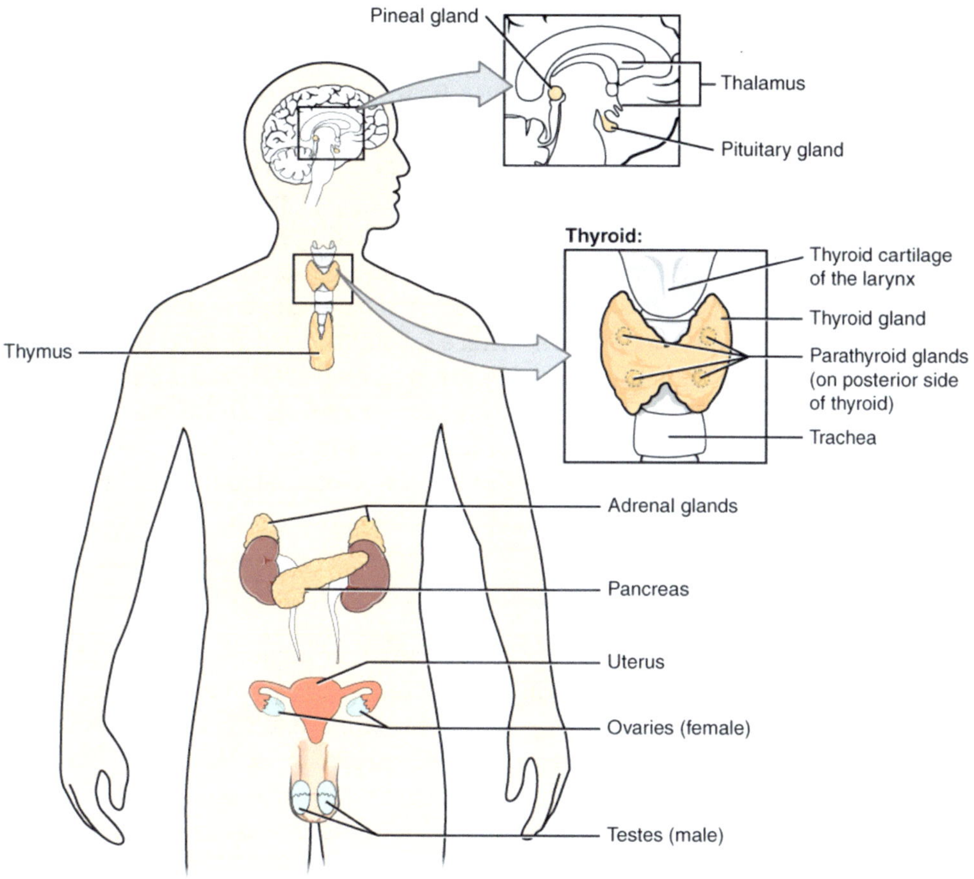

Figure 1.7. Exocrine pancreas versus endocrine pancreas.

Source: By OpenStax College - Anatomy & Physiology, Connexions Web site. http://cnx.org/content/col11496/1.6/, Jun 19, 2013., CC BY 3.0, https://commons.wikimedia.org/w/index.php?curid=30148133

1.2.3. Role of Pancreatic Ducts

Pancreatic ducts lie at the center of the exocrine function of the pancreas, essentially responsible for delivering digestive enzymes and bicarbonate into the duodenum. The main pancreatic duct, or duct of Wirsung, extends from the tail to the head of the gland and merges with the common bile duct before emptying into the duodenum via the ampulla of Vater. The strategic anatomical position ensures that pancreas secretions counterbalance bile from the liver to ensure an optimal digestive process. The ductal system's architecture, in the shape of a tree-like system of small ducts, ensures efficient passage of pancreatic juice, determining the overall effectiveness of nutrient absorption in the intestines. Understanding this structural pattern is key to deciphering the complex control mechanisms of enzyme secretion and regulation, serving as a foundation for the pancreas physiology (Dolenšek et al., 2017). Regulation of the exocrine secretion via the pancreatic ducts is highly regulated by both neural and hormonal stimuli. Pancreatic duct lining cells are specialized for bicarbonate excretion, which is critical in neutralizing gastric acid in the incoming chyme in the duodenum. This bicarbonate-enriched fluid, as well as digestive enzymes released from acinar cells, plays a significant role in supplying an optimal pH environment for effective enzymatic function. Hormones such as secretin and cholecystokinin play a critical role in modulating rates of excretion from ductal and acinar cells, indicating how highly integrated the hormonal control of pancreatic duct function is. Appreciations of these regulatory mechanisms emphasize the role of pancreatic ducts not just as passive conduits but as active contributors to digestive physiology (Dolenšek et al., 2017). Pathological mechanisms in pancreatic ducts have significant clinical implications, both on digestive function and health in general. For instance, mechanisms like pancreatitis or pancreatic duct obstruction can impede pancreatic juice transport, leading to raised ductal pressure and autodigestion of pancreatic tissue. Obstruction over a period of time can lead to complications such as steatorrhea, where fat malabsorption occurs due to the absence of digestive enzymes reaching the intestine. Research into ductal pathophysiology is essential, as it emphasizes the clinical relevance of duct dysfunction and its ability to lead to more diffuse digestive disease. Recognition of the role of pancreatic ducts in health and disease emphasizes the importance of complete understanding within the specialty of gastroenterology.

1.3. Endocrine Function of the Pancreas

The endocrine function of the pancreas is regulated primarily through clusters of cells named the islets of Langerhans. The islets contain several hormone-secreting cells including alpha cells, beta cells, delta cells, and PP cells that secrete glucagon, insulin, somatostatin, and pancreatic polypeptide, respectively. Among these, insulin and glucagon are of major importance in glucose homeostasis and metabolism. Insulin, secreted from beta cells, is responsible for glucose entry into tissues, while glucagon, secreted from alpha cells, counteracts the action of insulins by stimulating gluconeogenesis and glycogenolysis in the liver. This delicate balance of secretion keeps blood glucose within a narrow physiological range, indicative of the pancreas's central role in metabolic control as well as overall endocrine function. The coordination of pancreatic endocrine response is not only regulated by the hormonal signals but also by the intricate nervous system relationships. Thus, in particular, the autonomic nervous system controls pancreatic hormone secretion in accordance with physiological demands. The vagus nerve plays a special role, as it carries parasympathetic signals that stimulate insulin release during feeding, complementing nutrient utilization. On the other hand, sympathetic stimulation, mainly through thoracic spinal cord connections, can inhibit insulin release during stress, illustrating the close interaction of the nervous and endocrine systems in the maintenance of metabolic homeostasis. Experiments on the innervation of pancreatic islets suggest that some preganglionic fibers are resistant to disease damage like diabetes, illustrating the strength and resilience of these regulatory networks (Horst et al., 1984). New findings on pancreatic vasculature development, specifically lymph and blood vessel development, underscore the importance of these systems in the maintenance of endocrine functions of the pancreas. In embryonic development, studies have shown that blood and lymphatic vessels develop intricate networks around the islets of Langerhans, ensuring proper blood supply and delivery of nutrients for hormone production and release (Roost et al., 2014). The interconnection between vascularity and endocrine function highlights one critical area of pancreatic physiology where the supporting architecture is not just essential for function but also for future regenerative treatments for diseases such as diabetes. As we further elucidate pancreatic vascular development, it opens the door to new approaches to the restoration of insulin secretion and better management of metabolic disease (Figure 1.8).

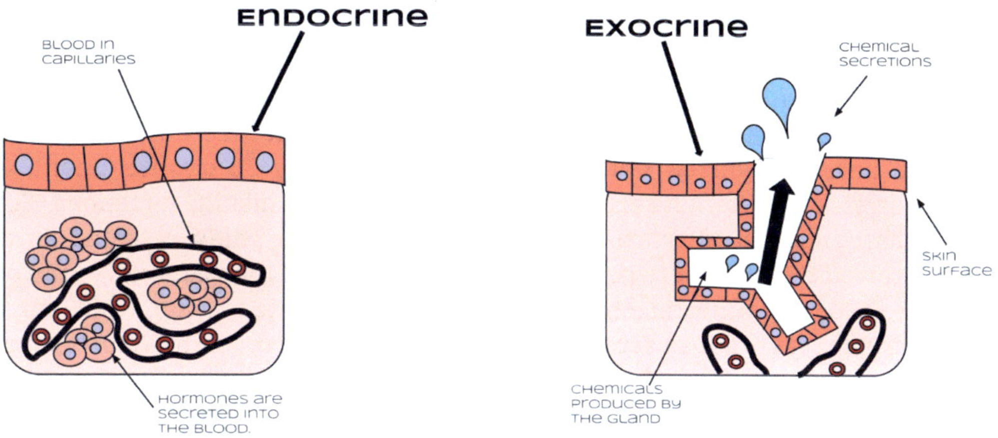

Figure 1.8. Endocrine and exocrine function of the human pancreas.

Source: By Mntrue15 - Own work, CC BY-SA 4.0, https://commons.wikimedia.org/w/index.php?curid=40658021

1.3.1. Hormones Produced by the Pancreas

The pancreas plays a crucial role in regulating metabolism through the secretion of a range of hormones from its endocrine activity, primarily the islets of Langerhans. Of these, insulin and glucagon play the most critical roles, with insulin mediating tissue uptake of glucose and glucagon mediating the release of glucose into the blood. The fine balance ensures the regulation of blood sugars, representative of the pancreas's crucial role in metabolic homeostasis. Derangement of the balance can lead to metabolic diseases such as diabetes mellitus, in which the fine balance between insulin and glucagon is lost. The function of the hormones is further supported by emerging insights that reveal profound interconnections between endocrine function and overall health, in particular when considering conditions such as pancreatic inflammation or trauma to exocrine and endocrine function, leading to resultant complications, such as type 3c diabetes, as well described by contemporary literature (Valente et al., 2024). In addition to insulin and glucagon, the pancreas secretes somatostatin and pancreatic polypeptide, adding a further dimension of regulation to the endocrine system. Somatostatin inhibits the secretion of insulin and glucagon, thus serving as a modulator that fine-tunes these hormone's effect on blood sugar levels. This multifaceted function underscores the pancreas's complex abilities in regulating energy balance in the body. Pancreatic polypeptide, primarily with regulation of gastric motility and exocrine secretion, reflects the pancreas functional dichotomy, as it interacts with its exocrine function to optimize digestive processes. In the larger context of the gastrointestinal tract, these hormones play a role in highlighting the function of the pancreas not only in metabolism but also in digestion, as outlined in the anatomy and physiology of the gastrointestinal tract (Burch et al., 2021). The function of the pancreatic hormones is an echo of a multicellular regulatory process that is well justified to ensure physiological homeostasis. Changes in the secretion of hormones can have significant metabolic consequences, thus stressing the need for maintaining pancreatic health. Advances in understanding the interrelationship of pancreatic function and metabolic disease have recognized potential avenues for the control of diabetes and exocrine pancreatic insufficiency. As researchers continue to explore the interrelationship between the hormonal processes and gastrointestinal health, it is evident that the pancreas is not an accessory organ but an integral member of both endocrine and exocrine systems. Further understanding of the pancreas functions and hormone secretion, therefore, may lead the way to improved diagnostic and therapeutic modalities for linked diseases, which is essential in the improvement of patient outcomes and the effective control of chronic disease (Valente et al., 2024).

1.3.2. Regulation of Blood Glucose Levels

Regulation of blood glucose levels is a critical physiological process emphasizing the pancreas's vital function in maintaining homeostasis. The pancreas is composed of clusters of cells known as the islets of Langerhans, which contain the hormone-secreting beta cells involved in the production of insulin. The primary function of insulin is to allow glucose to enter cells, thus lowering blood sugar levels following the intake of food. Conversely, during a decrease in blood glucose levels, pancreatic alpha cells secrete glucagon, a hormone that triggers the activation of glycogenolysis and gluconeogenesis by the liver, increasing blood glucose levels. This intricate interaction between insulin and glucagon demonstrates how the body can gain glucose homeostasis within a narrow physiological range of values in order to prevent both hyperglycemia and hypoglycemia. Recent studies on the role of the pancreas have enlightened extrapancreatic mechanisms involved in glucose regulation. For instance, studies have demonstrated the fact that combined extracts of *Vernonia amygdalina* and *Gongronema latifolium* could mimic the effect of insulins. In streptozotocin-induced diabetic Wistar rats, infusion of extracts resulted in a significant decrease in serum glucose levels following 28-day treatment, which was comparable to insulin injections. Surprisingly, the histological study revealed an impressive regeneration of the islet cells of the pancreas in the extract-treated group, which implies a new therapeutic approach to diabetes management that would complement current insulin treatment. Such findings emphasize the intricate nature of blood sugar regulation involving both hormonal and herbal components and can shed more light on diabetes therapy. Moreover, the body's ability to modify its glucose-regulating mechanisms depends on a wide range of factors, including diet, exercise, and stress.

Insulin sensitivity is the essence of the efficacy of tissue glucose metabolism, and lifestyle can be determinative in setting it. Exercise has been found to enhance insulin sensitivity, with increased glucose uptake and protection against the development of insulin resistance. In contrast, stress raised in the long term leads to elevated levels of cortisol, which can cause raised blood glucose through its effects to increase gluconeogenesis and block glucose entry into muscle and fat tissue. Knowledge of these mechanisms is fundamental to the creation of a complete set of interventions to maintain blood glucose within the normal range, particularly in those at risk of metabolic disease, and in reasserting the central role of lifestyle and pancreatic physiology in glucose homeostasis (Figure 1.9).

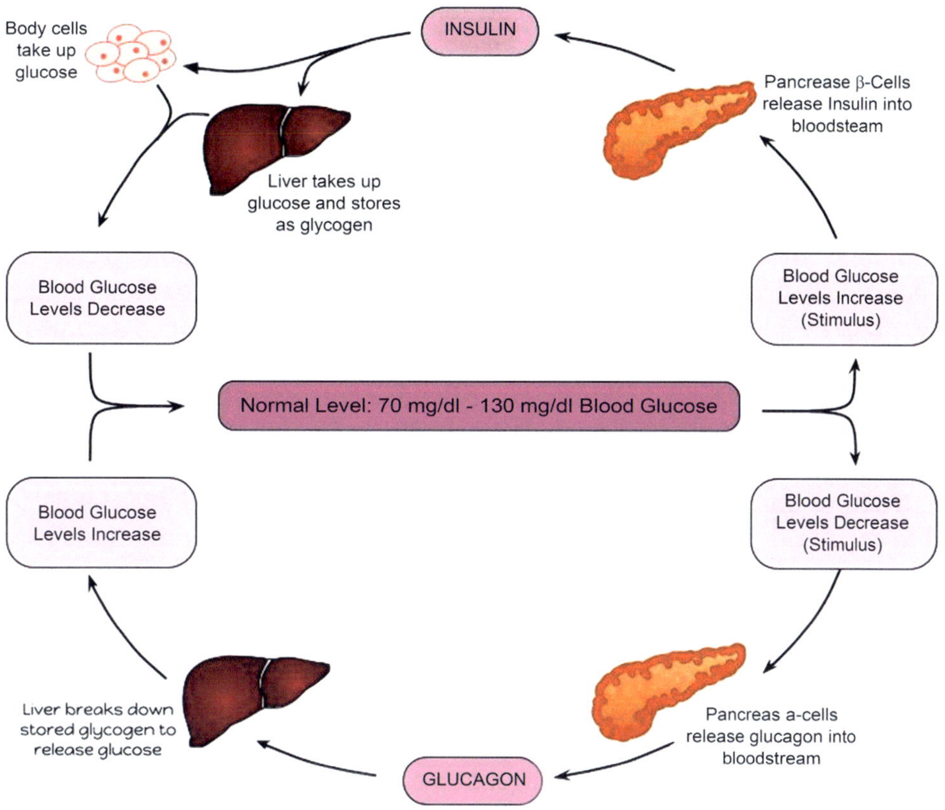

Figure 1.9. Regulation of blood glucose levels.

Source: By Carogonz11 - Own work, CC BY-SA 4.0, https://commons.wikimedia.org/w/index.php?curid=130403735

1.3.3. Impact of Endocrine Dysfunction (e.g., Diabetes)

The consequences of endocrine dysfunction, particularly diabetes, significantly alter the anatomy and physiology of the pancreas. In diabetic patients, the pancreatic islets, which secrete insulin, are exposed to various degrees of dysfunction. This is either through autoimmune destruction, as in the case of Type 1 diabetes, or through insulin resistance and consequent loss of beta-cells, which is characteristic of Type 2 diabetes. The consequences of the diseases do not stop at impaired glucose metabolism but extend to the structural integrity of the pancreas. Research has demonstrated that chronic hyperglycemia may trigger inflammatory processes and metabolic derangements within pancreatic tissues (Khan et al., 2024). These may, in the long run, lead to pancreatic fibrosis and disruption of islet architecture, further impairing the organs' capacity to regulate blood sugar balance. Identification of such morphologic alterations is crucial in informing therapeutic strategies and interventions in the treatment of diabetes. Even more importantly, endocrine dysfunction in diabetes has consequences on the overall physiological roles of the pancreas. Compromised insulin secretion not only affects glucose but may also compromise other important hormones, including glucagon and somatostatin. Dysfunction of these hormones further complicates metabolic derangements, leading to complications in the form of hyperglycemia and cardiovascular risk. Recent studies have demonstrated that surgical procedures, such as in the case of severe obesity and diabetes, may trigger morphological changes within the pancreatic tissue. For instance, short bowel syndrome models have recorded an impressive increase in the mass and size of pancreatic islets through beta-cell proliferation due to surgical alteration in the digestive tract (Pérez-Arana et al., 2015). Such observations underscore the plasticity of the pancreas under certain conditions, showing the interaction of surgical methods, regulation of hormones, and general pancreatic integrity. Additionally, diabetes management through pharmacologic treatment illustrates the complex interaction between the drug and pancreatic function. Recent data regarding simvastatin, a commonly prescribed cholesterol-lowering medication, have illustrated its significant influence on pancreatic histomorphology. Simvastatin administration in preclinical models has resulted in severe pancreatic inflammation and biochemical marker shifts, i.e., decreased serum amylase concentrations and elevated alkaline phosphatase concentrations (Khan et al., 2024). Such unwanted effects must be judiciously weighed, particularly in diabetic patients who are probably on multiple medications. The understanding of the interaction between pharmacologic treatments and pancreas structure and function can guide improved clinical practice and aid in the creation of therapies that maintain pancreatic integrity and treat endocrine dysfunction appropriately.

1.4. Exocrine Function of the Pancreas

The exocrine role of the pancreas plays a primary role in enabling efficient digestion, served primarily by the secretion of pancreatic juice. Pancreatic juices contain digestive enzymes like amylase, lipase, and proteases, which are responsible for the digestion of carbohydrate, fat, and protein, respectively. Secretion is prompted by the ingestion of food since availability of nutrients in the small intestine triggers a cascade of neural and hormonal events leading to the release of pancreatic fluid. The enzymes are secreted by specialized cells known as acinar cells and transported through a duct system to the duodenum. This intricate system demonstrates the character of pancreatic exocrine function in supplying nutrient absorption and metabolic balance of the body. Besides enzymes, pancreatic juices have high concentrations of bicarbonate, providing neutralization of gastric acid entering the small intestine. This is aimed at enabling optimal pH for enzyme function to ensure digestion processes are efficiently conducted. Research conducted by Mellanby and others has indicated that bile has the ability to stimulate secretions of pancreatic juice; however, it is not the principal stimulus for enzymatic secretion in all cases. Instead, pancreatic exocrine cell responsiveness to diet components continues to be the most significant determinant of volume and effectiveness of secretion. Additional research demonstrates varied responses to bile and suggests that effects could be dependent upon species and experimental conditions, as demonstrated by results of Ivy & Lueth and Thomas & Crider (Riepl et al., 1992). An understanding of dynamics of the exocrine pancreas also involves comprehension of interaction between its vascular systems, ensuring delivery of vital nutrients and hormones. Pancreatic blood and lymph vessel development is required to support its exocrine function. As per human pancreatic organogenesis research, angiogenesis and lymphangiogenesis are primordial events which are initiated early in gestation and are essential in order to provide pancreatic cells with proper blood supply and effectively remove waste products. Such vascularization supports the proper secretion and activity of pancreatic enzymes, which are essential for digestion. Thus, a complete understanding of the exocrine function of the pancreas should take into account such anatomical and physiological interactions (Roost et al., 2014) (Figure 1.10).

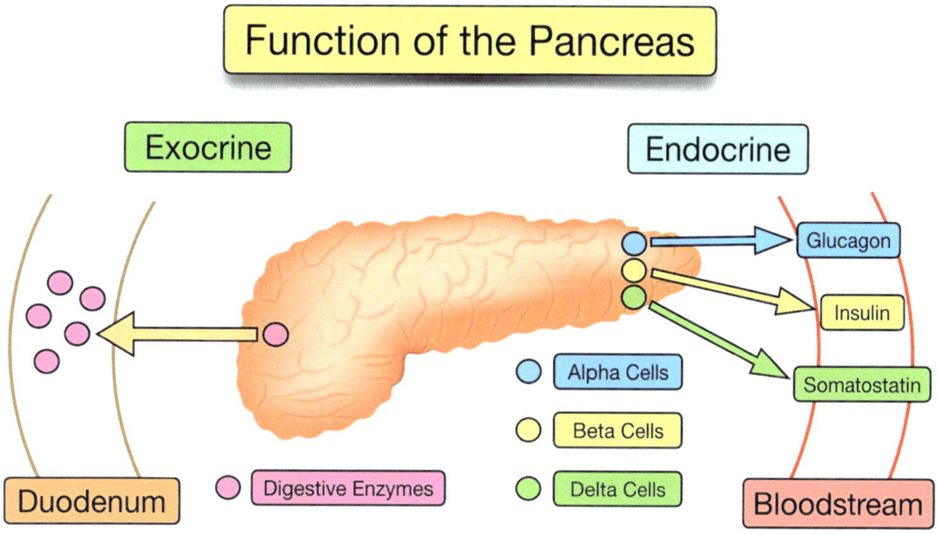

Figure 1.10. Function of the pancreas.

Source: https://external-content.duckduckgo.com/iu/?u=https%3A%2F%2Fimages.squarespace-cdn.com%2Fcontent%2Fv1%2F5e48489da899cd09424943db%2F3e1b4ea6-b4bd-441d-bbd7-29a8d6e3e1da%2Fpancreas-function-digestive-endocrine-insulin.jpeg&f=1&nofb=1&ipt=c4f1007 3dc59475abad2bf007162a33049b9ef70c9214dec45513244bc7bc274.

1.4.1. Production of Digestive Enzymes

The pancreas takes the lead in secreting digestive enzymes that hydrolyze the macromolecules into nutrients that are absorbed in the gastrointestinal tract. The organ uses specialized cells known as acinar cells for synthesizing and secreting enzymes into the gastrointestinal tract. The enzymes include amylase, lipase, and proteases. Amylase is used for the digestion of carbohydrates, lipase for fat digestion, and proteases like trypsin and chymotrypsin for protein digestion. The enzymes are secreted under tightly controlled conditions and mostly as a response to hormonal stimuli, like cholecystokinin (CCK) and secretin, released upon food entering the small intestine. The process ensures enzymes are activated at the optimal time and location to prevent premature digestion of the pancreas itself and permit optimal nutrient absorption in the next digestive cycle. The pancreatic enzymes function uniquely to ensure maximum efficiency in the emulsification and hydrolysis of complex food molecules. For instance, the action of bile salts secreted by the liver enables the action of lipase by emulsifying fats, which maximizes enzymic action on the surface. Each enzyme functions optimally at particular pH ranges; for instance, the proteolytic enzymes are optimal in alkaline conditions in the duodenum. Interestingly, research shows pancreatic function adjusts to dietary adaptations, displaying an evolutionary benefit under fluctuating feeding regimes. Developmental phases in other animals, such as the ballan wrasse, display the importance of digestive enzyme maturation as related to feeding habits, demonstrating how digestive potential evolution goes hand in hand with food availability (Norland et al., 2022). The ongoing action of digestive enzymes over changing environmental conditions demonstrates an impressive adaptive measure. For example, in certain bat species during winter, digestive enzymes like amylase and chitinases remain active even with compromised feeding opportunities. Such physiological adaptation allows for sporadic feeding, ensuring nutrient acquisition under conditions of scarcity (Maxinová et al., 2017). This shows the significance of digestive enzyme synthesis not only in nutrient assimilation but also in ecological stability in organisms. The proficiency with which the pancreas can synthesize and regulate such enzymes shows its role in maintaining overall metabolic health, nutrient homeostasis, and the ability of the organisms to withstand changing environments, ultimately showing its inherent role within the gastrointestinal system (Figure 1.11).

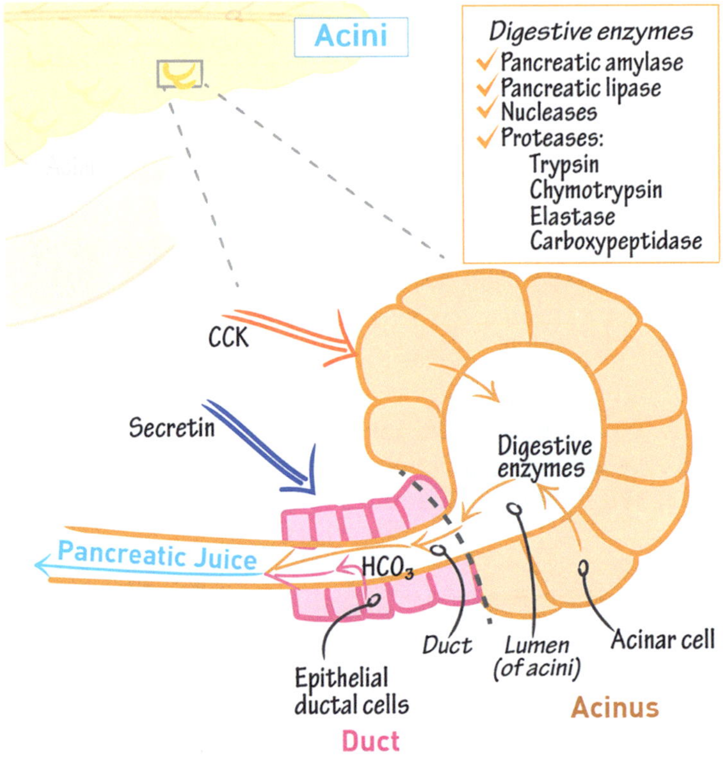

Figure 1.11. Production of digestive enzymes.

Source: https://gobudwig.com/wp-content/uploads/2021/05/1620-1528386266614-991x1024.png.

1.4.2. Role in Digestion and Nutrient Absorption

The pancreas plays a central role in the digestion and absorption of nutrients by virtue of its exocrine and endocrine dual functions. As an exocrine gland, it secretes a sequence of digestive enzymes, such as amylase, lipase, and proteases, which play a central role in the digestion of carbohydrates, fats, and proteins respectively. With the arrival of food in the duodenum, the pancreas secretes these enzymes into the intestinal lumen, where they promote digestion. Interestingly, as early as 1926, Mellanby demonstrated that the addition of bile to the duodenum elicits secretion of pancreatic juice, enhancing efficiency in digestion. The coordination of the pancreas with the biliary apparatus shows the significance of their combined role in eliciting stimulation of nutrient breakdown and absorption during digestion (Riepl et al., 1992). Besides the secretion of enzymes, the pancreas has the role of secreting bicarbonate ions, which neutralize gastric acid that finds its way to the small intestine. Neutralization plays a central role in creating an optimal pH environment for digestive enzymes to effectively carry out their roles. Without bicarbonate secretion, acidic contents from the stomach would interfere with enzymatic activity, thereby inhibiting digestion and nutrient absorption. Furthermore, controlled bicarbonate secretion is finely regulated by hormonal stimuli, such as secretin, in response to acidic chyme in the duodenum. This regulatory role demonstrates how the pancreas is not only charged with the secretion of digestive enzymes but also has a central role in ensuring physiological conditions for nutrient absorption (Hartoyo & Iriyanti, 2017). The role of the pancreas in digestion is even more critical when the complex interplay of its secretions with gut microbiota and food components is considered. It has been identified through research that the content of pancreatic juice can be determined by dietary compounds, thereby impacting gut health as well as the presence of nutrients. To illustrate, synbiotic application in animal feed has proven to be influential on the process of digestion as well as on gastrointestinal health, but research has shown that some levels have little effect on organ weight or efficiency of nutrient processing (Hartoyo & Iriyanti, 2017). This interaction showcases the interactive nature of the digestive system and emphasizes the pancreas's central role of enabling not just the chemical digestion of food, but the subsequent absorption of vital nutrients, leading to overall wellness and health.

1.4.3. Disorders Related to Exocrine Function (e.g., Pancreatitis)

Exocrine pancreas disorders, including pancreatitis, are daunting clinical problems and highlight the paramount role of this organ in the maintenance of digestive health. Pancreatitis can conveniently be categorized into two broad categories, acute and chronic. Acute pancreatitis is classically heralded by acute abdominal pain, nausea, and vomiting, secondary to pancreatitis, and may be caused by etiologies such as gallstones or alcohol binge. The pathophysiology is marked by premature activation of digestive enzymes within the pancreas, with resultant autodigestion and destruction of the tissue. Chronic pancreatitis is marked by progressive fibrosis and ductal obstruction, usually secondary to chronic alcoholism or hereditary etiologies, and can result in permanent damage and loss of exocrine function. These disorders not only impair digestion but can also profoundly impair metabolic processes, highlighting the pancreas's multifaceted role in the maintenance of health. Recent literature highlights the role of pancreas transplantation as an emerging treatment modality for disorders of exocrine function, especially in situations where standard management is suboptimal. Pancreas transplantation has been reported to have good outcomes in the restoration of endocrine and exocrine function, especially for patients with chronic pancreatitis or cystic fibrosis, from literature. With advances in surgical technique and immunosuppressive regimens, the success rates of these operations have improved appreciably in the last decade. Patients with pancreas transplantation for exocrine disorders have comparable survival rates to those with diabetes mellitus, attesting to the effectiveness of this intervention in improving quality of life and restoring critical body functions. Nevertheless, cautious attention to operative risk and the subtleties of long-term immunosuppression remain key to transplant decision-making and underscore the importance of intensive patient education and support. Furthermore, there is a growing body of evidence to suggest that the inter-relationship between exocrine dysfunction and neonatal health needs to be the focus of future research endeavors. For instance, research into pancreatic function in full-term neonates with perinatal pathology has demonstrated gross changes in exocrine secretory function and neonatal hypoxia is postulated as a causative agent in subsequent gastrointestinal disease. The research demonstrated differential enzyme activity, such as amylase and lipase activity, with the result in respect to the severity of the perinatal pathology. Such evidence points to the susceptibility of the pancreas in early life and questions long-term consequences for gastrointestinal function in affected infants. Resolution of these matters by early identification and intervention may be able to minimize the risk of chronic pancreatic disease, and an integrated approach to neonatal management and follow-up in at-risk populations is thus emphasized (Kuryk et al., 2024) (Figure 1.12).

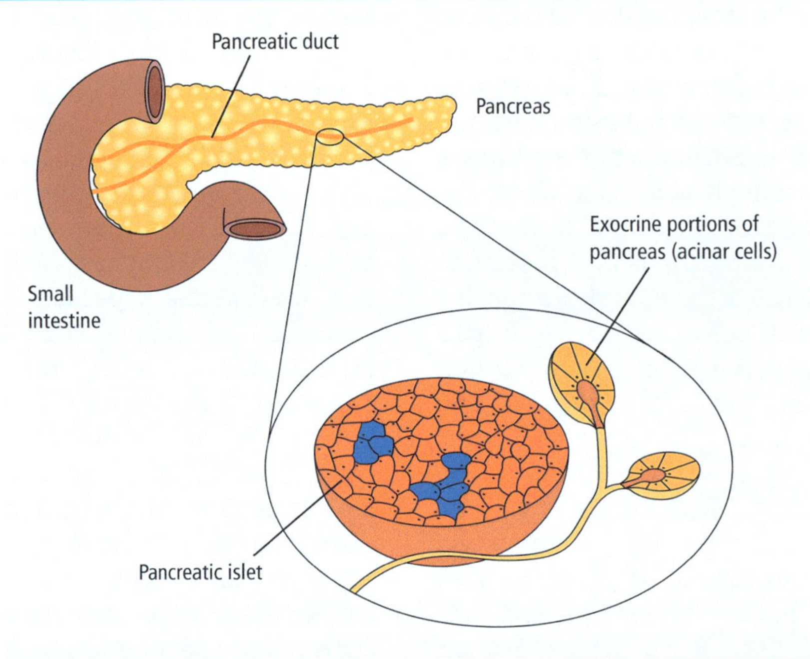

Figure 1.12. Pancreatic exocrine dysfunction.

Source: https://wchh.onlinelibrary.wiley.com/cms/asset/5e46eba5-15ee-453b-bed5-ee5ed187a1c2/pdi2118-fig-0001-m.jpg.

1.5. Blood Supply and Innervation

The pancreas, an extremely vital organ in the human body, has a rich blood supply and complex innervation that is critical to its functioning and regulation. The organ is richly vascularized, with blood being provided by the splenic artery, gastroduodenal artery, and superior mesenteric artery. The extensive blood supply is not only beneficial in the provision of blood supply to the pancreatic tissue but also in the provision of hormones and enzymes into the blood. Besides this, blood vessel organization within the pancreas is associated with functional anatomy, ensuring exocrine and endocrine elements are perfused optimally. The unique vascular organization ensures the optimal exchange of nutrients and metabolic by-products, crucial in maintaining the homeostasis and overall physiological function, as described in pancreas physiology literature (Dolenšek et al., 2017). Pancreatic innervation is an important determinant of functional integrity, controlling the balance of hormonal release through complex neural circuits. The autonomic nervous system, comprising sympathetic and parasympathetic fibers, plays a very crucial role in the modulation of pancreatic function. While sympathetic nerves modulate the majority of blood flow into the gland by innervating the vascular smooth muscle, parasympathetic innervation is critical to stimulate the secretion of digestive enzymes. Interestingly, current research reveals a difference in human and murine islet biology, including patterns of innervation, suggesting that human islets are less dependent on cholinergic input than their murine counterparts. It suggests that the functional role of neural regulation and vascular interactions is highlighted by species-specific features, modifying our understanding of pancreatic physiology (Rodriguez-Diaz et al., 2012). An appreciation of the relationship between innervation and blood supply to the pancreas is of great importance for physiology and disease. Conditions such as diabetes mellitus readily demonstrate the implications of altered pancreatic function controlled by vascular and nervous factors. The Langerhans islets with endocrine cells responsible for the secretion of hormones are supplied with a specialized blood supply strictly controlled to ensure sufficient release of hormones into the systemic circulation. The converse relationship with neural signals, in contrast, implies that a changed innervation could result in ineffective glucose regulation and amplify diseases such as diabetes. Recent research demonstrates the role of vascular and neural interactions in the islets and suggests that therapies aimed at these mechanisms may be of particular importance in normalizing diabetic patients' function (Dolenšek et al., 2017). As advances in technology and knowledge develop, the explanation of these mechanisms will enhance our understanding of the pancreas function in diabetes and the regulation of metabolism (Figure 1.13).

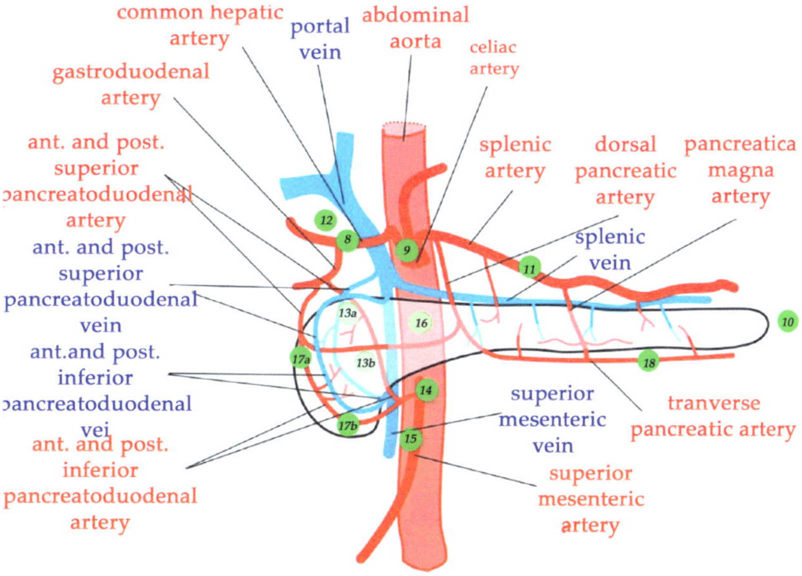

Figure 1.13. Pancreas blood supply anatomy.

Source: Dolenšek J, Pohorec V, Rupnik MS, Stožer A. Pancreas Physiology [Internet]. Challenges in Pancreatic Pathology. InTech; 2017. Available from: http://dx.doi.org/10.5772/65895s

1.5.1. Vascular Supply to the Pancreas

The vascular supply of the pancreas is critical to its complex functions, exocrine and endocrine. The major arterial supply is provided by branches of the celiac trunk and the superior mesenteric artery, with a special role played by the splenic artery. As these arteries divide, they offer a double supply of blood to the head and the body of the pancreas. In particular, the pancreaticoduodenal arteries, a branch of the gastroduodenal artery, supply the head and the anterior segment of the pancreas. This double supply by the celiac trunk and the superior mesenteric artery delivers nutrients and removes waste products efficiently, sustaining the metabolic activity of the organ. Familiarity with this vascular pattern also helps us to understand the pancreas physiological functions and points to its susceptibility to vascular-related pathological processes (Dolenšek et al., 2017). Apart from arterial supply, venous drainage also plays a vital role in the vascular anatomy of the pancreas. Venous blood is drained by the splenic vein and the superior mesenteric vein, which finally drains into the hepatic portal vein. This pattern ensures that pancreatic digestion products are carried well to the liver for processing before distribution into the systemic circulation. The intricate venous network is a support system to the arterial supply, pointing to the role of hemodynamics in ensuring the well-being of the pancreas. Interference with this vascular drainage system has dire consequences, such as pancreatitis or the development of varices. The venous system is thus not a passive organ but an active player in the overall function of the pancreas and the regulation of metabolic load (Gerussi et al., 2024). Furthermore, the reliance of vascular supply on pancreatic function is emphasized by the organs autoregulatory mechanisms. Pancreatic blood supply is able to compensate to meet metabolism demand, with the potential for enhanced perfusion during digestive activity when maximum enzyme secretion is present. This autoregulation is crucial for both exocrine activities, involving high volumes of blood flow for digestive enzyme secretion, and endocrine activities, particularly the secretion of hormones like insulin and glucagon from the islets of Langerhans. Through these processes, researchers can make use of therapeutic solutions that account for conditions like pancreatic insufficiency and diabetes, where vascular supply is impacted. Knowledge of the vascular network provides valuable information regarding the complexity of the pancreas anatomy and physiology, positioning the organ to take its place in the sphere of importance in metabolic regulation and digestive function (Dolenšek et al., 2017) (Figure 1.14).

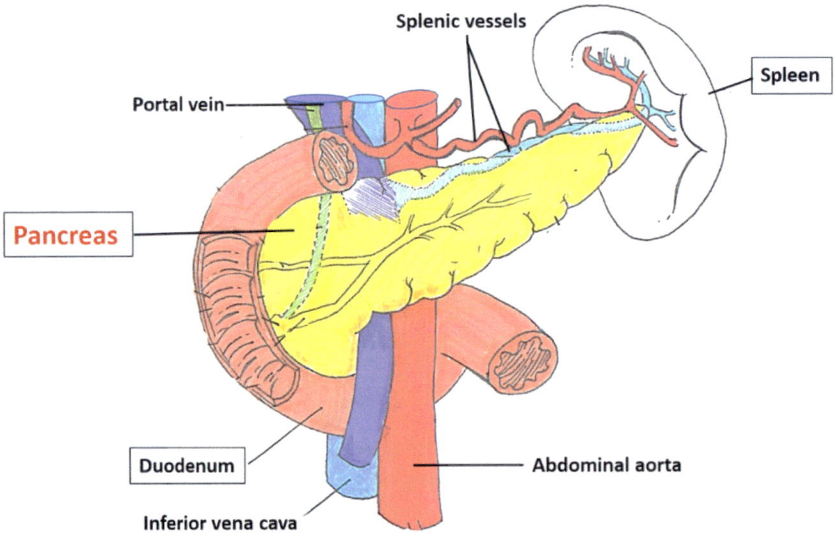

Figure 1.14. Vascular supply to the pancreas.

Source: https://www.anatomyqa.com/wp-content/uploads/2017/05/location-of-pancreas.png.

1.5.2. Nerve Supply and Its Significance

The pancreas, a highly complex organ of the abdominal cavity, is extensively innervated by nerves that play a key role in its physiological function. The innervation of the pancreas is primarily from the autonomic nervous system, consisting of sympathetic and parasympathetic fibers. The fibers regulate pancreas functions, including the secretion of digestive enzymes and hormones. The sympathetic fibers originate from the celiac plexus, inhibiting the secretion of glucagon and insulin, thus having a regulatory effect on blood glucose. Conversely, the parasympathetic fibers, primarily of vagus nerve origin, activate pancreatic secretions required for digestion. The double innervation creates the central balance achieved by the nervous system depending on physiological demand, with a focus on the role of nerve supply in pancreas function (Dolenšek et al., 2017). The significance of nerve supply goes beyond the anatomical importance; it highlights how nerve tracts have an effect not just on pancreatic function but also on overall metabolic homeostasis. Changes in these nerve tracts can lead to profound physiological consequences, such as defective insulin secretion, a feature of diseases like diabetes mellitus. Because the pancreas is responsive to neural stimulation, it modulates its secretion of insulin and glucagon to maintain glucose homeostasis. Dysregulation of this nerve connection may lead to metabolic disease. Therefore, neuroanatomy and physiology must be considered in an integrated manner, allowing for a greater understanding of how and why pancreatic function is disrupted in disease states. This interconnectedness sets the central position of nerve supply in the maintenance of metabolic balance and sets the stage for potential therapeutic interventions in the management of pancreatic dysfunction (Porro & Richards, 2017). Besides, the significance of nerve supply to the pancreas is further demonstrated in the context of stress response. Stress induces the sympathetic nervous system to cause the release of catecholamines, which consequently inhibit the release of insulin, hence stimulating glycogenolysis, a function significant in the increase of blood glucose levels. This physiological response demonstrates the pancreas function as not just a digestive organ but also a significant aspect of the general response of the body to stress. Clinical evidence has also demonstrated that chronic stress can induce dysregulations in the functioning of the pancreas, and hence the significance of the concept of nerve supply in health and disease. Implications of treatment extend beyond the treatment of pancreatic disease to the general interplay of nerve signaling in the adaptive response of the body to external insult. The intricate interaction of the pancreas and its nerve supply thus becomes significant in the maintenance of systemic homeostasis and points to the complex function of the organ in human physiology (Dolenšek et al., 2017).

1.5.3. Interaction with the Autonomic Nervous System (ANS)

The pancreas, a central organ in the regulatory metabolic homeostasis, demonstrates a multifaceted interaction with the ANS and plays a central role in its functioning. The autonomic nervous system consists of the sympathetic and parasympathetic divisions, both of which innervate the pancreas to control its endocrine and exocrine functions. This intricate neural interaction plays a central role in controlling the secretion of hormones, such as insulin and glucagon, which play a crucial role in the metabolism of glucose. The research shows that the sympathetic fibers play an important regulatory function in the blood perfusion to the islets of Langerhans, controlling the secretion of hormones into the circulation, and the parasympathetic fibers are more involved in the triggering of insulin release in response to states of nutrient consumption. This double innervation indicates the sensitivity of the pancreas to the state of body metabolism and its dependence on the ANS for the optimal physiological regulation (Proshchina et al., 2018). The interaction between pancreatic function and autonomic nervous activity becomes more significant in the context of several metabolic diseases. For instance, diabetes mellitus, the failure of the pancreas to effectively control insulin levels may lead to severe health diseases. Research shows human pancreatic islets have diverse innervation patterns compared to mice, and this may indicate a probable difference in their functional dynamics. Human islets are less responsive to direct parasympathetic input, as they can secrete acetylcholine as a paracrine signal to control their response to elevated glucose levels, indicating a complex interaction between the local and systemic mechanisms of signaling (Rodriguez-Diaz et al., 2012). These findings indicate the manner in which autonomic differences in innervation may influence diseases such as diabetes, possibly altering therapeutic interventions to normalize pancreatic function. Knowledge of the interaction of the autonomic nervous system with the pancreas provides insightful information about the organ's physiology and its participation in metabolic derangements. Research on the reinnervation process of islet grafts and vascularization emphasizes the ANS's involvement in functional recovery following transplantation. As shown with experiments on the use of cutting-edge imaging platforms, the neural input during engrafting is critical for the restoration of the islets microenvironment, implying that autonomic signaling is required for ideal function (Proshchina et al., 2018). This not only emphasizes the need for further research on how autonomic influences shape the endocrine topography of the pancreas but also suggests potential clinical applications, primarily in the creation of targeted therapies for diabetes and other related diseases, that rely on the intricate interaction of neural and hormonal interactions in pancreatic physiology.

1.6. Clinical Significance of the Pancreas

The pancreas is a central organ of both the exocrine and endocrine systems with profound implications for digestive and metabolic functions. As an endocrine organ, the pancreas regulates blood glucose levels via the excretion of hormones such as insulin and glucagon, illustrating how pancreatic dysfunction results in diseases such as diabetes mellitus. As an exocrine organ, its function is the secretion of digestive enzymes such as amylase, lipase, and proteases, respectively, involved in carbohydrate, fat, and protein digestion. It is paramount to appreciate the diverse functions and clinical implications of the pancreas in disease management for pancreatic impairment, and therefore the rationale for ongoing research and medical education within the field. The intricate interaction of these functions warrants the clinical significance of the pancreas as a central organ with implications for not only individual health outcomes but also public health concerns such as metabolic disorders. Pancreatic dysfunction clinically results in numerous pathologies such as pancreatitis, pancreatic cancer, and diabetes, each varying in complexity in diagnosis and management. For instance, acute pancreatitis is typically induced by gallstones or chronic alcoholism, leading to inflammation destroying exocrine and endocrine functions. Research such as that illustrated in Khan et al. (2024) illustrates how pharmacological agents such as simvastatin induce pancreatic inflammation, illustrating the rationale for the appreciation of drug interactions and side effects that affect pancreatic function. Also, pancreatic cancer is extremely insidious, with the tendency to present late in the stages of the disease due to initial nonspecific symptoms. Early screening and appreciation of risk factors are paramount in optimizing patient outcomes, further illustrating the rationale for an appreciation of pancreatic anatomy and physiology in the clinical arena. Integration of sex- and gender-based medicine (SGBM) into pancreatic health clinical expertise enhances patient-centered care essential for optimal treatment. Evidence has shown striking contrasts in the presentation and course of pancreatic disease according to sex- and gender-related factors, as identified in the results of Ludwig et al. (2020). This informs decisions on more personalized treatment plans, enhancing therapeutic outcomes and patient satisfaction. Aside from that, awareness of the underrepresentation of sociocultural factors in medical school curricula can enhance healthcare professionals' capacity to address the heterogeneity of their patients' needs. Overall, clinical relevance of the pancreas extends beyond its anatomical and physiological roles since future developments in research and educational programs will shape the future of pancreatic health as well as its influence on global health outcomes (Figure 1.15).

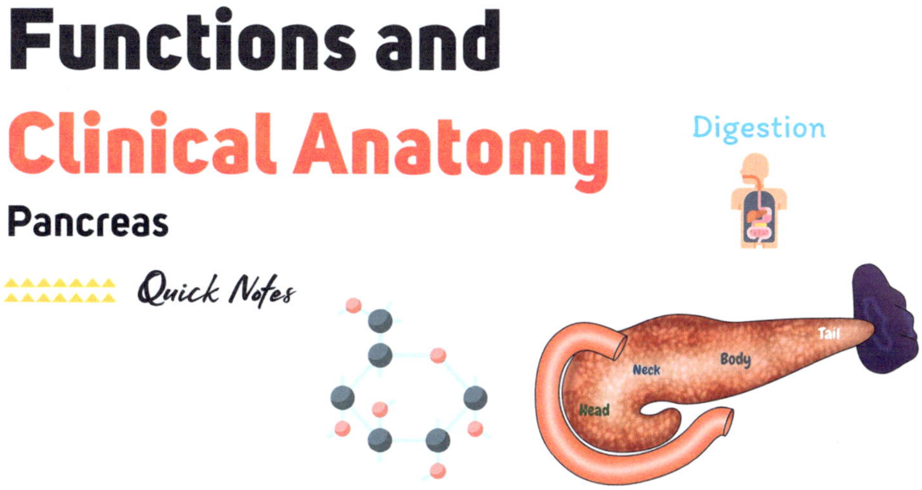

Figure 1.15. Functions-and-clinical-anatomy of pancreas.

Source: https://alpha.uscreencdn.com/assets/621/player_image/2007422/221219-QN-04-Functions-and-Clinical-Anatomy-PLAYER.1671640331.jpg.

1.6.1. Common Diseases Affecting the Pancreas

The pancreas is a critical organ of the digestive and endocrine system, and thus is susceptible to a wide range of diseases, the most common among them are pancreatitis, diabetes mellitus, and pancreatic cancer. Acute pancreatitis with acute inflammation of the pancreas is usually due to gallstones or alcohol. The signs and symptoms are acute abdominal pain, nausea, and vomiting, and thus need immediate medical attention. Conversely, chronic pancreatitis is due to chronic inflammation, leading to permanent damage to pancreatic tissue. The conditions impair insulin production and can result in the development of diabetes mellitus, wherein the body's response to insulin is poor, further impairing metabolic processes and subjecting patients to other diseases. Diabetes mellitus bears a close association with pancreatic failure, and it predominantly manifests itself in the form of Type 1 and Type 2 diabetes. Type 1 diabetes is an autoimmune disorder wherein the immune system of the body targets the insulin-secreting beta cells of the pancreas. Conversely,

Type 2 diabetes usually manifests itself due to insulin resistance, usually caused by lifestyle and obesity. As discussed in recent studies, there is a very close correlation between long-standing diabetes and an increased predisposition towards the development of pancreatic diseases such as pancreatitis and pancreatic cancer. Additionally, as the pancreas is unable to regulate glucose levels, it can be subjected to histological changes, e.g., fatty infiltration and fibrosis—these, in turn, can grossly impair its overall activity (Khan et al., 2024). Pancreatic cancer, a very virulent neoplasm, is very difficult to diagnose and treat as it usually manifests itself in its symptom-free early stages. The disease is usually most commonly linked with chronic pancreatitis, diabetes mellitus, and familial factors. Clinical research highlights that certain biomarkers can suggest pancreatic cancer but become apparent late in the course of the disease (Caro et al., 2011). With the progression of the cancer, typical symptoms are unexplained weight loss, jaundice, and pain in the abdomen. The interaction of pancreatic function, cancer pathology, and body balance necessitates additional studies of the development of effective diagnostic and therapeutic approaches in pancreatic diseases. Understanding the mechanisms of such diseases is essential for the design of preventive strategies and improved patient outcomes.

1.6.2. Diagnostic Methods for Pancreatic Disorders

Pancreatic disease diagnosis is a multifaceted process, integrating multiple diagnostic methods to evaluate pancreatic health in detail. Conventional imaging methods, including ultrasound (US), computed tomography (CT), and magnetic resonance imaging (MRI), yield information on structural pathology, including tumors, cysts, and pancreatitis. These imaging methods, although essential in the detection of anatomical defects, might be short of information on pancreas functional capacity. Functional tests, most notably, those that measure exocrine function, are therefore important in comprehensive diagnosis. Quantification of enzyme secretion and function can lead to early detection of chronic pancreatitis, wherein function is impaired with normal imaging findings. Such a multimodal process not only improves the diagnostic accuracy but also guides treatment strategies as much as to the pancreas pathology. Recent developments in the diagnostic process have improved the accuracy of pancreatic function estimation. One such important method is the short endoscopic secretin test, determining bicarbonate secretion following secretin stimulation. This test has been shown to have promise in detecting exocrine pancreatic insufficiency as well as in conventional methods, aided by its sensitivity and specificity in clinical evaluation. Automated biochemical analysis, including the measurement of amylase and lipase concentration in duodenal juice samples, has also made diagnostic processes easier, with quick results available to clinicians. Comparison between automated and manual analysis indicates the accuracy of these newer methods, warranting their application in routine clinical practice for diagnosis of pancreatic disorders (Erchinger, 2018). Overall, these developments are an integral part of the diagnostic management of pancreas dysfunction and disease. However, histological examination is also a cornerstone in the diagnosis of pancreatic disease, particularly in the detection of underlying pathological alterations. Traditional thin-section histology, despite being commonly practiced, is limited in the visualization of the complex three-dimensional interactions of pancreatic tissue. Novel breakthroughs in hydrogel techniques have bridged such limitations and enabled high-throughput volumetric interrogation of the pancreatic sample. Such novel methods enable a greater insight into pancreatic development and innervation, with a specific interest in disease setting. Comparative studies with special emphasis on the advantages of intact-tissue techniques over conventional techniques demonstrate their potential to complement clinical diagnosis and research data in the setting of pancreatic pathologies. As our understanding of pancreatic anatomy and physiology continues to grow, so does the necessity to apply diverse diagnostic techniques to enable accurate and effective treatment of pancreatic disease (Hsueh et al., 2017) (Figure 1.16).

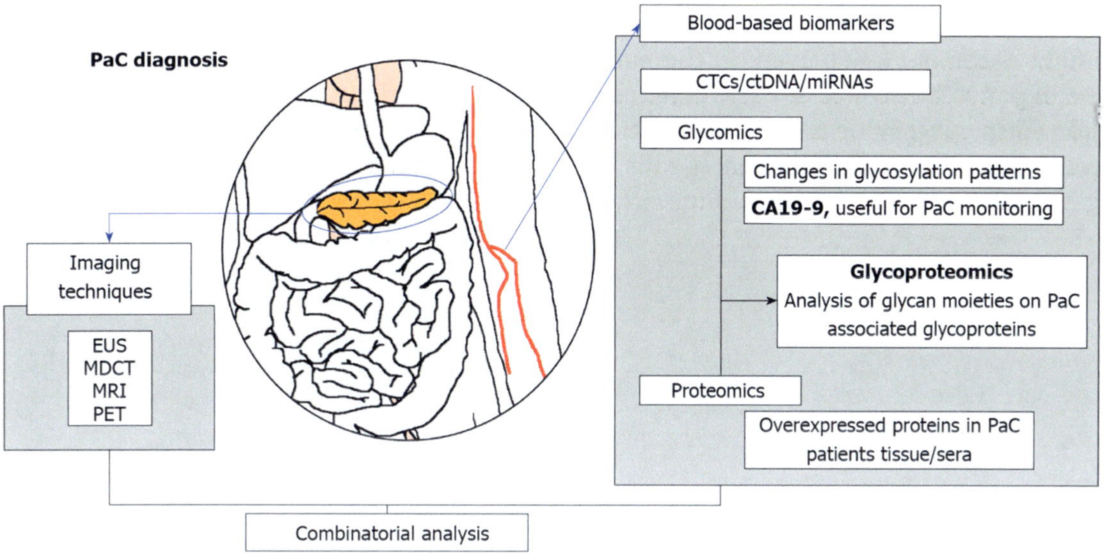

Figure 1.16. Diagnostic methods for pancreatic disorders.

Source: https://www.researchgate.net/publication/326032591/figure/fig1/AS:644348257505289@1530636004582/Overview-of-pancreatic-cancer-diagnosis-methods-imaging-techiques-and-the-exisiting-and.png.

1.6.3. Treatment Options and Management Strategies

Effective management and treatment of pancreatic disorders, such as pancreatic cancer, involve a multidisciplinary approach. The first approach may be surgical resection, such as the Whipple procedure, for the removal of the neoplasm and the surrounding tissue. This is normally the best approach for localized neoplasms, enhancing the chance of long-term survival. Nevertheless, patients are normally diagnosed late due to the pancreas's deep anatomical location, and therefore surgical alternatives become complicated. Supportive therapy such as chemotherapy or radiation may thus be required to treat unresectable neoplasms. For instance, combined therapy with chemotherapeutic drugs such as FOLFIRINOX or gemcitabine and nab-paclitaxel has been promising in enhancing survival in metastatic disease, thus the need for early diagnosis and intervention to enhance outcomes in affected individuals (Silva et al., 2024). Palliative therapy is also necessary in the treatment of pancreatic cancer, especially in unresectable neoplasms. The approach primarily aims at enhancing the quality of life through the relief of symptoms and psychological complications that arise during treatment. Relief of pain, nutritional support, and psychosocial support are critical elements of an overall approach. Patients also benefit from the new therapies such as targeted drug treatment or immunotherapy, which are proving to be potential alternatives to standard chemotherapeutic regimens. The therapies are customized to the patient, thus the need for personalized medicine in the treatment of pancreatic disorders. As understanding of the pancreas's complex function increases, so also the need for innovative treatment approaches that match patient-specific needs and clinical environments. Lastly, enhancement of the diagnostic approaches greatly influences the treatment of pancreatic diseases. Endoscopic ultrasound (EUS) and magnetic resonance cholangiopancreatography (MRCP) are increasingly becoming key players in the early diagnosis of pancreatic cancers. Early diagnosis allows for early surgery or the administration of adjuvant therapy, which is advantageous in altering the course of the disease. Biomarker studies are also being pursued to identify non-invasive screening devices, enabling improved monitoring and management of high-risk groups. Incorporating genetic testing with biomarkers can also affect treatment strategies by selecting candidates for targeted therapy. Such a combined strategy allows practitioners to individualize management options based on the disease stage and overall patient status with the ultimate goal of improving survival and improving the quality of life of the patients (Silva et al., 2024).

A CLOSER LOOK

IMPORTANCE OF UNDERSTANDING PANCREATIC ANATOMY AND PHYSIOLOGY

A lucid understanding of pancreatic anatomy and physiology is the key to clinical practice and the advancement of medical science. The pancreas is a critical organ with a twin role of endocrine and exocrine function, secreting hormones like insulin and glucagon and digestive enzymes required for the absorption of nutrients. By understanding the structural features and functional mechanism of the pancreas, medical professionals can recognize pathological changes that can occur in many diseases, affecting the management of diabetes and pancreatitis, for example. Additionally, a deep understanding of pancreatic histomorphology, as evidenced by studies indicating pancreatic health changes with the effect of a medication like simvastatin, offers insights into the interconnection between anatomical structure and physiological function (Luiten et al., 1984).

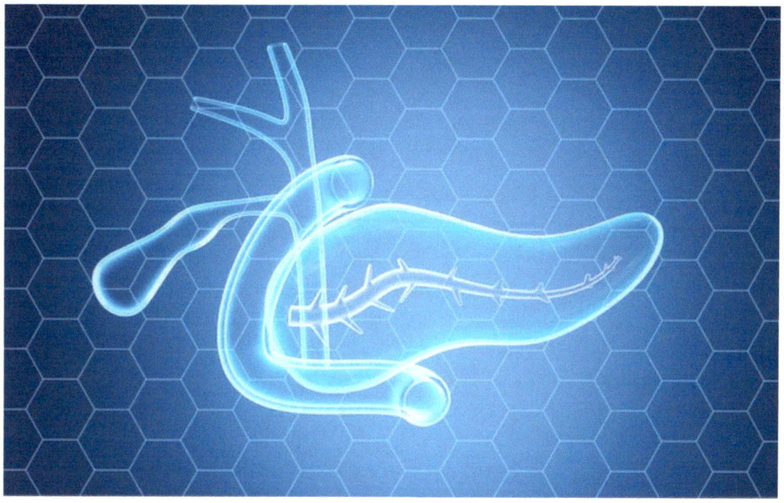

Source: https://img.freepik.com/premium-photo/human-pancreas-gall-bladder-organ-model-3d-rendering_778569-5640.jpg?w=900.

Thus, understanding the underlying anatomy and physiology enhances diagnostic skills and therapeutic interventions. Understanding pancreatic anatomy goes beyond the identification of its components; it entails respect for the complexity of its Functional Unit, such as acinar and ductal cells, and vascular and neural supply. The extensive review of pancreatic development and microstructure is integral to an understanding of how changes in these systems may have implications for clinical practice. For example, the coordination of enzyme secretion, regulated by local and systemic control, is intimately associated with the glands anatomical structure. The study of systematic investigation of the physiological mechanisms demonstrates mechanisms controlling pancreatic juice secretion, which plays a vital role in the digestion of carbohydrates, proteins, and fats. Such detailed information allows correlating with dysfunctions specific dysfunctions and structural changes, thus a profound understanding of various pancreatic diseases. In addition, deep knowledge of pancreatic physiology is vital to understanding the clinical presentation of pancreatic dysfunction. Abnormal levels of pancreatic enzymes in serum are a biochemical marker for pancreatitis or pancreatic cancer. An example is the work on serum amylase and alkaline phosphatase alterations emphasizing the role of such enzymes as indicators of pancreatic function or dysfunction. Furthermore, the adoption of an integrated concept of the pancreas allows for the integration of clinical cases with physiological and anatomical data, which provides increased clinical understanding. In addition to directing therapeutic maneuvers, an integrated approach directs research studies aimed at elucidating the pathophysiology of pancreatitis with a view to improving gastroenterology patient outcomes (Figure 1.17).

SUMMARY

In studying the complex anatomy and multi-dimensional physiology of the pancreas, it is quite clear that the organ is central to homeostasis in the human body. The pancreas is an endocrine as well as an exocrine gland, secreting essential hormones like insulin and glucagon and digestive enzymes. This duality highlights its importance, especially in the prevalence of metabolic diseases like diabetes. Studies, for example, the study that identified the regenerative capacity of herbal extracts on pancreatic tissue, reveal how interventions could facilitate the recovery of pathological processes and thus re-spark interest in therapeutic interventions that could capitalize on the pancreas's intrinsic capabilities (Akpaso et al., 2011). Thus, studying the anatomy of the pancreas and how it responds to different stimuli can provide insights into new treatments for disorders in its functioning. Further, the structural development of the pancreas, especially vascularization, is of crucial importance to its physiological functions. The complex blood and lymphatic systems are essential in maintaining pancreatic activity and facilitating successful metabolic regulation. Evidence reveals that by gestational weeks 17–22, blood and lymphatic networks are well established, which suggests that the pancreas is pre-sensitized to its endocrine function during early development. This highlights the importance of vascular integrity and the transport of nutrients and hormones in maintaining pancreatic health and function (Roost et al., 2014). Thus, as scientists continue to deconstruct the complexity of pancreatic development and function, it could very well lead to revolutionary approaches in regenerative medicine and therapy for pancreatic disease. Lastly, a comprehensive understanding of the anatomy and physiology of the pancreas not only enhances our understanding of its critical functions but also informs clinical practice and therapeutic interventions. As more information comes to be known, for instance, regarding pancreatic repair and regeneration, it opens the way for more future research on the mechanistic processes of such processes. The information derived from existing studies, particularly those conducted on the impact of various interventions on the pancreas's health, highlights the need for further extending our therapeutic interventions in diabetes management and pancreas insufficiency (Akpaso et al., 2011). Hence, future research on this unique organ continues to be imperative to improve patient outcomes and further medical knowledge.

The pancreas, a vital organ of the human body, is a dual endocrine and exocrine gland and a vital part of digestion and glucose metabolism. Anatomically, the pancreas is made up of four primary regions: the head, body, tail, and the pancreatic duct, which is a vital part of secreting digestive enzymes into the small intestine. These digestive enzymes, such as amylase, lipase, and proteases, play a vital role in the digestion of carbohydrates, fats, and proteins, respectively. The endocrine part, which is mainly organized in clusters referred to as the islets of Langerhans, plays a role in hormonal secretion, which secretes insulin and glucagon, influencing blood sugar levels. The complex interaction between the two functions makes the pancreas vital in the maintenance of homeostasis in the body and places it at the forefront of controversies regarding metabolic diseases. Surgical treatment of obesity and type 2 diabetes mellitus poses implications for pancreas anatomy and physiology. For example, studies show that severe changes in the digestive system have a severe impact on the function of the pancreas. Research shows that severe alteration of the digestive system has a severe impact on the function of the pancreas. Research shows that short bowel syndrome (SIC), through massive intestinal resection, results in significant alterations in pancreatic islet morphology and beta-cell dynamics. Specifically, the adaptation mechanism following SIC results in an increased relative area and size of pancreatic islets, which is due to beta-cell proliferation mechanisms. This evidence implies direct alteration of pancreatic health by surgical alteration, which demonstrates the organ's responsiveness to severe anatomical alteration during procedures such as gastric bypass or biliopancreatic diversion. The identification of such adaptability guides clinical practices in the management of pancreatic metabolic disorders and highlights the importance of total comprehension of pancreatic physiology after surgery (Pérez-Arana et al., 2015). The intricacy of the pancreas's interaction with other physiological systems also highlights the organ's complexity and central role in health. Pancreatic secretion of hormones not only controls glucose metabolism but also responds to other hormones and signaling pathways in the body. For instance, glucagon is counterbalanced by insulin to keep blood glucose in a very narrow range, as evidence of the fine tuning needed to sustain metabolic balance. Additionally, the endocrine pancreas is regulated by nutrients from digestion, with evidence suggesting that intestinal hormones stimulate pancreatic adaptation after alterations in nutrient flow (Seidel & Ernst, 2012). Such multiplex interaction highlights the pancreas's profound role in overall metabolism and health, as justification for ongoing research on the role of the pancreas in medical disorders, particularly those with metabolic dysregulation.

KEY TERMS FROM THIS CHAPTER

Keywords	Abdominal cavity	Autonomic Nervous System
Bicarbonate excretion	Bicarbonate secretion	Bicarbonate-enriched fluid
Blood flow	Blood sugar levels	Blood supply
Celiac plexus	Chronic pancreatic disease	Diabetes mellitus
Digestive and metabolic functions	Digestive enzyme secretion	Duodenal papilla
Endocrine dysfunction	Endocrine gland	Gastrointestinal system
Human body	Magnetic resonance imaging (MRI)	

References

1. Riepl, R. L., & Lehnert, P. (1992). The role of bile in the regulation of exocrine pancreatic secretion. *Scandinavian journal of gastroenterology*, *27*(8), 625–631. https://doi.org/10.3109/00365529209000130 (accessed on 26 May 2025).
2. Pérez-Arana, G., Camacho-Ramírez, A., Segundo-Iglesias, M. C., Lechuga-Sancho, A. M., Sancho-Maraver, E., Aguilar-Diosdado, M., & Prada-Oliveira, J. A. (2015). A surgical model of short bowel syndrome induces a long-lasting increase in pancreatic beta-cell mass. *Histology and histopathology*, *30*(4), 479–487. https://doi.org/10.14670/HH-30.479 (accessed on 26 May 2025).
3. Porro, L. B., & Richards, C. T. (2017). Digital dissection of the model organism Xenopus laevis using contrast-enhanced computed tomography. *Journal of anatomy*, *231*(2), 169–191. https://doi.org/10.1111/joa.12625 (accessed on 26 May 2025).
4. Akpaso, Mfon I., Item J. Atangwho, Amabe Akpantah, Victor A. Fischer, Anozeng O. Igiri, and Patrick E. Ebong. 2011. "Effect of Combined Leaf Extracts of Vernonia Amygdalina (Bitter Leaf) and Gongronema Latifolium (Utazi) on the Pancreatic β-Cells of Streptozotocin-Induced Diabetic Rats". *Journal of Advances in Medicine and Medical Research* 1 (1):24-34. https://doi.org/10.9734/BJMMR/2011/215.(accessed on 26 May 2025).
5. Carpino, G., Renzi, A., Cardinale, V., Franchitto, A., Onori, P., Overi, D., Rossi, M., Berloco, P. B., Alvaro, D., Reid, L. M., & Gaudio, E. (2016). Progenitor cell niches in the human pancreatic duct system and associated pancreatic duct glands: an anatomical and immunophenotyping study. *Journal of anatomy*, *228*(3), 474–486. https://doi.org/10.1111/joa.12418 (accessed on 26 May 2025).
6. Hsueh, B., Burns, V., Pauerstein, P. *et al.* Pathways to clinical CLARITY: volumetric analysis of irregular, soft, and heterogeneous tissues in development and disease. *Sci Rep* **7**, 5899 (2017). https://doi.org/10.1038/s41598-017-05614-4 (accessed on 26 May 2025).
7. Silva FFVe, Ballini A, Di Domenico M, Padín-Iruegas ME. The Complexity of the Pancreatic Lymphatic System and the Key Role of Para-Aortic Lymph Node Metastasis in Pancreatic Cancer Prognosis Prediction: A Comprehensive Review. *Anatomia*. 2024; 3(2):124-135. https://doi.org/10.3390/anatomia3020010 (accessed on 26 May 2025).
8. Proshchina AE, Krivova YS, Leonova OG, Barabanov VM, Saveliev SV. Development of Human Pancreatic Innervation [Internet]. Autonomic Nervous System. InTech; 2018. Available from: http://dx.doi.org/10.5772/intechopen.77089 (accessed on 26 May 2025).
9. Beebe, L., Hesse, D., & Massey, A. (2019). *UGA Anatomy and Physiology 2 Lab Manual* (3rd ed.). https://core.ac.uk/download/217306575.pdf (accessed on 26 May 2025).
10. Burch, J., & Collins, B. (2021). Anatomy and physiology of the gastrointestinal tract. In *Oxford Handbook of Gastrointestinal Nursing*. https://www.semanticscholar.org/paper/b39466ebf77424b07806967a164e04a3e2713522 (accessed on 26 May 2025).
11. Roost, M. S., van Iperen, L., de Melo Bernardo, A., Mummery, C. L., Carlotti, F., de Koning, E. J., & Chuva de Sousa Lopes, S. M. (2014). Lymphangiogenesis and angiogenesis during human fetal pancreas development. *Vascular cell*, *6*, 22. https://doi.org/10.1186/2045-824X-6-22 (accessed on 26 May 2025).

12. Carroll, J. P. (1930). *Physiology of the Pancreas* [Master's thesis, Boston University]. https://open.bu.edu/bitstream/2144/8191/1/physiologyofpanc00carr.pdf (accessed on 26 May 2025).
13. Gerussi, T., Graïc, J.-M., Orekhova, K., Cozzi, B. & Grandis, A. (2024) Vascularization of the gastrointestinal tract of the bottlenose dolphin (*Tursiops truncatus*, Montagu 1821). *Journal of Anatomy*, 244, 628–638. Available from: **https://doi.org/10.1111/joa.13989** (accessed on 26 May 2025).
14. Porzionato, A., Fenu, G., Rucinski, M., Macchi, V., Montella, A., Malendowicz, L. K., & De Caro, R. (2011). KISS1 and KISS1R expression in the human and rat carotid body and superior cervical ganglion. *European journal of histochemistry : EJH*, *55*(2), e14. https://doi.org/10.4081/ejh.2011.e14 (accessed on 26 May 2025).
15. Dolenšek J, Pohorec V, Rupnik MS, Stožer A. Pancreas Physiology [Internet]. Challenges in Pancreatic Pathology. InTech; 2017. Available from: http://dx.doi.org/10.5772/65895 (accessed on 26 May 2025).
16. Ensing, M., Paton, R., Speel, P. H., & Rada, R. (1994). An object-oriented approach to knowledge representation in a biomedical domain. *Artificial intelligence in medicine*, *6*(6), 459–482. https://doi.org/10.1016/0933-3657(94)90025-6
17. Erchinger, F. G. (2018). A short endoscopic Secretin test for the diagnosis of chronic pancreatitis [Doctoral dissertation, University of Oslo]. https://core.ac.uk/download/479084989.pdf (accessed on 26 May 2025).
18. Seidel, M. E., Ernst, C. H. (2012). Trachemys Agassiz Sliders. Catalogue of American Amphibians and Reptiles 891, 1-17.(accessed on 26 May 2025).
19. Gruessner, R. W. G., Laftavi, M., Pankewycz, O. G., & Gruessner, A. C. (2024). Pancreas transplantation for the treatment of pancreatic exocrine disorders. *Journal on Surgery, 5*(2), 45–51. https://www.semanticscholar.org/paper/f71069a118b9ad746e4b06298e26b520a91442bc (accessed on 26 May 2025).
20. Hartoyo, B., & Iriyanti, N. (2017). Effect of Symbiotic supplementation in feed on Tegal male duck's internal organs. https://core.ac.uk/download/287241337.pdf (accessed on 26 May 2025).
21. uang, A. S., Mohindroo, C., & Weinreb, R. N. (2016). Aqueous Humor Outflow Structure and Function Imaging At the Bench and Bedside: A Review. *Journal of clinical & experimental ophthalmology*, *7*(4), 578. https://doi.org/10.4172/2155-9570.1000578
22. Khan, H. G., Khan, M. M., Kiani, M. R. B., Kundi, M. A., et al. (2024). Statin-induced changes in rat pancreatic tissue: A histological and biochemical perspective. *Journal of Histological Research*. https://core.ac.uk/download/616940510.pdf (accessed on 26 May 2025).
23. Ludwig, S., Nauman, A. T., Regitz-Zagrosek, V., & Schluchter, M. D. (2020). Quantitative and qualitative analysis on sex and gender in preparatory material for national medical examination in Germany and the United States. *BMC Medical Education, 20*(1), 1–12. https://core.ac.uk/download/288114323.pdf (accessed on 26 May 2025).
24. Maxinová, E., Šustr, V., & Uhrin, M. (2017). Digestive enzymes in *Rhinolophus euryale* (Rhinolophidae, Chiroptera) are active also during hibernation. *Folia Zoologica, 66*(2), 123–131. https://core.ac.uk/download/286139279.pdf (accessed on 26 May 2025).
25. Norland, S., Rønnestad, I., & Sæle, Ø. (2022). Developmental stages of the ballan wrasse from

first feeding through metamorphosis: Cranial ossification and the digestive system. *Journal of Fish Biology, 101*(6), 1355–1374. https://core.ac.uk/download/534453807.pdf (accessed on 26 May 2025).

26. Rodriguez-Diaz, R. (2012). *Regulation of Human Pancreas Hormone Secretion by Autonomic Innervation* (Doctoral dissertation, University of Miami). https://core.ac.uk/download/70340024.pdf (accessed on 26 May 2025).

27. Zhou Y, Sun B, Li W, Zhou J, Gao F, Wang X, Cai M and Sun Z (2019) Pancreatic Stellate Cells: A Rising Translational Physiology Star as a Potential Stem Cell Type for Beta Cell Neogenesis. Front. Physiol. 10:218. doi: 10.3389/fphys.2019.00218 (accessed on 26 May 2025).

28. Luiten, P. G., ter Horst, G. J., Koopmans, S. J., Rietberg, M., & Steffens, A. B. (1984). Preganglionic innervation of the pancreas islet cells in the rat. *Journal of the autonomic nervous system, 10*(1), 27–42. https://doi.org/10.1016/0165-1838(84)90065-1 (accessed on 26 May 2025).

29. Tonetti, L. (2017). The discovery of lymphatic system as a turning point in medical knowledge: Asali, Pecquet and the end of hepatocentrism. *History of Medical Science, 34*(1), 67–76. https://core.ac.uk/download/144472986.pdf (accessed on 26 May 2025).

30. Valente, R., Coppola, A., Scandavini, C., Halimi, A., Magnusson, A., Lauro, A., Sotirova, I., et al. (2024). Interactions between the exocrine and the endocrine pancreas. *Journal of Clinical Medicine, 13*(1), Article 120. https://www.semanticscholar.org/paper/553f75ccae395169cae9c7e26bf129479ad4fe71 (accessed on 26 May 2025).

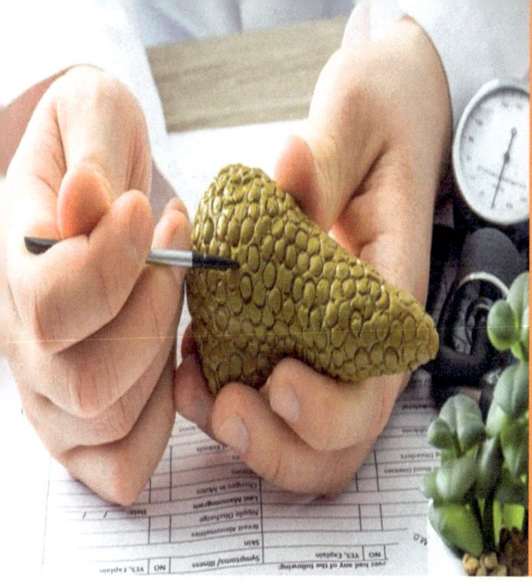

Chapter 2

DIAGNOSTIC MODALITIES IN PANCREATIC DISEASES

Contents

Introduction

The pancreas is a central organ in digestion and glucose metabolism, and therefore its health is essential for general well-being. Nevertheless, pancreatitis and pancreatic cancer, among other pancreas-related diseases, are major causes of morbidity and mortality globally. The difficulty in diagnosing pancreatic diseases is in their frequently nonspecific symptomatic presentation and intricate anatomy of the pancreas. The most vital challenge, therefore, is the development of effective diagnostic modalities. Following the history of these diagnostic modalities not only emphasizes the technological advancement of medical imaging but also points towards the significance of early detection in patient outcome improvement. It is vital to gain a profound understanding of these diagnostic modalities since early and correct diagnosis has an important role in deciding the management plan in pancreatic disease patients. In the clinical setting, there are several imaging modalities used in the assessment of pancreatic diseases, each with different strengths and weaknesses. These include US, CT, and MRI, which are the common modalities used today, each with an important role in the provision of information on the pancreas. For example, ultrasound can be the initial imaging modality due to its accessibility and absence of ionizing radiation; however, it is limited in obese or gassy individuals. On the other hand, CT scans produce high-quality cross-sectional images, which are priceless in tumor staging and complicated cases. In addition, MRI is best in the discrimination of solid and cystic lesions and follow-up of disease extension. Emphasis on the multimodality approach ensures that clinicians have a full set of diagnostic tools at their fingertips for precise diagnosis and tailored management of pancreatic pathologies (Scialpi et al., 2016). The combination of these imaging modalities provides a multi-dimensional approach to assessing pancreatic diseases, which ultimately translates to better patient care. Radiologists and physicians must collaborate to accurately interpret imaging results and consider them in the overall clinical context. Technical innovations in imaging modalities, such as the development of contrast-enhanced MRI and multidetector-row CT (MDCT), allow for the progressively more detailed visualization of pancreatic anatomy and associated tumors. These advances have the potential to revolutionize the diagnostic process and treatment of pancreatic disease. Moreover, continued research remains necessary in optimizing such diagnostic machines and their integration into clinical pathways. The goal remains the same: facilitating the healthcare provider to make timely and accurate diagnoses, thereby improving prognostic outcomes in patients with pancreatic disease (Copeland et al., 2020) (Figure 2.1).

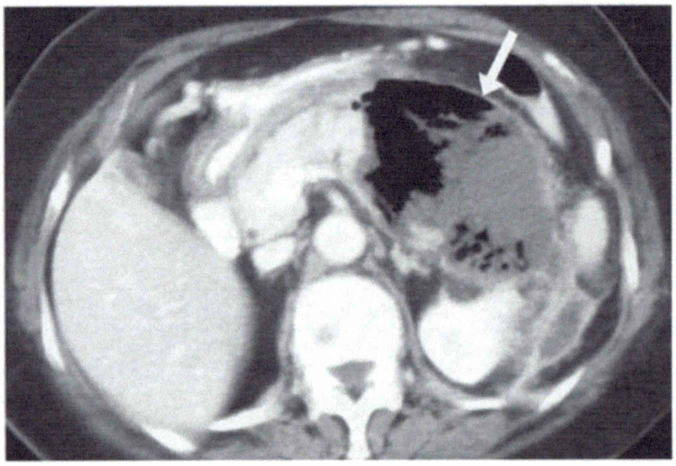

Figure 2.1. Diagnosis of pancreatic diseases.

Source: https://external-content.duckduckgo.com/iu/?u=https%3A%2F%2Fradiologykey.com%2Fwp-content%2Fuploads%2F2020%2F07%2F10-1055-b-002-85518_c002_f038.jpg&f=1&nofb=1&ipt=0f81a74bf68104a436fa3e9ded94b159704b8b310b976697316fe8cdfe0a150e.

Overview of Pancreatic Diseases

With the range of pancreatic diseases, it is important to note the range of conditions that impact this critical organ. The pancreas plays a role in digestion and endocrine secretions, and pancreatic diseases can have a significant effect on overall health. Among the more prevalent disorders are acute and chronic pancreatitis, defined by inflammation of the pancreas, frequently secondary to etiologies such as alcohol and gallstones. In the acute form, the inflammation may be abrupt and severe with complications such as necrosis of the pancreas or failure of systemic organs.

Chronic pancreatitis, however, is a slow process that can cause permanent alterations leading to diabetes or insufficiency of the pancreas. The range of presentations of these diseases requires having an advanced knowledge base to facilitate proper diagnostic and therapeutic approaches, paving the way for further study into advanced diagnostic techniques. Pancreatic cancer, and most particularly pancreatic ductal adenocarcinoma, is one of the most lethal of the pancreatic diseases, with its aggressive course and poor prognosis. Early detection continues to be a major challenge in the face of the usually asymptomatic presentation and non-specific symptoms, which are frequently mimicked by less severe diseases. Because of the insidious course, many patients present late, greatly restricting the choices for treatment. Recent developments in imaging techniques, such as endoscopic ultrasound and magnetic resonance imaging, have become increasingly valuable for earlier detection, allowing healthcare practitioners to detect lesions that are not visible with conventional imaging. Additionally, the role of specific biomarkers in the diagnosis and surveillance of pancreatic cancer is taking center stage. Through the integration of these modalities of diagnosis, clinicians can enhance early detection and management, and greatly enhance patient outcomes in this fatal disease (Caplin et al., 2017). Furthermore, pancreatic neuroendocrine tumors (PNETs) constitute a special category of pancreatic disease characterized by their unique biology and clinically heterogeneous behavior. These tumors are indolent or aggressive in nature, with a propensity to pose diagnostic and therapeutic challenges. Treatment of PNETs is frequently multidisciplinary in nature, given their rarity and the intricacy of their treatment. Because these tumors can secrete hormones, specialized biochemical tests are essential for accurate diagnosis, with the utilization of advanced imaging technologies like PET scans. Given their heterogeneity, treatment strategies for PNETs must be tailored to the patient profile, with an emphasis on personalized medicine. This also underscores the importance of developing organized care pathways and treatment networks to deliver comprehensive care to patients with pancreatic disease, with all aspects of management from diagnosis to therapy carefully coordinated (Copeland et al., 2020) (Figure 2.2).

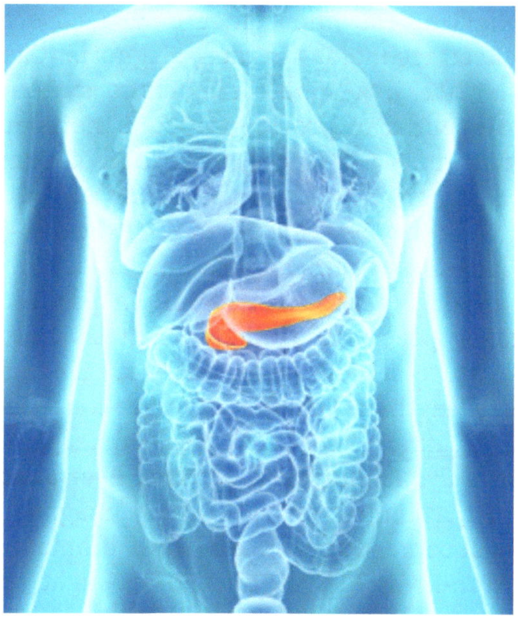

Figure 2.2. Pancreatic disease.

Source: https://external-content.duckduckgo.com/iu/?u=https%3A%2F%2Fstatic.wixstatic.com%2Fmedia%2F394550_7a33fc6b038b4a6e99d33bc8062f6325~mv2.jpg%2Fv1%2Ffill%2Fw_700%2Ch_834%2Cal_c%2Cq_85%2FPancreatic%2520Disease.jpg&f=1&nofb=1&ipt=8576ddaeac31ba83d2d36554754568b52cfc5e7c46134649b034f3b8bc6fdf79.

Importance of Accurate Diagnosis

Precise diagnosis in pancreatic diseases is essential due to the complex nature and multi-factorial pathophysiology of these diseases. As the pancreas is involved in a variety of body functions, misdiagnosis may result in inappropriate therapy and unhealthy outcomes. Diagnosis of pancreatic disorders is typically a concurrent synergy of imaging tests, biochemical tests, and clinical evaluation. For example, diagnosis of pancreatic cancer over benign pancreatic cysts necessitates advanced radiological tests such as MRI and CT scans. Moreover, absence of appropriate diagnostic tools, the diagnosis of pancreatic neuroendocrine neoplasms may be delayed or misdiagnosed, highlighting the importance of expertise and advanced technology in their diagnosis (Caplin et al., 2017). A robust diagnostic system is thus essential to provide targeted therapeutic interventions and enhance patient outcomes. More importantly, the importance of precise diagnosis is not confined to single cases but has long-term health implications for resources and management of resources. In pancreatic diseases, precise and timely diagnosis has the potential to prevent unnecessary surgeries and reduce lengths of hospital stay, with consequent lower healthcare costs. In disease management such as Cystic Fibrosis associated liver disease (CFLD), reliance on traditional diagnostics may become suboptimal; new biomarkers and non-invasive tests must be brought in to enhance diagnostic precision (Hage et al., 2013). The synergy of tests, for example, transient elastography and specific serum markers, is an important advance in preemptive management strategies. Therefore, attributing significance to precise diagnostic procedures not only enhances single-case patient management but is essential to optimize healthcare resources and enhance overall public health outcomes. Moreover, promoting a multidisciplinary approach highlights the importance of precise diagnoses in the optimal management of pancreatic diseases. Multidisciplinary teamwork among various specialists, including gastroenterologists, radiologists, and pathologists, ensures thorough patient assessment and treatment planning. Such teamwork is particularly important in the management of the complexities of pancreatic disease, whose overlapping symptoms and signs can challenge clinical judgment. A customized approach to the development and implementation of diagnostic modalities has the potential to develop coordinated networks, optimizing patient flows through timely referral and specialist input (Caplin et al., 2017). A specific focus on accurate diagnosis ensures continued education and application of new technologies, ultimately leading to better patient outcomes and management strategies. In summary, accuracy in diagnostic procedures cannot be overstated since it constitutes the foundation of successful therapy and enhanced patient care.

2.1. Common Pancreatic Diseases

Pancreatic diseases are a collection of conditions that have a potentially significant impact on both pancreatic function and overall health. Most prevalent among these are pancreatic adenocarcinoma, chronic pancreatitis, and pancreatic neuroendocrine tumors. Chronic pancreatitis entails chronic inflammation and fibrosis of the pancreas, followed by chronic abdominal pain, malabsorption, and diabetes mellitus. Alternatively, pancreatic adenocarcinoma is characterized by late diagnosis, aggressive behavior and poor prognosis. Diagnostic modalities for such a disease are usually imaging modalities like magnetic resonance imaging (MRI) and computed tomography (CT) and biochemical markers. Advancements more recently emphasized the importance of treating diseases like pancreatic neuroendocrine tumors in a multidisciplinary manner, due to the need for individualized treatments and the different diagnostic requirements (Caplin et al., 2017). Cystic fibrosis (CF) also has complications involving the pancreas, such as cystic fibrosis-associated liver disease (CFLD), occurring in approximately 30% of CF patients. As prevalent as it is, surprisingly little effective routine diagnostic modality for CFLD has been reported. Increased serum protein profiling provided new avenues for the identification of experimental biomarkers for the detection of CFLD with higher specificity. Research has identified proteins like TIMP-4 and Endoglin showing significant changes in CFLD patients compared to non-liver disease patients. Coupling with transient elastography, a non-invasive imaging modality, to such biomarkers has provided high diagnostic accuracy for CFLD, thus enhancing sensitivity and predictability in test patients (Hage et al., 2013). The intersection of these pancreatic illnesses—with chronic pancreatitis potentially leading to pancreatic cancer, and the impact of cystic fibrosis further complicating pancreatic function, illustrates the significance of comprehending the diagnostic paradigms of the illnesses. The intersection of imaging tests and biomarkers not only allows for early diagnosis but also is an important factor in the successful management of the illnesses. Because each type of pancreatic illness has unique pathological features, there must be ongoing research toward establishing diagnostic criteria and new emerging paradigms of treatment. New research must be done to formulate standardized protocols that can be used in clinical care, where patients can be offered correct diagnosis as well as concomitant timely and appropriate management (Figure 2.3).

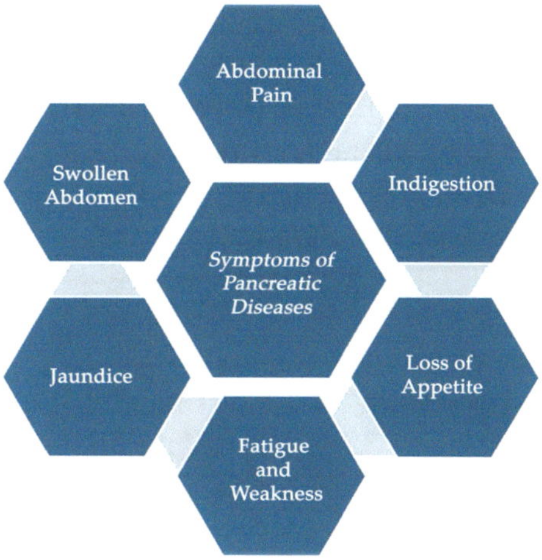

Figure 2.3. Common pancreatic diseases.

Source: https://external-content.duckduckgo.com/iu/?u=https%3A%2F%2Fwww.ckbhospital.com%2Fwp-content%2Fuploads%2F2024%2F11%2FPancreatic-Diseases.png&f=1&nofb=1&ipt=d924afe10414cad0165abc20dc7e64ceaa5ae300fbc1add2bf58c622d278472a.

2.1.1. Acute Pancreatitis

The diagnostic workup in acute pancreatitis is important because of the severe complications and complex presentation of the disease. This inflammatory disease of the pancreas has a multitude of clinical presentations, most commonly abdominal pain, vomiting, and anorexia. Laboratory investigation is important when planning a differential diagnosis; for example, increased serum level of pancreatic amylase and lipase is commonly seen with pancreatitis. These markers can be misleading in the sense that extrapancreatic diseases can alter their concentration, and the clinical picture is all the more interesting. In the dog, an increased concentration of canine pancreatic lipase immunoreactivity (cPLI) has been found to yield diagnostic information, especially when pancreatitis should be excluded from other gastrointestinal or hepatic system diseases. Such diagnostic complexities indicate that one should employ a multi-modal strategy while evaluating patients with suspected acute pancreatitis. Besides clinical presentation and laboratory investigation, imaging modalities also have an important role to play in the diagnosis of acute pancreatitis. Radiography and ultrasound are two of the most commonly employed modalities that help in understanding pancreatic morphology and complications. Ultrasound is especially helpful because it enables real-time imaging of the pancreas and adjacent structures. It helps in the detection of peritoneal effusion, necrosis, or development of an abscess in acute pancreatitis complications. Also, a retrospective study emphasized the importance of cytological examination of bile aspirated through cholecystocentesis, which showed infectious agents in a high percentage of cases, thus establishing a relationship between biliary disease and pancreatic pathology (Peters et al., 2015). This finding not only highlights the role of imaging in acute presentation but also the importance of evaluating other systems that can affect the diagnosis and management of pancreatic disease. The multifactorial pathogenesis of acute pancreatitis necessitates a holistic diagnostic process with a combination of modalities. While conventional biomarkers such as serum amylase and lipase are useful, a lack of reliability in cases of extrapancreatic disease can render diagnosis difficult. New evidence supports the use of specific lipase assays, such as cPLI, as being more reliably correlated with the disease, and thus validating diagnostic accuracy (Hulsebosch et al., 2015). Furthermore, awareness of the limitations of specific markers enables clinicians to estimate the overall pancreatic health status. Therefore, an integrative diagnostic process involving clinical assessment, laboratory investigations, and imaging studies is essential for the effective management and treatment of acute pancreatitis. With ongoing research in the field, the prospect of more specific diagnostic criteria becoming available may herald more positive patient outcomes (Figure 2.4).

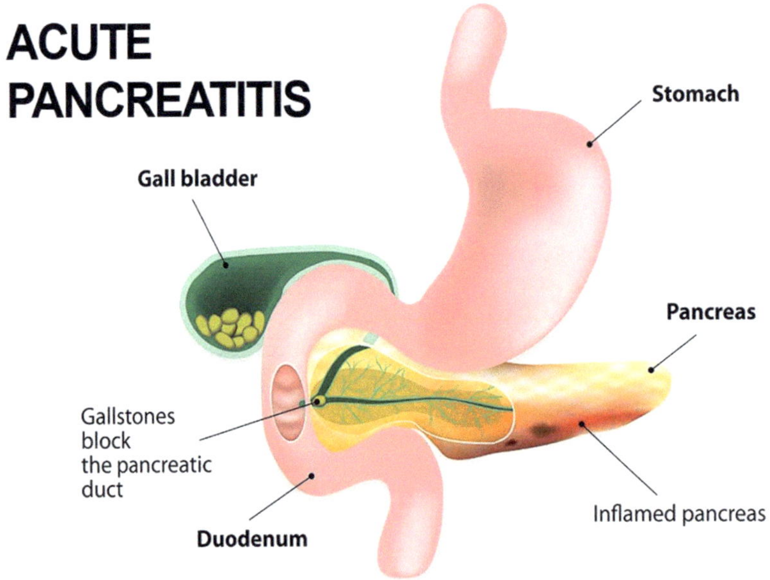

Figure 2.4. Acute pancreatitis.

Source: https://external-content.duckduckgo.com/iu/?u=https%3A%2F%2Fwww.stepwards.com%2Fwp-content%2Fuploads%2F2017%2F01%2Facute-pancreatitis-diagram.jpg&f=1&nofb=1&ipt=babdb11a7975e140610f7b506352e8624b2d7a4cd1dffa29adf4bc75a6c9a373.

2.1.2. Chronic Pancreatitis

Chronic pancreatitis is characterized by repeated inflammation of the pancreas leading to irreversible damage and altered architecture of pancreatic tissue. The disease typically presents in the form of recurrent abdominal pain, malabsorption, and diabetes mellitus due to pancreatic parenchymal destruction. Although it may be secondary to acute pancreatitis, alcoholism is the most common etiology of chronic pancreatitis and is the etiology of chronic loss of pancreatic function. Chronic pancreatitis is also a multisystem disease requiring an arsenal of diagnostic modalities to establish its nature and severity. Imaging modalities such as ultrasound, CT, and MRI play a pivotal role in imaging pancreas inflammation, calcifications, and architectural changes, which are pivotal in precise diagnosis and management plans of the affected patients. Of the various diagnostic modalities utilized for chronic pancreatitis, MRI has been found to be an extremely valuable modality. Research has proven MRI to be highly accurate in diagnosis with the ability to differentiate between benign and malignant pancreatic lesions. Since certain management strategies need to be instituted based on the nature of the pathology, this is important. MRI, for instance, can be used to identify chronic changes in the pancreas that may be missed by less sensitive imaging modalities and thus enable proper medical or surgical treatment. MRI also correctly diagnoses the presence of complications of chronic pancreatitis such as pancreatic pseudocysts or biliary obstructions, further establishing its role in the diagnostic algorithm of pancreatic diseases (Tripalo-Batoš et al., 2011). Apart from imaging modalities, cytological examination of pancreatic fluid and bile also provides valuable information regarding chronic pancreatitis. Cholecystocentesis, for instance, enables the collection of bile, which can be cytologically analyzed. This approach identifies infectious agents and inflammatory cells, providing additional information that can be correlated with imaging and clinical presentation. In a study involving canines and felines, cytology was found to possess diagnostic utility, with microorganisms detected in a high percentage of the specimens. Integration of cytological information with imaging has the potential to add rigidity to the chronic pancreatitis diagnostic algorithm and allow integrated evaluation of related pancreatic and biliary disease (Peters et al., 2015). The use of a multimodal diagnostic approach, therefore, not only enhances the sensitivity of diagnosing chronic pancreatitis but also informs optimal management guidelines.

2.1.3. Pancreatic Cancer

Pancreatic cancer diagnosis is a difficult task due to the deep anatomical location of the organs and the often asymptomatic presentation of the disease in the initial stage. The newer imaging modalities such as CT, MRI, and endoscopic ultrasound (EUS) have completely revolutionized the detection of pancreatic malignancies. CT is superior in showing pancreatic mass and metastatic disease, while MRI provides better soft tissue contrast for differentiating pancreatic structures and lesions. EUS is highly useful for obtaining fine-needle aspiration (FNA) for histological diagnosis, which is the sine quo non of definitive diagnosis. As the biology of pancreatic cancer continues to evolve, optimization of these imaging modalities will be the key to enhancing detection rates, especially in high-risk patients who may otherwise remain undetected until the disease reaches an advanced stage. In addition to conventional imaging, innovative biomarker research is also a rapidly evolving field for the early diagnosis of pancreatic cancer. Serum levels of tumor markers such as carbohydrate antigen 19-9 (CA 19-9) have been shown to be useful in facilitating diagnosis and monitoring disease progression. While rising levels of CA 19-9 can suggest pancreatic cancer, it is not disease-specific and can lead to false-positive tests in other conditions. Its utility as a stand-alone diagnostic tool, therefore, is restricted. According to current guidelines, the combination of

CA 19-9 with imaging studies would enhance the precision of diagnosis. Additionally, research on the progress in liquid biopsy techniques is ongoing that could potentially allow the detection of circulating tumor DNA (ctDNA) and other biomarkers of pancreatic cancer and thus provide a less invasive test for early detection than conventional techniques (Lykoudis et al., 2019). Pancreatic cancer treatment necessitates a multidisciplinary approach due to the heterogeneity and complexity of the disease. This is most applicable to pancreatic neuroendocrine neoplasms, which are unique therapeutic challenges and need individualized therapeutic approaches. Patient health status and individual tumor biology-based individualized therapies often need a multidisciplinary team of pathologists, radiologists, medical oncologists, and surgeons to optimize outcomes. Recent studies indicate that this collaborative approach can significantly improve therapeutic efficacy and patient survival rates (Caplin et al., 2017). The integration of specialized biochemical tests and radiological investigations into clinical protocols may also streamline the diagnostic procedure, and thus treatment regimens can be optimized. Organized healthcare provision with specialization in the treatment of pancreatic disease can thus make resource management more effective and ultimately become a platform for optimizing patient care in this challenging area (Figure 2.5).

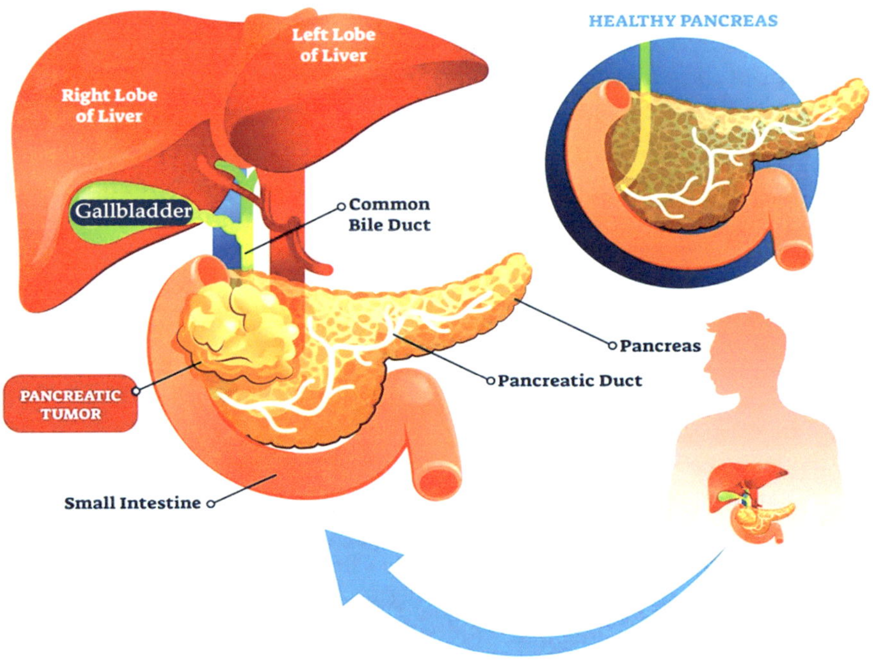

Figure 2.5. Pancreatic-cancer.

Source: https://blog.medicaresolutions.com/wp-content/uploads/2019/11/Pancreatic-cancer-illustration.jpg.

2.2. Traditional Diagnostic Techniques

Diagnosis of pancreatic diseases has long been dependent on traditional diagnostic techniques, which are an integral part of clinical practice. Among these techniques, imaging modalities such as ultrasound, CT, and MRI are the cornerstones in providing detailed anatomical details. These techniques facilitate the evaluation of structural pathologies of the pancreas, including tumors, cysts, or signs of pancreatitis. For instance, CT scans hold valuable significance with high sensitivity in the detection of pancreatic masses and the determination of disease progression or complications. Though these traditional techniques provide valuable information, these are typically subject to confirmation by more invasive techniques such as endoscopic and laparoscopic procedures, which are additional risks to the patients and cause complications if not carried out with caution. In the last decade or so, endoscopic techniques, particularly EUS, have been at the forefront of pancreatic disease diagnostics. EUS offers real-time imaging and tissue sampling through fine-needle aspiration, which is invaluable in the diagnosis of pancreatic malignancies. Symposia such as the one organized by the National Institute of Diabetes and Digestive and Kidney Diseases highlighted the process of standardization of EUS techniques and the improvement in the accuracy of sampling pancreatic lesions (Lee et al., 2017). This has far-reaching consequences for the identification of the disease in the early stage, since obtaining the correct diagnosis can permit timely intervention and potentially improved outcomes for the patients. EUS also allows the evaluation of complex pancreatic structures that may not be properly evaluated with traditional imaging, thereby increasing overall diagnostic accuracy. In spite of advancements in imaging technology and interventions such as EUS, the integration of these traditional techniques with newer diagnostic agents is an area of research interest in clinical fields. As highlighted in recent literature, the convergence of molecular imaging techniques with conventional methods can facilitate an improved understanding of disease mechanisms and response to treatment (Ding et al., 2012). Convergence is particularly relevant in pancreatic cancer when nonspecific symptoms complicate early diagnosis. Through the investigation of the biodistribution of novel imaging agents and their pharmacokinetics, investigators aim to further refine the diagnostic process and develop customized treatment processes. Therefore, the application of both conventional and new methods can significantly improve the quality of patient care in pancreatic disease, with improved diagnostic sensitivity and therapeutic responsiveness (Figure 2.6).

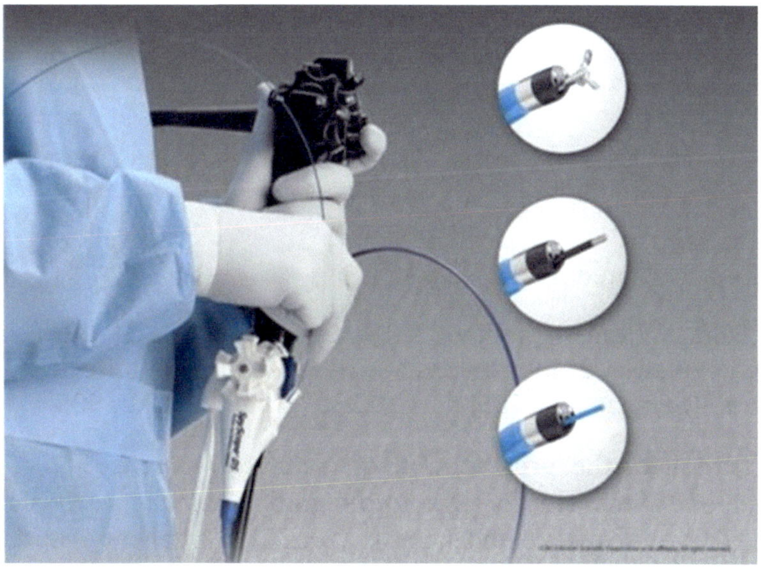

Figure 2.6. Advanced diagnostic methods for biliary tract and pancreatic diseases.

Source: https://top1cdn.top1health.com/cdn/am/93491/225120.jpg.

2.2.1. Physical Examination and Patient History

Physical examination and correlation with patient history are crucial in early diagnostic evaluation of pancreatic diseases. Careful patient history provides information on risk factors such as family history, lifestyle, and previous medical history, including pancreatitis or gallbladder disease. These historical findings guide clinicians to possible etiologies of pancreatic dysfunction and follow-up investigations to be optimized. On physical examination, clinicians must assess abdominal tenderness and distension, and signs of systemic involvement such as jaundice or weight loss, to suggest underlying pancreatic disease.

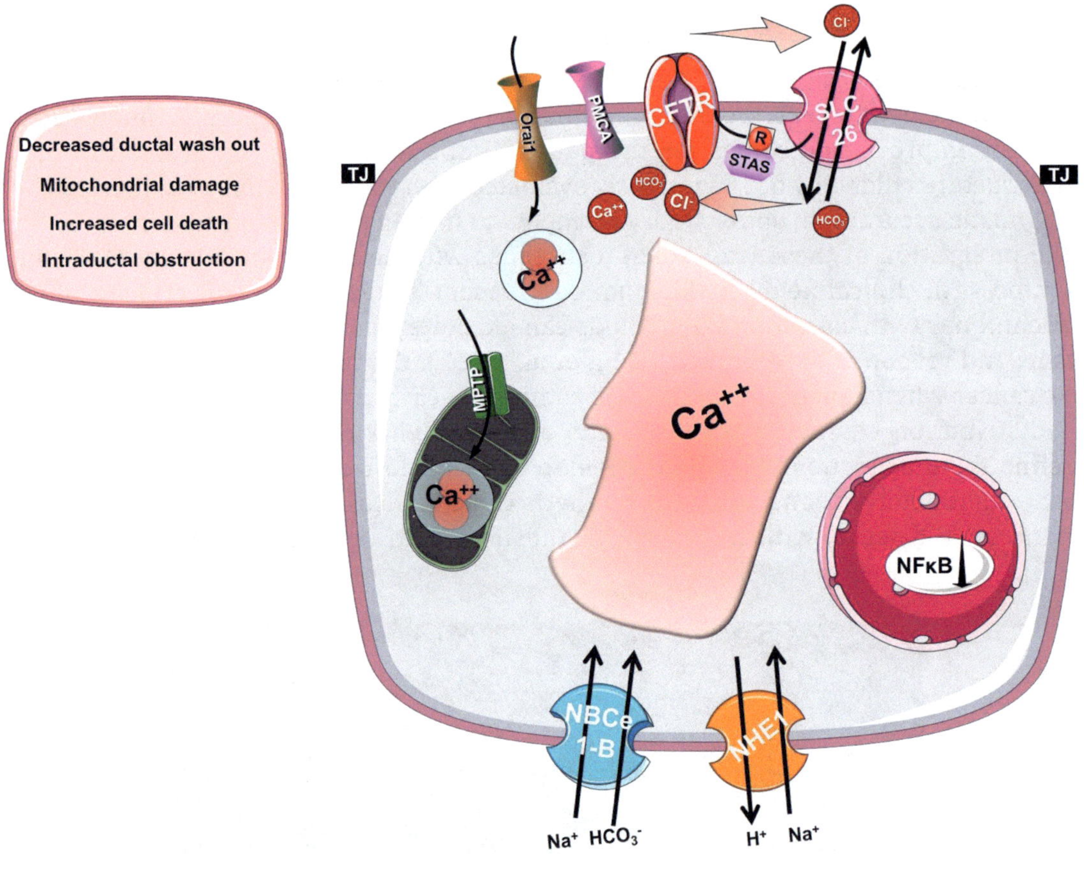

Figure 2.7. Cystic fibrosis-related liver disease.

Source: Madácsy T, Pallagi P and Maleth J (2018) Cystic Fibrosis of the Pancreas: The Role of CFTR Channel in the Regulation of Intracellular Ca2+ Signaling and Mitochondrial Function in the Exocrine Pancreas. Front. Physiol. 9:1585. doi: 10.3389/fphys.2018.01585.

Notably, identification of the presentation of pancreatic diseases in multicultural patient populations, and indeed in the elderly, can significantly enhance early detection efforts and therapeutic gain, such that this aspect of diagnosis is a crucial component of optimal patient care. The diagnostic utility of physical examination is maximized by correlation with directed patient history. For instance, in adolescent and adult CFLD, identification of patient history can identify factors for more advanced pancreatic disease. Recent data has pointed to specific serum proteins as markers in the diagnosis of diseases such as CFLD, again to establish the premise that history and physical examination can shed light on subsequent assessment tools, such as transient elastography. The inclusion of physical examination findings with patient history can therefore reveal abnormalities in liver function and pancreatic status, to facilitate an accelerated and enhanced diagnosis. When clinicians acknowledge the patient's history and physical status as an integrated, global construct, this significantly enhances their diagnostic skills. In addition, identification of the subtleties of patient history is particularly significant in high-risk populations such as the elderly, who present with uncharacteristic symptoms. Acute pancreatitis among the elderly has been established to manifest differently from their younger counterparts through less severe pain and non-specific gastrointestinal signs. This variation requires a vigilant clinical evaluation aided by an excellent patient history to avoid misdiagnosis or unwarranted delay. In urgent situations, clinicians need to remain vigilant for subtle presentations of acute pancreatitis, complementing the evaluation process through historical assessment and physical examinations. A broad strategy to establish a diagnosis not only streamlines the identification of pancreatic abnormalities but also facilitates a patient-oriented approach in treating these multi-factorial illnesses effectively, as demonstrated in recent studies in the elderly population (Stefanov, 2024) (Figure 2.7).

2.2.2. Blood Tests and Biomarkers

The role of blood tests and biomarkers in the diagnosis of pancreatic disease has gained prominence, particularly in discriminating between such diseases as pancreatitis and pancreatic cancer. Blood tests can detect elevated levels of certain enzymes, such as lipase and amylase, which are typically associated with inflammation of the pancreas. However, recent studies reveal that such biomarkers are not always an indicator of the severity of pancreatic damage or incidence of extrapancreatic diseases, and hence the interpretation of results is challenging. For instance, certain conditions such as acute renal injury may lead to spurious elevations of such biomarkers, thereby compromising the sensitivity of diagnosis. Therefore, the use of blood tests must be informed by understanding the underlying disease and biological states to enable clinicians to differentiate between primary pancreatic disease and other conditions that are likely to simulate pancreatic pathology, as reported in studies on pancreatic enzyme behavior in renal failure (Hulsebosch et al., 2015). Another recent approach to the diagnosis of pancreatic disease assessing new biomarkers that would enhance early detection and treatment outcomes. Pancreatic ductal adenocarcinoma (PDAC) presents daunting challenges to early diagnosis, typically presenting at advanced stages, significantly lowering survival rates, according to studies. New studies reveal the potential of ctDNA, protein biomarkers, and microRNA profiles as potential markers for early detection. Detection of such biomarkers can lead to more sensitive screening regimens that significantly enhance patient outcomes by enabling early intervention (Resnek et al., 2018). Thus, their translation to clinical application can revolutionize the paradigm of diagnosis of pancreatic disease from a reactive to a preventive approach, and ultimately, enhance the prognoses of these patients. Though optimistic, the utilization of blood tests and biomarkers as a standard part of diagnostic protocols for pancreatic disease is still riddled with problems that need addressing. Foremost among them are standardization and validation of biomarkers, which are in varied phases of investigation and application in the clinic. While several putative biomarkers have been identified, no conclusive panels or platforms for screening in a noninvasive manner have been proven. Extensive testing will be required to establish the specificity and sensitivity of these biomarkers in varied groups of patients to determine their clinical utility. As translation research advances, the generation of useful biomarker panels can be a key to the alteration of the paradigm of control of pancreatic disease, and therefore, larger multicenter studies must be performed to validate these promising strategies in detail (Vaccaro & Resnik, 2018) (Figure 2.8).

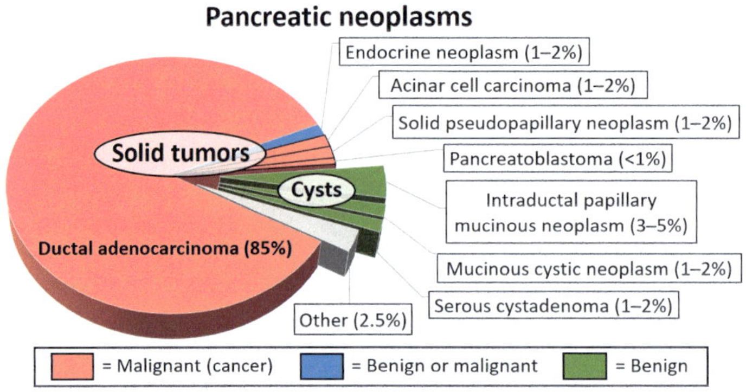

Figure 2.8. The pancreatic ductal adenocarcinoma (PDAC).

Source: By Mikael Häggström, M.D. Author info- Reusing images- Conflicts of interest:NoneMikael Häggström, M.D. - Own work using:Wang, Y (2011). "Diffusion-weighted MR imaging of solid and cystic lesions of the pancreas.". Radiographics 31 (3): E47-64. DOI:10.1148/rg.313105174. PMID 21721197., CC0, https://commons.wikimedia.org/w/index.php?curid=122380612

2.2.3. Imaging Techniques: X-Rays and Ultrasounds (US)

The use of imaging modalities like X-rays and ultrasounds is crucial in the diagnosis and treatment of pancreatic disease. X-rays, despite being a ubiquitous tool in medical imaging, have limitations in their ability to image soft tissues, such as the pancreas. Yet, they can be used to identify complications related to pancreatic disease, such as calcifications that may reflect chronic pancreatitis. Furthermore, advances in imaging technology have enabled better visualization of the pancreas, particularly when X-rays are used in combination with contrast media. This combination improves the specificity of diagnoses and assists in the evaluation of pancreatic masses, indicating the value of X-rays as an adjunct tool in diagnostic protocols for pancreatic disease. While X-rays are not perfect, their value to the overall diagnostic strategy is invaluable, particularly in emergencies where quick assessments are vital. Ultrasound imaging has become a valuable modality in the diagnosis of pancreatic disease, providing real-time imaging without the hazards of ionizing radiation. This imaging modality is particularly valuable in the evaluation of pancreatic morphology and perfusion, and as such, is a first-line imaging choice in many clinical situations. Using high-frequency sound waves, ultrasound can detect abnormalities like pancreatic cysts, tumors, and inflammation to assist in the diagnosis of conditions like pancreatitis and pancreatic cancer. The real-time imaging capability of ultrasounds also makes them useful for guided procedures, including aspirations or biopsies, further increasing their clinical value. Studies have shown that the sensitivity of ultrasounds can be greater in the detection of some pancreatic lesions than X-rays, and therefore, establishes its place as a valuable imaging technique in the diagnostic tool kit for pancreatic diseases. Thus, the wide availability and non-invasive nature of ultrasounds render them highly beneficial in acute and chronic conditions as well. In the context of the diagnostic case of pancreatic diseases, the combination of X-rays and ultrasounds is highly apparent. While both modalities have strengths and weaknesses, combined use in complementary situations provides a comprehensive evaluation of pancreatic diseases. For instance, while X-rays might provide evidence of calcific changes typical of chronic pancreatitis, ultrasounds highly excel in evaluation of the soft tissue structures and possible neoplasms. Also, ongoing advancements in imaging modalities are creating the opportunity for more multimodal investigation, taking the best of both modalities. Such progress is critical in resolving difficult diagnostic questions in the context of pancreatic diseases, as they lead to more accurate and timely interventions. Lastly, the combination of X-rays and ultrasounds in the context of an overall diagnostic strategy ensures that clinicians can maximize patient outcomes to the best, in alignment with the trends in personalized medicine observed in the context of pancreatic diagnostics (Cunha et al., 2014; Rogers et al., 2015).

2.3. Advanced Imaging Modalities

The development of newer imaging modalities has revolutionized the diagnostic landscape of pancreatic disease, particularly in differentiating between benign and malignant disease. Clearly, modalities like MRI and CT have become first-line imaging modalities, with excellent visualization of the anatomy of the pancreas and pathology. Indeed, MRI provides better soft-tissue contrast, which enables the detection of subtle lesions beyond the imaging capacity of other modalities. Moreover, the use of Multi-Detector CT has enhanced image acquisition time, enabling comprehensive evaluation of pancreatic tumors, size, location, and vasculature involvement. These modalities are the basis for early detection and successful management, enabling multidisciplinary management that is paramount in optimizing patient outcomes in the management of pancreatic disease (Caplin et al., 2017). Besides MRI and CT, EUS also has a role in the diagnostic armamentarium of pancreatic diseases. EUS is particularly useful in the assessment of small lesions that may not be optimally characterized by other imaging modalities. It enables fine-needle aspiration biopsy, which enables histopathological diagnosis with minimal invasiveness. The fact that imaging of the pancreas is performed with an endoscopic modality enables EUS to have real-time high-resolution imaging that is crucial in assessing conditions like pancreatic adenocarcinoma or neuroendocrine tumors. Moreover, it enables the segregation of different types of cysts, enabling clinical decision-making effectively. EUS inclusion in the diagnostic pathway is a classic example of the need to utilize advanced imaging modalities to ensure accuracy and provide individualized treatment options for pancreatic disorders (Stieber et al., 2008). The inclusion of recent developments in imaging modalities also saw the use of molecular imaging and personalized biomarkers, further reflecting the complexity of pancreatic diseases. Techniques such as Positron Emission Tomography (PET) allow for functional imaging capable of detecting metabolic activity observed in tumors, differentiating malignant from benign processes on the basis of their pattern of glucose use. Furthermore, the application of serum biomarkers such as CA19-9 demonstrates synergistic utility when utilized in conjunction with advanced imaging modalities. The evidence available demonstrates that the Access (R) GI Monitor assay is highly accurate for diagnosing pancreatic cancer, once again highlighting the utility of careful assessment utilizing both laboratory and imaging findings (Stieber et al., 2008). These advances not only enhance diagnostic accuracy but also allow for individualized treatment regimens, making management of pancreatic disease more effective and patient-centered (Figure 2.9).

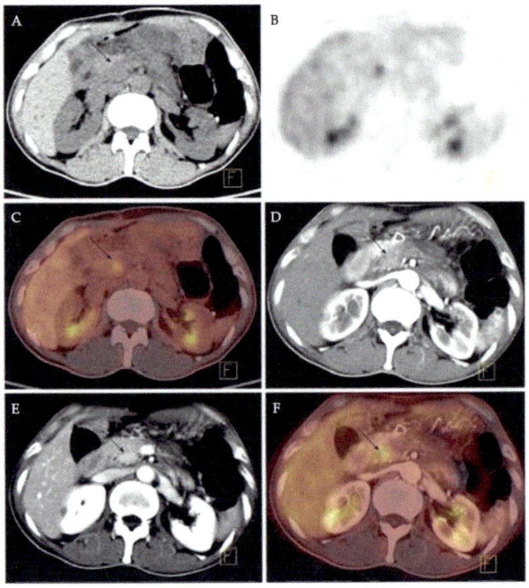

Figure 2.9. A 46-year-old female patient with repeated upper abdominal pain.

Source: https://f6publishing.blob.core.windows.net/01d89a16-51fb-4bb7-aa12-f25012b2ed83/WJG-21-2988-g001.jpg.

2.3.1. Computed Tomography (CT) Scans

CT scanning is one of the most valuable imaging tools in the assessment of pancreatic disease, particularly in the identification of tumors and determination of tumor extent. This imaging tool uses X-ray technology to produce cross-sectional images of the body with exquisite detail, allowing clinicians to visualize the pancreas with great definition. Its value is exemplified in the case of pancreatic cancer, where staging appropriately is imperative to treatment and prognosis. Over-reliance on CT, however, is not without boundaries; evidence shows that numerous patients are subjected to unnecessary surgical interventions due to the misinterpretation of tumor resectability based on CT imaging alone (Tamburrino et al., 2016). It is thus essential to acknowledge the limitations of CT while, at the same time, utilizing its diagnostic benefit to optimize patient outcomes in the treatment of pancreatic disease. While CT scans are still the gold standard for initial assessment, adjunct imaging technologies are increasingly being touted to improve diagnostic precision and reduce adverse surgical outcomes. MRI, EUS, and PET, for instance, can provide helpful information on tumor involvement with adjacent structures and potential metastases that may not be seen with a CT scan. Current evidence suggests that in some instances, these alternative imaging tools can prevent patients from unnecessary laparotomies due to misestimation of tumor spread based on CT imaging alone (Tamburrino et al., 2016). Furthermore, the addition of CT with these newer imaging tools may define tumor resectability, thus guiding clinicians to more individualized and relevant therapy. This multi-faceted approach is imperative in an arena where the costs of misdiagnosis can translate into pertinent patient morbidity. The integration of new imaging modalities within the diagnostic algorithm for pancreatic disease is a testament to the need for ongoing evaluation of the efficacy of each modality. For example, the systematic review of pancreatic cancer diagnosis protocols revealed significant variability within the diagnostic performance of different tests to ascertain resectability. Such variability is a testament to the need for the application of evidence-based guidelines and consensus clinical expertise to optimize diagnostic protocols. With the use of a platform that supports a variety of imaging modalities, the healthcare provider is well placed to accurately ascertain a patient's disease stage, hence the informed discussion of treatment. Ultimately then, as new diagnostic technology continues to emerge, their prudent application will become more essential in developing improved outcomes for patients with pancreatic disease.

2.3.2. Magnetic Resonance Imaging (MRI)

MRI is a key diagnostic imaging modality in the diagnosis and management of pancreatic disease. As part of a multimodality approach, MRI supplements the other imaging modalities like US and CT, which are primarily focused on the differentiation of solid and cystic tumors of the pancreas. The unique advantages of MRI enable it to provide clear views of anatomy, thereby allowing for a more accurate evaluation of pancreas parenchyma, ducts, and adjacent soft tissues. Such accuracy is significant in the diagnosis of pancreatic lesions and the staging of tumor. Moreover, the non-invasive nature of MRI and the absence of ionizing radiation make it a modality of choice in some clinical settings, particularly when repeated scans are required for follow-up of disease or evaluation of response to treatment (Scialpi et al., 2016). Among the advantages of MRI in the evaluation of pancreatic disease is the capacity to provide high-contrast images of soft tissue structures, thereby enabling the characterization of pancreatic lesions. Multiparametric MRI enables enhanced differentiation of various tumor types ranging from benign cysts to malignant carcinomas. The modality is not only required in primary diagnosis but also follow-up because it can direct the clinician on the best strategies for intervention. MRI has the capacity to detect tissue composition and blood flow changes, thereby providing insight into tumor biology and behavior. As an imaging problem-solving modality, MRI fills the gap left behind by other imaging modalities, thereby its indispensable nature in complex cases of pancreas pathology (Scialpi et al., 2016). MRI is also a key modality in developing theranostics—a science that is founded on simultaneous diagnosis and therapy of diseases, particularly cancers. The integration of molecular imaging techniques with MRI enables clinicians to quantify the biodistribution and pharmacokinetics of therapeutic agents in pancreatic tumors. This application is critical in the planning of treatment protocols for individual patients since it reflects the extent to which a drug reaches the target site. The quantitative MRI values not only direct the treatment process but also provide essential information to enable further drug development and therapeutic effectiveness to be evaluated. Application of MRI to diagnose and treat pancreatic diseases thus goes beyond the conventional imaging techniques and provides a cornerstone in modern medical practice for diseases with multiple factors.

2.3.3. Endoscopic Ultrasound (EUS)

EUS has emerged as a cornerstone diagnostic tool in the evaluation of pancreatic diseases, particularly in identifying lesions and assessing their characteristics. With its high-resolution imaging capabilities, EUS provides real-time visualization of the pancreas, bile ducts, and surrounding structures. This modality enhances the clinician's ability to detect subtle abnormalities that traditional imaging techniques, such as CT, may overlook. For instance, EUS is particularly adept at identifying small pancreatic tumors, cysts, and the local invasion of surrounding tissues, which are critical for planning appropriate surgical interventions. Notably, studies have shown that EUS significantly increases the accuracy of resectability assessments compared to CT alone, thereby reducing the incidence of unnecessary laparotomies, a common complication arising from misdiagnosis during initial imaging evaluations (Tamburrino et al., 2016). The diagnostic utility of EUS extends beyond mere visualization; it also encompasses FNA, which allows for cytological evaluation of suspicious pancreatic masses. This capability is invaluable in differentiating benign from malignant lesions, particularly in cases where imaging findings are inconclusive. The precision of EUS-FNA comes from the close proximity of the endoscope to the lesion, facilitating targeted sampling without the need for invasive surgical procedures. Although the sensitivity and specificity of EUS in determining unresectable diseases have been reported to be appreciably high, debates regarding its routine application in patients with resectable pancreatic cancer still exist due to variations in diagnostic practices and interpreting results (Tamburrino et al., 2016). Thus, the integration of EUS into the diagnostic pathway is not without its complexities and necessitates further investigation and standardization. Techniques to enhance the efficacy of EUS are ongoing relentlessly, as attested by collaborative workshops to bridge gaps in research. These workshops underscore the necessity for the establishment of multicenter consortia to facilitate more significant data collection and analysis in the setting of pancreatic disease. Standardization of EUS protocols and the development of purpose-designed equipment for therapeutic intervention are also pertinent to optimize patient benefit. Early diagnosis of pancreatic disease at high risk underscores the therapeutic value of EUS in preclinical prevention of malignancy before clinical disease. With the ever-changing spectrum of pancreatic disease diagnostic modalities, EUS is at the forefront, leading the charge forward to further diagnostic and therapeutic advances in the treatment of complex pancreatic disease (Figure 2.10).

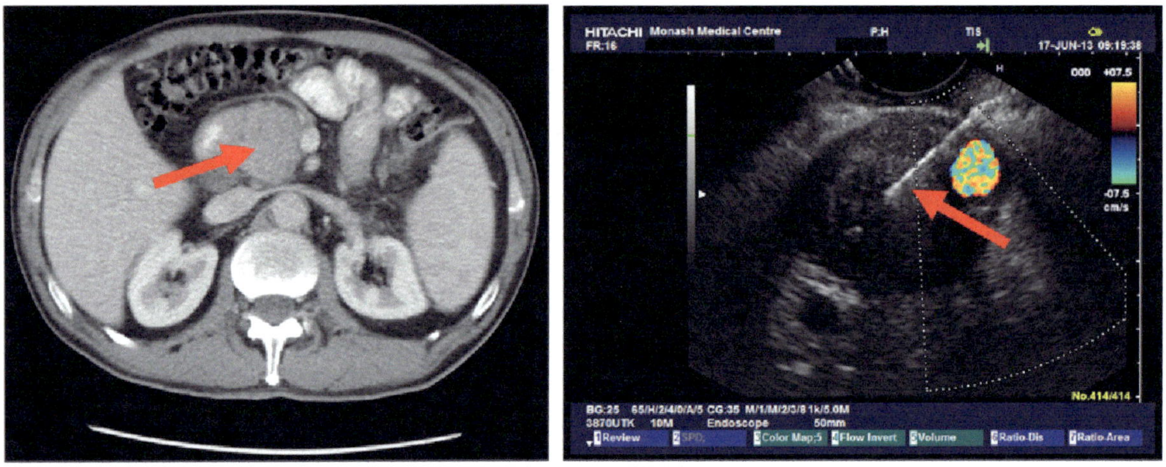

Figure 2.10. Endoscopic ultrasound (EUS) in pancreatic cancer.

Source: https://external-content.duckduckgo.com/iu/?u=https%3A%2F%2Fai2-s2-public.s3.amazonaws.com%2Ffigures%2F2017-08-08%2F750641cf958b78b28c2369d7b10659dea65b98f2%2F6-Figure1-1.png&f=1&nofb=1&ipt=4b4e853cf8e25e39c2e8739a7e0743791c603f0609233201d954f2e61f1ea45f.

2.4. Biopsy Techniques

Among various diagnostic modalities employed to evaluate pancreatic diseases, biopsy techniques are most critical in final diagnosis and management planning. Primarily, endoscopic ultrasound-guided fine-needle aspiration (EUS-FNA) has become the preferred method of sampling pancreatic lesions. Not only does the technique provide access to lesions hitherto considered inaccessible, but it is also less likely to be complicated by percutaneous biopsies. Furthermore, EUS-FNA is sensitive in the diagnosis of a broad range of pancreatic diseases ranging from malignancy to extramedullary plasmacytoma, thereby allowing for prompt and appropriate planning of therapy based on histological diagnosis. Reliability of tissue diagnosis cannot be overstressed since it determines therapeutic interventions that would significantly influence patient morbidity and mortality rates, especially in the discrimination between surgical candidates and those needing chemotherapeutic regimens (Miljkovic' et al., 2012). Advances in EUS technology have generated controversy regarding the standardization of biopsy performance. Important research gaps were identified at a National Institute of Diabetes and Digestive and Kidney Diseases workshop, with emphasis being placed on the need for multicenter large trials in further development of EUS imaging and sampling techniques dedicated to pancreatic diseases (Lee et al., 2017). By having standardized protocols, clinicians can render a more uniform interpretation of EUS findings and promote uniformity of tissue sampling practices. Such measures are of particular significance in the setting of variable presentation of pancreatic lesions, which can mimic each other in imaging studies. Furthermore, the prolongation of training of endoscopists and the involvement of pathologists in the biopsy procedure maximizes the accuracy of diagnosis and minimizes complications such as malignant seeding, which has been a problem with conventional biopsy methods (Miljkovic' et al., 2012). With the medical sciences advancing towards more improved diagnosis modalities, the collaboration between researchers and clinicians remains the motivating force for developing advances in biopsy techniques. Ongoing research in new technologies, such as the use of new imaging machines and better sampling accessories, is aimed at improving the safety and efficiency of therapeutic EUS procedures (Lee et al., 2017). This collaborative work is reflective of an increased awareness that early detection and accurate diagnosis are the cornerstones to dealing with aggressive pancreatic diseases adequately. Through the creation of an interdisciplinary model of detection of the most important imaging features and optimization of sampling strategies, medical experts can better manage the intricacies of pancreatic lesions. The future of pancreatic disease management hinges on the harmonization of these new diagnostic modalities and biopsy techniques, ultimately maximizing patient outcomes in this intricate area (Figure 2.11).

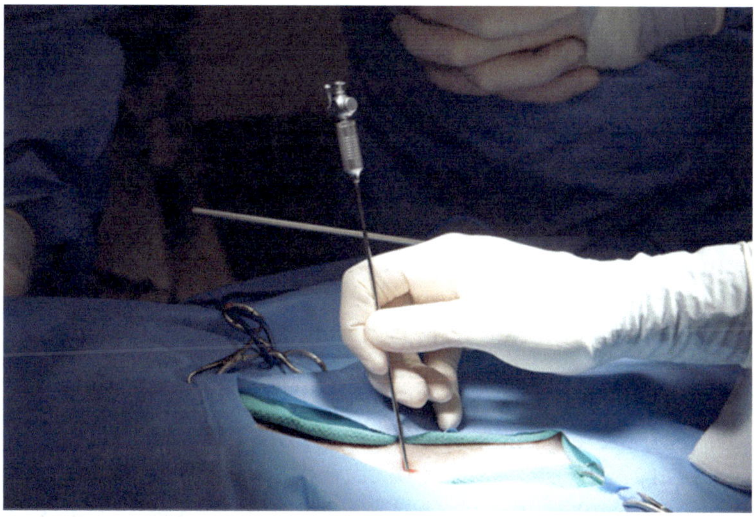

Figure 2.11. Pancreatic biopsy.

Source: https://files.brief.vet/migration/gallery/22466/prop-panc-bx-step-2-2-22466-gallery.png.

2.4.1. Fine-Needle Aspiration Biopsy (FNA)

FNA is now a vital tool in the diagnosis of pancreatic disease, especially in the discrimination between malignant and benign lesions. The process is minimally invasive and entails the use of a thin needle to aspirate cellular tissue from suspected pancreatic masses, which may then be analyzed for cytology. Among the advantages of FNA is that it is relatively complication-free compared to surgical biopsies and the potential to provide rapid diagnostic results. Furthermore, success with FNA is greatly enhanced by the use of imaging modalities, such as EUS, which offers high-quality images of pancreatic tissue. This facilitates precise lesion localization, thus maximizing sampling and diagnostic yield. The role of FNA is not simply one of straightforward diagnosis; it is of critical importance in guiding therapy, especially in severe disease such as pancreatic tumors. Accurate identification of the nature of the tumor dictates whether or not a patient undergoes surgical therapy, chemotherapy, or palliative therapy. For instance, the ability to distinguish pancreatic adenocarcinoma from other illnesses, including extramedullary plasmacytoma, can significantly change patient outcomes. For pancreatic plasmacytoma, accurate tissue diagnosis permits the selection of less aggressive therapy, including chemotherapy and radiation, in preference to risky surgical therapy. The implication of accurate tissue characterization by FNA may lead to decreased morbidity and mortality and emphasize the significance of expertise in this diagnostic tool, especially in gastroenterologists and oncologists. Despite its value, the use of FNA is not controversy-free and poses challenges. Controversy in the use of needle gauge selection and the use of the stylet during aspiration has contributed to the controversy of optimal procedural regimen. Ongoing research on the application of contrast agents in enhancing the efficacy of EUS-FNA is offering real-time imaging and possibly enhanced diagnosis. With ongoing development in EUS technology, FNA will become even more sophisticated, meeting the need for accurate and dependable diagnostic tools in the event of pancreatic disease. Ongoing education of practitioners with the most current techniques will be crucial, particularly with the potential for more complicated pancreatic pathology and the need for accurate diagnosis to direct successful treatment protocols (Miljkovic' et al., 2012; Berzin et al., 2014).

2.4.2. Core Needle Biopsy (CNB)

CNB has been a valuable diagnostic tool in the evaluation of pancreatic disease. The integrative modality offers greater acquisition of tissue specimens than FNA, thereby enhancing the diagnostic yield and the possibility of histologic assessment of pancreatic lesions. Core needle biopsy is particularly valuable in differentiating between various tumor types, for example, benign and malignant lesions, and is useful in the planning of suitable therapy. The need for obtaining accurate pathology of pancreatic lesions cannot be overstated, in that misdiagnosis results in inappropriate therapy and resultant patient morbidity. As imaging modalities like EUS have improved, CNB has gained immense popularity in that it allows the sampling of targeted lesions that would otherwise be difficult to accurately assess, thereby making the process of diagnosis easier in the management of pancreatic disease (Lee et al., 2017). The value of core needle biopsy in the pancreatic environment is further demonstrated by recent evidence that it can enhance diagnostic accuracy over practice. For example, the combination of EUS and CNB not only enhances tissue characterization accuracy but also supplies critical information on tumor staging and grading. This multimodal modality has been invaluable in several clinical environments, for example, lesions that are complicated by surrounding anatomical structures or where imaging results are indeterminate. Further, CNB's ability to yield larger specimens means that accurate assessment of cellular architecture and tumor microenvironment is possible, factors that are critical to determining the appropriate treatment protocols. As research pushes the limits of CNB applications, it is more and more apparent that this technique lies at the heart of the creation of individualized treatment plans among patients with pancreatic cancer (Takahashi et al., 2009). Despite its advantages, the application of core needle biopsy is not complication-free. Infection and bleeding complications are potential and must be carefully balanced in the diagnostic process of pancreatic disease. Operator competence and experience are also vital to the success of the procedure; inadequate sampling can lead to false-negative diagnoses and repeated procedures. For this reason, standard practice and guideline development in the application of CNB is needed to minimize risks and maximize its benefits. Research continues to aim to optimize the technique, e.g., the application of high-technology imaging technology and advanced needle designs. In the end, the inclusion of core needle biopsy in an integrated diagnostic strategy enhances pancreatic disease assessment accuracy and has a pronounced impact on patient outcomes in this difficult clinical environment (Lee et al., 2017) (Figure 2.12).

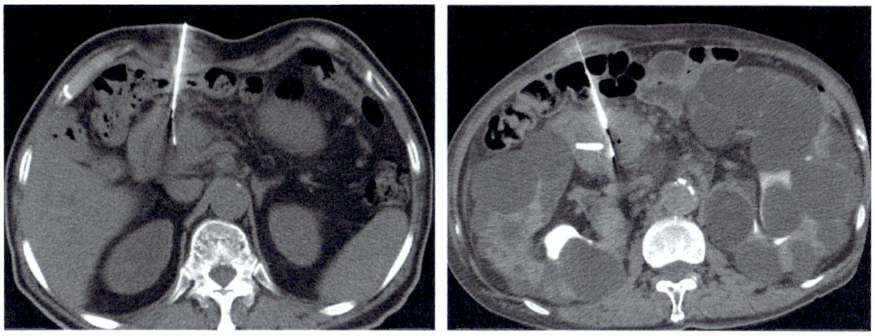

(a) (b)

Figure 2.12. CT-guided pancreatic biopsy using trans-intestinal approach: (a) trans-colonic, and (b) trans-jejunal routes.

Source: https://www.clinicalradiologyonline.net/article/S0009-9260(16)00105-7/fulltext.

2.4.3. Endoscopic Biopsy Procedures

Endoscopic biopsies are a crucial innovation in the diagnostic arsenal of pancreatic disease, especially in the workup of suspicious lesions within the pancreas. Through the use of EUS, doctors can make precise images of the pancreas, and abnormal masses that might be malignant can be detected. FNA or biopsy methods can then be employed to obtain tissue samples of the mass directly. This minimally invasive process reduces morbidity in the patient compared to conventional surgical biopsies, and accurate histopathological diagnosis can be made. Endoscopic biopsies can also yield precious information regarding the character of the lesion—benign or malignant—and enable the formulation of a specific treatment protocol. Endoscopic biopsy procedures are therefore, a crucial intervention in the early detection and treatment of pancreatic disease. The application of endoscopic biopsy methods has forced a rethinking of conventional diagnostic methods, and the impact on the differentiation between each of the pancreatic lesions has been significant. Current research illustrates the benefit of EUS-guided FNA in differentiating intrapancreatic accessory spleen from non-functional neuroendocrine tumors (NF-NETs) and other pancreatic masses, a differentiation that is crucial to the advisability of surgical treatment. As highlighted by research on false positives and subsequent misdiagnosis, such as in the case of 68Ga-Dotatoc uptake for pancreatic NET but subsequently found to be IPAS, accuracy in diagnostics becomes absolutely critical (Lancellotti et al., 2019). Such misdiagnosis highlights the risk involved in the sole use of imaging study alone in the absence of corroborative evidence available by histologic examination by endoscopic biopsy procedures. In addition to the increased diagnostic accuracy, future research using endoscopic methods is opening doors to innovation in the therapeutic management of pancreatic disease. Annual workshops, funded by the National Institute of Diabetes and Digestive and Kidney Diseases, have emphasized the most significant research gaps and the need to standardize EUS procedures for the most prevalent pancreatic diseases (Lee et al., 2017). With this collective effort comes the goal of not only improving the sampling of pancreatic lesions but also the development of specialized devices that make the procedure safer and more efficient. By bridging these gaps, the medical community can ensure that endoscopic biopsy remains at the cutting edge of diagnostic and therapeutic interventions, ultimately translating into improved patient outcomes in pancreatic diseases (Figure 2.13).

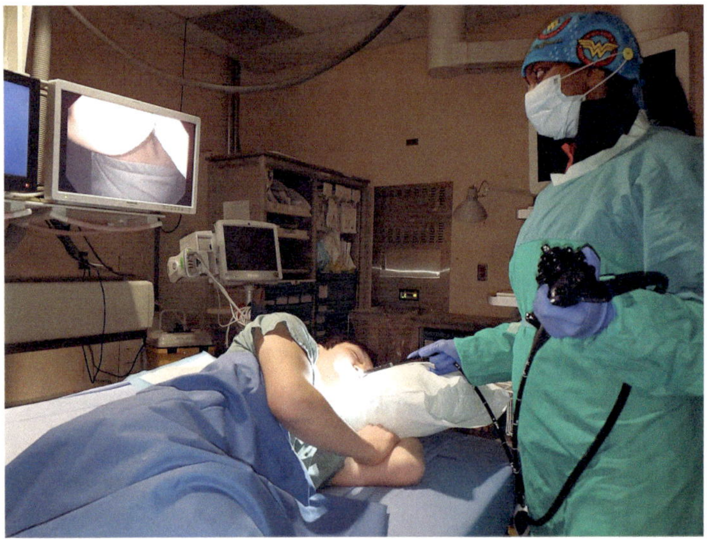

Figure 2.13. Endoscopy biopsy pancreas.

Source: By Samir - Own work, CC BY-SA 4.0, https://commons.wikimedia.org/w/index.php?curid=101875193

2.5. Emerging Diagnostic Technologies

The evolution of diagnostic technology forms the focal point in addressing the complexity of pancreatic diseases. Emerging technologies such as EUS have greatly enhanced the visualization and evaluation of lesions within the pancreas. Through being a minimally invasive equipment, EUS allows for the observation of pancreatic tissue and surrounding structures more intimately, hence facilitating early detection of malignancy. The application of EUS in the diagnosis of pancreatic adenocarcinoma is particularly relevant, as it can potentially enhance the staging process and guide therapeutic intervention. In the face of controversies regarding the appropriateness of EUS for various clinical presentations, the evidence suggests that more studies are needed to optimize its use in clinical practice as well as the validity of pancreatic disease diagnostics (Berzin et al., 2014). Thus, continued investigation of EUS and other imaging modalities is necessary in optimizing diagnostic accuracy and patient care. Additionally, the promise of nanotechnology and its applications in diagnostic clinical practice continues to be an exciting area of development, particularly for pancreatic diseases. Nano-enabled imaging agents facilitate improved detection at cellular and molecular levels critical for the sensing of early pancreatic conditions. These advanced agents enhance contrast and signal detectability in imaging processes, which helps in better localization of pancreatic tumors. Further, the use of nanoparticles in therapeutic strategies, such as targeted drug delivery, can facilitate enhanced traditional diagnostic processes by forming a self-sustained loop of diagnosis and treatment. The combination of nanotechnology and diagnostics not only expands the spectrum of diagnostic modalities but also offers prospective ways for the effective management of pancreatic diseases and optimizing therapeutic results with personalized therapy (Shariati et al., 2019). Liquid biopsies are among the new-generation technologies that also mark a paradigm shift in monitoring and pancreatic disease diagnosis. With analysis of circulating tumor cells and circulating tumor DNA, liquid biopsies are a minimally invasive substitute for traditional tissue biopsies. Liquid biopsy can lead to the early identification of pancreatic cancer biomarkers and the timing so critical to increasing survival. Beyond this, the versatility of liquid biopsy workflows allows real-time monitoring of disease and response to treatment, thus enabling personalized therapy. With continued study of the optimization of liquid biopsy technologies, their application to routine clinical practice will inevitably transform the treatment of pancreatic disease. Lastly, advances in diagnostic technology promise a new era of precision medicine, in which interventions are individualized to meet the specific needs of individual patients and improve overall awareness and treatment of pancreatic disease (Figure 2.14).

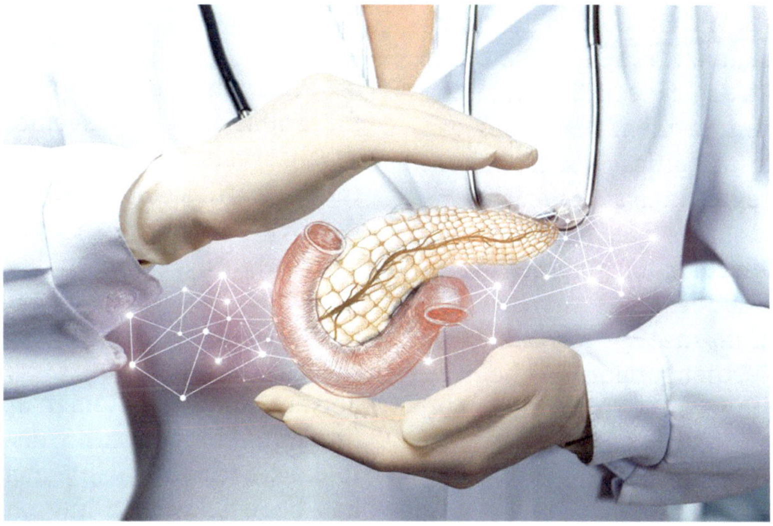

Figure 2.14. Emerging diagnostic technologies of pancreati-diseases.

Source: https://thisquarterly.sg/wp-content/uploads/2020/10/know-about-pancreati-diseases-01-1024x682.jpg.

2.5.1. Molecular Imaging Techniques

Molecular imaging techniques play a central role in the diagnosis and treatment of pancreatic pathology and serve as a bridge between conventional imaging technologies and new therapeutic approaches. They comprise a number of various techniques, including PET, single-photon emission computed tomography (SPECT), and optical imaging, which allow for the visualization of biological processes at the cellular and molecular levels. Molecular imaging can identify pancreatic tumors and shed light on their biology using targeted biomarkers and radiolabeled probes, enabling early intervention in the clinic. Such advancements in molecular imaging technologies hold the power to revolutionize diagnostic practice for pancreatic disease, with increasingly targeted therapy plans taking into consideration the patient's own pathology and disease course. One of the most important advantages of molecular imaging is that it can quantitatively evaluate drug biodistribution and pharmacokinetics in pancreatic disease. Techniques such as PET and SPECT are capable of localizing and quantitating radioisotope-labeled nanoparticles and other delivery vehicles for drugs, thereby informing therapeutic choices and patient outcomes. This is particularly significant in the field of theranostics, in which the treatment and diagnostic roles are combined to most effectively treat cancer. The imaging data correlation with treatment responses can provide insights into the efficacy of treatment and track disease progression, so interventions remain timely and appropriate. With ongoing advancements in molecular imaging, its use in everyday clinical practice holds the promise to optimize the overall strategy for managing pancreatic disease. Further support for the need for molecular imaging comes from the need for advanced tools and new methodologies to optimize pancreatic disease diagnosis and treatment. A multicenter trials workshop sponsored by the National Institute of Diabetes and Digestive and Kidney Diseases highlighted the need for such trials with the ultimate aim of standardization of EUS techniques and optimal imaging characteristics for various pancreatic diseases (Lee et al., 2017). These partnerships point toward research gaps that molecular imaging can help bridge, including the identification of high-risk lesions before the development of macroscopically detectable disease. In addition, novel imaging modalities could enhance the application of therapeutic EUS procedures toward safe and effective pancreatic disease treatment. With evolving disciplines, the integration of molecular imaging into diagnosis programs will inevitably support clinical decision-making, ending up influencing improved outcomes in patients.

2.5.2. Liquid Biopsy Advancements

Emerging technologies in liquid biopsies have arrived as a very important aspect in the diagnostic modalities of pancreatic diseases, that is early detection and follow-up. Liquid biopsies allow one to analyze biomarkers in body fluid such as blood or urine, which is non-invasive and patient-friendly compared to traditional tissue biopsies. This technique has tremendous potential in pancreatic cancer, one of the most deadly cancers, where timely intervention is paramount. Through the identification of circulating tumor cells (CTCs) and ctDNA, liquid biopsies provide an opportunity to see genetic mutations that may decide targeted therapies. As observed in studies of other types of cancer, the versatility of liquid biopsy methods can be used within the area of pancreatic diseases to contribute immensely to personalized medicine and extend additional sophistication in the insight into cancer progression. The incorporation of new technologies, such as Surface-Enhanced Raman Spectroscopy (SERS), into liquid biopsy platforms further contributes to diagnostic ability in pancreatic disease. SERS has been shown to have high specificity and sensitivity for biomarker detection, and it is a revolutionary tool in cancer and oncology. Using highly sensitive analytical techniques, SERS enables the rapid identification of cancer cells and molecular profiling, which are pivotal for the effective management of pancreatic cancers. This is consistent with the rising need for non-invasive diagnostic approaches that can detect cancer at an earlier stage and will have a major impact on patient survival. SERS and microfluidics integration not only advances the accuracy of liquid biopsy but also promises easier integration within clinics, thus avoiding the challenges faced by the application of conventional diagnostic techniques in gastroenterology, particularly in pancreatic diseases. As exciting as liquid biopsy advancement is, some challenges of clinical validation as well as standardization of the approaches, particularly for pancreatic cancer, remain. While there exist biomarkers like CA19-9 that are used today, their limitations in sensitivity and specificity necessitate the creation of new biomarkers through liquid biopsy assays. Research has, therefore, identified several potential markers for cholangiocarcinoma, suggesting that these need to be further investigated in larger studies. The incremental progress towards the clinical use of these biomarkers necessitates further research and development. As liquid biopsies evolve, they could potentially not only be employed as a diagnostic tool but also as a monitoring tool for treatment and relapse follow-up, further optimizing the whole course of pancreatic disease management and patient care in the future (Ney et al., 2021) (Figure 2.15).

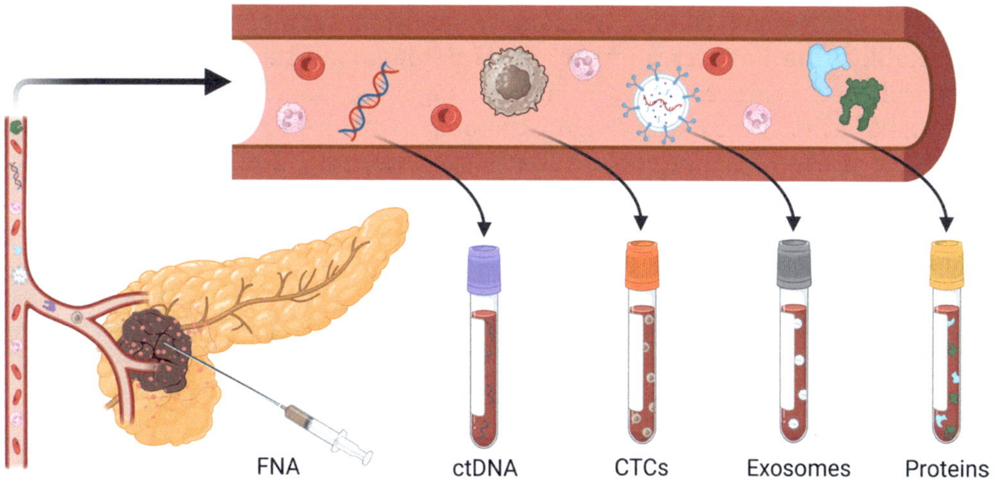

Figure 2.15. Liquid biopsy advancements.

Source: Munnings R, Gibbs P, Lee B. Evolution of Liquid Biopsies for Detecting Pancreatic Cancer. *Cancers*. 2024; 16(19):3335. https://doi.org/10.3390/cancers16193335

2.5.3. Artificial Intelligence (AI) in Diagnostic Imaging

The integration of AI in diagnostic imaging has revolutionized the treatment process for pancreatic ailments. Among the most notable advantages of AI technologies is that they are able to analyze complicated imaging data quicker and more precisely than previously possible. This capability enhances the detection and description of pancreatic lesions, which can be subtle and hence quite hard to detect using traditional methods of imaging. With clinicians relying more and more on AI for enhancing diagnostic accuracy, studies have indicated that AI solutions can attain a 99% accuracy rate in diagnosing malignancies, marking a revolutionary shift in clinical practice. Moreover, AI algorithms continue to improve themselves through iterative learning on vast data sets and therefore become better at detecting intricate patterns in imaging studies, which is needed for early and effective management of the patient in pancreatic pathology (Ozsahin et al., 2022). Apart from diagnosis, AI uses also extend beyond the detection of the condition; they are hugely engaged in prognostic evaluation as well as in planning the treatment for pancreatic ailments. With the application of natural language processing and machine learning algorithms, AI systems can combine data from patient history, imaging studies, and biomarker data, thereby allowing for personalized therapeutic strategies. For instance, AI can make the outcome of patients following surgery more predictable, thereby enabling clinicians to make data-based decisions that enhance the quality of care. The AI research explosion has also set off research efforts focused on leveraging big data analytics to produce precise predictive models that can potentially change patient pathways by refining preoperative optimization and individualized adjuvant treatment (McGivern et al., 2023). Along with this, the evolving landscape of AI applications in diagnostic imaging at the intersection of pancreatic disease raises key issues regarding the ethics dimension and the requirement for policy guidelines. Emphasis on transparency in AI algorithms is critical, as reliance on them necessitates true comprehension of their functioning limits, along with patient data bias. As clinical decisions are more and more being driven by AI technology, ongoing cooperation between healthcare professionals and technologists is necessary to ensure that developments supplement and do not replace clinical wisdom. In addition, further strong research studies will be needed to establish the long-term impact of AI deployment on patient outcomes, the quality of care, and overall healthcare costs. This multi-pronged approach will be vital in realizing the complete potential of AI for innovating diagnostic tools in the context of pancreatic diseases while maintaining patient safety (Ozsahin et al., 2022; McGivern et al., 2023).

A CLOSER LOOK

FUTURE IN PANCREATIC DISEASE DIAGNOSIS

With ongoing advances in medical diagnostic technology, future directions in pancreatic disease diagnosis will likely emphasize the integration of advanced imaging techniques with molecular biology. Traditional imaging techniques, such as CT and MRI, have been extremely valuable in the diagnosis of pancreatic diseases; however, their limitations necessitate innovative solutions. New imaging technologies, including functional imaging and hybrid modalities combining anatomical with molecular data, show great promise for providing an improved understanding of pancreatic pathologies. Specifically, the application of functional MRI or PET in conjunction with standard imaging improves pancreatic cancer diagnosis and allows more accurate estimation of disease staging, hence addressing the urgent need for improved diagnostic tools in this field. With imaging progress, the role of circulating biomarkers in diagnosing pancreatic disease is gaining greater significance. Current biomarkers, particularly those related to pancreatic cancer like CA 19-9, tend to be non-specific and insensitive, leading to challenges in early diagnosis and prediction. Circulating RNA and other multianalyte testing are promising to characterize the disease more efficiently. For instance, NETest demonstrates clinical utility by quantifying circulating transcripts that can potentially quantify tumor burden and activity and thus offer insight into response to therapy and monitoring of disease.

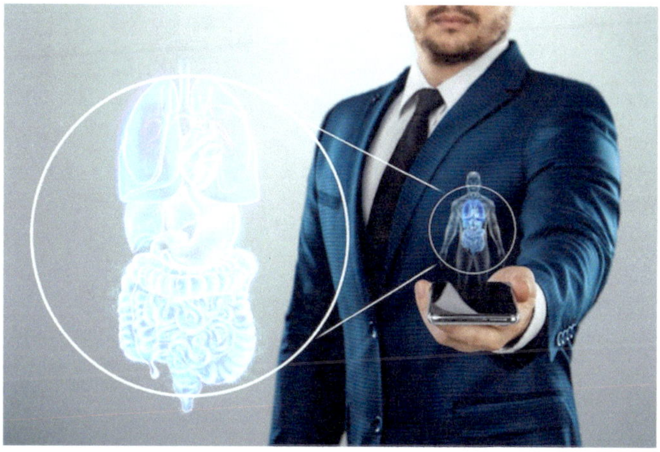

Source: https://img.freepik.com/premium-photo/holographic-projection-scannin-internal-organs-person-x-ray-phone_99433-5677.jpg?w=826.

Future diagnostic technologies will likely focus on combining these new biomarkers with imaging modalities to allow an integrated approach that enhances accuracy as well as speed of diagnosis of pancreatic disease. The push for an individualized approach to medicine will also lead the way in diagnostic modalities for pancreatic disease. Interdisciplinary collaboration between oncologists, radiologists, and molecular biologists will be important to formulate more targeted diagnostic criteria that deal with the heterogeneous nature of pancreatic disorders. Consensus panels, such as the multinational Delphi exercise involving experts in neuroendocrine neoplasms, underscore the importance of a multidisciplinary effort to identify and confirm new diagnostic models. Consensus noted circulating multianalyte RNA as a fertile area with which to advance existing diagnostic methods. As the practice changes, it will be important to guide the creation of clinico-biological tests that are capable of providing high-definition information about disease status and response to therapy to improve patient outcomes in pancreatic disease care (Patel & Oppenheimer, 2025) (Figure 2.16).

SUMMARY

In highlighting the most important findings in the field of pancreatic disorders' diagnostic modalities, how accurate and timely diagnosis of pancreatic disorders significantly enhances patient outcomes is evidently clear. With emphasis on a comparison of the various imaging techniques, such as CT, MRI, and PET, the diagnostic accuracy field is seen to be a complex one. Every modality is particular to its strengths and limitations, and practitioners are compelled to include patient-specific factors and clinical situations in making the optimal diagnostic approach. For instance, 68-Ga-Dotatoc PET/CT has been recognized as the gold standard for discriminating neuroendocrine tumors from non-neoplastic conditions such as an intrapancreatic accessory spleen (IPAS) (Lancellotti et al., 2019). Such precise diagnosis not only assists in creating effective treatment plans but also prevents improper surgical intervention. Moreover, the advent of new biomarker studies can potentially revolutionize the detection of pancreatic disease, particularly in complex cases where imaging alone might be inadequate. Biomarkers have been discovered in recent studies that possess the ability to increase diagnostic sensitivity and specificity for conditions like CFLD, which is prevalent among cystic fibrosis patients but often underdiagnosed due to a lack of periodic sensitive diagnostic methods (Hage et al., 2013). The significant upregulation of proteins like TIMP-4 and Endoglin among CFLD patients points toward the role of serum biomarkers alongside routine imaging methods. This development accentuates the importance of prospective research to validate these new biomarkers and develop standardized protocols to integrate them into clinical practice, which can result in better and less invasive diagnostic regimens. As a final remark, the evaluation of pancreatic disease diagnostic modalities not only represents the current capability of present technology but also paves the way for future possibilities. A comprehensive strategy using imaging with potential serum biomarkers may lead to improved diagnostic efficacy and patient care. The dynamic process of the modalities is meant to highlight the necessity for coordination among specialists, researchers, and clinicians across disciplines to make the best use of the modalities. Though further research elucidates the intricate dynamics between serum biomarkers and the pathology of pancreatic disease, stakeholders must ensure these findings are integrated into clinical practice guidelines. This commitment can ultimately reshape the diagnostic model, offering the promise of better patient care and outcomes in the case of pancreatic diseases.

Diagnosis of pancreatic illnesses has also come a long way, and the key takeaway here is to use more than one diagnostic modality to get reliable results. General imaging modalities like CT and MRI are extremely useful in terms of understanding pancreatic morphology as well as pathology. For example, CT scans are very good at detecting pancreatic masses and inflammatory lesions, while MRI gives superior visualization of soft tissue contrast and the vascular system. Imaging modalities are employed as a first point of investigation to determine the requirement of further exploration of visualized abnormalities. With diagnostic accuracy being of paramount significance, imaging results are supplemented by clinical presentations when formulating an appropriate management strategy. In addition to imaging, biochemical investigations also have a crucial role in the diagnosis of pancreatic disorders, particularly endocrine-related disorders. Pancreatic cancer and pancreatitis may lead to biochemical marker alterations, which may indicate the development of disease. Specifically, in the context of acute pancreatitis, serum levels of amylase and lipase are typically elevated and will distinguish this condition from other gastrointestinal diseases. Further, new evidence has also explored the possibility of some biomarkers of pancreatic disease, such as

TIMP-4 and Endoglin, within liver disease in cystic fibrosis. These biomarkers show encouraging results in refining diagnostic accuracy and highlight the necessity for further study to identify valid and specific markers of pancreatic pathologies (Hage et al., 2013). Innovation in modality also highlights the necessity for multidisciplinary management of pancreatic diseases. A combination of imaging, laboratory tests, and specialized techniques facilitates a complete understanding of the patient's condition. For instance, the application of EUS and FNA allows for cytological evaluation of pancreatic lesions to further narrow down the diagnostic process. Additionally, this multi-modality can involve interdisciplinary collaboration among gastroenterologists, radiologists, and pathologists to ensure maximum patient outcomes. This multi-disciplinary strategy is particularly crucial in the management of complicated diseases such as pancreatic neuroendocrine neoplasms, wherein this may facilitate personalized therapy planning based on the unique characteristics of each tumor (Caplin et al., 2017). The continuous development of diagnostic modalities should thus be given priority to enhance the accuracy and efficiency of pancreatic disease diagnosis and management.

KEY TERMS FROM THIS CHAPTER

- Abdominal pain
- Central organ
- Circulating tumor cells (CTCs)
- Cystic fibrosis (CF)
- Medical community
- Pancreatic cysts
- Biopsy Techniques
- Chronic inflammation
- Clinical environment
- Cystic fibrosis-associated liver disease (CFLD)
- Multifactorial pathogenesis
- Pancreatic diagnostics

References

1. Ney, A., Garcia-Sampedro, A., Goodchild, G., Acedo, P., Fusai, G., & Pereira, S. P. (2021). Biliary Strictures and Cholangiocarcinoma - Untangling a Diagnostic Conundrum. *Frontiers in oncology*, *11*, 699401. https://doi.org/10.3389/fonc.2021.699401 (accessed on 26 May 2025).
2. Lykoudis, P. M., Partelli, S., Muffatti, F., Caplin, M., Falconi, M., Fusai, G. K., & RARECARENet Working Group (2019). Treatment challenges in and outside a specialist network setting: Pancreatic neuroendocrine tumours. *European journal of surgical oncology : the journal of the European Society of Surgical Oncology and the British Association of Surgical Oncology*, *45*(1), 46–51. https://doi.org/10.1016/j.ejso.2017.08.019 (accessed on 26 May 2025).
3. Ambrosini, V., Baum, R. P., Bodei, L., Kidd, M., et al. (2016). Imaging and biomarkers in gastroenteropancreatic neuroendocrine tumor disease management. https://core.ac.uk/download/199417681.pdf Oberg, K., Krenning, E., Sundin, A., Bodei, L., Kidd, M., Tesselaar, M., Ambrosini, V., Baum, R. P., Kulke, M., Pavel, M., Cwikla, J., Drozdov, I., Falconi, M., Fazio, N., Frilling, A., Jensen, R., Koopmans, K., Korse, T., Kwekkeboom, D., Maecke, H., ... Modlin, I. M. (2016). A Delphic consensus assessment: imaging and biomarkers in gastroenteropancreatic neuroendocrine tumor disease management. *Endocrine connections*, *5*(5), 174–187. https://doi.org/10.1530/EC-16-0043 (accessed on 26 May 2025).
4. Lee, L. S., Andersen, D. K., Ashida, R., Brugge, W. R., Canto, M. I., Chang, K. J., Chari, S. T., DeWitt, J., Hwang, J. H., Khashab, M. A., Kim, K., Levy, M. J., McGrath, K., Park, W. G., Singhi, A., Stevens, T., Thompson, C. C., Topazian, M. D., Wallace, M. B., Wani, S., ... Singh, V. K. (2017). Endoscopic Ultrasound and Related Technologies for the Diagnosis and Treatment of Pancreatic Disease - Research Gaps and Opportunities: Summary of a National Institute of Diabetes and Digestive and Kidney Diseases Workshop. *Pancreas*, *46*(10), 1242–1250. https://doi.org/10.1097/MPA.0000000000000936 (accessed on 26 May 2025).
5. Scialpi, M., Reginelli, A., D'Andrea, A., Gravante, S., Falcone, G., Baccari, P., Manganaro, L., Palumbo, B., & Cappabianca, S. (2016). Pancreatic tumors imaging: An update. *International journal of surgery (London, England)*, *28 Suppl 1*, S142–S155. https://doi.org/10.1016/j.ijsu.2015.12.053(accessed on 26 May 2025).
6. Stieber, P., Molina, R., Gion, M., Gressner, A., Troalen, F., Holdenrieder, S., Auge, J. M., Zancan, M., Wycislo, M., & Jarrige, V. (2008). Alternative antibody for the detection of CA19-9 antigen: a European multicenter study for the evaluation of the analytical and clinical performance of the Access GI Monitor assay on the UniCel Dxl 800 Immunoassay System. *Clinical chemistry and laboratory medicine*, *46*(5), 600–611. https://doi.org/10.1515/CCLM.2008.126 (accessed on 26 May 2025).
7. Lancellotti, F., Sacco, L., Cerasari, S., Bellato, V., Cicconi, S., Ciardi, A., Muttillo, E. M., Feola, T., Caronna, R., & Chirletti, P. (2019). Intrapancreatic accessory spleen false positive to 68Ga-Dotatoc: case report and literature review. *World journal of surgical oncology*, *17*(1), 117. https://doi.org/10.1186/s12957-019-1660-2 (accessed on 26 May 2025).
8. McGivern KG, Drake TM, Knight SR, Lucocq J, Bernabeu MO, Clark N, Fairfield C, Pius R, Shaw CA, Seth S, Harrison EM. Applying artificial intelligence to big data in hepatopancreatic and biliary surgery: a scoping review. *Art Int Surg*. 2023;3:27-47. http://dx.doi.org/10.20517/ais.2022.39 (accessed on 26 May 2025).

9. Berzin, T. M., & Trindade, A. J. (2014). *Clinical Controversies in Endoscopic Ultrasound*. https://core.ac.uk/download/28948200.pdf (accessed on 26 May 2025).

10. . Takahashi, Y., Irisawa, A., Bhutani, M. S., Hikichi, T., Takagi, T., Shibukawa, G., Wakatsuki, T., Imamura, H., Sato, A., Sato, M., Ikeda, T., Suzuki, R., Obara, K., Hashimoto, Y., Watanabe, K., & Ohira, H. (2009). Two Cases of Retroperitoneal Liposarcoma Diagnosed Using Endoscopic Ultrasound-Guided Fine-Needle Aspiration (EUS-FNA). *Diagnostic and therapeutic endoscopy, 2009*, 673194. https://doi.org/10.1155/2009/673194

11. Peters, L. M., Glanemann, B., Garden, O. A., & Szladovits, B. (2016). Cytological Findings of 140 Bile Samples from Dogs and Cats and Associated Clinical Pathological Data. *Journal of veterinary internal medicine*, *30*(1), 123–131. https://doi.org/10.1111/jvim.13645 (accessed on 26 May 2025).

12. Busse, R., Ferch, M., Fuchs, S., Grössmann, N., et al. (2019). Evidence-based indications for the planning of PET or PET/CT capacities are needed. https://core.ac.uk/download/287885302.pdf (accessed on 26 May 2025).

13. Caplin, M., Falconi, M., Fusai, G. K., Lykoudis, P. M., et al. (2017). Treatment challenges in and outside a specialist network setting: Pancreatic neuroendocrine tumors. https://core.ac.uk/download/168403284.pdf (accessed on 26 May 2025).

14. Shariati, M., Willaert, W., Ceelen, W., De Smedt, S. C., & Remaut, K. (2019). Aerosolization of Nanotherapeutics as a Newly Emerging Treatment Regimen for Peritoneal Carcinomatosis. *Cancers*, *11*(7), 906. https://doi.org/10.3390/cancers11070906

15. Copeland, L. I. B. T., James, D., Duinkerken, M. S. I., Kelsey, G., et al. (2020). *Jefferson Digital Commons Quarterly Report: January–March 2020*. https://core.ac.uk/download/299811518.pdf (accessed on 26 May 2025).

16. Hulsebosch, S. E., Palm, C. A., Segev, G., Cowgill, L. D., Kass, P. H., & Marks, S. L. (2016). Evaluation of Canine Pancreas-Specific Lipase Activity, Lipase Activity, and Trypsin-Like Immunoreactivity in an Experimental Model of Acute Kidney Injury in Dogs. *Journal of veterinary internal medicine*, *30*(1), 192–199. https://doi.org/10.1111/jvim.13806

17. Cunha, L., Mathé, D., Metello, L. F., Szigeti, K., et al. (2014). The role of molecular imaging in modern drug development. https://core.ac.uk/download/47140757.pdf (accessed on 26 May 2025).

18. Tamburrino, D., Riviere, D., Yaghoobi, M., Davidson, B. R., & Gurusamy, K. S. (2016). Diagnostic accuracy of different imaging modalities following computed tomography (CT) scanning for assessing the resectability with curative intent in pancreatic and periampullary cancer. *The Cochrane database of systematic reviews*, *9*(9), CD011515. https://doi.org/10.1002/14651858.CD011515.pub2 (accessed on 26 May 2025).

19. Ding, H., & Wu, F. (2012). *Image Guided Biodistribution and Pharmacokinetic Studies of Theragnostic*. https://core.ac.uk/download/81626143.pdf (accessed on 26 May 2025).

20. Uzun Ozsahin, D., Ikechukwu Emegano, D., Uzun, B., & Ozsahin, I. (2022). The Systematic Review of Artificial Intelligence Applications in Breast Cancer Diagnosis. *Diagnostics (Basel, Switzerland)*, *13*(1), 45. https://doi.org/10.3390/diagnostics13010045 (accessed on 26 May 2025).

21. Patel, M., & Goldberg Oppenheimer, P. (2025). Advancements in cancer diagnostics: integrating surface-enhanced Raman spectroscopy and microptofluidics for precision and versatility. *Applied Spectroscopy Reviews.* Advance online publication. https://doi.org/10.1080/05704928.2025.2465394 (accessed on 26 May 2025).

22. Hage, L., Kügler, M., Menendez Menendez, K., Naehrlich, L., et al. (2013). *Serum Proteome Profiling Identifies Novel and Powerful Markers of Cystic Fibrosis Liver Disease.* https://core.ac.uk/download/12175519.pdf (accessed on 26 May 2025).

23. Khanna, A. K., Tiwary, Satyendra K., Kumar, Puneet, Pancreatic Pseudocyst: Therapeutic Dilemma, *International Journal of Inflammation*, 2012, 279476, 7 pages, 2012. **https://doi.org/10.1155/2012/279476**

24. Miljković, M., & Senadhi, V. (2012). *Use of Endoscopic Ultrasound in Diagnosing Plasmacytoma of the Pancreas.* https://core.ac.uk/download/619642399.pdf (accessed on 26 May 2025).

25. Vaccaro MI, Resnik R. Translational Pancreatology. New Approaches in the Development of Novel Biomarkers as Screening Methodologies for Pancreatic Cancer. J Transl Gastroenterol Clin Hepatol. 2018 Feb;1(1):101 (accessed on 26 May 2025).

26. Rogers, C. (2015). *Radiological Perspective of The Formation of Pressure Ulcers–A Comparison of Pressure and Experience on Two Imaging Surfaces.* https://core.ac.uk/download/603206223.pdf (accessed on 26 May 2025).

27. Stefanov, Y. (2024). *Diagnosis and Treatment of Acute Pancreatitis in Adult Patients.* Proceedings - Symposium "Alumni Club and Friends" - April, 5-6, 2024. https://core.ac.uk/download/622091523.pdf (accessed on 26 May 2025).

28. Tripalo-Batoš, A., Šverko, A., Krušlin, B., Mustapić, M., Marotti, M., & Bekavac Bešlin, M. (2011). Korelacija između slikovnog prikaza magnetskom rezonancijom i histopatologije u diferencijaciji bolesti gušterače. *[Correlation Between MRI Imaging and Histopathology in Differentiation of Pancreatic Diseases].* https://core.ac.uk/download/14446684.pdf (accessed on 26 May 2025).

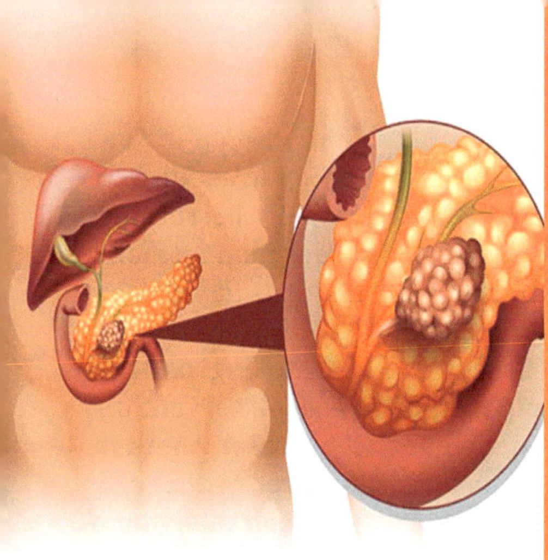

Chapter 3

ACUTE PANCREATITIS

Contents

Introduction

Acute pancreatitis is an acute and severe inflammation of the pancreas that typically arises secondary to multiple underlying etiologies such as gallstones, alcohol consumption, or metabolic disease. Acute pancreatitis may present with a wide range of symptoms, ranging from intense abdominal pain to vomiting to nausea, which can lead to significant morbidity. Over the last few decades, the incidence of acute pancreatitis has been increasing, and it remains a significant concern for physicians. Healthcare providers should understand the etiology, pathophysiology, and management of this disease in detail to treat the clinical characteristics of acute pancreatitis optimally. Furthermore, as genetic factors and treatment protocols are researched, more attention is given to individualized treatment to further accommodate each patient, providing improved outcomes and a higher understanding of the complexity of conditions (Klimenko et al., 2024). Diagnosis of acute pancreatitis is often made challenging by the presence of overlapping symptoms with other gastrointestinal diseases. Serum amylase and lipase concentrations, imaging tests such as CT scans, and endoscopic ultrasound to determine the severity of the illness as well as potential complications, are some of the routine diagnostic methods. Grading of the severity of acute pancreatitis is critical as it guides management methods and potential interventions. Based on recent findings, infected necrosis is a key driver for treatment protocols, corroborating an endoscopic step-up approach for localized pancreatic necrosis patients (Klimenko et al., 2024). Furthermore, what is essential in improving patient outcomes and minimizing complications is the recognition of the importance of early intervention and precise diagnosis, emphasizing the importance of a thorough diagnostic process. Another significant characteristic of acute pancreatitis is its association with pancreatic cancer, which can manifest as an unusual presenting symptom. Such an association highlights the necessity of vigilant diagnostic workup to identify pancreatic malignancies in their early stage in the setting of acute pancreatitis. The initial evaluations must try to exclude common causes such as gallstones and alcohol, as well as search for potential neoplasms through the use of advanced imaging modalities and tumor markers. Early recognition of pancreatic cancer in such patients is crucial; it allows for initiating effective treatment modalities that can significantly enhance prognosis and quality of life. Hence, the complex interdependence between acute pancreatitis and pancreatic cancer highlights the need for close patient follow-up and targeted screening algorithms to avoid the risk of overlooking malignant processes during acute attacks (Figure 3.1).

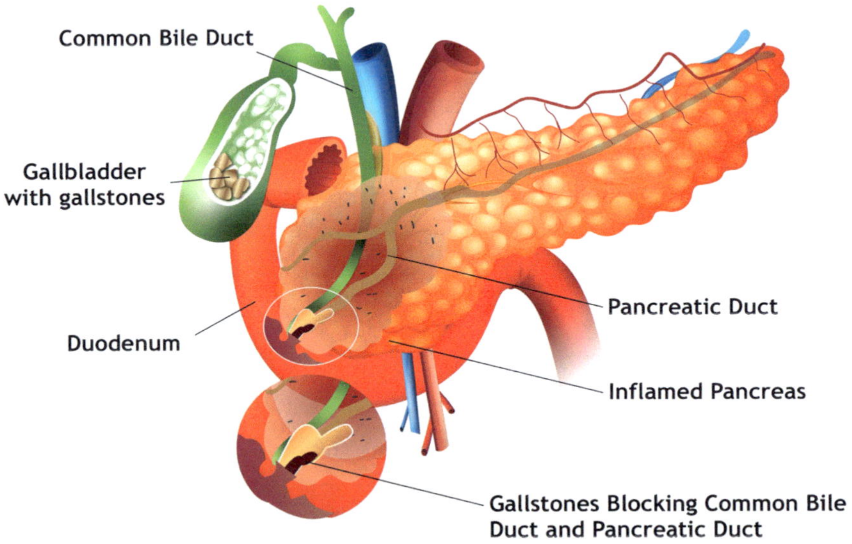

Figure 3.1. Acute pancreatitis (AP) caused by gallstones.

Source: https://www.statpearls.com/pictures/getimagecontent/22474.

Definition of Acute Pancreatitis (AP)

AP is an acute pancreatitis inflammation that may cause different serious complications if it is not treated in time. It is characterized by the early activation of pancreatic enzymes, which cause autodigestion of the pancreatic tissue. The etiology of inflammation is via multiple etiological sources such as gallstone disease, chronic pancreatitis, and excessive alcohol consumption, certain drugs, and metabolic disturbances like hyperlipidemia. The acute attack of this disease typically appears as severe pain in the abdomen, vomiting, nausea, and sometimes even systemic presentations like fever and tachycardia. Identification of the pathophysiology of acute pancreatitis is crucial for early intervention and diagnosis, as rapid intervention can make a significant difference in patient prognosis. The pathophysiology of acute pancreatitis is an inflammatory cascade initiated by the premature activation of digestive enzymes within the pancreas. This undesirable enzymatic action can lead to tissue damage, inflammation, and systemic involvement with organ failure. Diagnosis is typically clinical and laboratory investigation, e.g., serum testing of pancreatic enzymes like lipase and amylase. An increase in their levels is indicative of pancreatic damage and forms a key part of establishing the condition. However, it is important to consider the setting of other diseases, in that elevated lipase may be observed under other conditions, for instance, with renal injury, and this complicates the clinical course of acute pancreatitis (Hulsebosch et al., 2015, 2018). Supportive therapy, such as intravenous fluid resuscitation, analgesia, and nutrition, along with treatment of the cause, often controls acute pancreatitis. When gallstones are an underlying cause, surgery may be needed to remove the stones and restore bile duct flow. Further investigation is also important in terms of identifying predictive markers as well as potential preventative measures. The commonality of acute pancreatitis and the varied presentations indicate a need for clinical and general population awareness. Such knowledge can lead to early diagnosis and enhance the prospects for those who are affected, demonstrating the value of further research into this complicated disease.

Importance of Understanding the Condition

A full understanding of acute pancreatitis is critical, since the disease's incidence has been rising and potentially severe. Current studies indicate that the incidence of acute pancreatitis is progressively elevated, with doubled or tripled frequencies compared to the 1970s. Approximately 25% of acute attacks are severe, with necrotizing histologic injury that threatens survival. A mean mortality of about 10% points to not only the severity of the condition but also the need for targeted research and intervention strategies. The pathophysiology of acute pancreatitis needs to be well understood in order to develop specific medical treatments since the current treatment modalities are still largely supportive. This understanding can ultimately be translated into better outcomes for patients and inform clinical practice, as treatment for a more prevalent disease becomes better. Moreover, the complex etiology of acute pancreatitis necessitates a multi-pronged approach to its investigation and treatment. Advances in molecular biology and animal models have allowed researchers to examine the earliest acinar events leading to this disease. With the help of transgenic mice models and gene deletion methods, scientists are unraveling the intricate pathways to the inflammatory response, with proteins interacting along the path of the initiation of the disease. This type of research is invaluable in that it yields insights that can be translated into clinical therapies in the human population. Understanding these molecular mechanisms has the potential to uncover some biomarkers and therapeutic targets, thus opening a window of opportunity for new treatment protocols, yet to be established. Laboratory advances have the potential to significantly alter the clinical picture of acute pancreatitis. Lastly, current research into the inflammatory mechanism of acute pancreatitis reflects its interdependence with chronic forms. Earlier evidence pointed to the role of alternatively activated macrophages in chronic pancreatitis, and more recent evidence may elucidate the acute form. The understanding of signaling pathways in macrophages, such as those involving IL-4 and IL-13, illuminates the complex inflammatory pancreatic milieu. The study of pancreatic stellate cell roles as mediators in both the acute and chronic forms adds to the picture of pancreatic disorders. By identifying and treating pathways that are involved in the disease process, researchers can develop novel therapeutic approaches aimed at limiting fibrosis and improving patient control in acute pancreatitis and its complications, ultimately enhancing the quality of life for patients (Figure 3.2).

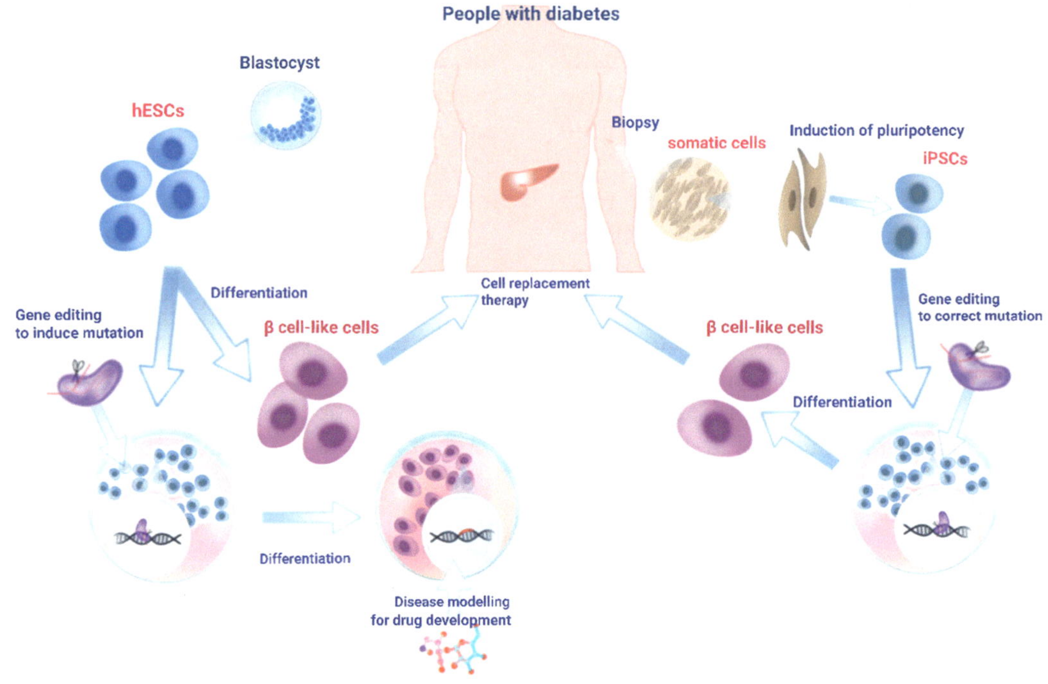

Figure 3.2. Functional genomics in pancreatic β cells.

Source: Hu M, Cherkaoui I, Misra S and Rutter GA (2020) Functional Genomics in Pancreatic β Cells: Recent Advances in Gene Deletion and Genome Editing Technologies for Diabetes Research. Front. Endocrinol. 11:576632. doi: 10.3389/fendo.2020.576632

3.1. Anatomy and Physiology of the Pancreas

The pancreas, an upper abdominal organ that plays a vital role, is unique as it is both an endocrine and an exocrine gland with a major role in digestion and glucose utilization. The organ is anatomically divided into four portions: the head, neck, body, and tail, with its widespread ductal system facilitating the release of digestive enzymes. The exocrine component consists of acinar cells responsible for secreting digestive enzymes, including amylase, lipase, and proteases, that are needed to break down carbohydrates, fats, and proteins, respectively. Regulated secretion by acinar cells is intimately linked to the ductal cells, which modify the pancreatic juice composition for effective digestion. An appreciation of this anatomical and functional organization is required to appreciate conditions such as acute pancreatitis, where inflammation can disrupt normal secretory processes to have significant clinical effects (Vrolyk et al., 2025). In acute pancreatitis, the physiology of the pancreas becomes relevant because of the organ's response to injury and stress. The pathophysiologic mechanisms resulting in acute pancreatitis most frequently involve the premature activation of pancreatic enzymes, which can culminate in autodigestion of the pancreas. This derangement not only leads to pancreatitis but also has systemic effects, which can culminate in complications such as acute lung injury and organ dysfunction. Acute necrotizing pancreatitis has been reported to trigger a violent inflammatory response, characterized by the invasion of immune cells into the pancreas and the consequent formation of pro-inflammatory cytokines. This cascade of inflammation is pivotal in disease severity as well as complications from disease, hence making understanding pancreatic physiology critical in diagnosing and managing acute pancreatitis effectively (Vrolyk et al., 225). Furthermore, the closeness of structures adjacent to the pancreas causes the development of acute pancreatitis, as its proximity to other crucial organs could dictate the course and management of the disease. In particular, the pancreas is closely related to the duodenum, bile ducts, and major vascular structures. In acute pancreatitis, the inflammatory process can be extended to surrounding neighboring organs and cause secondary complications such as biliary obstruction or vascular thrombosis. Secondly, awareness of the anatomical location enables the clinician to assess and avoid complications, as well as formulate interventions such as imaging studies or surgery if needed. The intricate relationship between the pancreas and other organs highlights the importance of detailed knowledge of its anatomy and physiology, enhancing patient care and treatment planning for acute pancreatitis (Dolenšek et al., 2017) (Figure 3.3).

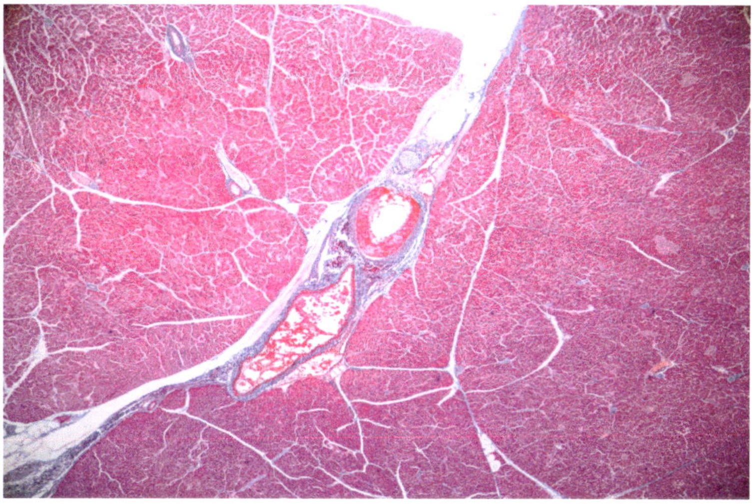

Figure 3.3. The tissue of the pancreas is an organ of the digestive system and an endocrine organ.

Source: https://devcell.bio.uci.edu/wp-content/uploads/sites/9/2019/06/Pancreas-Tissue.jpeg.

3.1.1. Location and Structure of the Pancreas

The pancreas is a critical gland located in the retroperitoneal space that extends along the posterior abdominal wall. It lies behind the stomach in a horizontal position and is bordered anteriorly by the duodenum and posteriorly by large vessels like the aorta and inferior vena cava. This location is significant since anatomical relationships of the pancreas can influence surgical complications and outcomes, particularly in surgical procedures like the Whipple resection. Understanding the complex anatomy of the pancreas, comprising the head, body, and tail, is important in comprehending conditions such as acute pancreatitis. The head of the pancreas is in close association with the duodenum, while the body and tail extend towards the spleen, highlighting the organ's multi-planar interactions within the abdominal cavity (Ajmera et al., 2020). This intricacy highlights the importance of proper anatomical knowledge in diagnosis and surgery. The pancreas is elaborately constructed with both exocrine and endocrine functions. The exocrine component, constituting the larger portion of the organ, is in charge of producing digestive enzymes and bicarbonate secreted to the duodenum for digestion.

The endocrine portions, however, consist of the islets of Langerhans secrete hormones like insulin and glucagon into the bloodstream. This dual function underlines the importance of the pancreas not just in digestion but also in metabolic regulation. The harmony of structure and function comes into singular prominence in the context of acute pancreatitis, where inflammation of pancreatic tissue disrupts the organ's digestive and hormonal functions. Pancreatic duct failure, located within the structure of the organs, can lead to enzyme backup and subsequent autodigestion of the pancreas itself, aggravating the condition (Kelly et al., 1963). Additionally, anatomical variations of the pancreatic duct system are key to understanding the pathogenesis of acute pancreatitis. The complicated branching network and possible anatomical variations can affect the susceptibility of duct obstruction or damage, which in turn may induce inflammation. Studies have established that damage to pancreatic ducts can cause serious postoperative complications, making recovery from acute pancreatitis more complicated (Kelly et al., 1963). The intimate relationship of the pancreas with structures in close proximity, like the common bile duct and major blood vessels, also affects operative maneuvers and the likelihood of perioperative complications. A clear knowledge of pancreatic anatomy not only benefits the management of acute pancreatitis but also steers surgeons from damaging delicate structures during surgery (Ajmera et al., 2020). Hence, familiarity with the location and arrangement of the pancreas is fundamental to preventing and managing this condition (Figure 3.4).

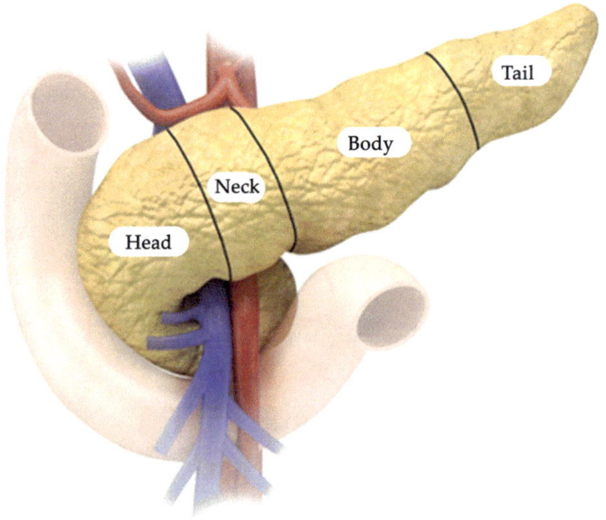

Figure 3.4. Pancreas anatomy is uncinate.

Source: https://radiologykey.com/wp-content/uploads/2016/09/A303228_1_En_7_Fig2_HTML.gif.

3.1.2. Functions of the Pancreas in Digestion

The pancreas has significant functions in digestion, primarily as an exocrine organ. The pancreas releases digestive enzymes such as amylase, lipase, and proteases, which are essential for carbohydrate, fat, and protein digestion, respectively. Enzymes are released into the duodenum after food reaches the small intestine to facilitate digestion. This enzyme activity is responsible for the breakdown of complex nutrients into a simpler form to be maximally absorbed by the blood. In acute pancreatitis, however, premature activation of such enzymes within the pancreas itself would initiate autodigestion of pancreatic tissue and may result in inflammation and tissue damage. Awareness of the exocrine function of the pancreas is important since malfunction will also make digestion, and indeed the overall metabolic status of the patient suspected to or diagnosed with acute pancreatitis, complicated. Moreover, the pancreas plays a crucial regulatory function by controlling the pH of the intestines contents through the secretion of bicarbonate. The pancreas releases sodium bicarbonate into the small intestine to neutralize the stomach acid in the chyme to create the best environment for the digestive enzymes to function best. Defective secretion of bicarbonate during an attack of acute pancreatitis can lead to digestive complications and aggravate the condition. The disturbance of this regulating mechanism can augment acidity in the intestinal lumen, which can result in reduced enzyme activity and faulty nutrient absorption. Further, the inflammatory reaction initiated during acute pancreatitis can modulate bicarbonate transport, highlighting the highly cooperative relationship between pancreatic function and gastrointestinal wellbeing in the affected patients. Lastly, the role of diet cannot be ignored when one thinks about pancreatic function during digestion and in disease states like acute pancreatitis. There is evidence to suggest that high-fiber diets influence the health of patients suffering from pancreatic disease. More specifically, fiber intake has been shown to be associated with reduced incidence of pancreatic complications and improved intestinal barrier function due to its prebiotic effect. However, this interaction is complicated; whereas fiber may stabilize intestinal function, it may also inhibit the activity of pancreatic enzymes, particularly in patients with exocrine pancreatic insufficiency. The dual effects of fiber on digestion add emphasis to the importance of individualized dietary management, particularly in the treatment of acute pancreatitis, where it is essential to uphold enzyme function. Thus, dietary modifications should be included as part of the overall treatment strategy to address pancreatic health and gastric efficiency in patients with such conditions (Arnelo et al., 2017; Ribichini et al., 2019).

3.1.3. Role of the Pancreas in Endocrine Regulation

The pancreas plays a critical role in endocrine function through the secretion of hormones to maintain glucose homeostasis. The organ is made up of clusters of cells known as the islets of Langerhans, in which the beta cells synthesize insulin, a critical hormone that lowers blood sugar levels, and the alpha cells secrete glucagon to raise blood sugar levels when needed. This delicate regulation is vital to metabolic health, and disruption of this system can lead to diseases such as diabetes. Acute pancreatitis is also complicated by inflammation and damage to pancreatic tissue that can disrupt normal hormone secretion, exacerbating metabolic dysregulation. It has been shown that severe exacerbations of acute pancreatitis can impair insulin secretion and responsiveness, leading to hyperglycemia, which is a common complication in patients. So, not only is the pancreas critical for functions of digestion, but also critical to regulate endocrine functions to manage metabolism in health and disease. Understanding the interaction between inflammation and endocrine function within the pancreas sheds light on the pathogenesis of acute pancreatitis. During inflammatory attacks, as in those that occur with pancreatitis, islet cells of the pancreas may have abnormal amounts of insulin and glucagon. The promotion of signaling pathways, including those involved in Yes-associated protein (YAP) and transcriptional co-activator with PDZ-binding motif (TAZ), is implicated in both the pathology of pancreatic cancer and chronic pancreatitis, illustrating the complex response of the endocrine pancreas to injury. Specifically, YAP and TAZ expression levels are upregulated in activated stellate cells and may modulate the regenerative and dysplastic processes occurring within pancreatic tissues. These findings show that systemic and local inflammation are not only to blame for exocrine dysregulation but also for endocrine malfunction, therefore impacting the general metabolic status of the patient with acute pancreatitis (Morvaridi et al., 2015). The research further indicates that the susceptibility of the islets of Langerhans to inflammation and ischemia may be extremely different from the exocrine tissue of the pancreas. Ischemia/reperfusion (I/R) injury plays a central part in the inflammation of acute pancreatitis and pancreas transplantation. Experiments have shown that while exocrine tissue exhibits strong inflammatory responses in the form of leukocyte adhesion and edema following a prolonged period of ischemia, the islets of Langerhans are involved to a lesser extent, with fewer leukocyte interactions along with decreased inflammatory responses overall. This variation in vulnerability suggests that while acute pancreatitis has the potential to inflict widespread damage and inflammation, the relative resistance of the islets could be of value in offering suggestions for therapeutic measures aimed at sustaining endocrine function in the face of acute pancreatic damage (Preissler et al., 2010). Knowledge of these mechanisms is important for the design of integrated treatment regimens for acute pancreatitis, both exocrine and endocrine restitution (Figure 3.5).

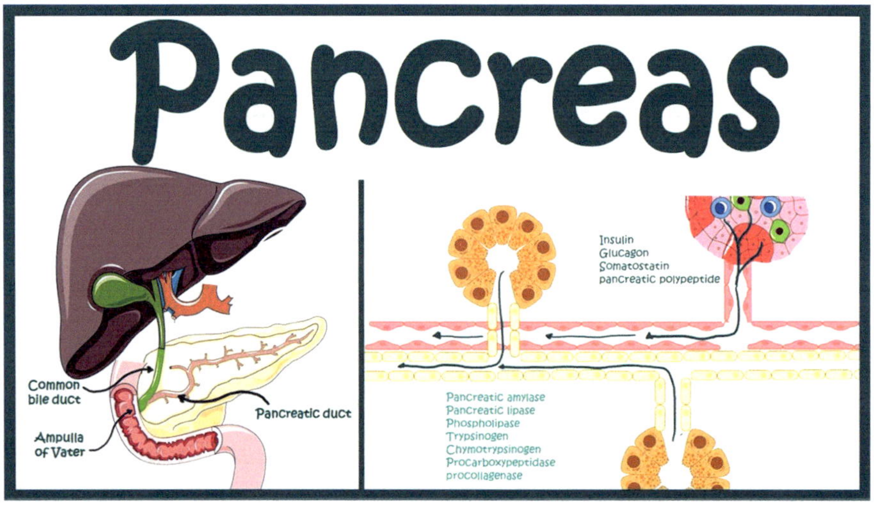

Figure 3.5. Endocrine function of the pancreas endocrine system.

Source: https://i.ytimg.com/vi/s5vjBr9PNeQ/maxresdefault.jpg.

3.2. Causes of Acute Pancreatitis (AP)

It is significant to identify the etiology of AP to prevent and handle the condition accordingly. The most frequent causes are alcohol excess and gallstone disease, which have a significant percentage in acute pancreatitis. Alcohol-induced pancreatitis is mostly caused by chronic alcohol use, which stimulates pancreatic digestive enzymes to result in inflammation. Gallstones may also obstruct the pancreatic duct, trapping digestive enzymes that can cause tissue damage. Either way, treatment to reverse these etiologies in the early stages can lessen the intensity of the disease as well as repeated attacks. Apart from alcohol and gallstones, there are lesser-known etiologies for acute pancreatitis, like genetic predisposition and some medications. Rare hereditary disorders, such as hereditary pancreatitis, possess significant risk factors that can lead to recurrent attacks of pancreatic inflammation. Several genetic mutations have been identified as participating in hereditary pancreatitis, including PRSS1 and SPINK1 gene mutations (Chaidos et al., 2020). Besides, several drug substances have been implicated in acute pancreatitis, including certain classes of medications like azathioprine and certain antibiotics. The extensive range of etiologic causes also demonstrates the necessity of comprehensive patient evaluation for the establishment and treatment of individuals' individual causes. Another significant etiologic reason for acute pancreatitis is systemic or infectious etiologies. Conditions such as hypertriglyceridemia with elevated circulating triglyceride levels can trigger acute pancreatitis due to the toxicity of fat metabolites to pancreatic tissue. In addition, infections, including viral infections like mumps or cytomegalovirus, can result in pancreatitis. While these causes are perhaps less well known than gallstones or alcohol, they should not be forgotten, particularly with noxious presentations of the disease. The complexity of acute pancreatitis highlights the necessity of a multi-factorial diagnostic process involving a comprehensive medical history, genetic testing, and appropriate imaging to cure and prevent this potentially life-threatening disease (Schmiegelow et al., 2016) (Figure 3.6).

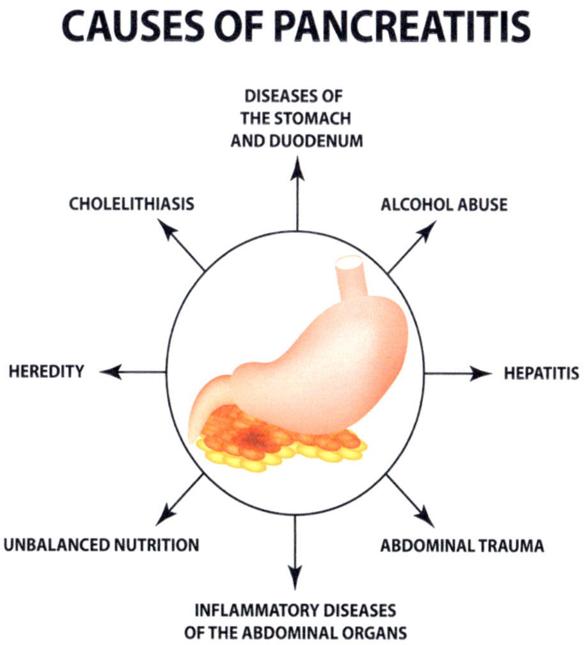

Figure 3.6. Causes-of-pancreatitis.

Source: https://cdn1.vectorstock.com/i/1000x1000/26/10/causes-of-pancreatitis-the-structure-vector-22642610.jpg.

3.2.1. Gallstones as a Primary Cause

The presence of gallstones is a significant precipitating factor in the development of acute pancreatitis. Gallstones, particularly when they migrate from the gallbladder into the common bile duct, can block the pancreatic duct. Blocking will cause increased pressure within the pancreas, ultimately leading to the early activation of digestive enzymes that destroy and inflame pancreatic tissue. Estimates suggest gallstones account for 40%–70% of the cause of acute pancreatitis, particularly in those populations with a higher incidence of cholelithiasis. Understanding pathophysiologic mechanisms linking gallstones to acute pancreatitis highlights effective management strategies to manage gallstone disease, as treating the etiology significantly reduces recurrence and complication rates from acute pancreatitis. Furthermore, gallstones can interact with the incidence of acute pancreatitis in any population, making it important the deliberate assessment in patients presenting with pain in the abdomen. The presentation may be an abrupt onset of severe epigastric pain, nausea, and vomiting, for which a work-up for gallstones can be prescribed. Magnetic resonance cholangiopancreatography (MRCP) and endoscopic retrograde cholangiopancreatography (ERCP) are valuable diagnostic modalities that can help in the diagnosis of obstructive gallstones. Beyond the acute inflammation process, gallstones can also be responsible for complications such as pancreatic necrosis or abscess formation that further complicate the clinical presentation. Therefore, establishing an explicit diagnostic process is essential in the management of early intervention, especially where gallstones are determined to be the proximate cause of acute pancreatitis. It is also crucial to keep in mind that while gallstones are accountable for a considerable proportion of acute pancreatitis, other rare causes must never be excluded. For instance, certain medications, such as atypical antipsychotics such as olanzapine, have been implicated in acute pancreatitis, usually in the context of concomitant metabolic derangements such as hyperlipidemia. In some cases, however, the drug-pancreatitis connection may not be so readily apparent, rendering careful patient histories as well as ongoing monitoring of metabolic parameters useful. Although gallstones remain a major cause of acute pancreatitis, doctors should always be attentive to the possibility of other etiologies and not miss the implication of pharmacologic agents in causing pancreatic inflammation. It is only by integrating this comprehensive outlook that the patient outcome can be maximized and the therapeutic intervention rendered more focused and efficient in the treatment of acute pancreatitis, without n one-size-fits-all manner.

3.2.2. Alcohol Consumption and Its Effects

Consumption of alcohol has long been a proven risk factor for developing acute pancreatitis. Acute pancreatitis is an inflammatory process of the pancreas with various etiological causes, one of the major causes being excessive alcohol intake. It has been seen that excessive alcohol consumption can cause direct toxic damage to pancreatic cells, leading to inflammation and eventual damage. Moreover, the acute pancreatitis complications can be worsened by the ongoing consumption of alcohol, not only because it amplifies inflammatory reactions but also makes recovery more difficult. Therefore, heavy drinkers have a significantly higher risk of contracting acute pancreatitis and suffering serious health effects from this ailment, highlighting the importance of public awareness about alcohol use. In addition, alcohol use and acute pancreatitis are correlated with statistical evidence that indicates the probability of contracting this disease among alcoholics. Heavy alcohol consumption, which is over two drinks a day, was revealed to have increased risk for acute respiratory distress syndrome (ARDS), and the comorbid risk factors overlap with pancreatitis, namely smoking and pancreatitis. This study examined 1,422 residents and found that, after controlling for confounding variables, a history of heavy drinking was linked with elevated risk (odds ratio 2.9) for ARDS development, showing the broader picture of excessive drinking (Thakur et al., 2009). These results suggest that similar mechanisms could be at the back of both the pathological processes of ARDS and acute pancreatitis and indicate that more research is needed to understand their association. Aside from this, chronic pancreatitis, which is usually caused by prolonged alcoholism, can cause serious complications such as diabetes mellitus type 3c, a secondary cause of pancreatic insufficiency. This occurs when the pancreas cannot secrete insulin due to injury of its exocrine tissue and is particularly prevalent in individuals who have had a history of chronic alcoholism. A patient study of 261 patients established that patients with chronic pancreatitis exhibited a characteristic risk pattern of developing secondary diabetes, and both body mass index as well as imaging studies revealed high rates of comorbidities (Diaconu et al., 2018). The cross-talk between alcohol intake and chronic pancreatitis serves to underscore the necessity of dealing with alcohol consumption not only to prevent pancreatitis but also to prevent the long-term consequences of its effect on pancreatic function and the other metabolic consequences that result from their interaction (Figure 3.7).

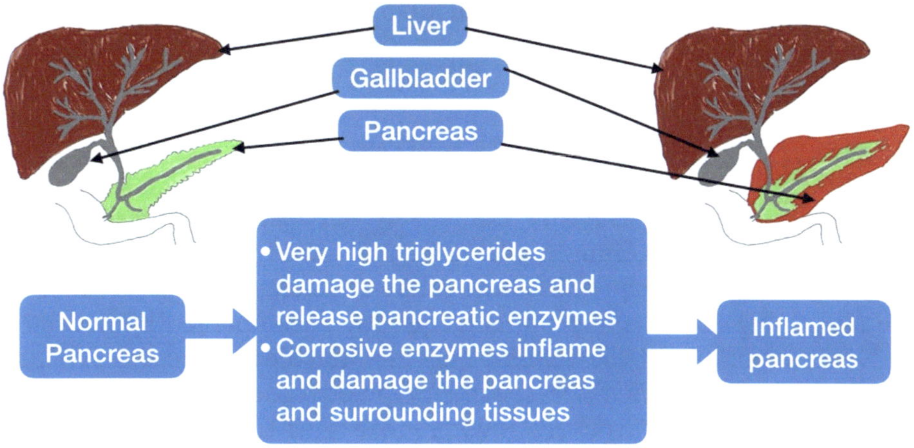

Figure 3.7. Alcoholic pancreatitis.

Source: https://patienteducationmd.com/wp-content/uploads/alcoholic-pancreatitis-768x402.jpg.

3.2.3. Other Contributing Factors (e.g., Medications, Infections)

In addition to the traditionally accepted causes, such as gallstones and alcohol consumption, acute pancreatitis can also occur due to a variety of other causes, including drugs and infections. Certain drugs, particularly those classified as nonsteroidal anti-inflammatory drugs (NSAIDs), diuretics, and antibiotics, have been linked with the onset of acute pancreatitis. Notably, the risk is accentuated by chronic exposure and some drug interactions, prompting healthcare providers to exercise restraint when administering these drugs to patients who have other risk factors. This relationship is important to comprehend because it allows for more integrated management plan that not only addresses the initial diet and lifestyle changes needed but also manages and monitors the pharmacologic agents inducing this multifactorial condition (Khan et al., 2024). Infections are also a dire but often overlooked characteristic of acute pancreatitis. Several infections, particularly viral infections like mumps and cytomegalovirus, can cause pancreatitis either by direct infection of the pancreatic cells or by inducing an inflammation process. This dual mechanism underscores the importance of detecting infectious agents among pancreatitis-symptomatic patients, given the fact that early detection and treatment administration of such infections can potentially stop the development of the disease. The association between infection and pancreatitis necessitates clinicians to keep in mind a wide variety of etiologies upon diagnosing and treating this potentially lethal disease, reminding us that acute pancreatitis does not solely arise from lifestyle issues or anatomical abnormalities (Wu et al., 2023). Nor should the role of metabolic disorders be discounted when in the context of acute pancreatitis. Conditions such as hyperlipidemia and hypercalcemia can predispose to acute pancreatitis by mechanisms that disrupt normal pancreatic function. Elevated levels of triglycerides, for instance, can induce lipid peroxidation and inflammation of the pancreas and lead to acute attacks. Hypercalcemia also causes necrosis of the pancreas by precipitation of calcium salts in the pancreatic ducts and subsequent gland dysfunction. As science increasingly unearths the environmental and genetic etiology of susceptibility to such metabolic disturbances, clinicians are urged toward the adoption of an organ systems-oriented prevention and treatment plan. This underscores the complexity of acute pancreatitis, in which a unified understanding several causative factors is central to successful management and improved patient outcomes (Khan et al., 2024).

3.3. Symptoms and Diagnosis

Acute pancreatitis symptoms can also vary immensely between patients, making it challenging to provide an accurate diagnosis. Common presentations are severe upper epigastric pain that is most commonly described as a sharp, immediate sense of intense discomfort that can be referred to the back. The classic-dependent symptom is frequently accompanied by nausea, vomiting, and loss of appetite. Most significantly, the patient may also have evidence of systemic stress in the form of fever and tachycardia, which are secondary presentations of the inflammatory process with the pancreas. All healthcare workers must realize that the clinical presentation of acute pancreatitis can be quite similar to other abdominal diseases and hence, diagnosis becomes more difficult. It can lead to complications, particularly in special groups, such as pregnant women, where mortality could be extremely high, with rates being reported at up to 11.6%–18.7%, since it is also associated with both fetal and maternal mortality (Tang et al., 2024). Acute pancreatitis diagnosis usually includes a combination of clinical assessment, laboratory investigation, and imaging studies. The initial evaluation begins with an appropriate history and physical, noting abdominal pain and other systemic complaints. Serum markers such as amylase and lipase are important, with rising levels having the ability to diagnose inflammation of the pancreas. These results may not necessarily be sensitive or specific, though, and therefore further tests are required. Imaging studies such as abdominal ultrasound or computed tomography (CT) scans are also highly valuable in diagnosing gallstones or complications like necrosis. The integration of laboratory and imaging results allows clinicians to classify the severity of the disease appropriately. Research emphasizes the requirement for a robust diagnostic framework, particularly in identifying risk factors such as hyperlipidemia, which is currently understood to be the primary etiology of acute pancreatitis attacks (Chikatipalli et al., 2024). Despite evolving diagnostic parameters, patient management procedures still require optimization. The application of dynamic nomogram models has also been found to be promising in terms of improving the predictability for risk detection of acute pancreatitis, particularly in specified populations like pregnant women. Various variables like levels of triglyceride, body mass index, and inflammatory markers are taken into account during assessment by such models. Clinicians can be aided by these models in prioritizing intervention and management of care. Furthermore, understanding the interactions between different risk factors and complications such as pancreatic necrosis or systemic infections is crucial in enhancing overall patient outcomes. Thus, the integration of advanced diagnostic tools and medical knowledge is required for the early detection and optimal management of acute pancreatitis, ultimately reducing morbidity and mortality risk factors associated with this multifactorial disease (Chikatipalli et al., 2024; Tang et al., 2024) (Figure 3.8).

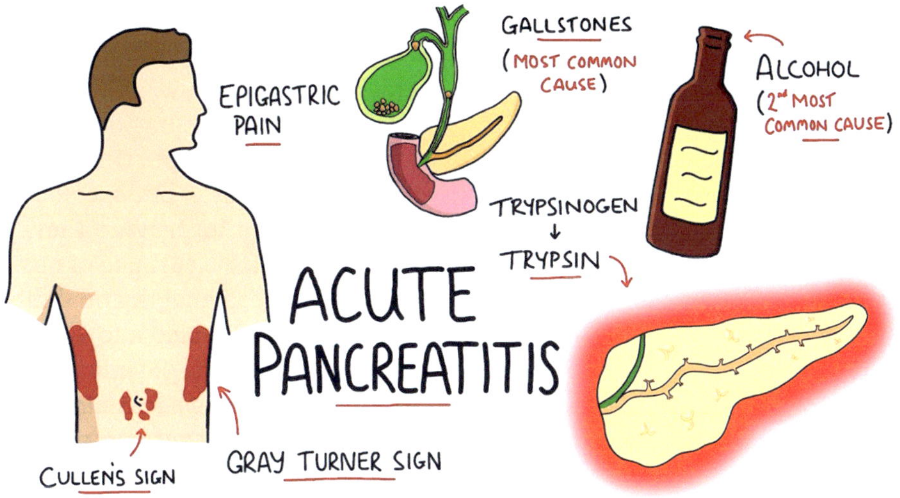

Figure 3.8. Acute pancreatitis signs and symptoms.

Source: https://i.ytimg.com/vi/5kYClavXZgE/maxresdefault.jpg.

3.3.1. Common Symptoms of Acute Pancreatitis (AP)

AP is characterized by a range of signs and symptoms that are typically acute in onset and could be of diverse intensity. The most typical symptom is agonizing abdominal pain, which is often presented as a stabbing or piercing pain. The pain tends to begin in the upper abdomen and diffuse into the back or shoulders, making patients uncomfortable and unable to recover. Furthermore, the pain is also accompanied by nausea and vomiting in some of the patients, adding to the overall discomfort. These gastrointestinal manifestations can further lead to dehydration and electrolyte imbalance, which require urgent medical attention to stabilize the patient's condition. As the symptoms become more severe, there is also a risk of having systemic manifestations such as fever and tachycardia, indicative of a heightened inflammatory response. Thus, early detection of these symptoms is critical in the proper management of acute pancreatitis and in preventing worsening complications. Apart from pain and nausea, tenderness of the abdomen upon examination is a significant symptom of acute pancreatitis. The rigidity or guarding that patients have upon palpitation of the abdomen signifies an inflammation of the pancreas and the surrounding tissues. Bloating or fullness is also complained of by some individuals as a result of interference with normal digestive function. Besides, some patients also present with changes in their bowel movements, such as diarrhea or oily stools, a situation known as steatorrhea, due to an impairment of digestive enzyme secretion. Such symptoms indicate the important role of the pancreas in digestive and endocrine functions since acute pancreatitis stops it from functioning normally and generates overall health complications. Early identification of such symptoms may diagnose the condition and implement appropriate treatment measures. The clinical presentation of acute pancreatitis can be masked by underlying disease or polypharmacy in the elderly on occasion. On occasion, medications such as doxycycline have been known to cause drug-induced acute pancreatitis, which can complicate diagnosis due to the broader spectrum of symptoms that can simulate other gastrointestinal illnesses (Goldin et al., 2024). Older patients typically experience difficulty in recognizing distinctive patterns of symptoms because of their complex medical history and background drugs. Ultimately, recognition of symptoms of acute pancreatitis, such as severe pain, nausea, and changes in bowel habits, becomes most crucial for healthcare professionals. Recognition of less frequent etiologies, such as drug-related etiology, can result in better intervention approaches and outcomes for patients, especially among vulnerable populations at risk for polypharmacy (Yrkm, 2024).

3.3.2. Diagnostic Tests and Procedures

Diagnostic tests and studies are critical in the diagnosis and management of acute pancreatitis. History and physical examination are most often the initial steps in the evaluation, with abdominal pain and gastrointestinal symptoms being the predominant signs. Other diagnostic modalities need to be employed to ascertain the diagnosis and the severity. Serial blood measurements are done to measure levels of enzymes, notably amylase and lipase, which are classically elevated in acute pancreatitis. C-reactive protein (CRP) has also been utilized as a marker to show the degree of inflammation and guide clinical decisions regarding the form of treatment to follow, as seen in Jokić et al. (2012). Apart from that, imaging studies like CT and ultrasound are utilized for observing pancreatic architecture, detecting complications, and diagnosing likely etiologies such as biliary calculosis. In acute pancreatitis, diagnosis is more than just labeling the condition. Diagnostic tests play an essential part in monitoring the course of the disease and response to treatment. The application of non-invasive imaging modalities, i.e., MRCP, has become more important in assessing the anatomy of biliary-pancreatic trees, particularly in suspected choledocholithiasis. Endoscopic procedures may also be needed to provide therapeutic options, such as ERCP for clearance of obstructing stones. Combined, these imaging modalities not only aid in diagnostics but also allow for the anticipation of complications to permit instant treatment to be administered as necessary to prevent further impairment, as discussed in Rošić (2011). Even though laboratory and imaging evaluations are included in the diagnostic management of acute pancreatitis, they should be implemented according to prescribed protocols to ensure maximum effectiveness. It is essential that clinicians adhere to evidence-based standards in the realms of diagnosis accuracy and therapy, not only routine tests, but also advanced techniques when necessary. For instance, acute pancreatitis complications such as pancreatic necrosis or the formation of an abscess may necessitate advanced imaging or even biopsy in certain scenarios to manage the patient clinically effectively. The rational use of diagnostic facilities also avoids unnecessary interventions that do not improve patient outcomes, thereby reducing healthcare costs. In summary, the multi-dimensional strategy in diagnosing acute pancreatitis is essential to ensuring maximum patient care and promoting recovery trends, in support of the need for ongoing research and reformulation of existing protocols, such as in Jokić et al. (2012), Rošić (2011) (Figure 3.9).

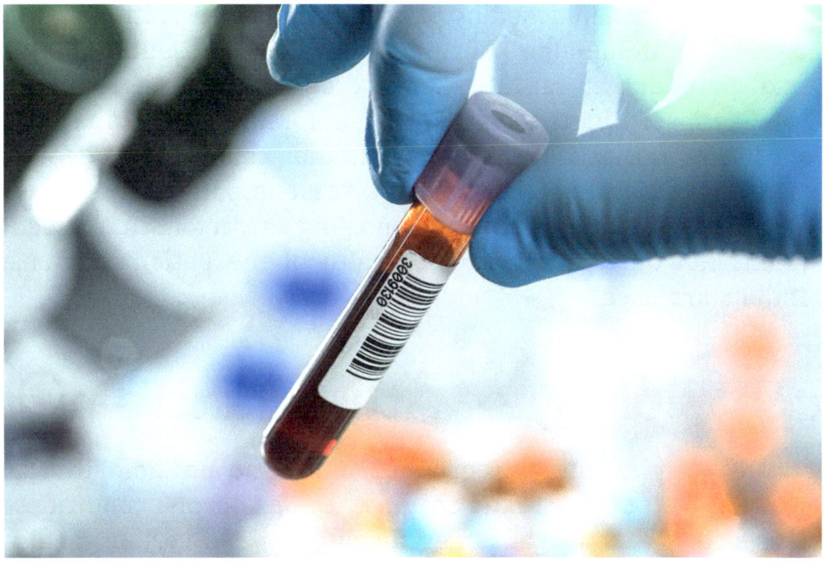

Figure 3.9. Diagnostic tests and procedures of acute pancreatitis.

Source: https://www.verywellhealth.com/thmb/g8wDy4eNL77YCQRdVLO4M7aFJtM=/1500x0/filters:no_upscale():max_bytes(150000):strip_icc()/GettyImages-1339206392-2cc6872c9fd64603bbc3e4a27631188d.jpg.

3.3.3. Differentiating Acute Pancreatitis (AP) from Other Conditions

AP differentiation from other conditions is critical for effective treatment and the best patient outcome. One of the greatest challenges for differentiation is identifying clinically mimicking presentations that can masquerade as acute pancreatitis, such as cholecystitis, peptic ulcer disease, and mesenteric ischemia. Overlapping symptoms—primarily abdominal pain, nausea, and vomiting, are prone to misdiagnosis if accurately evaluated. Ultrasound and CT imaging can be employed to assist the clinician in detecting characteristic acute pancreatitis findings, such as free fluid in the peritoneum or changes in pancreatic shape. However, a side-by-side comparison of findings on these modalities is necessary to rule out other conditions that mimic acute abdominal pain. A multifactorial approach with complete patient history and laboratory investigation will thus have to be employed in a bid to acquire an appropriate diagnosis and subsequent management plan. Laboratory testing continues to play an important role in the differential diagnosis of acute pancreatitis. Increased serum amylase and lipase concentrations are traditionally believed to be related to inflammation of the pancreas, but they are not pathognomonic for pancreatitis. Other conditions like acute cholecystitis and peptic perforating ulcers may also manifest with raised pancreatic enzymes, thereby complicating diagnosis. There is emerging evidence on the use of other biomarkers, such as procalcitonin (PCT), to enhance diagnostic accuracy in critically ill patients. This is all the more so since PCT has been found to be more specific and sensitive when distinguishing between systemic inflammatory response syndrome (SIRS) and conditions like sepsis, thereby assisting clinicians in differentiating acute pancreatitis from infections that may have a similar presentation (BalcI et al., 2002). The use of these new diagnostic methods decreases the risk of misdiagnosis and facilitates intervention on time. Autoimmune pancreatitis is a significant condition that must be ruled out from acute pancreatitis due to its typical presentation and therapeutic approaches. It can be mimicked by pancreatic cancer, resulting in unjustifiable surgery unless properly diagnosed. Autoimmune pancreatitis tends to present with obstructive jaundice and severe abdominal pain, and it can be encountered in the background of elevated serum immunoglobulin G (IgG4) levels, particularly Type 1 autoimmune pancreatitis (Azzopardi et al., 2014). Acute response to corticosteroid therapy is another characteristic feature. The physicians thus should retain a strong suspicion of this benign disease in patients with classical presentation of pancreatitis, particularly if the case has atypical imaging characteristics. Effective discrimination among these conditions not only preserves the health of the patient but ensures appropriate therapeutic interventions are used.

3.4. Pathophysiology of Acute Pancreatitis (AP)

AP pathophysiology is a complex interplay of biochemical and physiological pathways triggered largely by premature activation of pancreatic enzymes. Under normal conditions, the enzymes are not activated, but risk factors such as gallstones, alcoholism, and certain medications can induce premature enzyme activation in the pancreas. The premature activation results in autodigestion of the pancreatic tissue, inflammation, necrosis, and, if not treated, systemic illnesses. In inflammation, various pro-inflammatory cytokines are secreted that augment the local damage and are also responsible for the resolution of an SIRS.

The identification of distinct biochemical markers has evolved over time, but further research is needed to establish the precise mechanisms behind triggering and perpetuating these injurious cascades in AP (Wang et al., 2024). Mitochondrial uncoupling protein 2 (UCP2) is one of the leading actors within the pathophysiologic landscape of pancreatic diseases, including acute pancreatitis. UCP2 has been shown to have regulatory roles for oxidative stress and inflammatory responses, both crucial in AP pathology. Its overexpression in pancreatic tissue indicates that alterations to the function of UCP2 would have sweeping implications. The latest data show that UCP2 may play a role as a central control factor, controlling not only the inflammatory pathways but also the metabolic derangements in pancreatic pathology. Its action gives some clues to the therapeutic targets that would be capable of preventing the progression of acute pancreatitis. Increased research into the regulatory pathways of UCP2 may help shed light on its specific functions in the disease pathophysiology and, ultimately, in new therapeutic strategies (Wang et al., 2024). Coagulopathy is an integral part of the pathophysiology of acute pancreatitis and has direct effects on patient outcomes and making clinical decisions more complex regarding the disease. The activation of the coagulation cascade as a result of pancreatic injury leads to the production of thrombin, mainly caused by the tissue factor on activated monocytes. This leads to microvascular thrombosis and subsequent tissue ischemia, an important component of multi-organ dysfunction, which is a major concern in AP cases.

The equilibrium between fibrinolysis and coagulation is key; pro-inflammatory cytokines increase dysfunction in the protein C system, leading to inhibited fibrinolytic activity. The ensuing coagulopathy can range from minor coagulation test abnormalities to life-threatening conditions like disseminated intravascular coagulation and highlights the significance of intervention for the treatment of this aspect of acute pancreatitis more vigorously (Figure 3.10).

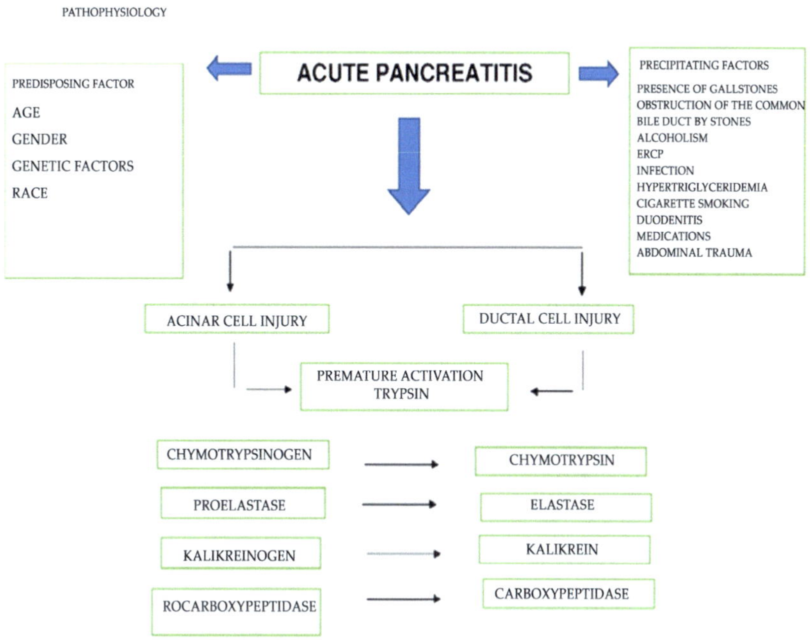

Figure 3.10. Pathophysiology of acute pancreatitis.

Source: https://d20ohkaloyme4g.cloudfront.net/img/document_thumbnails/33b79ecd56003834bc563bd893d8fe7c/thumb_1200_927.png.

3.4.1. Mechanisms of Pancreatic Injury

The pathophysiology of pancreatic injury in acute pancreatitis is multifactorial and primarily revolves around the process of autodigestion, wherein the activated pancreatic enzymes begin to break down pancreatic tissue itself. This is a result of the premature activation of digestive enzymes, which in their inactivated form exist inside the acini of the pancreas but become activated once they are released into the intestinal lumen. If these enzymes are activated too early, they might trigger a cascade of inflammation and thereby enhance the damage to tissues and also bring about necrosis. Other etiological factors which cause acute pancreatitis—anything from gallstones to alcohol intake in excess—might also contribute to dysfunction in enzyme secretion and pancreatic juice flow. Thus, the complexity of these mechanisms emphasizes the necessity of comprehensive research into the particular cellular and molecular mechanisms that dictate pancreatic damage in acute pancreatitis (Reddy et al., 2015). Additionally, the role of inflammatory mediators is crucial when it comes to pancreatic injury. Activation of inflammation pathways—namely the release of cytokines and chemokines, is accountable for amplifying tissue damage and systemic complications of acute pancreatitis. Through the process of inflammation, inflammatory cells invade pancreatic tissue, releasing pro-inflammatory cytokines such as interleukin-1 and tumor necrosis factor-alpha and inducing further inflammatory response. The cascade reactivity of inflammation not only results in local pancreatic injury but may also lead to systemic inflammatory responses, producing multiple organ failure, a common complication of severe acute pancreatitis. Clarification of these pathways is of critical significance, as effective modulation of inflammatory processes has potential therapeutic applications to avoid pancreatic damage and improve clinical outcomes in patients (Reddy et al., 2015). Emerging evidence defines the cross-talk between visceral adipose tissue and pancreatic damage, outlining a new aspect of the pathophysiology of acute pancreatitis. Studies show that in acute pancreatitis, visceral adipose tissue gets exposed to massive stress and damage, driven by lipolytic activity of adipocytes. Specifically, pancreatic lipase has the ability to hydrolyze triglycerides within this adipose tissue, releasing excess nonesterified fatty acids (NEFAs). These NEFAs can enhance locally produced inflammation as well as contribute to organ failure, further enhancing the severity of acute pancreatitis. Remarkably, knockout mice models have demonstrated that removing pancreatic triglyceride lipase (PNLIP) offers a protective mechanism against adaptive lipolysis and associated pancreatic acinar injury. Consistent with the complex inter-relationships between pancreas and adipose tissue, there is a significant area for research that enlightens potential therapeutic avenues to contain pancreatic injury and associated complications in acute pancreatitis (Figure 3.11).

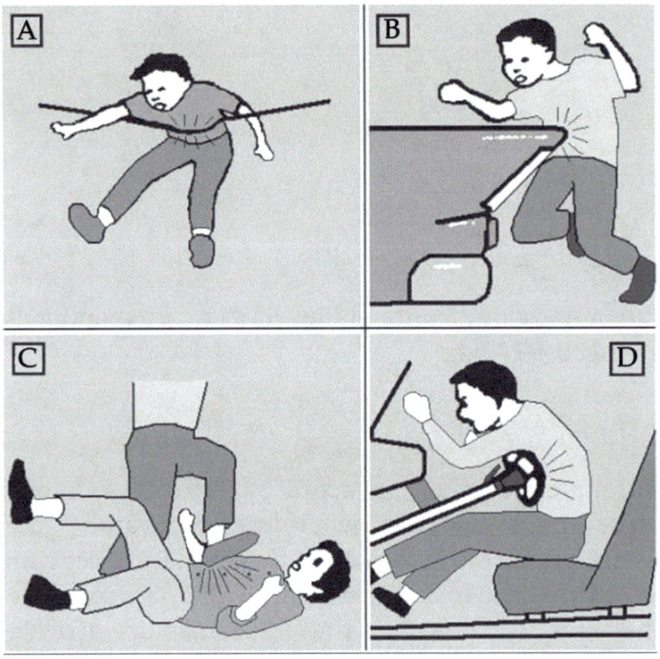

Figure 3.11. Common-mechanisms-of-pancreatic-injury.

Source: https://www.researchgate.net/profile/Stanislaw-Stawicki/publication/23679082/figure/fig3/AS:667781117808143@1536222118794/Common-mechanisms-of-pancreatic-injury-A-Application-of-direct-linear-pressure-to-the.jpg.

3.4.2. Inflammatory Response and Complications

The inflammatory response of acute pancreatitis is a complex and multifaceted process that develops as the body attempts to wall off the autodigestive injury. The injury to the pancreas initially activates the immune system, releasing pro-inflammatory cytokines and chemokines that have the ability to further intensify tissue inflammation and necrosis. As the disease progresses, this localized inflammatory response can then become systemic, leading to fulminant complications such as SIRS and multiple organ failure. Detection and control of these complications are significant because they greatly influence patient outcomes and recovery times. Poor management of the inflammatory response can open the door for secondary infection, further complicating patient care and requiring more intense interventions. The therapeutic potential of nutrition in acute pancreatitis is underscored by its impact on the inflammatory process and complications. There is evidence that specific dietary maneuvers, including fiber addition, can reduce the frequency of pancreatic necrosis and infection by stabilizing the intestinal barrier and immune modulation. In acute pancreatitis patients, it has been correlated that dietary prebiotic fortification is followed by decreased SIRS rates and hospitalization duration, enabling more effective treatment outcomes. Yet, with caution, it should be noted that excessive fiber intake is absorbed by the pancreas, hampering the enzyme activity and complicating nutritional support for patients who have exocrine pancreatic insufficiency. Thus, the ratio of food constituents is paramount to ensure optimal recovery while minimizing risks of inflammatory processes inherent in the disease (Ribichini et al., 2019). Wherever dietary support is necessary, particularly in patients unable to receive oral intake, parenteral nutrition (PN) may prove a life-saving measure. Evidence has demonstrated that the addition of immunonutrients such as glutamine and omega-3 fatty acids to PN solutions effectively prevents complications of acute pancreatitis. Evidence has established that parenteral immunonutrition significantly reduces infectious complications as well as hospital stay days and therefore improves patient prognosis. The treatment not only addresses the acute nutritional deficiencies encountered by the patients but also modulates the inflammation associated with the disease process. Due to the dual focus on inflammation and therapeutic diet, the incorporation of immunonutrition into clinical management is an interesting option in the process of recovery and mitigating the detrimental effects of acute pancreatitis (Jafari et al., 2015).

3.4.3. Impact on Other Organ Systems

The impact of acute pancreatitis, however, is not only within the pancreatic organ but also takes a tremendous toll on other organ systems. Precisely, the pathologic process of necrosis and inflammation in acute pancreatitis can play a role in the development of SIRS, which can overwhelm other systems of the body. The inflammatory mediators spilled from the damaged pancreas can precipitate changes in gut permeability, resulting in the translocation of bacteria and endotoxins to the circulation. This may cause complications such as sepsis, and thus present an important challenge in the management of patients with acute pancreatitis. Secondarily, the resulting SIRS may initiate multisystem organ failure, predominantly in the respiratory and cardiovascular systems, and leading to increased morbidity and mortality in the affected patients. Early recognition and treatment, along with monitoring of organ function, assume great significance since systemic complications arise following the initial pancreatic injury. The cardiovascular system is the most vulnerable to the effects of acute pancreatitis. Throughout the course of the disease, excessive fluid loss can occur, which is largely due to third-space sequestration of fluid in the abdomen. This can lead to hypovolemia and decreased cardiac output, complicating the patient's clinical condition. Also, augmented intra-abdominal pressure due to edema can interfere with venous return, forming a vicious circle of compromised perfusion and organ dysfunction. The relationship between cardiovascular dysfunction and intra-abdominal hypertension (IAH) has been established, with a suggestion that early interventions to treat IAH could be a means of avoiding its consequences. The realization of the complicated association between acute pancreatitis and cardiovascular complications enables clinicians to develop a proper management plan to correct these essential problems and improve patient outcomes (Keulenaer et al., 2015). The renal system is yet another organ system that is influenced markedly by acute pancreatitis, in this case, through the development of acute kidney injury (AKI). The cause of AKI developing in an acute pancreatitis case is most frequently a result of a variety of factors including hypovolemia, nephrotoxicity of circulating inflammatory mediators, and systemic infection influence. Elevated cytokine and other inflammatory markers may be the culprit for renal vasoconstriction and reduced glomerular filtration. A double whammy of therapy-induced fluid overload and underlying renal impairment demands careful monitoring to prevent exacerbation. Studies have proven not just that AKI worsens the prognosis in patients with acute pancreatitis but also that it has the potential to reverse the overall course of recovery. Understanding the effect of acute pancreatitis on renal function is crucial in the planning of individual therapeutic regimens that will serve to protect renal integrity under proper therapy for the pancreatic disease (Schäfer et al., 2005) (Figure 3.12).

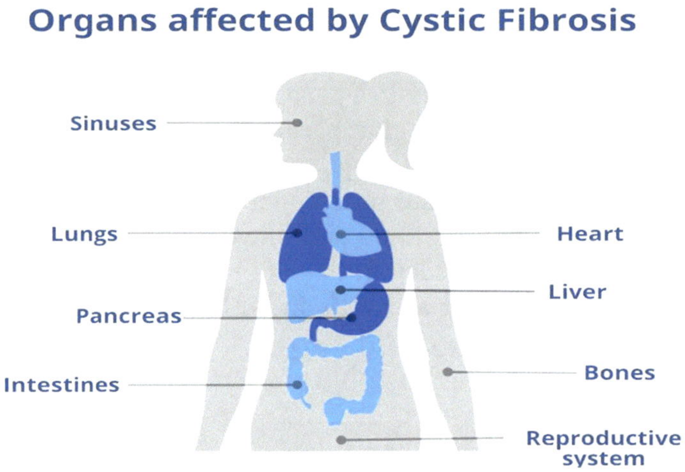

Figure 3.12. Organs-affected by cystic fibrosis.

Source: https://www.cysticfibrosis.gr/wp-content/uploads/2024/04/CF-Organs-affected-eng.jpg.

3.5. Treatment Options

Management of acute pancreatitis largely depends on the severity of the condition. Mild conditions may be managed by conservative treatment with rest provided to the pancreas to enable it to recover, intravenous fluid resuscitation, and pain relief. All these are important and are the initial measures in the management of acute pancreatitis because they minimize the complications such as IAH and pancreatic damage. In more severely affected patients, especially those with signs of organ failure, intra-abdominal pressure monitoring becomes even more critical. Rising intra-abdominal pressure can further aggravate the condition, leading to even more serious complications. Treatment in the end is focused on managing the symptoms and addressing any cause, such as gallstones or excessive drinking, that may have led to the acute pancreatitis attack. Where conservative therapy fails or there is widespread necrotizing pancreatitis, additional, more invasive intervention may be required. Surgery, for instance, necrosectomy, may be required to remove necrotic tissue from the pancreas and around the pancreas. Beyond symptom relief, this measure greatly reduces the risk of infection and systemic complications. Where intra-abdominal collections occur, interventions like percutaneous drainage successfully alleviate IAH. These measures are critical in restraining further deterioration of the patient's condition and are capable of improving overall results. Patients must be well evaluated to determine the ideal timing and mode of surgical management, balancing the risks of surgery against the benefit of relief of symptoms. Having been successful with the acute phase, long-term dietary and lifestyle modifications are subsequently addressed to avoid recurrence. Patients are most consistent in being advised to follow a low-fat diet, limit alcohol intake, and discontinue any suspected dietary precipitants. Educating the patient about the disease and possible future complications is also a significant aspect of managing patients. Follow-up and observation are also required, especially in those with chronic pancreatitis developing as a complication of an initial attack. Treatment modalities might include pharmacotherapy, for example, enzyme replacement therapy in patients with malabsorption and nutritional deficiencies. All these aspects have to be treated comprehensively, and the importance of prevention through lifestyle modification in long-term management protocols in patients with a history of acute pancreatitis (Figure 3.13) becomes evident.

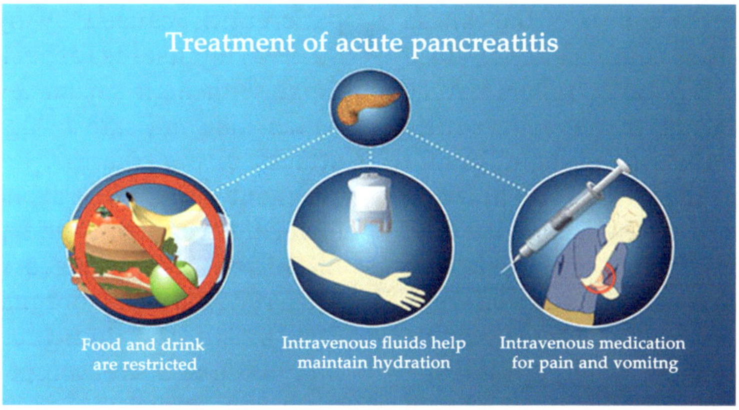

Figure 3.13. Management and treatment of acute pancreatitis.

Source: https://external-content.duckduckgo.com/iu/?u=https%3A%2F%2Fwww.animatedpancreaspatient.com%2Fen-pancreas%2Fslides%2Fmanagement-and-treatment-of-acute-pancreatitis%2Fapp02-slides-ch5_slide_06%24jpg&f=1&nofb=1&ipt=ec987498265593f8163c380d1da49c27feed199e2ecca7188bc10c118c7fcc63.

3.5.1. Initial Management and Supportive Care

The management of acute pancreatitis is initially all about the provision of proper supportive therapy to prevent complications and promote recovery. After being diagnosed, the initial management often involves fluid resuscitation, considering that significant fluid shifts typically occur as a response to inflammation. Intravenous fluid administration plays an important role in maintaining hemodynamic stability and ensuring perfusion to vital organs. Electrolyte monitoring is equally important, as derangement can lead to further complications. The Korean Pancreatobiliary Association (KPBA) stresses the importance of individualized fluid management in their guidelines, pointing out that early and cautious fluid resuscitation is the cornerstone in the management of acute pancreatitis (Schäfer et al., 2005). It aims not only to avoid potential organ failure but also to favor the patient's overall course of improvement. Of similar concern in the initial management regimen is also taking into account dietary modification, depending on the condition of the patient. In mild pancreatitis, oral nutrition may be resumed quickly, often starting with clear liquids and advancing as tolerated. In patients with more severe pancreatitis, they are usually NPO (nothing by mouth) for a longer period to allow healing of the pancreas. The new guidelines point out that nutritional support in the form of enteral feeding or parenteral nutrition can be crucial to the preservation of metabolic needs during this period (Schäfer et al., 2005). The gradual reintroduction of nutrition not only facilitates recovery but also prevents the complications of extended starvation and tissue catabolism. In the recovering patient, ongoing supportive care becomes increasingly essential in managing the course of the illness and preventing potential complications. Close monitoring for signs of systemic inflammatory responses is essential, as acute pancreatitis can predispose individuals to potentially life-threatening conditions like pancreatic necrosis and infection. Utilization of the Delphi method for refining current supportive care guidelines knowledge makes clinical practice more effective by making the management techniques utilized evidence-based and universally applicable. Moreover, enabling a team-based approach among healthcare professionals allows for an integrated care strategy, to the advantage of both immediate and ultimate outcomes in acute pancreatitis patients. Lastly, thorough initial management and supportive care underpin recovery and significantly reduce morbidity from this problematic condition.

3.5.2. Medications and Their Role in Treatment

Treatment of acute pancreatitis may need a multidisciplinary approach and drug therapy holds the key in regulating symptoms and pathogenesis. Intravenous fluid resuscitation is the first line of treatment in most cases in order to stabilize the hydration status of the patients and maintain electrolytes. Following stabilization, targeted pharmacological therapy, i.e., analgesics for pain, is required for patient comfort and will significantly contribute to improving recovery outcomes. In some cases, medications like octreotide and ulinastatin can be prescribed to block pancreatic secretions and thereby lessen the load on the diseased pancreas. These therapies, while supportive, need to be administered carefully after consideration of the contraindications and side effects, particularly when the patient's illness is already complicated by other concurrent medical conditions, e.g., pregnancy, in which treatment is restricted (Schäfer et al., 2005). Lipid-lowering drugs like fenofibrate and ezetimibe have also come to play a significant role as adjuncts to treat severe acute pancreatitis caused by hypertriglyceridemia. Such drug use is especially highlighted in those with high serum levels of triglycerides, which may indicate a high risk for recurrent attacks of pancreatitis. In a clinical case of a pregnant patient, intravenous hydration, lipid-lowering treatment, and pancreatic secretion inhibition were successfully used with no recurrence during pregnancy (Schäfer et al., 2005). The case indicates the importance of individualized treatment where the benefit from the utilization of some medications is weighed against potential hazards, especially in vulnerable populations. Proper integration of such therapeutic drugs into patient management plans can lead to improved outcomes under the paradigm of acute pancreatitis. Apart from the pharmacologic modalities for the early acute stage, the treatment of complications such as pancreatic pseudocysts necessitates innovation in medical management. Traditional long-standing surgical methods were the norm; however, advanced endoscopic techniques provided a gateway toward less invasive options with favorable results. Endoscopic ultrasound-guided drainage is able to treat pancreatic pseudocysts safely with minimal risks of open surgery complications and improved patient welfare. Drainage can be achieved using plastic stents, with clinical trials demonstrating their effectiveness as well as a cost-saving method compared to higher-end devices like lumen-apposing metal stents. This active cycle of drug abuse and procedural treatment highlights the imperatives of treatment alternatives to be integrated with both clinical efficacy and economic considerations in the management of acute pancreatitis (Figure 3.14).

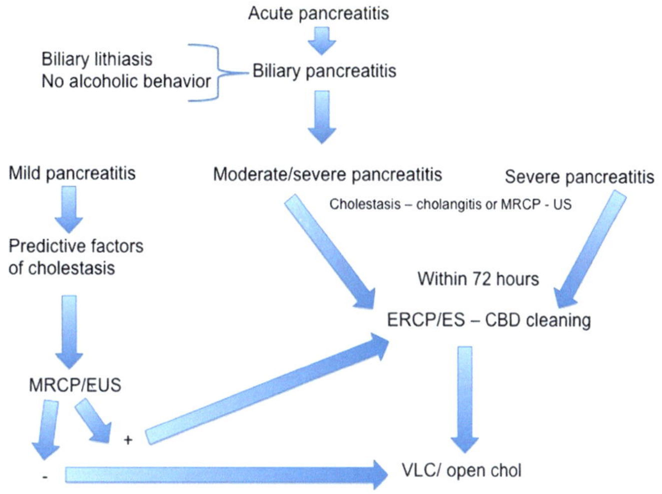

Figure 3.14. Role of surgery in the treatment of pancreatitis and its complications.

Source: Neri, V. (2015). Role of Surgery in the Treatment of Pancreatitis and Its Complications. InTech. doi: 10.5772/58932

3.5.3. Surgical Interventions for Severe Cases

Surgical procedures in the management of acute pancreatitis are reserved as a second option for only severe cases when conservative measures fail to provide relief from complications. Patients with signs of severe illness may develop various complications, including necrotizing pancreatitis, pancreatic abscess, or infection, that need surgical evaluation. Surgical treatment can be categorized into open surgery and minimally invasive treatments, based on the patient's condition and the extent of pancreatic damage. Timely intervention is crucial since delay has the potential to complicate patient outcomes. Early surgery is typically linked with less morbidity and mortality, highlighting the need for rapid assessment and intervention strategies. In such cases, imaging studies and clinical evaluation ultimately guide the surgical intervention, highlighting the need for a multidisciplinary team to achieve optimal care. Of the specific surgical interventions that may be utilized, necrosectomy is an important procedure for the management of infected pancreatic necrosis. Necrosectomy involves the debridement of necrotic pancreatic tissue and is usually reserved as a treatment option if percutaneous drainage is not effective. Different studies indicate that necrosectomy is effective in decreasing infection and allowing for healing, thus enhancing patient outcomes with acute pancreatitis. The choice between laparoscopic and open necrosectomy is still a target for future research, with the laparoscopic procedure having been associated with reduced hospital stay and less postoperative pain. However, despite these advances, the technical nature of the surgical procedure makes it demand substantial experience, as there may be a risk of complications like hemorrhage, organ failure, and further infection, emphasizing the need for careful preoperative planning as well as postoperative monitoring. Aside from necrosectomy, additional surgical interventions can also be entertained in cases where complications like abscesses arise. Percutaneous drainage techniques are popular as less invasive interventions, especially in the treatment of pancreatic collections and abscesses. However, if these interventions fail, more definitive surgery might be required. The significance of the management of IAH within these operating environments cannot be overemphasized, as elevated intra-abdominal pressure has the potential to result in post-surgical complications. Knowledge of IAH and its implications enables early intervention to prevent abdominal compartment syndrome. With an increasing understanding of surgical approaches and the complexity of severe acute pancreatitis, the integration of various approaches is required to deliver the best patient outcomes and improve overall survival (Ribichini et al., 2019; Keulenaer et al., 2015).

3.6. Complications of Acute Pancreatitis

Complications of acute pancreatitis are multifactorial and potentially greatly affect outcomes in the patient. Among these, pancreatic necrosis is a particularly serious form, characterized by the death of pancreatic tissue due to enzymatic autodigestion. The disease can potentially lead to severe systemic inflammatory responses and sepsis, and it is challenging to treat the patient clinically.

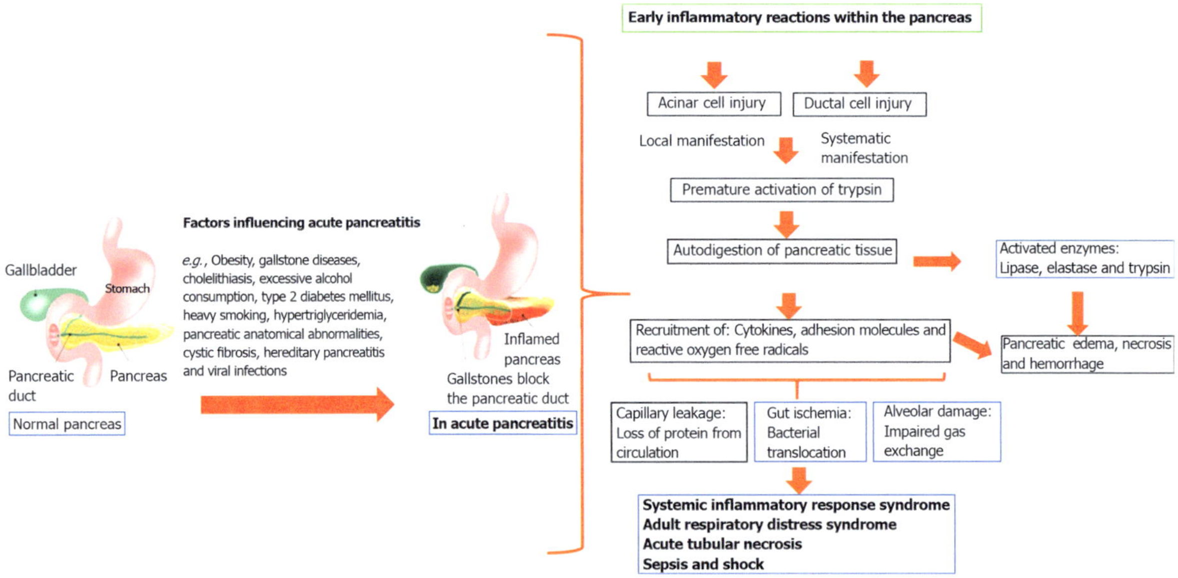

Figure 3.15. Gut microbiome in acute pancreatitis.

Source: https://f6publishing.blob.core.windows.net/c812492c-0015-468b-9ac5-8803f80fb385/WJG-27-5019-g001.png.

The death rates in necrotizing pancreatitis can be exceedingly high if not managed, and the need for immediate identification and intervention is paramount. Additionally, associated complications like abscess formation or organ failure with necrosis mandate more aggressive interventions and longer stays. Prompt identification and proper therapeutic management are essential in preventing these complications and enhancing patient prognosis for acute pancreatitis. Another major complication is the development of pancreatic encephalopathy, a rare but serious complication seen in acute pancreatitis, particularly in its severe presentations. Pancreatic encephalopathy is a neurologic complication that is associated with high mortality and is beset with significant diagnostic and therapeutic challenges. The pathophysiology is still not completely understood, but it underscores the multifactorial interaction between systemic inflammation, cerebral hypoperfusion, and deranged metabolism in acute pancreatitis. Recent reports have brought to attention the importance of timely management, drawing attention to the fact that prompt intervention can improve the prognosis of patients presenting with this complication. Increased awareness of pancreatic encephalopathy signs and in-depth knowledge about possible interventions are critical in clinical practice since they can have a significant impact on morbidity and mortality rates among severely compromised patients (Constantin et al., 2014). In addition, patients with diseases such as inflammatory bowel disease may have unique complications when they acquire acute pancreatitis. The evidence indicates that acute pancreatitis may occur either as an extraintestinal manifestation of inflammatory bowel disease or as a side effect of drugs, thus complicating clinical presentations. Despite the commonality between the two conditions, evidence shows that prognostic factors and complications are largely the same as those of patients with acute uncomplicated pancreatitis. This finding is a tribute to the need for strict evaluation and evidence-based management strategies that do not compromise patient care by the additional burden of inflammatory bowel disease. Nonetheless, the higher risk of infection and special consideration for treatment in immunosuppressed patients justify the necessity for personalized care in such cases (Kornélia et al., 2022) (Figure 3.15).

3.6.1. Local Complications (e.g., Pseudocysts, Necrosis)

Acute pancreatitis can potentially be complicated by several local complications, none of which are more important than pseudocysts and pancreatic necrosis regarding their impact on patient outcome. Pseudocysts are fluid-filled cysts that may be found within the pancreas or even within the surrounding tissues in the setting of acute inflammation via the enzymatic digestion of pancreatic tissue. While the majority of pseudocysts resolve spontaneously without intervention, symptomatic or larger cysts may require drainage due to associated risks of infection, abdominal pain, or bowel obstruction. Sound management is warranted because a pseudocyst can signal a complicated clinical course, and if monitored improperly, can lead to further sequelae. Pancreatic necrosis is another serious complication of acute pancreatitis, which can become infected and contribute exponentially to the mortality and morbidity.

Necrosis refers to tissue death caused by a cutoff in the supply of blood and the furious inflammatory response that acute pancreatitis causes. Infarction of the necrotic tissue poses a critical concern, which often requires early surgical intervention or complex endoscopic procedures. Minimally invasive techniques, such as percutaneous and endoscopic drainage, have been encouraging. The study shows that these approaches can effectively cure vast necrotic fields without the necessity for more invasive procedures, thus being a valuable change in the therapeutic regimen of highly involved patients. Early treatment is critical in the management of acute pancreatitis's local complications, particularly in complications of pancreatic encephalopathy, complicating the clinical presentation. Evidence calls for early diagnostic and treatment strategies to be adopted to avert complications of severe acute pancreatitis. Where infections do occur, as is the case with necrotic tissue, percutaneous and endoscopic therapy combined has been known to enhance recovery odds, reducing dependence on surgery (Constantin et al., 2014). With the evolution in medicine, there is a need for more study of treating such complications in order to further improve patient outcomes and expand the body of knowledge regarding the process of this multifaceted disease (Constantin et al., 2014).

3.6.2. Systemic Complications (e.g., Organ Failure)

Acute pancreatitis is predominantly linked with the risk of systemic complications, and organ failure represents a primary concern that can significantly diminish patient outcomes. Inflammation caused by pancreatic injury establishes distant effects throughout the body, impairing the functioning of multiple organ systems. This phenomenon is important in defining the severity of acute pancreatitis because it diverts attention away from localized pathology to systemic compromise of health. Research has established that some of the complications, such as cardiovascular impairment and respiratory insufficiency, commonly arise as a result of the inflammatory mediators released in acute pancreatitis attacks and therefore require close clinical observation and early intervention in impaired patients (Constantin et al., 2014). Triglyceride levels and systemic acute pancreatitis complications have been emphasized in recent studies. Elevated serum triglycerides (TG) are found to be linked with greater severity of the disease and increased risk of organ failure. In a cohort study, patients whose TG was more than 200 mg/dL had significantly greater respiratory, renal, and cardiovascular failure, with persistent and multiple organ failure. This correlation highlights the significance of monitoring and managing triglyceride levels early on at the diagnosis of acute pancreatitis so that at-risk individuals can be identified (Hidalgo et al., 2022). Hence, the measurement of TG levels can be a valuable prognostic marker in the clinical management of the condition. Early identification and intervention for systemic complications are essential to improve the outcomes among patients with acute pancreatitis. Prompt management approaches can greatly reduce the incidence of organ failure, subsequently enhancing recovery rates and reducing death. Studies have shown that earlier interventions are crucial, citing the importance of initiating forceful fluid resuscitation and monitoring for evidence of organ dysfunction. Equally important is an urgent response to complications such as pancreatic encephalopathy, although rare, presents a formidable challenge in management, which could be life-saving (Constantin et al., 2014). Therefore, a comprehensive strategy involving both early diagnosis and complete management of systemic complications must be adopted to ensure the optimum treatment of the patient in acute pancreatitis.

3.6.3. Long-Term Effects and Recurrence

The effects of acute pancreatitis are of long-term duration and tend to recur in their attacks, making patient management complicated. From research, acute pancreatitis, particularly alcoholic pancreatitis, is highly prone to recurrence, with successful readmission rates varying between 43% after the first year of initial treatment. This resulting high recurrence rate is undesirable because of the risk of continued damage to pancreatic tissue, eventually leading to chronic pancreatitis, more severe complications and an inferior quality of life for victims. The synergism of alcohol diseases with other psychosocial factors, such as tobacco use, makes this condition worse, with most patients demonstrating evidence of alcohol use disorder and complications, complicating the process of recovery and further treatment (Li et al., 2025). Metabolic conditions also play a key role in the determination of long-term outcomes of patients following acute pancreatitis events. Interestingly, stress hyperglycemia has also proven to be an important predictor of short-term outcomes. Its potential for long-term health consequences, including the onset of diabetes, reminds us that more work is needed in this area. Among non-diabetic patients who have an acute insult, a high proportion of those with stress hyperglycemia go on to develop evidence of diabetes, indicating a very important relationship between early acute attacks and chronic metabolic disease. While stress hyperglycemia itself does not seem to be connected with the recurrence of pancreatitis or with the progression to chronic diseases of this kind, its role in the long-term management of pancreatic function should not be overstated, stressing the importance of routine diabetes screening among patients with post-acute pancreatitis (Zhang et al., 2024). Understanding the long-term consequences and recurrence tendencies of acute pancreatitis is essential for developing preventive strategies and therapeutic modalities. Recurrence of acute attacks not only imposes a further burden on healthcare facilities but also exerts a significant psychological as well as physical effect on the patients. With the administration of proper follow-up care through lifestyle modification, education to the patient on the dangers of future alcohol use, and continued monitoring for metabolic derangements like diabetes, healthcare providers can better manage the long-term consequences of the disease. Research must continue to advance our understanding of acute pancreatitis pathophysiology, with a focus on recurrence determinants and probability of chronic disease progression, to improve outcomes for the individual (Li et al., 2025) (Figure 3.16).

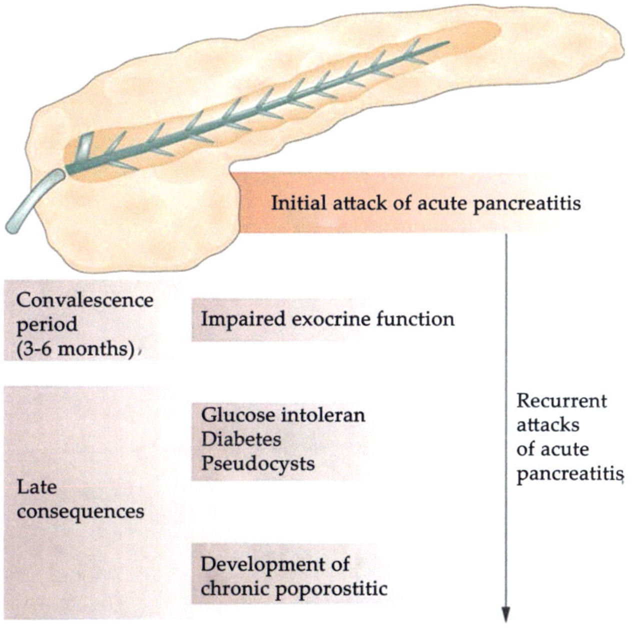

Figure 3.16. Acute pancreatitis: risk of recurrence and late consequences of the disease.

Source: https://media.springernature.com/full/springer-static/image/art%3A10.1038%2Fnrgastro.2009.106/MediaObjects/41575_2009_Article_BFnrgastro2009106_Fig1_HTML.jpg.

A CLOSER LOOK

EARLY RECOGNITION AND TREATMENT OF ACUTE PANCREATITIS

Early diagnosis and management of acute pancreatitis are very important determinants that largely impact the outcomes of patients. The early detection of this disease enables proper therapeutic management, which can reduce the risk of major complications and offer better recovery opportunities. Acute pancreatitis, which is inflammation of the pancreas, is a rapidly progressing condition that can result in systemic complications if not managed. Hence, clinicians must be vigilant while assessing symptoms such as severe abdominal pain, nausea, and vomiting, as these may be indicators of this fatal condition. Early initiation of diagnostic procedures, which include ultrasonography and laboratory tests, is essential in arriving at an accurate diagnosis and subsequent proper management options that can greatly reduce morbidity and mortality due to pancreatitis. In the veterinary field, the complexities of acute pancreatitis mandate prompt treatment to ensure optimal outcomes.

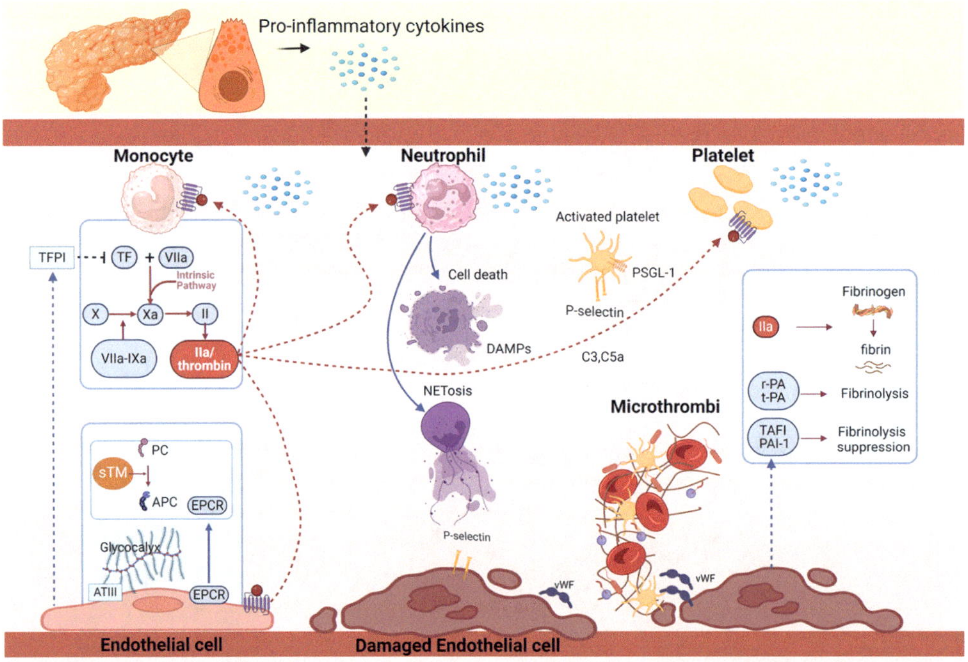

Source: https://www.researchgate.net/publication/385789314/figure/fig1/AS:11431281290288346@1731565323548/Pathophysiology-of-coagulopathy-in-acute-pancreatitis-The-activation-of-coagulation-by_Q320.jpg

As in the case of dogs and cats, the diagnosis of acute pancreatitis is very difficult because of the heterogeneity of clinical presentation and due to the inherent limitations of imaging modalities such as abdominal radiography and computed tomography. Early recognition is thus a must so that definitive treatments such as fluid therapy and nutrition therapy can be instituted at the earliest. These treatments not only address symptoms but also monitor the progression of the disease, which in most instances results in additional health complications or even pet death. Prognosis in animals that are admitted with acute pancreatitis varies based on their status at admission; hence, early diagnosis is an essential factor in altering the direction of their recovery. Understanding acute pancreatitis pathophysiology has also stressed the necessity of early therapeutic management. Excess alcohol consumption has been found to be a significant risk factor for acute pancreatitis because it compromises normal pancreatic function and induces stress in the endoplasmic reticulum (ER) of pancreatic acinar cells. Such a compromise can lead to cell injury and defective proteostasis, exacerbating the condition. Early detection allows intervention that can restore normal pancreas function, with diet and medication targeted to decrease inflammation. By addressing these early causes before complications arise, medical staff can truly enhance the quality of life and outcome for these patients drastically. Early detection and effective treatment pathways are therefore important in managing acute pancreatitis effectively (Waldron et al., 2018) (Figure 3.17).

SUMMARY

The management of acute pancreatitis is a multifaceted approach addressing both short-term clinical requirements and long-term sequelae of the illness. Central to the treatment plan is the management of the etiologic factors themselves, whether gallstones or alcohol use. Identification and elimination of these causative factors can exert a significant effect on preventing recurrent attacks and complications. Moreover, the need for a reflective diet regimen in recovery cannot be overstated. In particular, supplementing with dietary fiber can potentially be crucial in stabilizing intestinal barrier functions, thereby reducing rates of undesirable outcomes such as necrosis and systemic inflammatory responses, as identified by recent evidence (Ribichini et al., 2019). This management feature brings into focus the balance between clinical outcomes and nutrition in patients with acute pancreatitis. Furthermore, the cross-talk between acute pancreatitis and other systemic diseases also becomes meaningful in the context of treatment. The interplay between pancreatic inflammation and cardiovascular status, for instance, is better valued, and studies show that syndromes like Takotsubo cardiomyopathy can occur secondary to acute abdominal catastrophes (Gould et al., 2020). This shows the severity of acute pancreatitis, where the outcome is not only confined to the digestive system but also requires a holistic monitoring system. Clinicians must employ an interprofessional approach in terms of the assessment and management of potential complications. This global consideration not only facilitates successful management but also promotes patient safety and outcomes in the long run. Lastly, the conclusion drawn via current knowledge of acute pancreatitis underscores the quintessential role of personalized patterns of care based on the unique patient's special clinical situation. The heterogeneity of the illness ensures that one method may not suit all, and therefore, careful scrutiny of each individual case becomes extremely important. Future research needs to continue investigating the etiopathogenesis of inflammation and healing, as well as emerging dietary options. These innovations are aimed at enhancing the management of acute pancreatitis, thereby reducing the payload of the disease on healthcare systems and patients. In essence, while the challenges posed by acute pancreatitis are monumental, an evidence-based practice that is well-informed has the likelihood of improved patient-centered care modalities.

For acute pancreatitis, a deep understanding of the disease's etiology and clinical presentation is essential. Acute pancreatitis is most importantly characterized by sudden-onset inflammation of the pancreas and typically occurs as a consequence of gallstones, chronic consumption of alcohol in excess, or particular medications. This inflammatory process can lead to numerous complications, like necrotizing pancreatitis, which can further raise the intensity of the disease and result in systemic inflammatory responses. The clinical presentation may be very diverse, and the presenting symptoms are usually abdominal pain, nausea, and vomiting. Identification of these symptoms is critical to early diagnosis and treatment since untreated acute pancreatitis can result in high morbidity or mortality due to complications such as multiorgan failure and infection. Observational studies have shown that numerous factors influence the course of acute pancreatitis, such as the severity of the initial attack and the presence of comorbid illnesses. The assessment of severity is most often performed with scoring systems such as the Ranson criteria or the APACHE II score to evaluate clinical parameters to help predict outcomes. Furthermore, in patients with more severe forms of pancreatitis, early detection of IAH can be significant. IAH is perhaps best recognized as a significant cause of organ dysfunction in critically ill patients, for example, with acute pancreatitis.

Identification and appropriate control of IAH are essential since it can have a profound impact on the worldwide clinical course and may require fluid management and patient positioning (Schmiegelow et al., 2016). It has also been stressed through research that early intervention in terms of nutrition is essential in the management of acute pancreatitis. In the past, total bowel rest was administered to patients, but more recent guidelines suggest early enteral feeding, which has been shown to enhance recovery while minimizing complications. Nutrition plays a key role in maintaining gastrointestinal integrity and preventing systemic infection, which is given utmost importance in conditions of inflammatory diseases like acute pancreatitis. In addition, containment of the potential toxic effects of therapeutic agents is necessary for maximizing treatment protocols. Utilization of universal definitions for these toxic effects will help clinicians measure treatment safety and efficacy accurately. Through ongoing advances in the discipline, the use of multimodal approaches will be essential in improving the outcome of acute pancreatitis patients (Schmiegelow et al., 2016).

KEY TERMS FROM THIS CHAPTER

- Acute kidney injury (AKI)
- C-reactive protein (CRP)
- Electrolytes
- Enzymatic autodigestion
- Gene deletion methods
- Glucose utilization
- Inflammatory process
- Acute pancreatitis symptoms
- Cytomegalovirus
- Endocrine restitution
- Enzymes
- Gland dysfunction
- Infectious etiologies
- Intra-abdominal hypertension (IAH)

References

1. Waldron, R. T., Su, H. Y., Piplani, H., Capri, J., Cohn, W., Whitelegge, J. P., Faull, K. F., Sakkiah, S., Abrol, R., Yang, W., Zhou, B., Freeman, M. R., Pandol, S. J., & Lugea, A. (2018). Ethanol Induced Disordering of Pancreatic Acinar Cell Endoplasmic Reticulum: An ER Stress/Defective Unfolded Protein Response Model. *Cellular and molecular gastroenterology and hepatology*, *5*(4), 479–497. https://doi.org/10.1016/j.jcmgh.2018.01.001
2. Addiss, D. G., Fenwick, A., Jourdan, P. M., & Lamberton, P. H. L. (2018). Soil-transmitted helminth infections. https://core.ac.uk/download/96884381.pdf (accessed on 26 May 2025).
3. Ajmera, R., Kokandakar, H. R., Muneza, S., Nilkanth, S., & Boralkar, A. K. (2020). Surgical pathology of Whipple pancreaticoduodenectomy: A 3-year experience at a tertiary cancer care center of Marathwada region of India. *5*, 69–78. https://www.semanticscholar.org/paper/1cee98713b5ddce173cfa4cd9815c85882a1a868 (accessed on 26 May 2025).
4. Hidalgo, N. J., Pando, E., Alberti, P., Vidal, L., Mata, R., Fernandez, N., Gomez-Jurado, M. J., Dopazo, C., Blanco, L., Tasayco, S., Molero, X., Balsells, J., & Charco, R. (2022). Elevated Serum Triglyceride Levels in Acute Pancreatitis: A Parameter to be Measured and Considered Early. *World journal of surgery*, *46*(7), 1758–1767. https://doi.org/10.1007/s00268-022-06533-w (accessed on 26 May 2025).
5. Thakur, L., Kojicic, M., Thakur, S. J., Pieper, M. S., Kashyap, R., Trillo-Alvarez, C. A., Javier, F., Cartin-Ceba, R., & Gajic, O. (2009). Alcohol consumption and development of acute respiratory distress syndrome: a population-based study. *International journal of environmental research and public health*, *6*(9), 2426–2435. https://doi.org/10.3390/ijerph6092426
6. Arnelo, U., Haas, S. L., Löhr, J. M., Martin, I., et al. (2017). Pancreatic exocrine insufficiency after bariatric surgery. https://core.ac.uk/download/188827229.pdf (accessed on 26 May 2025).
7. Jafari, T., Feizi, A., Askari, G., & Fallah, A. A. (2015). Parenteral immunonutrition in patients with acute pancreatitis: a systematic review and meta-analysis. *Clinical nutrition (Edinburgh, Scotland)*, *34*(1), 35–43. https://doi.org/10.1016/j.clnu.2014.05.008 (accessed on 26 May 2025).
8. Schmiegelow, K., Attarbaschi, A., Barzilai, S., Escherich, G., Frandsen, T. L., Halsey, C., Hough, R., Jeha, S., Kato, M., Liang, D. C., Mikkelsen, T. S., Möricke, A., Niinimäki, R., Piette, C., Putti, M. C., Raetz, E., Silverman, L. B., Skinner, R., Tuckuviene, R., van der Sluis, I., ... Ponte di Legno toxicity working group (2016). Consensus definitions of 14 severe acute toxic effects for childhood lymphoblastic leukaemia treatment: a Delphi consensus. *The Lancet. Oncology*, *17*(6), e231–e239. https://doi.org/10.1016/S1470-2045(16)30035-3 (accessed on 26 May 2025).
9. Azar, R., Jonnalagadda, S., Kerr, T. A., Prakash, C., et al. (2007). *Pancreatitis Following Olanzapine Therapy: A Report of Three Cases*. https://core.ac.uk/download/83101025.pdf (accessed on 26 May 2025).
10. Azzopardi, N. (2014). *The Great Pretender: Autoimmune Pancreatitis*. https://core.ac.uk/download/46602519.pdf (accessed on 26 May 2025).
11. Ribichini, E., Stigliano, S., Rossi, S., Zaccari, P., Sacchi, M. C., Bruno, G., Badiali, D., & Severi, C. (2019). Role of Fibre in Nutritional Management of Pancreatic Diseases. *Nutrients*, *11*(9), 2219. https://doi.org/10.3390/nu11092219 (accessed on 26 May 2025).

12. BalcI, C., Sungurtekin, H., Gürses, E., Sungurtekin, U., & Kaptanoglu, B. (2003). Usefulness of procalcitonin for diagnosis of sepsis in the intensive care unit. *Critical care (London, England)*, *7*(1), 85–90. https://doi.org/10.1186/cc1843

13. Constantin VD, Carâp A, Socea B, Bobic S. Pancreatic Encephalopathy—A Rare Complication of Severe Acute Biliary Pancreatitis. *Journal of Mind and Medical Sciences*. 2014; 1(1):40-51. https://doi.org/10.22543/2392-7674.1005 (accessed on 26 May 2025).

14. Reddy, B. S., Bonigala, S. D., & Pandy, V. (2015). Role of endogenous peptides and enzymes in the pathogenesis of acute pancreatitis: A review. *Tropical Journal of Pharmaceutical Research*, *14*(7), 1305-1310. https://doi.org/10.4314/tjpr.v14i7.26 (accessed on 26 May 2025).

15. Borbásné Farkas, K., Boros, E., Czakó, L., Dohos, D., Erőss, B. M., Hegyi, P., et al. (2022). *Inflammatory Bowel Disease Does Not Alter the Clinical Features and The Management of Acute Pancreatitis: A Prospective, Multicenter, Exact-Matched Cohort Analysis*. https://core.ac.uk/download/552510548.pdf (accessed on 26 May 2025).

16. Boyanov N, Milinich N, Shtereva K, Madzharova K, Tufkova S, Penkova-Radicheva M, Radicheva D, Shopov N. Cost-Effectiveness in Alternative Treatment Options for Pancreatic Pseudocysts. *Reports*. 2024; 7(2):38. https://doi.org/10.3390/reports7020038(accessed on 26 May 2025).

17. Chaidos, C., Georgiou, E., Polydorides, M., Tsikopoulos, K., et al. (2020). Endoscopic transgastric drainage of pancreatic pseudocyst in hereditary pancreatitis: A case report. https://core.ac.uk/download/287177177.pdf (accessed on 26 May 2025).

18. Chawla, A., Habtezion, A., Hsieh, M. H., Murali, R., et al. (2015). *Alternatively Activated Macrophages Promote Pancreatic Fibrosis in Chronic Pancreatitis*. https://core.ac.uk/download/323077813.pdf.

19. Chikatipalli, R., Mohammad, A. B., & Nelavala, A. (2024). A prospective study on assessment of risk factors, clinical characteristics and outcomes of acute pancreatitis in a tertiary care center. *International Journal of Clinical Pharmacokinetics and Medical Sciences*. https://www.semanticscholar.org/paper/e18d5b2db81125d3fccd40ee781bfea5910dc614 (accessed on 26 May 2025).

20. Hulsebosch, S. E., Palm, C. A., Segev, G., Cowgill, L. D., Kass, P. H., & Marks, S. L. (2016). Evaluation of Canine Pancreas-Specific Lipase Activity, Lipase Activity, and Trypsin-Like Immunoreactivity in an Experimental Model of Acute Kidney Injury in Dogs. *Journal of veterinary internal medicine*, *30*(1), 192–199. https://doi.org/10.1111/jvim.13806Daminet, S., Hesta, M., Paepe, D., & Saunders, J. (2010). Acute pancreatitis in dogs and cats: Medical imaging, biopsy, treatment and prognosis. https://core.ac.uk/download/55845908.pdf (accessed on 26 May 2025).

21. De Waele, J. J., Ejike, J. C., Leppäniemi, A., De Keulenaer, B. L., De Laet, I., Kirkpatrick, A. W., Roberts, D. J., Kimball, E., Ivatury, R., & Malbrain, M. L. (2015). Intra-abdominal hypertension and abdominal compartment syndrome in pancreatitis, paediatrics, and trauma. *Anaesthesiology intensive therapy*, *47*(3), 219–227. https://doi.org/10.5603/AIT.a2015.0027 (accessed on 26 May 2025).

22. de Oliveira, C., Khatua, B., Noel, P., Kostenko, S., Bag, A., Balakrishnan, B., Patel, K. S., Guerra, A. A., Martinez, M. N., Trivedi, S., McCullough, A., Lam-Himlin, D. M., Navina, S., Faigel, D. O., Fukami, N., Pannala, R., Phillips, A. E., Papachristou, G. I., Kershaw, E. E., Lowe, M. E., ... Singh,

V. P. (2020). Pancreatic triglyceride lipase mediates lipotoxic systemic inflammation. *The Journal of clinical investigation, 130*(4), 1931–1947. https://doi.org/10.1172/JCI132767 (accessed on 26 May 2025).

23. Morvaridi, S., Dhall, D., Greene, M. I., Pandol, S. J., & Wang, Q. (2015). Role of YAP and TAZ in pancreatic ductal adenocarcinoma and in stellate cells associated with cancer and chronic pancreatitis. *Scientific reports, 5*, 16759. https://doi.org/10.1038/srep16759

24. Diaconu, C. C., Diculescu, M., Ditu, G., & Hainarosie, R. (2018). Pancreatogenesis type 3C diabetes. https://core.ac.uk/download/216809675.pdf (accessed on 26 May 2025).

25. Dolenšek, J., Pohorec, V., Rupnik, M. S., & Stožer, A. (2017). Pancreas physiology. https://core.ac.uk/download/322428900.pdf (accessed on 26 May 2025).

26. Preissler, G., Massberg, S., Eichhorn, M. E., Waldner, H., Loehe, F., Winter, H., & Messmer, K. (2010). Islets of Langerhans are protected from inflammatory cell recruitment during reperfusion of rat pancreas grafts. *European surgical research. Europaische chirurgische Forschung. Recherches chirurgicales europeennes, 44*(3-4), 192–200. https://doi.org/10.1159/000302732 (accessed on 26 May 2025).

27. Goldin, M. R., Petry, R., & Goyal, P. (2024). Doxycycline-associated acute pancreatitis: A rare adverse effect of a commonly prescribed antibiotic. *BMJ Case Reports, 17*(9). https://www.semanticscholar.org/paper/58fd040c8c6f94dfd3fb53e360d19770210e19b1 (accessed on 26 May 2025).

28. Gould, K., Miller, S., & Moll, J. (2020). An Early Holiday Surprise: Cholecystitis Wrapped in Takotsubo Cardiomyopathy. *Clinical practice and cases in emergency medicine, 4*(2), 137–141. https://doi.org/10.5811/cpcem.2020.1.45474Ren, J., Li, X., Sun, J., Han, M., Yang, G. Y., Li, W. Y., Robinson, N., Lewith, G., & Liu, J. P. (2015). Is traditional Chinese medicine recommended in Western medicine clinical practice guidelines in China? A systematic analysis. *BMJ open, 5*(6), e006572. https://doi.org/10.1136/bmjopen-2014-006572 (accessed on 26 May 2025).

29. Jiang, R., Gao, C., Bai, J., Li, A., Wang, X. H., Cao, F., & Li, F. (2024). Progress in the diagnosis and treatment of pancreatic cancer with acute pancreatitis as the initial symptom. *Zhonghua Wai Ke Za Zhi (Chinese Journal of Surgery), 62*(10), 973–977. https://www.semanticscholar.org/paper/ea8261b21ba6e4b96b79c7b9e6b101aa8e7f3d32 (accessed on 26 May 2025).

30. Jokić, R., & Milošević, P. (2012). [Acute pancreatitis in children]. *Medicinski Pregled, 65*(1–2), 69–71. https://www.semanticscholar.org/paper/d89aaae4e95412cf9fcb20789f1492208ac66361 (accessed on 26 May 2025).

31. Kelly, T., & Troyer, M. L. (1963). Pancreatic ducts and postoperative pancreatitis. *Archives of Surgery, 87*, 614–618. https://www.semanticscholar.org/paper/3af62a83cbe11806b09bb147f93a7cca3deffec0 (accessed on 26 May 2025).

32. Khan NN, Alnowaisser LN, Alomari AM, Asiri AA, Alharbi NA, Bayazeed KA, Jadaan NS, Alalyani RG, Alanazi SN, Algheryafi SS. Risk Factors and Management of Acute Pancreatitis; A Systematic Review. https://www.ijmdc.com/?mno=180065 [Access: May 15, 2025]. doi:10.24911/IJMDC.51-1701812193

33. (accessed on 26 May 2025).

34. Klimenko, A. V., & Klimenko, V. M. (2024). *Modern Trends in Diagnosis and Treatment of Acute Pancreatitis (Based on the 56th Meeting of the European Pancreatic Club, Santiago de*

Compostela, Spain, June 26–29, 2024). Herald of Pancreatic Club. https://www.semanticscholar.org/paper/656101b8dd527ac80cc77511d41516c90eccfaab (accessed on 26 May 2025).

35. Li, H., Tan, X., Li, J., & Zhang, Q. (2025). New Progress in the Study of Pathogenesis of Alcoholic Pancreatitis. *Digestion*, *106*(3), 212–226. https://doi.org/10.1159/000542548(accessed on 26 May 2025).

36. Li, L., Tan, Q., Wu, X., Mou, X., Lin, Z., Liu, T., Huang, W., et al. (2024). Coagulopathy and acute pancreatitis: Pathophysiology and clinical treatment. *Frontiers in Immunology, 15*. https://www.semanticscholar.org/paper/57a5ba3bc59d2835b209e1052b3047d85b6c133b (accessed on 26 May 2025).

37. Liu, P., Zhao, P., Zhao, T., & Yu, L. (2025). Pharmacological treatment of hypertriglyceridemia-induced acute pancreatitis during pregnancy: A case report and literature review. *Medicine, 104*. https://www.semanticscholar.org/paper/1e421f57dc1ec43f8dbaf2bac8a09845d6458d82 (accessed on 26 May 2025).

38. Meining, A., Umgelter, A., Baron, R., Beger, H. G., Bradley, E. L., Branum, G., et al. (2009). Infected necrosis in severe pancreatitis–Combined nonsurgical multi-drainage with directed transabdominal high-volume lavage in critically ill patients. https://core.ac.uk/download/16432292.pdf (accessed on 26 May 2025).

39. Hallberg, P., Hallberg, E., & Amini, H. (2004). Acute pancreatitis following medical abortion: Case report. *BMC women's health*, *4*(1), 1. https://doi.org/10.1186/1472-6874-4-1

40. Rošić, N. (2011). Rational drug use in acute pancreatitis: Case report. *3*, 29–35. https://www.semanticscholar.org/paper/7ad38c67180ae1f5521bbb7324276bdb3a8e7fe7 (accessed on 26 May 2025).

41. Tang, X., Chen, Y., Huang, S., Jiang, J., Luo, B., Ren, W., Zhou, X., Shi, X., Zhang, W., Shi, L., Zhong, X., & Lü, M. (2024). Acute Pancreatitis in Pregnancy: A Propensity Score Matching Analysis and Dynamic Nomogram for Risk Assessment. *Digestive diseases and sciences*, *69*(6), 2235–2246. https://doi.org/10.1007/s10620-024-08415-8 (accessed on 26 May 2025).

42. Schäfer, C., Tietz, A. B., & Göke, B. (2005). Pathophysiology of acute experimental pancreatitis: lessons from genetically engineered animal models and new molecular approaches. *Digestion*, *71*(3), 162–172. https://doi.org/10.1159/000086138 (accessed on 26 May 2025).

43. Vrolyk, V. (2025). *Lung Inflammation Associated with Acute Necrotizing Pancreatitis in Dogs and Mice*. https://core.ac.uk/download/226148613.pdf (accessed on 26 May 2025).

44. Wang, K., Zhang, L., Deng, B., Zhao, K., Chen, C., & Wang, W. (2024). Mitochondrial uncoupling protein 2: A central player in pancreatic disease pathophysiology. *Molecular Medicine, 30*. https://www.semanticscholar.org/paper/40e0ce3fb30ba4c193493eccf823ff3eb6e72746 (accessed on 26 May 2025).

45. Wu, Z., Zong, K., Zhou, B., Yin, K., Zhang, A., & Li, M. (2023). Incidence and risk factors of postoperative acute pancreatitis after pancreaticoduodenectomy: A systematic review and meta-analysis. *Frontiers in Surgery, 10*. https://www.semanticscholar.org/paper/6d721f074fb7d8c4721ea3f85c21e7850664b46b (accessed on 26 May 2025).

46. Sai YRKM (2024) Understanding pancreatic disorders: Acute and chronic pancreatitis, pancreatic cancer and diabetes: A mini-review on a few of the most common pancreatic

disorders. Ann Pancreat Disord Treatm 6(1): 006-010. DOI: 10.17352/apdt.000012 (accessed on 26 May 2025).

47. Zhang, J., Wang, X., Lv, Y., Hou, J., Zhang, C., Su, X., & Li, L. (2024). Impact of stress hyperglycemia on long-term prognosis in acute pancreatitis without diabetes. *Internal and emergency medicine*, *19*(3), 681–688. https://doi.org/10.1007/s11739-023-03524-0 (accessed on 26 May 2025).

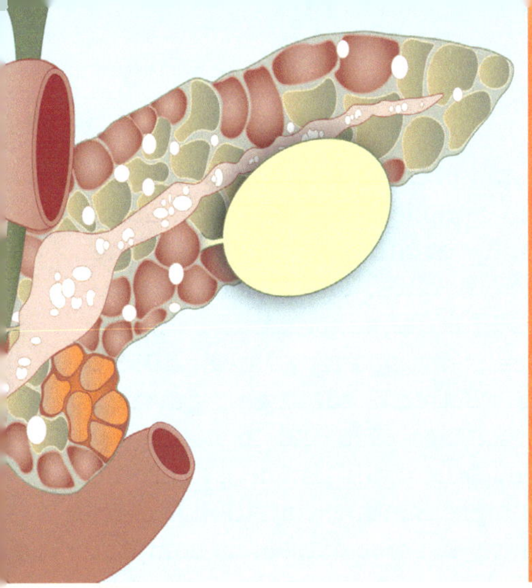

Chapter 4

CHRONIC PANCREATITIS

Contents

Introduction

Chronic pancreatitis (CP) is a severe clinical problem defined by recurring inflammation of the pancreas, leading to cumulative damage over time. CP is defined by endocrine and exocrine dysfunction and finally results in symptoms like chronic abdominal pain and malabsorption of nutrients. The etiology of chronic pancreatitis might be multifactorial and complex, typically spanning a range of etiologic factors such as alcoholism, hereditary predispositions, and autoimmune mechanisms. Of note is that this inflammatory disease does not exclusively take place among adults; there are certain forms, such as tropical calcific pancreatitis, that happen among children and young adults, a reflection of the inconsistent nature of its presentations and etiologies (Chowdhury et al., 1994). The importance of accurate diagnosis cannot be overemphasized since interventions begun in time may alleviate complications and improve the quality of life of the patient. Clinical presentation of chronic pancreatitis is variable in severity and duration set with symptoms important among which is chronic pain that can be debilitating in the majority of the patients. With the progression of the disease, the resulting morphological changes in the pancreatic tissue lead to the formation of complications like calcification and fibrosis of the pancreas. Gradual scarring may impair the ability of the pancreas to secrete digestive enzymes, which would further aggravate the malabsorption status. The disease course normally evolves over a period of a few years with repeated bouts of acute pancreatitis being an issue, risk of the development of diabetes mellitus, and risk of pancreatic malignancy (Dinesh, 2013). Identification of the disease course is crucial since it decides the treatment paradigms pursued in the management of pain and enzyme substitution therapy, which are essential to managing symptoms as well as the underlying disturbances in physiology. The best management of chronic pancreatitis is a multidisciplinary approach, combining pharmacologic therapy, nutritional care, and, in some cases, surgery. Pain management interventions frequently become extremely complex due to the progression of the disease and variability of patient responses to treatments. Currently, recent literature has explained the utility of imaging modalities such as MRCP and EUS in disease diagnosis and monitoring the progression of disease so that the clinician can personalize treatment that is best suited to each patient. Moreover, as chronic pancreatitis progressively evolves with time, the efficacy of enzyme replacement becomes a key factor for the restoration of digestive function and the alleviation of malabsorption symptoms. A clear understanding of the intricate interplay among these modalities of therapy can significantly maximize patient benefits and aid in the overall management of chronic pancreatitis (Figure 4.1).

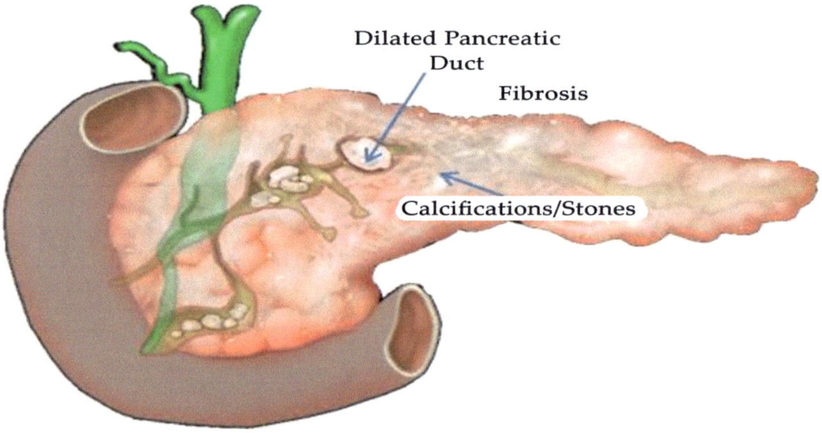

Figure 4.1. Chronic pancreatitis (CP).

Source: https://www.drchiragthakkar.com/wp-content/uploads/2020/04/fig1_5.jpg.

Definition of Chronic Pancreatitis (CP)

CP is defined as a chronic or recurrent inflammatory illness that induces progressive and irreversible morphological changes in the pancreas. With its disabling characteristics, the illness results in chronic abdominal pain and marked impairments in exocrine and endocrine pancreatic function. The irreversible nature of chronic pancreatitis distinguishes it from acute pancreatitis, wherein the former frequently includes reversible inflammation. According to Bornman et al. (2010), chronic pancreatitis's effect extends beyond the local inflammation alone, since it goes on to alter the function and structure of the pancreas over time, creating conditions that pose a danger to patients' quality of life. It is a disease that comes in many aspects and is worrying, especially due to its chronic symptoms and the additional complications it brings to diagnosis and management. Pain remains one of the hallmark symptoms of chronic pancreatitis, often impacting the physical and psychological condition of a patient. Pathogenesis of the disease is multifactorial, with alcoholism being the most prevalent cause of this disease in industrialized countries, and particularly in South Africa, where it is boosted by socio-economic factors. Chronic pancreatitis, as seen according to Bornman et al. (2010), is difficult for clinicians since it is experienced with clinical and pathological heterogeneity that complicates diagnosis and therapeutic control. The patient's pain is typically chronic and the intensity is changing, severely limiting daily activities and reducing the quality of life. Thus, a proper understanding of the disease is needed not just for appropriate medical treatment but also for managing the psychological and social dynamics of chronic pancreatitis. In managing chronic pancreatitis, there is a need to incorporate successful diagnostic and therapeutic strategies due to its complications. Various imaging methods, such as magnetic resonance cholangiopancreatography (MRCP) and endoscopic ultrasound (EUS), are important for estimating the disease's morphological alterations. These technologies allow for the detection of pancreatic duct blockage and other anatomical defects, hence guiding treatment options. Given that medical management usually represents the first line of intervention, as noted in Dinesh (2013), the combination of pain management interventions, enzyme replacement therapy, and potential surgical interventions remains key to overall care in individuals afflicted by this condition. It is essential to arrive at a multidisciplinary approach in a bid to improve patient outcomes and ensure holistic management of chronic pancreatitis, as clinical guidelines underscored in the literature (Figure 4.2).

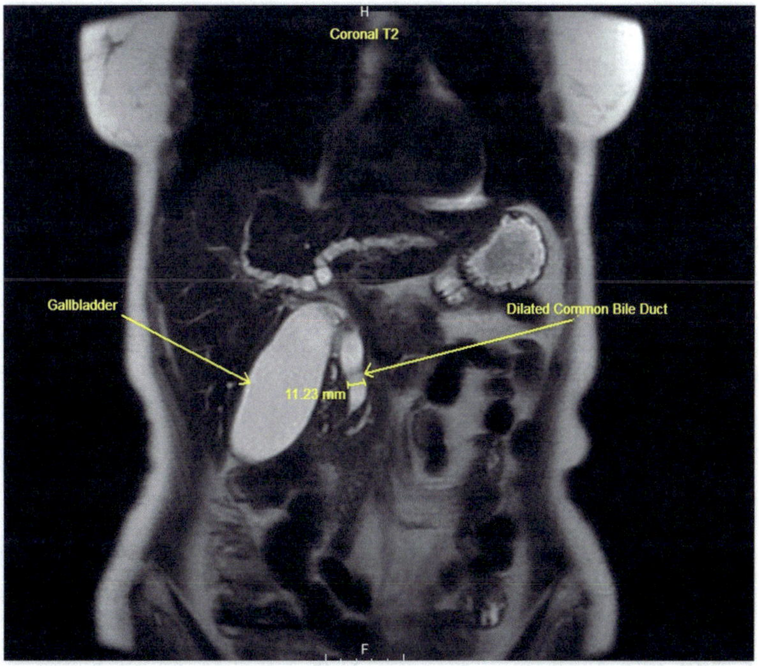

Figure 4.2. Magnetic resonance cholangiopancreatography (MRCP).

Source: https://greaterwaterburyimagingcenter.org/wp-content/uploads/2015/11/cbd.jpg.

Importance of Understanding the Condition

It takes a deep understanding of CP to maximize patient outcomes and to formulate treatment strategies. Clinicians must realize that CP is a complicated, multifaceted disease that not only inflicts severe physical pain but also seriously impairs patients' mental and emotional status. A realization of the nature of the disease can direct better pain management strategies, which remain an integral part of the treatment. Without a multifaceted understanding, treatment may be insufficient, and patients are vulnerable to ongoing pain and quality-of-life deterioration. Designing therapy aimed at CPs entails an understanding of CPs underlying mechanisms—affecting especially the calcification and fibrosis roles—to prevent disease advancement and construct interventions with patient-centered outcomes in mind. This deeper inquiry then provides a stage for cutting-edge research and clinical interventions that could transform the lives of individuals suffering from this debilitating illness (Abu-El-Haija et al., 2018). The intricacies surrounding the etiology of chronic pancreatitis, as it pertains to alcohol consumption, also highlight the importance of education and prevention initiatives. Alcoholic pancreatitis can be the initiating point for a cycle of acute flare-ups to chronic disease, and thus serves to highlight the need for early treatment and lifestyle modification (Ammann et al., 2009). By understanding the risk and progression of the disease, clinicians are then in a position to employ an educated dialogue with patients concerning alcohol consumption effects on pancreatic function, and the need for moderation or total abstinence. This strategy for education is crucial not only for patients but also for family members and support groups who might be extremely significant to patients' treatment adherence and life changes. In the end, anticipatory awareness of chronic pancreatitis facilitates a more holistic approach to patient care, perhaps reducing the prevalence of the disease and enhancing outcomes in terms of long-term management. Finally, the importance of valuing chronic pancreatitis is not just in the treatment of individual patients but also on a population health basis. The more individuals learn about the disease, the more research and funding are made available for the development of effective treatments. The historical underrepresentation of chronic pancreatitis in clinical literature has held progress back; thus, catalyzing action toward prioritizing research in pain management and therapeutics, as signaled by emerging mechanistic insight, is necessary (Abu-El-Haija et al., 2018). Such action can eventually translate into improved clinical guidelines and therapeutic paradigms that directly contribute to helping patients suffering from chronic pancreatitis. As stakeholders in the medical community rally around the need for greater awareness and understanding of this disease, the likelihood of improved care and better patient outcomes becomes more real. In so doing, the applicability of understanding of chronic pancreatitis resonates throughout individual patients and the healthcare setting as a whole.

4.1. Causes of Chronic Pancreatitis

Chronic pancreatitis is a multifactorial illness with many etiologic causes resulting in its development. Of these, alcohol is a potent cause responsible for a significant percentage of cases. Chronic and excessive alcohol consumption leads to inflammatory changes in the pancreas, demonstrated by recurrent attacks of pain and resultant fibrosis. This chronic damage has a tendency to cause loss of both exocrine and endocrine function, aggravating the clinical situation and contributing to the misery of the patients. In certain populations, in the young, non-alcoholic types such as tropical calcific pancreatitis are prevalent, wherein malnutrition and nutritional deficiencies are identified as primary etiologies for pancreatic damage, demonstrating the diverse armamentarium of etiologies that cause chronic pancreatitis (Chowdhury et al., 1994). In addition to diet and alcohol, genetic susceptibility also plays a significant role in the causation of chronic pancreatitis. Genetic mutations, particularly within the cationic trypsinogen gene (PRSS1), have been found to be significant risk factors that predispose patients to pancreatic injury. These mutations potentially lead to the preactivation of digestive enzymes within the pancreas, not only causing inflammation but also secondary fibrosis and calcification of pancreatic tissue. Hereditary pancreatitis with recurrent acute attacks developing into chronic disease over a period similarly emphasizes the importance of genetic background in explaining the disease course. Apart from these genetic factors, environmental mechanisms such as oxidative stress caused by free radicals complicate inflammatory processes in chronic pancreatitis (Chowdhury et al., 1994). Another pathogenetic factor in chronic pancreatitis is the participation of autoimmune mechanisms and recurrent acute pancreatitis attacks. Autoimmune pancreatitis, or inflammation caused by the immune system, can lead to chronic pancreatic damage if left untreated. It may, on occasion, be confused with other pancreatic disorders with similar symptoms. Furthermore, recurrent acute attacks can result in cumulative damage; even mild acute attacks have the potential to initiate a cascade of inflammatory processes that progress into chronic diseases. To effectively relieve pain and provide therapeutic intervention to those suffering from chronic pancreatitis, it is important to know these underlying mechanisms. Cumulatively, this discovery of various causes reflects the complexity of the disease and the necessity for a holistic and individualized treatment protocol (Dinesh, 2013) (Figure 4.3).

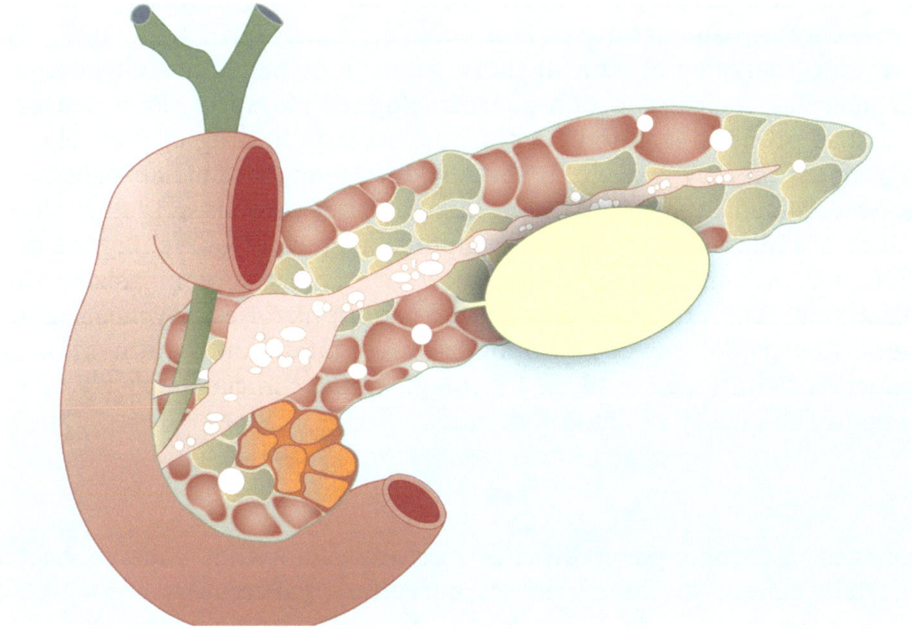

Figure 4.3. Causes of chronic pancreatitis (CP).

Source: https://external-content.duckduckgo.com/iu/?u=https%3A%2F%2Fueg.eu%2Fimages%2F748%2Fe49b8b4053df9505e1f48c3a701c0682_975_LARGE.png&f=1&nofb=1&ipt=a6afed19e4c7c28400614479145e22405923929485e5557c3bde745eea855d9d.

4.1.1. Alcohol Consumption

The association between alcohol consumption and chronic pancreatitis is a critical factor in identifying the etiology and progression of the disease. Alcohol is commonly identified as a significant risk factor for chronic pancreatitis, especially among Western populations. It induces an inflammatory response in the pancreas that triggers irreversible morphological changes in the long run. Such alterations damage the organ's normal function, resulting in incapacitating symptoms and complications, such as pain and malabsorption. Statistically, chronic alcoholism and chronic alcohol abuse are linked with a higher incidence of chronic pancreatitis, further highlighting the need to educate the general populace about the deleterious impact of alcohol on pancreatic function. The multifactorial etiology of the disease further suggests that while alcohol is the principal causative factor, other lifestyle and dietary factors may still have a potential influence on its impact, highlighting the use of integrated prevention and control measures. In chronic pancreatitis, socioeconomic determinants involved in alcohol consumption, particularly among vulnerable groups, should be addressed. For instance, in certain regions like South Africa, alcohol abuse is directly linked with chronic pancreatitis cases, particularly among the impoverished. Such groups tend to have other determinants like malnutrition and poor healthcare access, making treatment and prognosis challenging. The psychological effects of drug use are not just on the patients but also extend to their families and communities. Effective control, therefore, must be an answer to the connected issues of addiction and chronic disease, and this requires cooperation between healthcare professionals, social workers, and community organizations in planning combined support systems for the patients so that they are given both medical and psychological care where necessary. Management of pain in alcohol-induced chronic pancreatitis patients poses extremely challenging tasks. The debilitating and typically chronic character of pain in these subjects demands a multi-disciplinary strategy including both pharmacological and non-pharmacological measures. Pain can be alleviated by analgesics but is also prone to lead to addiction, particularly in drug or alcohol abusers. The use of enzyme replacement therapy is twofold: not only does it improve malabsorption, but it can also reduce pancreatic workload, in theory, avoiding inflammatory responses. Dietary changes, including alcohol abstinence, are important to manage symptoms and avoid worsening the disease. Detailed recommendations for such management strategies have emerged, emphasizing the requirement for individualized treatment modalities considering patient histories, psychosocial factors, and life change readiness (Bornman et al., 2010). Upon the recognition and treatment of the alcohol use and chronic pancreatitis interaction in all its complexities, clinicians can try to improve health outcomes as well as the quality of life in patients.

4.1.2. Genetic Factors

The role of genetics in chronic pancreatitis is a critical factor that underscores the severity of this disease. Certain genetic diseases, such as hereditary pancreatitis and cystic fibrosis, have been identified as primary etiologic agents for the onset of chronic pancreatitis. Gene mutations, particularly in the PRSS1 gene, have been found extensively in familial pancreatitis, leading to recurrent pancreatitis attacks that later become chronic inflammation. This susceptibility at the genetic level not only affects the timing but also the severity and course of pancreatic damage, highlighting the need for a better understanding of how genes interact with environmental risk factors. Interaction between genetic susceptibility and external influence can account for why some individuals become clinically manifest with chronic pancreatitis and others do not, and thus, further investigation into genetic testing as part of patient management models is warranted. Furthermore, the role of genes in calcium signaling and pancreatic secretory function is being investigated in chronic pancreatitis. For example, mutations in the calcium-sensing receptor gene have been identified as causing impaired calcium handling in pancreatic acinar cells, resulting in premature activation of digestive enzymes. The inappropriate activation can lead to inflammation followed by fibrosis of the pancreas. The interaction between genetic susceptibility and pathophysiological changes that arise in chronic pancreatitis evinces the intricacy of its etiology. Further, understanding such phenomena might provide insights into targeted therapies that may prevent or reverse the undesirable consequences of genetic mutations on pancreatic health and function, enhancing potential outcomes in patients. Finally, chronic pancreatitis's genetic profile is not only significant for explaining its cause but also for finding pain relief and enzyme replacement therapies. Genetic influence over the severity and character of pancreatic disease makes individually tailored modalities potentially more effective. Individuals with certain genetic mutations, for instance, can respond differently to standard enzyme replacement therapy, and so personalized treatment in terms of individual genetic profiles is essential. Besides, knowledge of the genetic predispositions implicated in chronic pancreatitis will aid in the prompt detection of at-risk individuals to intervene and prevent disease progression. Thus, ongoing research aiming towards the identification of the genetic cause of chronic pancreatitis will remain important for the enhancement of clinical management and therapeutic gain in this challenging disorder (Figure 4.4).

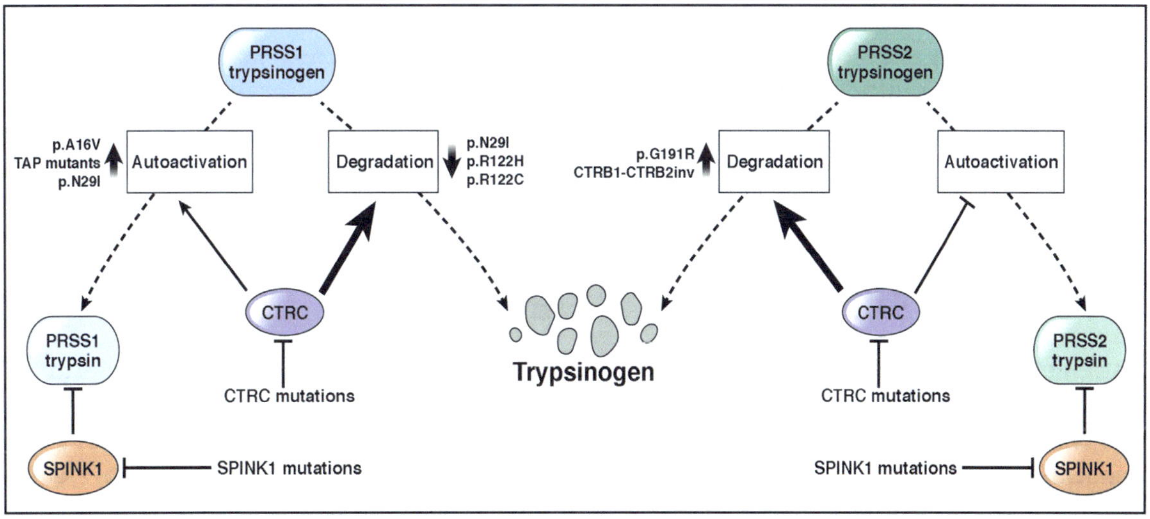

Figure 4.4. Pancreatitis-genetic-mutations.

Source: https://www.geneticlifehacks.com/wp-content/uploads/2023/06/pancreatitis-genetic-mutations.png.

4.1.3. Autoimmune Disorders

In the case of chronic pancreatitis, autoimmune disease is the most critical area to explore. Autoimmune pancreatitis (AIP) or a specific type of pancreas inflammation, is a condition where the immune system of the body mistakenly targets the pancreas and leads to significant organ dysfunction. AIP can be indistinguishable from radiological and clinical features of chronic pancreatitis caused by other causes, and thus, diagnosis and treatment can be difficult. The differential from typical chronic pancreatitis is mostly predicated on the pathologic immune-mediated process. Ultimately, the diagnosis of AIP not only alters the pancreatitis etiology but also enhances the therapeutic approach. Where autoimmunity is involved, immunosuppressive therapy becomes a cornerstone of management, in contrast to pain and enzyme replacement therapy normally administered in non-autoimmune pancreatitis patients with chronic pancreatitis, as supported by most clinical guidelines and research (Dinesh, 2013). Clinical importance in autoimmune pancreatitis is significant, particularly regarding course and presentation. AIP patients may develop recurrent abdominal pain and weight loss, indicative of pancreatic dysfunction. Notably, the condition can lead to fibrosis and calcification in severe cases, in the pattern of alcoholic or idiopathic chronic pancreatitis, but spread by different mechanisms of pathophysiology. Of special relevance, correct diagnosis of AIP is also crucial since it can affect the treatment program significantly, and therefore the role of sophisticated imaging techniques such as MRI and endoscopic ultrasound. These imaging technologies can map distinctive morphological changes within the pancreas that are attributed to autoimmune processes, making it possible to achieve timely and accurate diagnosis that forms the basis for effective clinical management (Bornman et al., 2010). The incorporation of immunologic insights in managing chronic pancreatitis can lead to improved outcomes. With autoimmune diseases, recognition of the immune system's role in disease pathogenesis guides therapeutic intervention beyond the conventional pain control and enzyme replacement. Systemic corticosteroids and other immunosuppressive drugs have become effective therapies for controlling the inflammatory process of AIP, thereby alleviating symptoms and avoiding further pancreatic damage. The convergence of autoimmune research and the standard management of chronic pancreatitis fosters a multidisciplinary care system, involving gastroenterologists, immunologists, and pain medicine specialists. Such an interprofessional approach fosters a total treatment plan, not merely symptom management but also long-term disease modification, and signifies enhanced patient care for chronic pancreatitis (Dinesh, 2013).

4.2. Progression of the Disease

The pathogenesis of chronic pancreatitis (CP) encompasses a sequence of pathological events resulting in irreversible damage to pancreatic tissue. The condition is believed to begin with bouts of acute inflammatory episodes, which, upon recurrence, lead to chronic inflammation. Chronic inflammation is sustained through a protracted inflammatory response, which triggers a variety of morphological alterations in the pancreas, including fibrosis and calcification formation, both of which severely impair pancreatic function. In CP, the irreversible nature of the changes represents a serious challenge to holistic management. Specifically, alcohol consumption is the most common cause in Western countries, leading to a unique disease course due to drug dependency, and the complexity of disease progression is further added (Chowdhury et al., 1994). In progressive chronic pancreatitis, progressive loss of exocrine and endocrine function occurs. Patients first come with abdominal pain, which gradually becomes disabling with the progression of the condition. Additionally, the chronic inflammatory state results in severe fibrosis, which obstructs the pancreatic ducts and results in malabsorption due to reduced secretion of enzymes necessary for digestion. In addition, there is a heightened risk of diabetes, in particular due to the destruction of insulin-producing cells, which marks the advent of conditions like fibrocalculous pancreatic diabetes (FCPD) (Chowdhury et al., 1994). This formation underscores the inter-relationship between morphological changes and dysfunction, further highlighting the importance of early diagnosis and treatment in the successful management of chronic pancreatitis. Lastly, the formation of chronic pancreatitis underscores the problematic nature of its clinical management. Patients normally encounter a range of complications related to the disease progression, varying from pain to significant nutritional deficit and metabolic disturbances. The chronic nature of the condition calls for holistic treatment involving pain relief management and enzyme replacement therapies. With the increasing progression of the disease, multidisciplinary treatment is increasingly essential in providing total treatment care to the patient for facilitating disease-specific management based on the presentation of the subject's complications and symptoms. Continuous research and updates clinically are essential in facilitating the changing management modalities in handling the complex presentations of this disabling disease (Bornman et al., 2010) (Figure 4.5).

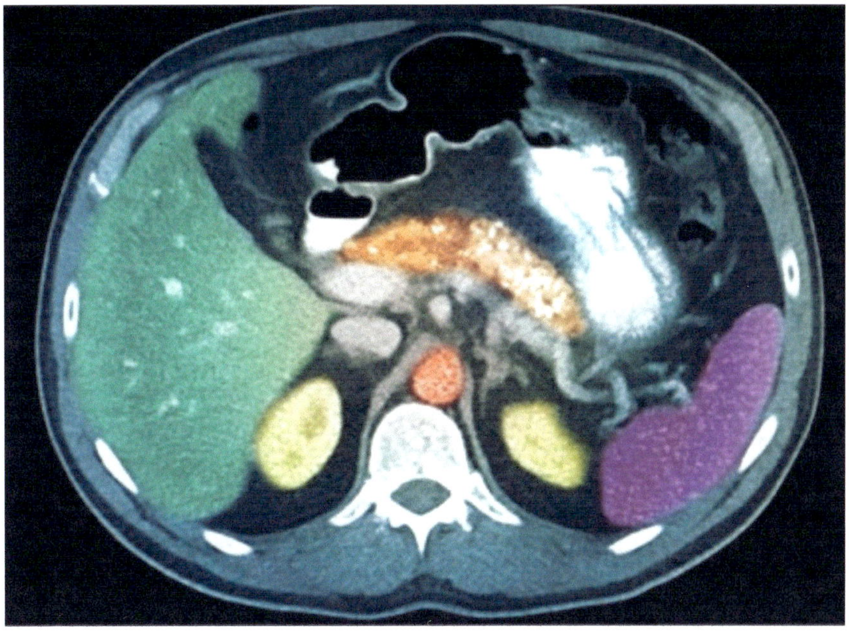

Figure 4.5. Chronic pancreatitis (CP): Challenging to diagnose.

Source: https://external-content.duckduckgo.com/iu/?u=https%3A%2F%2Fwww.gastroenterologyadvisor.com%2Fwp-content%2Fuploads%2Fsites%2F23%2F2019%2F08%2FChronic-Pancreatitis_SS_SS21261091-768x547.jpg&f=1&nofb=1&ipt=c81e416e3ce6e8101cc858f0a05112178b8d55205bdcd6c8a0409655c58eed7f.

4.2.1. Stages of Chronic Pancreatitis

The progression of chronic pancreatitis is typically described in various phases, each of which is characterized by some pathological changes and clinical manifestations. The disease begins with repeated abdominal pain and intermittent acute pancreatitis. Later, chronic inflammation leads to irreversible morphological changes of pancreatic tissue, ultimately causing fibrosis and calcification. The first phase is typically marked by acute inflammatory reactions, and which are accompanied by signs of nausea and epigastric pain, causing potential misdiagnosis. Early warning signs are crucial for early intervention to halt advancement. Repeated exacerbations propel the disease into advanced levels with increased tissue damage and the development of complications such as diabetes mellitus secondary to islet cell destruction and therefore necessitate careful monitoring and preventive management protocols for better patient outcomes (Chowdhury et al., 1994). In chronic pancreatitis, pancreatic calcifications characterize the second phase as a sign of advanced disease. These calcifications are likely to result from the deposition of calcium salts in dead tissue, followed by further loss of acinar cells. Such patients can present with chronic abdominal pain, steatorrhea, and weight loss due to malabsorption secondary to abnormal exocrine secretion. Calcifications can be detected using imaging tests, which also help determine the severity of the condition and the necessity of potential interventional therapy. The resulting chronic inflammation in this stage can lead to disruption of the integrity of pancreatic ducts and susceptibility to pancreatic duct obstruction or formation of a pseudocyst, for which a multi-disciplinary management plan, primarily by endocrinologists and gastroenterologists, is required to manage systemic complications (Bornman et al., 2010). The final stage of chronic pancreatitis is marked by massive fibrosis with loss of exocrine and endocrine functions. Such patients present here with intractable pain, crippling nutrient deficits, and the advent of diabetes, known as fibrocalculous pancreatic diabetes in certain circumstances, particularly where malnutrition is endemic (Chowdhury et al., 1994). The permanent changes emphasize the importance of the right measures for the relief of pain and for consideration being given to enzyme replacement therapy to facilitate digestion. Clinicians must function in these complications against the backdrop of individualized patient care, as pancreatitis is heterogeneous and complicated in nature. Investigation into the pathophysiology involving calcification and fibrosis has continued, with hopes for the identification of therapeutic targets, and this may hold the key to improved treatment options within this disorder of multifaceted nature (Bornman et al., 2010).

4.2.2. Symptoms and Diagnosis

Symptom awareness of chronic pancreatitis is important for early detection and management. Patients typically present with recurrent abdominal pain, predominantly epigastric in origin, that is stimulated by food intake or alcohol consumption. Pain often affects the patient's quality of life, such that it becomes difficult to carry out activities of daily living and results in significant psychological upset. With the progress of the disease, individuals may develop malabsorption, which results in weight loss and insufficiency of nutrients due to the loss of exocrine pancreatic function. In addition, complications occurring in later stages can lead to diabetes mellitus due to the impaired insulin secretion, thereby demonstrating the complex nature of symptoms of chronic pancreatitis and their impact on general health and quality of life (Bornman et al., 2010). Chronic pancreatitis diagnosis is a multi-dimensional process that involves the integration of clinical evaluation and high-end imaging. The detailed history and physical examination by the clinician set the proceedings in motion, aiming at symptomatology and etiological factors such as alcohol. Imaging technologies such as magnetic resonance cholangiopancreatography (MRCP), endoscopic ultrasound (EUS), and computed tomography (CT) play critical roles in making a diagnosis. Amongst them, MRCP is particularly useful in that it enables high specificity in visualizing pancreatic morphology and ductal anatomy so that changes corresponding to chronic pancreatitis can be identified by clinicians (Dinesh, 2013). As imaging technology advances, the accuracy of chronic pancreatitis diagnosis improves with time, allowing for earlier intervention and improved patient outcomes. Despite advances in diagnostic modalities, disparities still persist in clinical guidelines due to the heterogeneity of chronic pancreatitis. The diagnostic strategy recommended often utilizes both imaging and function tests, such as pancreatic function tests, to ascertain the extent of pancreatic damage and dysfunction. Clinical practice varies widely across regions depending on the prevalence of disease and the availability of diagnostic centers. For instance, in South Africa, cases of alcohol dominate and tailored recommendations emphasize the importance of the local settings in diagnosis and management strategies (Bornman et al., 2010). Consequently, the supply of up-to-date knowledge and resources to doctors remains central to enhancing the quality of care in patients with chronic pancreatitis (Figure 4.6).

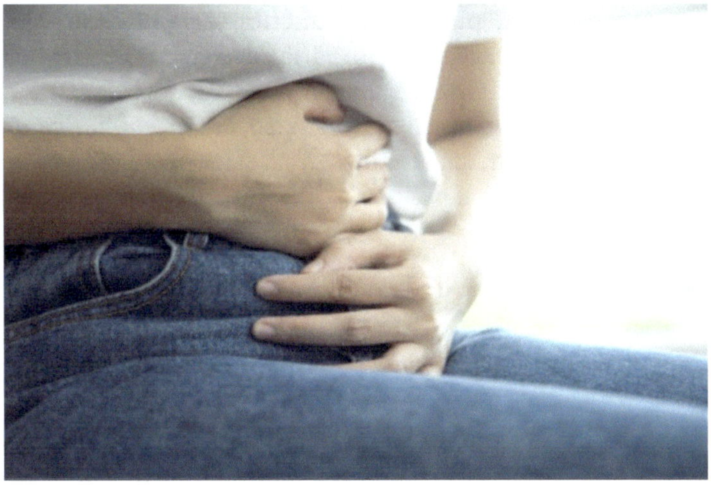

Figure 4.6. Pancreatitis: Signs and symptoms.

Source: https://encrypted-tbn3.gstatic.com/images?q=tbn:ANd9GcR--dU-hJGbghUznVaX97hOKGhkJq9pDsx8VLpd6BXRcragRq17.

4.2.3. Impact on Pancreatic Function

The impact of chronic pancreatitis on the function of the pancreas is dramatic, with the ongoing inflammatory process increasingly disrupting the structure of the pancreas. Pancreatic tissue in such a condition is increasingly substituted by fibrotic tissue, which impairs the organ's ability to secrete essential digestive enzymes and hormones. Such impairment is a regular cause of exocrine pancreatic insufficiency, with malabsorption of nutrients, loss of weight, and diarrhea. In addition, the destruction of the insulin-secreting beta cells can lead to diabetes, further complicating the clinical management of the patients. Patients with progressive disease can have greater distress and decreased quality of life due to nutritional deficits and metabolic abnormalities. Therefore, understanding how chronic pancreatitis alters pancreatic function is crucial to designing targeted therapeutic interventions to reverse these effects and improve patient outcomes (Abu-El-Haija et al., 2018; Parhiala et al., 2023). Furthermore, the association between osteoporosis, sarcopenia and chronic pancreatitis highlights the general effect on overall health and well-being. Exocrine pancreatic insufficiency patients are prone to malabsorption of nutrients, leading to deficiencies in vitamin D and calcium, which are essential for maintaining bone density. The morphological changes in the pancreatic tissue with progressive fibrotic scarring can impair the organ's ability to perform its regulatory functions, thus leading to metabolic imbalances. Sarcopenia, represented by loss of muscle strength and mass, can exacerbate the complications of nutrient absorption and physical function in such patients. Therefore, active management strategies through nutritional supplementation and close observation are needed to control such complications and improve the health conditions of chronic pancreatitis patients (Abu-El-Haija et al., 2018; Parhiala et al., 2023). Apart from exocrine and endocrine derangements, chronic pancreatitis tends to induce profound changes in pain patterns and control. The chronic pain in the abdomen experienced by the majority of patients, which is typically due to nerve damage and changes in the pancreatic tissue, becomes a point of emphasis in their therapy. Effective control of pain is necessary because, without it, pain can profoundly reduce the quality of life and impede the effectiveness of diet and medical treatments. The relationship between pancreatic function and chronic pain further defines the clinical presentation, with the development of potential cycles of weight loss and malnutrition as patients avoid alimentation due to anticipated discomfort. New treatments and pain management should not only focus on the relief of symptoms but also on the enhancement of recovery of the function of the pancreas and the general quality of life in patients (Abu-El-Haija et al., 2018; Parhiala et al., 2023) (Figure 4.7).

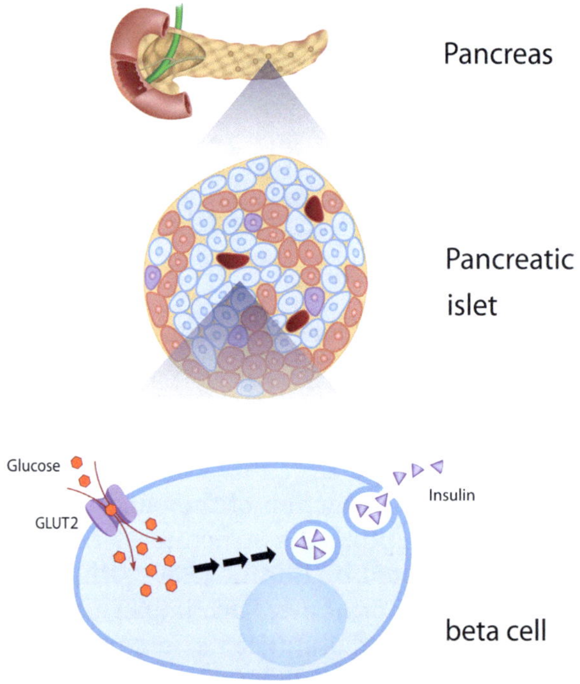

Figure 4.7. Insulin-producing beta cells.

Source: https://cfcdn.aerzteblatt.de/bilder/2019/07/img140084474.jpg.

4.3. Calcification in Chronic Pancreatitis

Calcification of chronic pancreatitis is a serious pathological feature that arises as a consequence of longstanding inflammation and injury to the pancreas. Pancreatic tissue ultimately develops necrosis and fibrosis, leading to calcified deposits in the gland. The calcifications can compromise normal pancreatic function and are typically associated with aggravated symptoms, particularly abdominal pain and malabsorption. The presence of calcium deposits is frequently related to the severity of the disease, which indicates ongoing cellular damage and inflammatory processes. Studies have confirmed that calcification can be exacerbated by nutritional aspects, such as malnutrition and some toxicities, underlining the etiological and pathogenic complexity of chronic pancreatitis, as in the case of tropical calcific pancreatitis, where pancreatic injury is critically mediated by malnutrition (Chowdhury et al., 1994). Furthermore, the calcification-induced structural alterations of the pancreas result in irreversible derangements of exocrine and endocrine functions, ultimately giving way to impaired hormone production and digestive enzyme secretion. Endocrine complications, such as diabetes mellitus, characteristically arise in patients with advanced disease due to loss of insulin-secreting beta cells. This is more common in fibrocalculous pancreatic diabetes, which one comes across often in the tropics, showing the wide range of presentation and complications of calcification of the pancreas (Chowdhury et al., 1994). Addressing these functions is crucial in the treatment of patient's health, as they are complaining of a decreased quality of life due to pain and metabolic imbalances, which require extensive treatment strategies that involve both pain management and enzyme substitution therapy. Imaging plays a pivotal role in diagnosing and assessing calcification of the pancreas. Techniques such as MRCP have become fore-frontal owing to their ability to delineate pancreatic morphology as well as identify calcifications with high specificity. Clinical experience has demonstrated MRCP to be superior to other imaging modalities, such as CT, in the demonstration of glandular structural change. Successful imaging is key to directing treatment strategies, particularly when chronic pancreatitis is complicated by obstructive complications that include calcifications. In short, mechanisms of calcification in chronic pancreatitis must be understood to allow early intervention and targeted treatment, with the ultimate long-term goal of preserving pancreatic function and enhancing patient outcomes despite this difficult disorder (Figure 4.8).

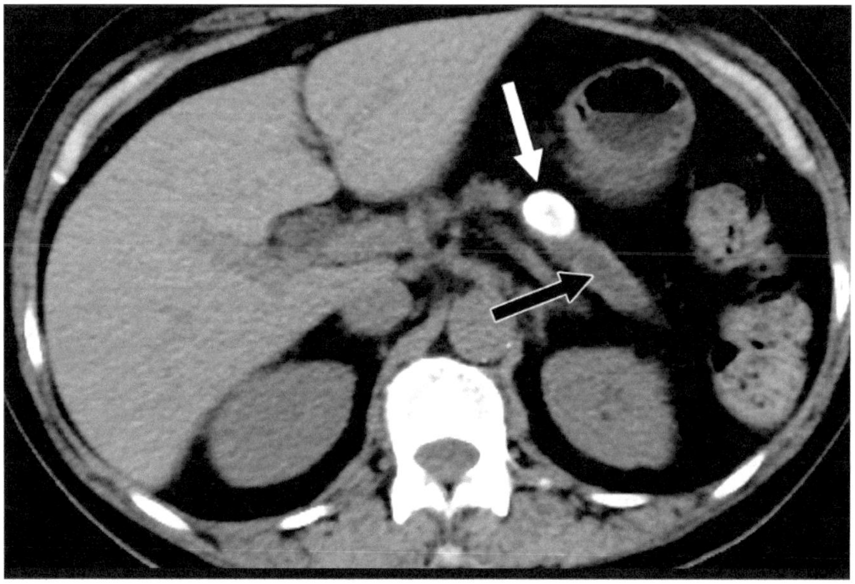

Figure 4.8. Pancreatic calcifications and calcified pancreatic masses.

Source: https://www.ajronline.org/cms/10.2214/AJR.17.17862/asset/images/large/07_17_17862_14.jpeg.

4.3.1. Mechanism of Calcification

The mechanism of calcification in chronic pancreatitis is a multifactorial process caused by recurrent pancreatitis and inflammation within the pancreas. Obstruction of the pancreatic duct in the early stages of the disease serves to accumulate digestive enzymes within the pancreas to digest pancreatic tissue. The process of digestion can cause necrosis and inflammation, ultimately resulting in calcium salt deposition. Over time, these deposits calcify through dystrophic calcification in the presence of normal serum calcium. Pathological calcification is the transformation of necrotic tissue into calcified substances, and this goes a long way to impair pancreatic function and cause complications like fibrosis and pain syndromes. Hence, enjoyment of this calcification process plays a central role in the management of the late stages of chronic pancreatitis and dealing with its debilitating consequences, including digestive deficiency and diabetes (Chowdhury et al., 1994; Dinesh, 2013). Moreover, the role of micronutrient shortages, particularly for tropical calcific pancreatitis, cannot be overstated. In risk areas of malnutrition, inadequate intake of essential nutrients like zinc, copper, and selenium can potentially exacerbate pancreatic injury and contribute to calcification. These deficiencies can potentially augment oxidative stress, leading to increased inflammation and additional tissue damage in the pancreas. As quoted evidence reveals, the interaction of malnutrition with environmental toxins, such as cyanogenic substances in certain diets, complicates the process (Chowdhury et al., 1994). The summation of such factors not only leads to structural changes in the pancreas through calcification but also produces sideropenic anemia and impaired glucose metabolism, aggravating the complication spectrum in chronic pancreatitis. Therefore, it is crucial that one should investigate the roles of nutrition factors as well as environmental factors while interpreting the mechanisms of calcification in such patients (Dinesh, 2013). Finally, calcification of the pancreas itself is crucial to pain management strategies as well as patient outcomes, generally in chronic pancreatitis. Calcified masses can be a contributor to the formation of strictures and pseudocysts, complicating further pancreatitis and causing persistent abdominal pain. Pain management strategies will then need to have an elaborate treatment plan with both medical and surgical as well as adjuvant therapies (Dinesh, 2013). Surgery, such as the Puestow procedure or Frey's procedure, may be warranted to decompress obstructing symptoms due to calcification. The challenge is then to be able to achieve adequate pain relief along with treatment of the underlying pathology of fibrosis and calcification. As imaging methods develop, which further our knowledge regarding pancreatitis evolution and calcifications behavior, clinicians can better individualize interventions, thus ultimately improving patients' quality of life in this chronic disease (Chowdhury et al., 1994) (Figure 4.9).

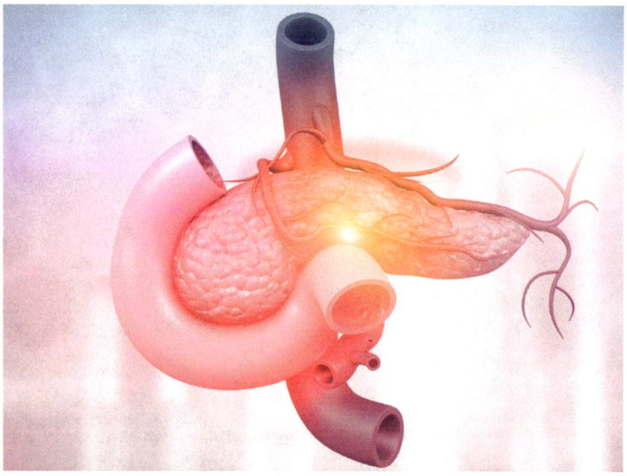

Figure 4.9. Protects acinar and ductal functions, and prevents the progression of chronic pancreatitis (CP).

Source: https://www.bioworld.com/ext/resources/Stock-images/Therapeutic-topics/Endocrine/Pancreas1.jpg?1712602217.

4.3.2. Diagnostic Imaging Techniques

Diagnosis and management of chronic pancreatitis demand the use of sensitive imaging modalities, which are essential to show structural and functional derangements of the illness. Among the widely used imaging techniques, abdominal ultrasonography, CT, and magnetic resonance imaging (MRI) stand out for their ability to create good images of the pancreas and surrounding structures. Abdominal ultrasound is often the initial imaging technique used due to its non-invasive nature and ready availability, and it may also be employed to assess pancreatic size and any potential cysts or calcifications that are suggestive of chronic pancreatitis. However, its failure to image deeper structures implies a requirement for supplementary imaging methods to confirm diagnoses and guide treatment in cases of suspected or confirmed pancreatitis, as recently noted in clinical controversy regarding the management of the disease (Stecca et al., 2023). Computed tomography is the gold standard for imaging of the gastrointestinal tract, greatly cherished for its superior sensitivity in detecting pancreatic architectural alterations, such as calcifications, ductal disturbances, and fibrosis typically seen in chronic pancreatitis. Computed tomography provides a cross-sectional view that allows the clinician to assess not just the pancreas but also the adjacent structures and complications, which may significantly influence the management of the patient. The advent of multidetector CT scanners has also further expanded the diagnostic capability, with rapid and extensive imaging that is helpful for identifying acute exacerbations to be identified quickly. Moreover, technical improvement in CT can diagnose chronic pancreatitis and pancreatic carcinoma, which are highly difficult to differentiate due to their identical presentations. These distinctions are significant since clinical nuances of pancreatitis progression were intended to provide meaning by ongoing studies (Yadav et al., 2018). Magnetic resonance imaging represents another useful diagnostic tool to include in the chronic pancreatitis arsenal when conventional modalities yield unclear findings. Offering increased soft tissue contrast, MRI is optimally equipped to illustrate the inflammatory changes and fibrosis characteristic of chronic pancreatitis. MRCP, specifically planned for pancreatic duct imaging, plays an important role in the evaluation of ductal anatomy and obstruction that may worsen symptoms. MRCP is non-invasive and significantly reduces patient exposure to ionizing radiation, an important consideration in the chronic disease state where serial imaging may be necessary. The information acquired using these imaging modalities is vital not only for the proper diagnosis but also for planning overall treatment plans from pain management to potential surgery, because the information about chronic pancreatitis evolves day by day with clinical experience and research (Stecca et al., 2023).

4.3.3. Clinical Implications of Calcification

The development of calcification in chronic pancreatitis is a significant clinical problem, as it typically represents a shift in pancreatic pathology and can adversely affect functional ability. Pancreatic calcifications are likely to be signs of a chronic inflammatory reaction that leads to insidiously progressive tissue loss. This pathologic change could complicate the management of patients because calcified pancreas tissue may cause obstructive phenomena or be implicated in the development of pancreatic exocrine insufficiency. These are complications that necessitate reconsideration of therapeutic strategies, such as pain management and enzyme replacement therapy. Understanding the clinical implications of calcifications is crucial in planning effective treatment strategies that consider both the structural and functional effects of chronic pancreatic disease. Moreover, calcification not only reflects the severity of the disease but is also predictive of progression to fibrosis. Fibrosis is an extremely useful prognostic factor in chronic pancreatitis patients, and calcified areas usually evolve into fibrotic lesions. Not only does this fibrotic transformation increase the risk of pancreatic cancer formation, but it also damages the organ's secretory function for digestive enzymes. The interaction among calcification, inflammation, and fibrosis points to the importance of close monitoring and timely management designed to counteract these changes. As indicated in research, the treatment of chronic pancreatitis should not only target symptoms but, more importantly, the involved pathophysiological pathways to calcification and related fibrosis, thus enhancing general patient outcomes (Mignogna, 2025). Further, research into therapeutic agents that have the ability to modulate calcification pathways is required to enhance patient treatment. For instance, particular drugs have been shown to be effective in altering the differentiation of monocytes to calcifying phenotypes and thereby indirectly alter calcification development in pancreatic tissue. These findings suggest that pharmacologic interventions, such as GLP-1 receptor agonists, could be beneficial in preventing vascular complications of chronic pancreatitis, particularly in diabetic patients at high risk for cardiovascular disease due to calcification (Etemad et al., 2005). Therefore, understanding the clinical relevance of calcification not only aids in the treatment of chronic pancreatitis but also offers promise for new therapies based on the biochemistry of this incapacitating disease (Figure 4.10).

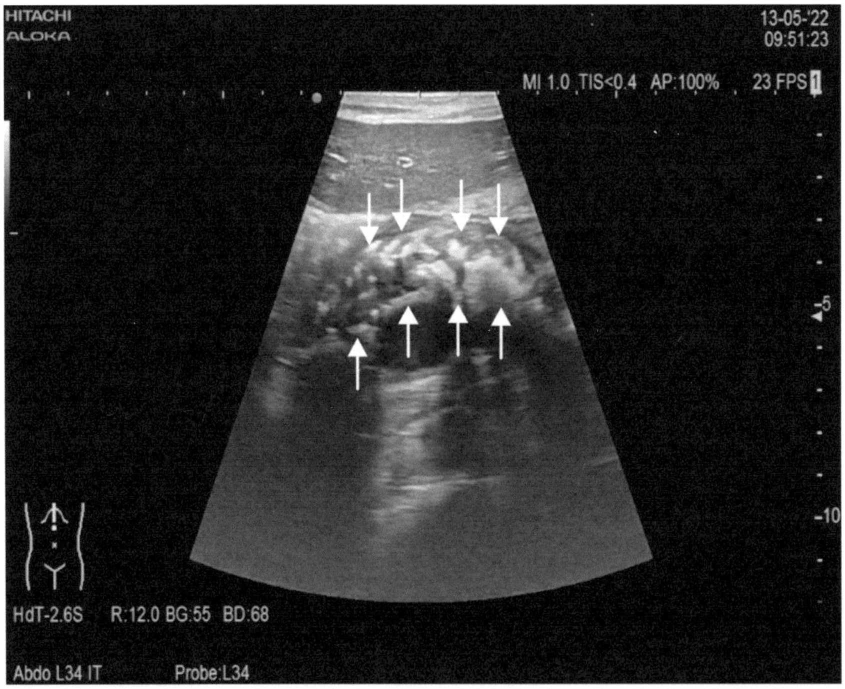

Figure 4.10. Pancreatic calcifications and pseudocyst revealed on a scan. White arrows: extensive pancreatic calcifications and pseudocysts.

Source: Marginean CM, Popescu M, Vasile CM, Stanciu M, Popescu IA, Biciusca V, Ciobanu D, Dobrescu A, Sandulescu LD, Bondari S, et al. Chronic Calcifying Pancreatitis Associated with Secondary Diabetes Mellitus and Hepatosplenic Abscesses in a Young Male Patient: A Case Report. *Gastroenterology Insights*. 2022; 13(3):305-312. https://doi.org/10.3390/gastroent13030031

4.4. Fibrosis and Its Consequences

The development of chronic pancreatitis usually culminates in the development of fibrosis, an unhealthy state in which normal pancreas tissue is replaced by fibrotic tissue. Fibrosis is a consequence of ongoing inflammation and cellular damage, leading to the irreversible morphological changes characteristic of chronic pancreatitis. It is not a matter of merely a reactive process to tissue injury, but forms a vicious circle of more inflammation and pain. The variability of fibrotic responses can significantly impair the exocrine and endocrine function of the pancreas, thereby aggravating the overall clinical picture of the disease. For example, fibrosis can cause pancreatic insufficiency, causing malabsorption and diabetes mellitus, which need assiduously managed interventions to restore the quality of life for patients and alleviate distress associated with these complications (Bornman et al., 2010). It is important to respect the interaction between fibrosis and pancreatitis because it highlights the multifactorial nature of pain management in such individuals. Abdominal pain, one of the features of chronic pancreatitis, can be exacerbated by entrapment of the pancreas and nerves by fibrosis (Prabu et al., 2011).

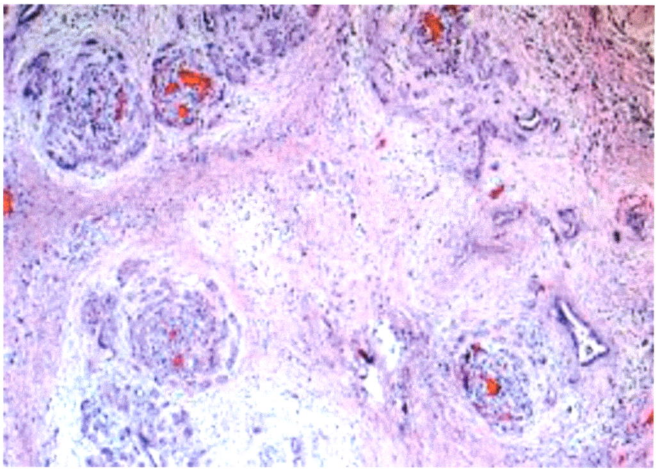

Figure 4.11. The fibrosis of chronic pancreatitis (CP).

Source: https://www.liebertpub.com/cms/10.1089/ars.2011.4079/asset/images/large/figure1.jpeg.

This recurrent and complex pain ultimately necessitates a thorough evaluation of pain management modalities, including both drug therapy and surgery. The subjectiveness of pain in this context of fibrosis stems from the requirement to tailor therapies to the patient's reaction and the etiology of their chronic pancreatitis. Physicians must pay particular attention to the interplay between fibrosis and pain sensation since both play an important role in determining a patient's treatment regimen and course of recovery. Apart from pain treatment, the presence of fibrosis also complicates matters in the form of nutritional support and enzyme replacement therapy. As the fibrotic tissue disrupts the normal functioning of the pancreas, patients usually develop exocrine deficiency, leading to malnutrition and impaired digestion. Enzyme replacement therapy becomes indicated; nevertheless, such therapy can be highly variable with respect to the degree of fibrosis. Individualized dosing regimens and ongoing adjustments according to clinical status and nutritional needs may be required in patients. Moreover, fibrosis interaction with nutrition management points to the necessity of providing treatment for chronic pancreatitis by a multidisciplinary team of gastroenterologists, dietitians, and pain specialists in an attempt to comprehensively address the multiple requirements of affected individuals (Bornman et al., 2010). Such interaction is pivotal in offering maximal outcomes under the multi-faceted challenges posed by fibrosis and its various repercussions (Figure 4.11).

4.4.1. Role of Fibrosis in Disease Progression

Fibrosis is a central process in the development of chronic pancreatitis, fundamentally altering the structure and function of pancreatic tissue. Recurrent inflammation in chronic pancreatitis leads to the deposition of extracellular matrix components, primarily collagen, that progressively replace normal pancreatic parenchyma. This fibrotic transformation results in the loss of both exocrine and endocrine functions, clinically presented as malabsorption and diabetes. The fibrotic process is not a passive consequence of damage but plays an active role in the disease process. Studies indicate that chronic inflammation is responsible for stimulating fibroblast activation, which leads to fibrosis and exacerbates pancreatic dysfunction, highlighting the urgent necessity for selective therapies targeting fibrosis modulation in the management of chronic pancreatitis (Chowdhury et al., 1994). Aside from its functional role, fibrosis in chronic pancreatitis has a direct correlation with the development of calcifications in the pancreas. Calcifications, often found by imaging techniques, are irreversible damage and are associated with an increased level of disease. Pancreatic stone creation may be a consequence of calcium deposits within the fibrotic tissue, i.e., within the stenotic ductal structures. When fibrosis progresses, fibrosis-induced ductal obstruction raises intra-ductal pressure and establishes a calcification-preferred microenvironment. This interaction not only makes managing the pain harder but can also be one of the factors that compel one to carry out more invasive procedures, once more rendering the recognition of an understanding of the fibrotic process in disease progression more crucial (Chowdhury et al., 1994). Fibrosis control is most important in chronic pancreatitis because it has a direct impact on the quality of life and long-term outcomes in the diseased patient. Pain control is particularly challenging with fibrosis because standard analgesic measures can be ineffective in the setting of pathologic changes. Fibrosis can produce an exaggerated sensitivity of pancreatic nerves to result in an increased perception of pain by patients. The current understanding of fibrogenesis offers promising therapeutic strategies, including antifibrotic therapy that can stop or even reverse pathologic remodeling. With further development in research, clinicians are advocating to adopt a multidisciplinary strategy for managing chronic pancreatitis, both symptomatically as well as addressing the fibrotic component to improve outcomes and quality of life (Bornman et al., 2010).

4.4.2. Histological Changes in the Pancreas

The histological changes within the pancreas resulting from chronic pancreatitis are both widespread and multifaceted. To begin with, inflammation triggers immune cell infiltration into the pancreatic parenchyma consisting of most frequently lymphocytes and macrophages. Infiltration is a continuous inflammatory process that disrupts normal pancreatic tissue architecture. Later on, repeated inflammatory attacks induce necrosis and fibrosis, where fibrous tissue replaces normal pancreatic cells to result in a general decline in exocrine and endocrine function. Acinar architecture is lost, which is crucial for the synthesis of enzymes, thus impairing digestion and metabolic control. Curiously, these changes set the stage for potential complications in the form of pancreatic insufficiency and diabetes mellitus, a reflection of the clinical significance of the histopathologic processes taking place in chronic pancreatitis, especially in the alcoholic setting, as stressed by Chowdhury et al. (1994). Chronic inflammation also leads to the formation of calcifications within the pancreatic tissue, a feature typical of chronic pancreatitis. These calcifications, typically initially identifiable on imaging modalities, are precipitated proteins and mineral deposits that have accumulated during the disease process. Microscopically, they can be identified with necrotic tissue and fibrosis, contributing to the overall desolation of pancreatic function. Tropical calcific pancreatitis, as reported by Chowdhury et al. (1994), involves a particular form of calcification, predominantly in children and young adults. These calcifications may lead to subsequent complications in the form of chronic pain and profoundly affect the quality of life. The chronic pain induced by these changes is a direct result of nerve involvement and the inflammatory environment, emphasizing the importance of appreciating these histological changes for effective pain management interventions. With more advanced levels of chronic pancreatitis, continuous fibrosis causes more widespread structural changes like islet cell damage that compromises insulin production. The direct correlation between histologic alterations and clinical symptoms becomes evident, as the integrity of both the exocrine and endocrine spaces is lost, patients may experience evidence of malabsorption and diabetes. Pancreatic architecture is changed, with strands of fibrosis demarcating areas of necrosis, ultimately taking on a calcified quality in imaging. Clinical practice guidelines identify the necessity of comprehensive management approaches that include these complications, as described in Bornman et al. (2010). The identification of pancreatic histological changes, therefore, not only aids the diagnosis of chronic pancreatitis but also personalization of successful pain relief and enzyme supplementation therapy capable of reversing the impact of pancreatic insufficiency (Figure 4.12).

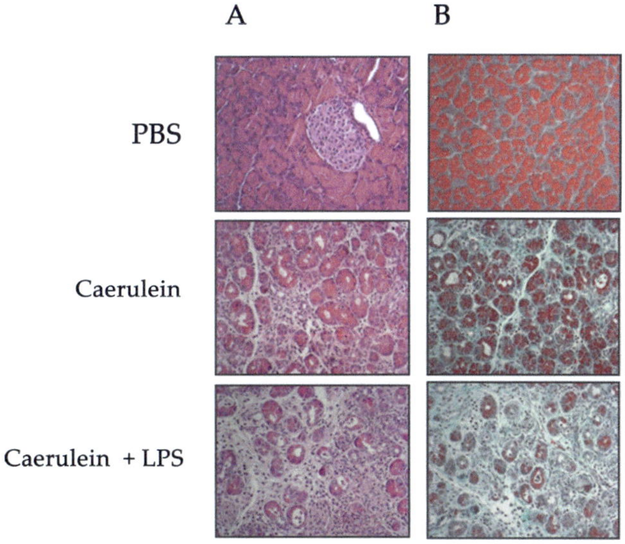

Figure 4.12. Histological changes of pancreatic tissue architecture after repetitive caerulein and combined caerulein-lipopolysaccharide (LPS) injections.

Source: Aghdassi, A.A., Mayerle, J., Christochowitz, S. et al. Animal models for investigating chronic pancreatitis. Fibrogenesis Tissue Repair 4, 26 (2011). https://doi.org/10.1186/1755-1536-4-26

4.4.3. Effects on Digestive Health

Chronic pancreatitis significantly alters gastrointestinal health by impairing the function of the pancreas to carry out its important exocrine roles. The inflammatory process accompanying this condition leads to endocrine and exocrine tissue destruction, which could ultimately lead to pancreatic insufficiency. Malabsorption of nutrients, weight loss, and nutritional deficiency are the typical presentations among chronic pancreatitis patients. This malabsorption may be observed as steatorrhea, with undigested fats in the stool indicating impaired digestive enzyme production. These gastrointestinal complications, if left unmanaged, can severely affect the quality of life, and medical interventions would be required to restore the optimal condition for digestion. Therefore, recognizing the relationship between digestive health and chronic pancreatitis is significant in developing effective therapeutic interventions for symptoms and nutritional care in affected patients (Prabu et al., 2011). Replacement enzyme therapy (ERT) is a critical treatment for patients with the digestive symptoms of chronic pancreatitis. While the disease progresses, the pancreas does not produce sufficient digestive enzymes, which subsequently results in the above malabsorption and complications. ERT attempts to replace the deficient enzymes so that better breakdown and assimilation of the nutrients by the intestine can be achieved. Not only does the treatment reverse steatorrhea, but it is also likely to enhance the overall nutritional intake and thus the nutritional status of the patient. Moreover, initiation of ERT early on guarantees better weight loss control and the avoidance of complications of malnutrition, ultimately increasing the patient's quality of life. These interventions stress the importance of a comprehensive approach to the management of chronic pancreatitis, particularly its adverse effects on gastrointestinal health (Bornman et al., 2010). In addition to enzyme replacement, dietary modifications are also crucial in the treatment of the digestive condition of chronic pancreatitis patients. A customized diet emphasizing low-fat intake can also prevent malabsorption symptoms and minimize gastrointestinal discomfort initiated by the disease. It is of critical significance that the patients collaborate closely with the medical team to develop a well-balanced diet regimen that can address their individual nutritional requirements and decrease the pancreas's workload. It is a multidisciplinary program involving not only dietary consultation but psychology as well, as it takes into account the psychological burden that chronic pancreatitis can impart on a person. These nutritional strategies, alongside enzyme replacement therapy, constitute a comprehensive treatment regimen that restores gastrointestinal function and promotes general well-being in patients with chronic pancreatitis. Therefore, active management of nutrition plays a crucial role in addressing the complex gastrointestinal challenges that come with this chronic disease (Prabu et al., 2011).

4.5. Pain Management Strategies

Effective pain control is a vital component of CP management, given the disease's infamous history of inducing crippling pain. A variety of therapeutic measures exists, ranging from pharmacologic intervention to lifestyle modification. Analgesics in the form of non-opioid drugs such as acetaminophen and nonsteroidal anti-inflammatory drugs (NSAIDs) are typically the initial steps in treating pancreatic pain. However, in extreme situations, opioids are indicated due to their ability to manage acute pain spells. Chronic use necessitates close monitoring to minimize the risk of dependence, particularly in populations with a high prevalence of alcohol-induced CP substance use disorders. Pain management strategies need explanation because, in the absence of accurate clinical practice guidelines, there is a need for a multidisciplinary treatment strategy, combining medical management and counseling psychology for optimal patient outcomes in CP (Bornman et al., 2010).

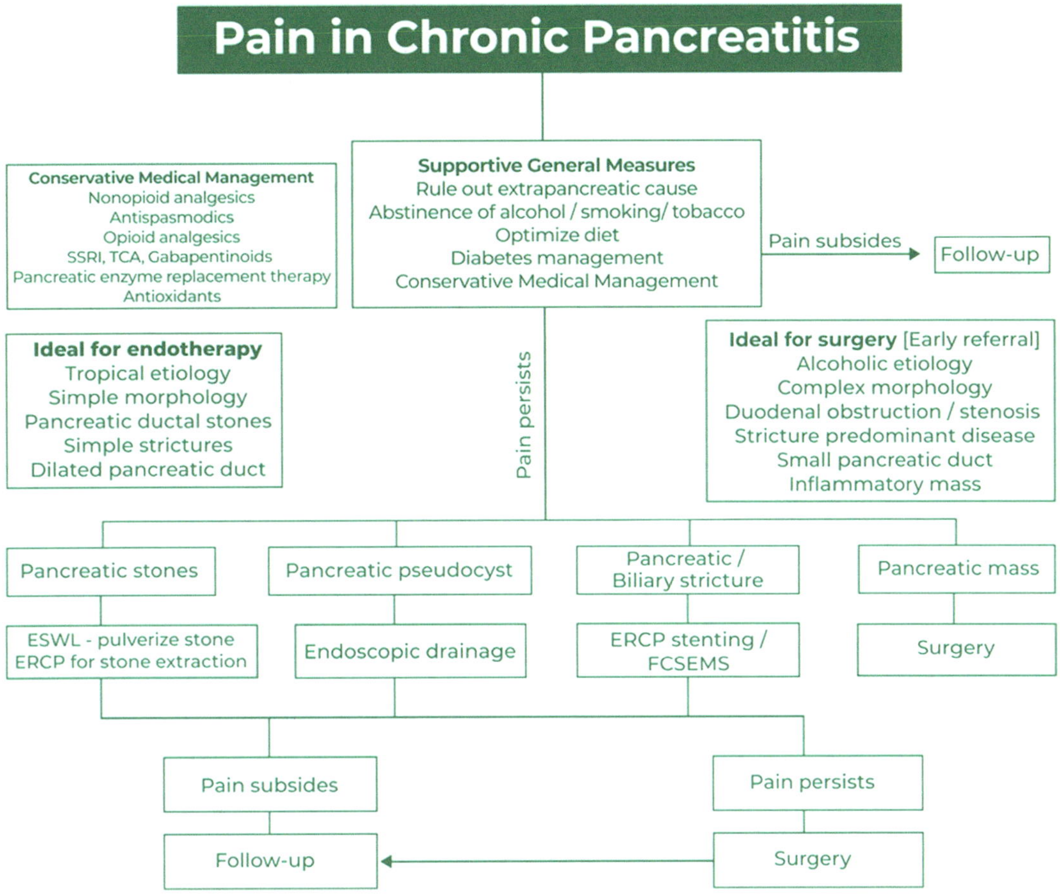

Figure 4.13. Pain in chronic pancreatitis.

Source: https://www.researchgate.net/publication/373951502/figure/fig1/AS:11431281204409070@1699759115111/Algorithm-for-management-of-pain-in-chronic-pancreatitis.png.

The addition of non-pharmacological interventions can complement the overall pain management plan for the patient with chronic pancreatitis. Non-pharmacological interventions are usually in the form of dietary modification, physical therapy, and cognitive-behavioral therapy (CBT), which have been promising for relief against chronic pain. Dietary modification is able to reduce pancreatic stress and may be complemented with low-fat diets that minimize the likelihood of exacerbating symptoms of pain. Physiotherapy can illustrate increasing mobility and pain reduction exercises, which enable patients to live an improved quality of life. CBT also equips patients with coping mechanisms for confronting the psychological effects of chronic pain, hence reducing perceived pain severity. The multifaceted nature of pain in CP emphasizes the use of an interrelated treatment plan incorporating conventional medical interventions and support systems (Bonariol et al., 2022). Interventional developments also provide reasonable alternatives for the treatment of chronic abdominal pain in CP patients. Endoscopic treatments, such as endoscopic retrograde cholangiopancreatography (ERCP), can help alleviate symptoms by treating complications, such as strictures and stones, which can exacerbate pain. Also, surgical options such as pancreatic resection may be explored in recalcitrant cases. The selected intervention needs to be individualized and performed based on an individual patient's specific anatomical and clinical condition, with special attention given to proper preoperative assessment. Coordination between gastroenterologists, pain specialists, and surgeons is needed to ensure that the chosen method aligns with both pain mitigation and control of the primary disease process. This integrative approach not only enhances pain management but also serves to improve the quality of life of patients (Bornman et al., 2010) (Figure 4.13).

4.5.1. Pharmacological Approaches

Pharmacologic management of CP is multifaceted, addressing both the symptomatic and pathologic manifestations of the illness. Control of chronic pain, a frequent and debilitating complaint voiced by the patient, is one of the fundamental elements of management. Therapy with NSAIDs and opioids is routine but must be employed cautiously with respect to side effects and addiction. Moreover, novel evidence underscores the application of adjuvant drugs, such as gabapentinoids or lidocaine patches, which can provide additive pain relief by targeting mechanisms of nerve pain. The selection of suitable pharmacological drugs is often patient-related and influenced by disease severity and patient tolerance to analgesic medication, necessitating an individualized approach in an attempt to maximize efficacy while minimizing risks. Besides pain management, pancreatic enzyme replacement therapy (PERT) is also crucial in managing maldigestion due to exocrine pancreatic insufficiency, a common complication of CP. Patients with this condition usually present with gastrointestinal symptoms, deteriorating nutritional and overall health status. PERT is responsible for replacing the deficient enzymes, allowing for fat, carbohydrate, and protein digestion, thus improving nutrient absorption and quality of life.

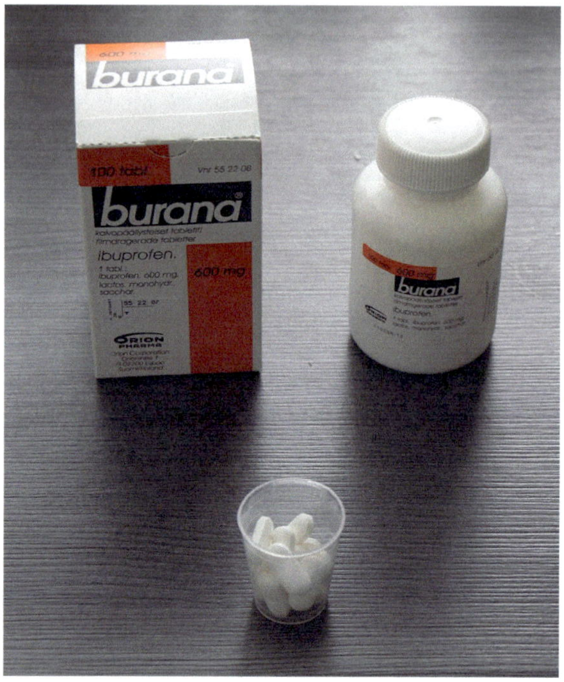

Figure 4.14. Pharmaceutical developments for chronic pancreatitis.

Source: By Styroks - Own work, CC BY-SA 4.0, https://commons.wikimedia.org/w/index.php?curid=79179911

The production of these enzymes has also become better, with enteric-coated preparations becoming the standard to ensure efficacy in the gut. Satisfactory responders to PERT may experience alleviation of symptoms and improvement in nutritional status, further highlighting the need for addressing enzyme deficiency, as well as pain, in a comprehensive treatment regimen for CP (Persano et al., 2023). Another pharmacologic management involves the treatment of inflammatory processes observed in chronic pancreatitis. Glucocorticoid therapy has been proposed in some cases to inhibit inflammation, though one must be careful in the use of these medications due to potential side effects. Additional research also shows that manipulation of gut microbiota by probiotics can be beneficial in lowering inflammation as well as enhancing overall pancreatic function. Current overviews suggest that early intervention with pharmacological interventions may shift the course of the disease and decrease the risk of complications like pancreatic calcification and fibrosis (Bonariol et al., 2022). With our increasing knowledge of CP, integration of specific pharmacological therapies can optimize disease control and patient outcomes, highlighting the complexity of therapy in chronic pancreatitis (Figure 4.14).

4.5.2. Non-Pharmacological Interventions

In managing the intricacies of chronic pancreatitis, the application of non-pharmacologic interventions takes center stage in symptom management and enhancing patients' quality of life. The interventions promote dietary management and lifestyle changes, which can reduce the debilitating nature of the disease. Nutritional therapy is of key importance, given that most of the patients suffer from malabsorption as a result of pancreatic insufficiency. An individualized diet with quality protein and sufficient caloric supply can possibly alleviate symptoms of malnutrition and support weight gain. Secondly, the importance of incorporating individualized meal planning based on the patient's diversified tolerance cannot be overemphasized. These dietary recommendations can potentially enhance the process of digestion and overall well-being and serve as a required foundation for comprehensive care in the treatment of chronic pancreatitis, as emphasized in the current literature on nutrition and diet in pancreatic disease (Persano et al., 2023).

Another vital non-drug measure relates to addressing the lifestyle factors contributing to the progression of chronic pancreatitis. Cigarette smoking and alcohol use reduction are particularly important since they are two of the largest risk factors for inducing pancreatic injury and inflammation. Such education is of utmost importance to empower the patient to make good decisions in their own health care. Healthcare provider facilitation, as well as the integration of, smoking cessation programs can help facilitate this process. Furthermore, physical activity is encouraged through active participation because physical activity is able to help with weight control and maximize metabolic processes. Facilitation of sustainable behavior through health professional support is able to encourage proactive living in the management of chronic pancreatitis and maximize clinical outcomes, as supported by integrated care standards (Bonariol et al., 2022). Finally, psychological counseling is usually overlooked but is crucial when dealing with chronic pancreatitis. The psychological burden of the emotional and physical challenges of the disease can lead to depression, anxiety, and decreased quality of life. Non-pharmacological interventions such as cognitive-behavioral therapy, mindfulness, and stress management techniques can help manage the condition in patients effectively. Integration of mental health interventions in the treatment plan not only allows for better control of emotions but also promotes adherence to dietary and lifestyle changes needed to control chronic pancreatitis. Clinicians in healthcare should therefore adopt an integrated approach that acknowledges the interdependence of physical and psychological well-being. Such an integrated strategy is vital for effective management and long-term wellness in patients with chronic pancreatitis, as noted in current healthcare debates (Persano et al., 2023).

4.5.3. Role of Palliative Care

Palliative care in the management of chronic pancreatitis is paramount since the disease further contributes to disabling symptoms and a significant reduction in quality of life. Palliative care has the purpose of eliminating pain and other distressing symptoms of chronic pancreatitis, including nausea, weakness, and weight loss. A major aspect of this approach is how patient-reported outcomes can be addressed so that patients are treated following what they want and need. In addition to other forms of treatment, effective palliative care not only aims to relieve physical symptoms but also to provide psychological and spiritual support such that patient management can become a more holistic experience. Early integration of palliative care into treatment protocols can dramatically improve overall patient well-being and can even lead to greater tolerance for therapy as patients accept the complexity of their disorder. Nutritional management of patients with chronic pancreatitis further emphasizes the role of palliative care. Since the disease is likely to lead to malabsorption and weight loss, healthcare professionals must enact measures that will ensure caloric intake. Interventions such as pancreatic enzyme supplementation, nutrition counseling, and administration of orexigenic medications can mitigate weight loss, ultimately maximizing patient outcomes (Hendifar et al., 2019). Palliative care places greater emphasis on the establishment of an integrated treatment plan that not only addresses physical symptoms but maximizes nutritional status. This is achieved by allowing patients to experience a quality of life less impaired, even when confronted with the many accompanying ailments of chronic pancreatitis and complications. Nutritional therapy placed as a priority achieves a significant impact on survival and overall health through palliative care. Finally, the multidisciplinary nature of palliative care in chronic pancreatitis demonstrates its efficacy when handling combined healthcare demands. Multidisciplinary care involving gastroenterologists, nurse practitioners, dietitians, and palliative care specialists is maximized for symptom control and enhanced patient satisfaction. Connecting clinics provide a valuable bridge for newly diagnosed patients through the timely provision of supportive therapy (Sreedharan et al., 2019). This model not only delivers information to patients about treatment and diagnosis but also provides a systematized support system in order to increase their quality of life. It enables proactive management of symptoms and prevention of complications, with the final outcome being a more holistic and rewarding health experience. By facilitating interdisciplinary collaboration, palliative care can become instrumental in the effective management of chronic pancreatitis.

4.6. Enzyme Replacement Therapy (ERT)

The role of ERT in the management of chronic pancreatitis is pivotal and multilateral because it is a direct response to the exocrine insufficiency caused by pancreatic damage. The therapy involves the administration of pancreatic enzymes to help the body digest food properly, an imperative that is in place when the pancreas is unable to produce enough enzymes. Chronic pancreatitis, with its consequent irreversible morphologic abnormalities frequently inducing pain and impairment, severely incapacitates digestion and absorption of nutrients (Chowdhury et al., 1994). The patients become malnourished, lose weight, and are associated with abdominal pain due to inadequate enzyme secretion. ERT is thus not only employed in alleviating these symptoms but also to maximize nutritional status in general, most importantly in healing and control of the disease. In particular, ERT is especially critical in patients with diseases such as fibrocalculous pancreatic diabetes that can arise due to chronic pancreatitis cases in conditions such as tropical calcific pancreatitis (Chowdhury et al., 1994). For such patients, enzyme replacements not only alleviate gastrointestinal manifestations but also reverse the metabolic sequelae of inadequate digestion, such as diabetes mellitus risk. The enzyme dosing is generally individualized based on the severity of the exocrine dysfunction and the patient's individual dietary requirements, illustrating the necessity of close control and professional evaluation to allow for optimal therapy. Individualization of treatment allows ERT to be significantly advantageous in enhancing the quality of life, minimizing the risk of malnutrition, and optimizing the effectiveness of overall disease management. Furthermore, ERT treatment is in line with the updated clinical practice guidelines that encourage multidisciplinary treatment of chronic pancreatitis (Bornman et al., 2010). In this case, doctors can employ the use of ERT as a component of comprehensive treatment that may include pain management and nutritional support. For example, the use of analgesics in conjunction with ERT provides a combined effect of treating both digestive enzyme deficiency and chronic pain. The combination of the approaches not only maximizes treatment efficacy but also adds evidence of the heterogeneity and complexity of chronic pancreatitis as a condition. Due to these complexities, ongoing clinical guidelines and studies will further evolve the ERTs role such that therapy continues to progress according to new evidence and patient needs, eventually enhancing clinical outcomes in this complex condition (Figure 4.15).

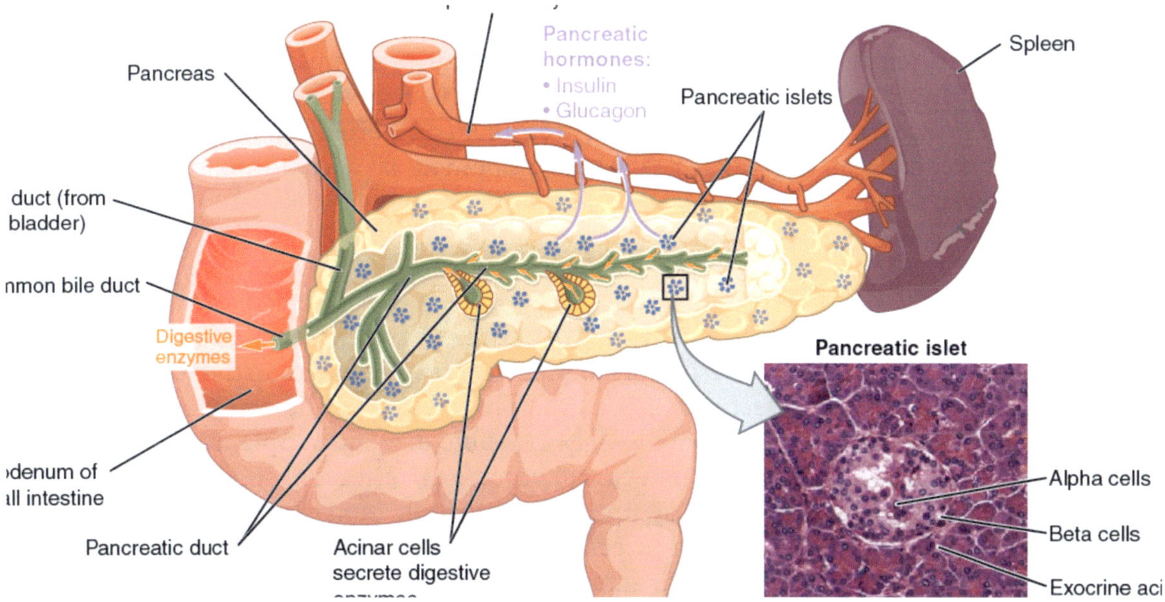

Figure 4.15. Activation of pancreatic enzymes.

Source: By OpenStax College - Anatomy & Physiology, Connexions Web site. http://cnx.org/content/col11496/1.6/, Jun 19, 2013., CC BY 3.0, https://commons.wikimedia.org/w/index.php?curid=30148155

4.6.1. Indications for Enzyme Replacement

Management of chronic pancreatitis is holistic, particularly in ERT. Patients with chronic pancreatitis experience exocrine pancreatic insufficiency in the majority of cases, with features of malabsorption of nutrients, weight loss, and steatorrhea. As the disease progresses, the pancreas becomes irreversibly morphologically damaged, leading to decreased production of digestive enzymes necessary for adequate digestion and absorption of fats and proteins. In such situations of patients with malabsorption symptoms or with abnormal fecal fat study results, ERT is subsequently an important component of the management regimen that allows enhanced nutrient absorption and quality of life. The incorporation of enzyme supplementation can greatly reduce gastrointestinal symptoms as well as reverse nutritional derangement that predominates in chronic pancreatitis (Bornman et al., 2010). The indications for enzyme replacement are particularly seen in the late stages of chronic pancreatitis, involving extensive exocrine and endocrine function loss, as explained in literature. As the process evolves, particularly when the underlying etiology is alcohol-related, the susceptibility to malnutrition increases, necessitating the use of pancreatic enzymes as a therapeutic approach. The decision to implement ERT is typically guided by clinical signs and symptoms such as abdominal pain, bloating, and weight loss, and diagnostic studies indicating poor pancreatic function. Moreover, the tailor-made delivery of enzymes can really benefit the patients in terms of relief and general nutritional status, hence placing ERT as a significant intervention at this juncture (Dinesh, 2013). Moreover, ERT should be regarded as a part of chronic pancreatitis multidisciplinary treatment. Not only is the knowledge of the physiological background of pancreatic insufficiency needed for its addition to protocols but also for the repeated monitoring of patient response to treatment. Constant monitoring through clinical evaluation and laboratory testing needs to be performed in order to modify enzyme dosing in a way that optimizes therapeutic benefit. As patients typically present with a complex array of symptoms, coordination among gastroenterologists, dietitians, and primary care physicians is critical for proper management. An integrated approach maximizes compliance with treatment in patients and facilitates long-term improvement in outcomes, making ERT a pivotal component in chronic pancreatitis treatment (Bornman et al., 2010).

4.6.2. Types of Enzyme Supplements

Enzyme supplements are now key components in the treatment of pancreatic exocrine insufficiency in chronic pancreatitis. They are primarily formulated to provide the digestive enzymes that the pancreas can no longer produce effectively due to the progression of the disease. PERT, a mixture of lipase, protease, and amylase, is the most widely available enzyme supplement. These enzymes facilitate patients to digest fats, proteins, and carbohydrates and, in turn, ensure the absorption of nutrients as well as prevent maldigestion symptoms. As chronic pancreatitis could lead to severe gastrointestinal distress and malnutrition, access to these supplements becomes imperative to maintain quality of life and nutritional health among victims (Phillips et al., 2021). The effectiveness of enzyme supplements in individuals with pancreatic insufficiency varies with a number of factors, such as enzyme type, dosage, and patient-specific requirements. Surprisingly, enteric-coated preparations are a popular choice as they protect the enzymes from gastric acid so that they get delivered at the correct site in the intestines. Additionally, some patients are supplemented with individualized enzyme regimens, particularly those whose counterparts have concomitant dietary restrictions or underlying malabsorption. Given the complexity of chronic pancreatitis, medical professionals must analyze each patient's case individually in order to provide the appropriate form and dosage of enzyme supplements in a bid to enhance their efficacy and secure positive health outcomes (Prabu et al., 2011). Lastly, patient education is the solution to the successful implementation of enzyme supplementation therapy as well. Patient awareness of proper use, potential side effects, and dietary inclusion of enzyme supplements can profoundly affect patient compliance and overall treatment success. Further, healthcare practitioners must also emphasize the necessity of monitoring and follow-ups in an overall care plan. Such a strategy not only treats the acute symptoms of maldigestion but also aids in the long-term control of chronic pancreatitis. Thus, enzyme replacement therapy is not just an option for treatment but an essential part of the overall management of chronic pancreatitis so that patients have healthier, better-balanced lifestyles (Prabu et al., 2011; Phillips et al., 2021) (Figure 4.16).

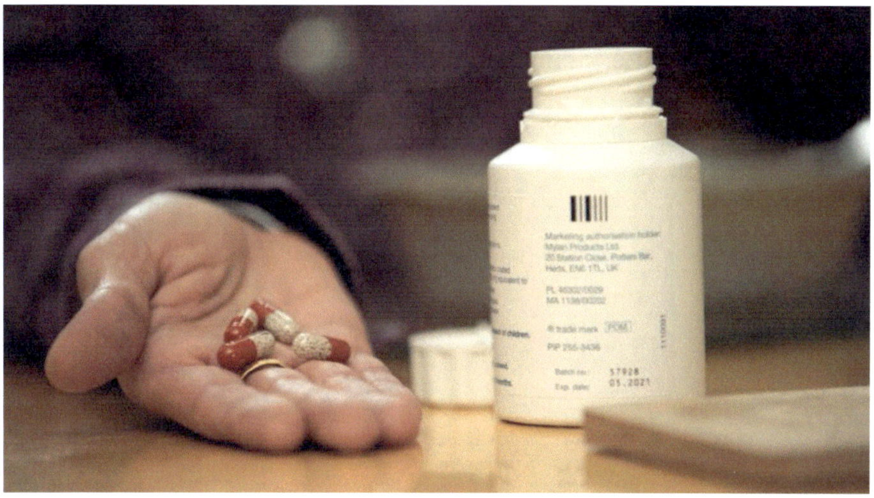

Figure 4.16. Pancreatic enzyme replacement therapy (PERT).

Source: https://external-content.duckduckgo.com/iu/?u=https%3A%2F%2Fwww.pancreaticcancer.org.uk%2Fwp-content%2Fuploads%2F2020%2F09%2FDSC04576-900x500-c-default.jpg&f=1&nofb=1&ipt=fdc11445491275b107f8c299a146b6f8754ed29e0f4879f0e16189d5c39ca333.

4.6.3. Benefits and Limitations of Therapy

In CP management, therapeutic options provide several benefits but are also discovered to possess identifiable constraints. Some of the most significant benefits of therapeutic management include pain relief and improvement in the quality of life (QoL) in instances of chronic pain associated with the disorder. Surgical interventions, while not frequently employed, have been promising to provide long-term pain reduction, decrease opiate pain medication usage, and enhance patient outcomes based on follow-up studies. This is significant, as the majority of CP patients struggle with debilitating symptoms that significantly impair their day-to-day function and overall quality of life. Successful treatment procedures, therefore, lead to a great improvement in both physical and mental health, underlining the necessity for meeting the needs of the patient as an entity. Therapy for pancreatitis is not, however, without its lacunae, which complicates the treatment aspect. One of the major limitations is the invasive nature of certain treatments, such as surgery or endoscopy, which carry high risks, including the results of complications from the treatment itself. These therapies may not be suitable for everyone, particularly those with severe comorbidities. Furthermore, heterogeneity in patients' reactions to these medications suggests that while some patients will experience significant relief, others will gain little or no benefits from similar therapies. This unpredictability highlights the importance of individual treatment modalities and careful clinical evaluation before selecting an appropriate therapeutic regimen. Moreover, adherence to conservative treatment protocols has both beneficial and harmful effects in the management of chronic pancreatitis. Non-operative therapies like nutritional support and replacement therapy with exogenous enzymes offer an avenue for optimal treatment of exocrine deficiency and improvement in gastrointestinal function without operative risk. However, these processes normally require continuous patient compliance and adjustments in lifestyle, which are challenging to ensure in the long term. More attention to patient education and follow-up support is crucial to obtain the best outcome of these therapies while combating the risk of noncompliance. Finally, a balance in understanding both therapeutic advantages and drawbacks is necessary to maximize the treatment of chronic pancreatitis, so that patient management continues to remain effective and customized.

A CLOSER LOOK

COMPREHENSIVE MANAGEMENT OF CHRONIC PANCREATITIS (CP)

Globally coordinating CP management is paramount due to the multi-faceted nature of the disease and its overall impact on the quality of life in patients. Coordination of the interrelationship between the inflammatory processes and the formation of related complications, such as calcification and fibrosis, needs to be handled by team care that addresses both symptoms and their cause. Lacking integrative management, patients typically suffer from ongoing pain and worsening function and can develop both exocrine and endocrine deficiency in the long term. Therefore, there is a need to configure treatment plans in the context of patient-oriented outcomes such that treatments not only relieve symptoms but also optimize well-being. Such a broad vision is able to bring new medications focused on the resolution of the various mechanisms of CP development, resulting eventually in improved management adjusted to the patient's requirements.

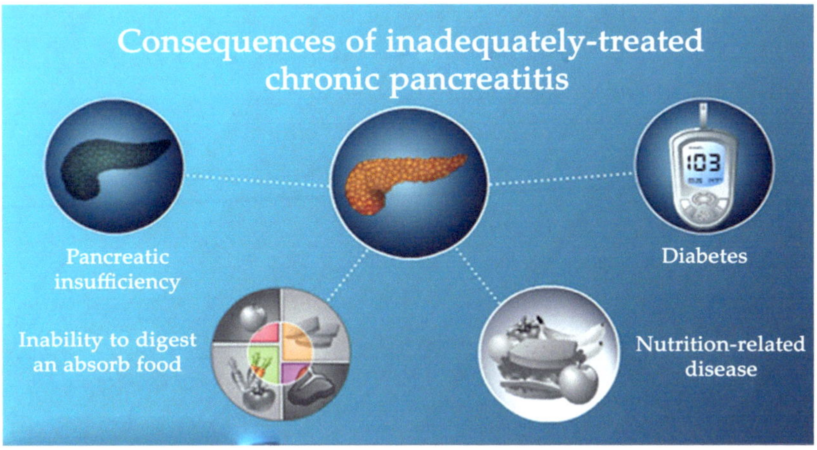

Source: https://external-content.duckduckgo.com/iu/?u=https%3A%2F%2Fwww.animatedpancreaspatient.com%2Fen-pancreas%2Fslides%2Fmanagement-and-treatment-of-chronic-pancreatitis%2Fapp02-slides-ch6_slide_05%24jpg&f=1&nofb=1&ipt=b92445b11ae6a665ba33c5ea06782ed3e8beaacbc9b472bb278b3bfdfad338e6.

Adequate diagnostics play a very significant role in the entire management of chronic pancreatitis. The disease, at its early stages, typically presents imprecise symptoms that delay timely and precise diagnosis. An aggressive diagnostic approach utilizing advanced imaging modalities, such as computed tomography and magnetic resonance cholangiopancreatography, is necessary for discriminating CP from other conditions of the gastrointestinal tract. In case of primary imaging that is inconclusive, endoscopic ultrasound can provide additional information about pancreatic pathology, thus helping patients access appropriate interventions. Additionally, the subtle onset of CP underscores the necessity of ongoing assessment and reassessment of patient status. Continuous monitoring not only enables clinicians to alter treatment plans effectively but also emphasizes the importance of preventive measures in minimizing the long-term effects. Early and precise diagnostics thus form the foundation of an effective management plan for patients suffering from chronic pancreatitis. Chronic pancreatitis pain control is a vital component of an entire care plan because of its strong impact on patient quality of life. Its treatment as a multifactorial issue demands knowledge of the disease course, with pain potentially transforming from episodic to chronic manifestations. Multimodal treatment, with both pharmacologic and lifestyle interventions, must be used to alleviate symptoms while avoiding any possible side effects. Emerging evidence has introduced promising treatments that could modify the pain course of CP, calling for future trials to confirm these novel measures. Furthermore, identifying the psychosocial determinants of chronic pain is crucial. The integration of psychological care into a treatment plan not only aids in managing pain but also supports adherence to medical advice and social support systems, ultimately enhancing patients' general coping strategy and level of life (Rodrigues-Pinto et al., 2019) (Figure 4.17).

SUMMARY

In summary, CP is a complex disease with characteristics of chronic inflammation, replacement of pancreatic tissue with fibrous tissue, and a continuum of complications such as pain and functional impairment. Knowledge of the diverse etiologies, especially alcohol, smoking, and idiopathic causes, is crucial for successful intervention and management. The etiological heterogeneity of CP requires a customized strategy taking into account the individualized etiology and clinical features in each patient. While the disease advances, it has a tendency to lead to widespread morphological changes that both endocrine and exocrine functions are severely impaired by, and therefore highlights the importance of early diagnosis and treatment. Raising awareness of the aforementioned factors can enhance patient outcomes and guide more effective treatment programs on how best to reduce the burden on both patients and healthcare systems (Bornman et al., 2010). Management of chronic pancreatitis should be multidisciplinary and involve both conservative and potential surgical interventions as appropriate. Initially, management of pain relief and lifestyle modification, including alcohol and cigarette smoking cessation, remains pivotal to the general treatment strategy. Additionally, enzyme replacement therapy in those patients with exocrine deficiency is key to preventing malnutrition and osteoporosis complications. The lack of precise guidelines in the majority of cases highlights the need for ongoing studies to develop evidence-based procedures. Specifically, data indicate that a considerable majority of patients continue dangerous habits even following diagnosis, highlighting the need for training programs to convey the long-term risks of CP (Parhiala et al., 2023). Ultimately, the prognosis for those with chronic pancreatitis is still dictated by many factors, including duration of disease, adherence to treatment protocols, and aggressive treatments. Recent literature suggests that surgery and endoscopy have the potential to provide dramatic symptomatic palliation and quality of life enhancement in select patients but are not necessarily indicated in all patients. It is also essential that healthcare providers remain vigilant to monitoring and management of the many complications of CP, such as osteoporotic fractures and sarcopenia. Through encouragement of a multidimensional treatment approach whereby both medical therapy and life modification are highlighted, practitioners have the potential to significantly affect the everyday experience of patients living with chronic pancreatitis, optimizing their quality of life and health overall (Bornman et al., 2010; Parhiala et al., 2023).

Chronic pancreatitis is typically characterized by chronic inflammation and permanent damage to the pancreas, hence presenting serious clinical issues. Chronic pancreatitis can be caused by multiple etiological factors, mainly alcohol consumption, which has been widely discussed regarding its initiation. According to recent studies, alcoholic pancreatitis can also be chronic in nature from its very inception, debasing the long-held understanding that only after repeated acute attacks does it become chronic. Histological examination of the patients has revealed that even presentations upon onset may have chronic lesions, and thus it is conceivable that the pancreas can be damaged before acute attacks, and thus needs advanced diagnosis and treatment measures (Cartmell, 2003). This observation helps to further emphasize the necessity of treating the causative factors for pancreatic injury, particularly in individuals who drink alcohol heavily. Furthermore, the pathogenic contribution of genetic factors towards chronic pancreatitis remains a topic of ongoing investigation. Investigations comparing polymorphisms in various genes, such as cytochrome P450 2E1, the key enzyme for alcohol metabolism, indicate that certain genetic forms provide a defense against the development of disease. In a controlled study, the prevalence of the polymorphisms was found to be lower in alcohol drinkers (Cartmell, 2003). Similarly, genetic processes appear to influence the inflammatory responses in the pancreas, such as the generation of prostaglandins and leukotrienes, which are linked with chronic inflammation and fibrotic changes. Notably, elevated concentrations of certain metabolites, i.e., 11β-PGF2a, have been correlated specifically with chronic pancreatitis and suggest that they can both act as biomarkers and as therapeutic targets. Chronic pancreatitis pain control is another critical aspect that significantly affects the quality of life of patients. There have been many therapeutic options, both medication and surgery, studied in an attempt to manage pain secondary to this chronic illness. Evolving knowledge of the disease has introduced novel measures that seek to reduce pain episodes, even in those with longstanding chronic pancreatitis (Ammann et al., 2009). In this instance, a multidisciplinary approach is essential, combining dietary control, enzyme replacement treatment, and pain management protocols specific to the patient has the potential to optimize results. Addressing the multifactorial nature of chronic pancreatitis allows practitioners to optimize patient management strategies, resulting in quality of life improvement and reduction of the disability of this debilitating condition.

KEY TERMS FROM THIS CHAPTER

Alcohol dominate
Autoimmune Disorders
Autoimmune pancreatitis (AIP)
Digestive health
Dysfunction
Enzyme therapy (ERT)
Genetic mutations
Palliative care
Alcoholism
Autoimmune mechanisms
Cell damage
Drug dependency
Endoscopic ultrasound (EUS)
Fibrocalculous pancreatic diabetes (FCPD)
Immunosuppressive therapy
Victims

References

1. Sreedharan, L., Kumar, B., Jewell, A., Banim, P., Koulouris, A., & Hart, A. R. (2019). Bridging clinic: The initial medical management of patients with newly diagnosed pancreatic cancer. *Frontline gastroenterology*, *10*(3), 261–268. https://doi.org/10.1136/flgastro-2018-101002 (accessed on 26 May 2025).
2. Ammann, R. W., Ammann, R. W., Morselli-Labate, A. M., Apte, M. V., Apte, M. V., Apte, M. V., Bachem, M. G., et al. (2009). *Alcoholic Pancreatitis: Pathogenesis, Incidence and Treatment with Special Reference to The Associated Pain*. https://core.ac.uk/download/pdf/8364065.pdf.
3. Abu-El-Haija, M., Gukovskaya, A. S., Andersen, D. K., Gardner, T. B., Hegyi, P., Pandol, S. J., Papachristou, G. I., Saluja, A. K., Singh, V. K., Uc, A., & Wu, B. U. (2018). Accelerating the Drug Delivery Pipeline for Acute and Chronic Pancreatitis: Summary of the Working Group on Drug Development and Trials in Acute Pancreatitis at the National Institute of Diabetes and Digestive and Kidney Diseases Workshop. *Pancreas*, *47*(10), 1185–1192. https://doi.org/10.1097/MPA.0000000000001175(accessed on 26 May 2025).
4. Bonariol, L., Caratozzolo, E., Colaut, F., Di Giacomo, A., et al. (2022). *Management of Acute and Chronic Pancreatitis*. https://core.ac.uk/download/551514001.pdf (accessed on 26 May 2025).
5. Bornman, P. C., Botha, J. F., Ramos, J. M., Smith, M. D., Van der Merwe, S., Watermeyer, G. A., & Ziady, C. C. (2010). Guideline for the diagnosis and treatment of chronic pancreatitis. *South African medical journal = Suid-Afrikaanse tydskrif vir geneeskunde*, *100*(12 Pt 2), 845–860. https://doi.org/10.7196/samj.4530 (accessed on 26 May 2025).
6. Rodrigues-Pinto, E., Caldeira, A., Soares, J. B., Antunes, T., Carvalho, J. R., Costa-Maia, J., Oliveira, P., Azevedo, R., Liberal, R., Bouça Machado, T., Magno-Pereira, V., & Moutinho-Ribeiro, P. (2019). Clube Português do Pâncreas Recommendations for Chronic Pancreatitis: Etiology, Natural History, and Diagnosis (Part I). *GE Portuguese journal of gastroenterology*, *26*(5), 346–355. https://doi.org/10.1159/000497388 (accessed on 26 May 2025).
7. Cartmell, M. T. (2003). *Genetic and Molecular Factors in The Aetiopathogenesis of Pancreatitis in Humans* [Doctoral dissertation]. https://core.ac.uk/download/29818592.pdf.
8. Chowdhury, R., Harada, H., Matsumoto, S., Mizushima, N., et al. (1994). *Tropical Calcific Pancreatitis: An Overview*. https://core.ac.uk/download/12529210.pdf (accessed on 26 May 2025).
9. Hendifar, A. E., Petzel, M. Q. B., Zimmers, T. A., Denlinger, C. S., Matrisian, L. M., Picozzi, V. J., Rahib, L., & Precision Promise Consortium (2019). Pancreas Cancer-Associated Weight Loss. *The oncologist*, *24*(5), 691–701. https://doi.org/10.1634/theoncologist.2018-0266
10. Dinesh, T. (2013). *To Evaluate the Efficacy of Diagnostic Modalities Used in Chronic Pancreatitis: Prospective Hospital-Based Observational Study* [Master's thesis]. https://core.ac.uk/download/235667945.pdf (accessed on 26 May 2025).
11. Phillips, M. E., Hopper, A. D., Leeds, J. S., Roberts, K. J., McGeeney, L., Duggan, S. N., & Kumar, R. (2021). Consensus for the management of pancreatic exocrine insufficiency: UK practical guidelines. *BMJ open gastroenterology*, *8*(1), e000643. https://doi.org/10.1136/bmjgast-2021-000643 (accessed on 26 May 2025).

12. Etemad, B., & Whitcomb, D. C. (2005). Chronic pancreatitis: Diagnosis, classification, and new genetic developments. *Gastroenterology & Hepatology*, *1*(2), 121–136. https://core.ac.uk/download/604620366.pdf (accessed on 26 May 2025).

13. Persano, M., Lisa Marcon, M., Paccagnella, E., Vigo, C., & Paccagnella, A. (2023). Dietary Interventions for Pancreatitis. IntechOpen. doi: 10.5772/intechopen.107319 (accessed on 26 May 2025).

14. Mignogna, C. (2025). *Pharmacological Intervention to Target the Procalcific Phenotypic Drift of Myeloid Cells: A Pilot Study*. https://core.ac.uk/download/638803506.pdf (accessed on 26 May 2025).

15. Parhiala, M. (2023). *Treatment of Chronic Pancreatitis*, Master's thesis. https://core.ac.uk/download/568276943.pdf (accessed on 26 May 2025).

16. Prabu, P. K. (2011). *Study of Calculus Pancreatitis* [Doctoral dissertation]. https://core.ac.uk/download/288215899.pdf (accessed on 26 May 2025).

17. Stecca, T., Nistri, C., Pauletti, B., Di Giacomo, A., Colaut, F., Ruperto, M., Caratozzolo, E., et al. (2023). Management of acute and chronic pancreatitis. In *IntechOpen eBooks*. https://doi.org/10.5772/intechopen.109115.

18. Yadav, D., Park, W. G., Fogel, E. L., Li, L., Chari, S. T., Feng, Z., Fisher, W. E., et al. (2018). PROspective Evaluation of Chronic Pancreatitis for Epidemiologic and Translational StuDies (PROCEED). *Pancreas, 47*(9), 1229–1238. https://doi.org/10.1097/MPA.0000000000001170.

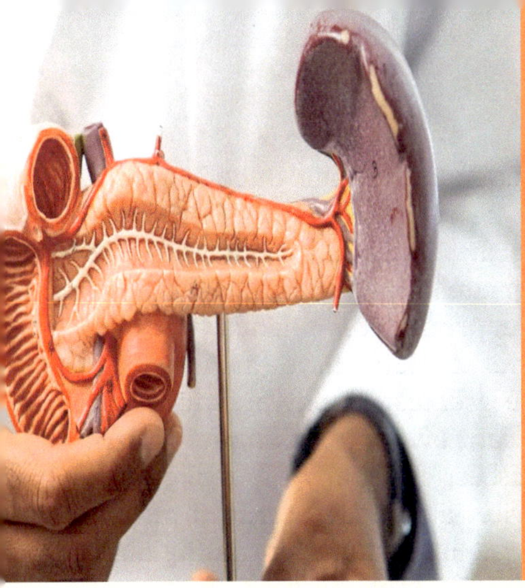

Chapter 5

CYSTIC NEOPLASMS OF THE PANCREAS

Contents

Introduction

The pancreas is often an overlooked organ, but it plays a significant role in digestion and glucose metabolism. Among the numerous pathologies that may affect this gland, cystic neoplasms are significant clinical lesions. They represent various types, such as serous and mucinous neoplasms, which possess specific characteristics and clinical features. Serous cystadenomas, by definition benign, typically possess a low risk of malignant transformation and are therefore reserved for resection only if symptomatic. Mucinous cystic neoplasms, due to their potential for producing invasive cancer, must have a more conservative approach to management due to their malignant predisposition. An understanding of the fundamental differences between these neoplasms is necessary in order to maintain a valid diagnosis and, more importantly, follow-up patient management. Over the past few years, there has been an exponential rise in the diagnosis and identification of intraductal papillary mucinous neoplasms (IPMN), mainly because of the advancement in imaging modalities. IPMNs are of pancreatic duct origin and exhibit mucin production with distension of the ductal system. Other classifications of IPMN include branch duct types that can be regarded as incidental and main duct types that are generally more aggressive. Determining the malignancy risk of IPMNs is crucial; there is a common understanding that "high-risk stigmata" or "worrisome features" may reflect a significantly elevated risk of pancreatic cancer. Hence, proper surveillance protocols and management cascades must align with these risk assessments to yield the optimal patient outcomes, as the evidence base for adhering to guidelines to the greatest extent practicable in clinical practice supports (Lawson et al., 2015). There has been recent evidence calling for urgent discrimination between the various cystic neoplasms of the pancreas, especially for malignancy potential and surveillance cascades. For example, the Fukuoka criteria provide a crucial outline for patient evaluation with branch duct IPMN that centers around the importance of finding high-risk stigmata in predicting pancreatic cancer risk. The evidence shows that the highest rates of cancer incidence occur among people who are in this high-risk category and therefore demand anticipatory surgical treatment (Azzopardi et al., 2014). Conversely, low-risk individuals can be managed using less aggressive strategies with an emphasis on individualized care based on each patient's risk assessment. As the area of pancreatic cystic neoplasms continues to evolve, sustained research and adherence to consensus recommendations will be key to further refining surveillance and treatment protocols in affected individuals (Figure 5.1).

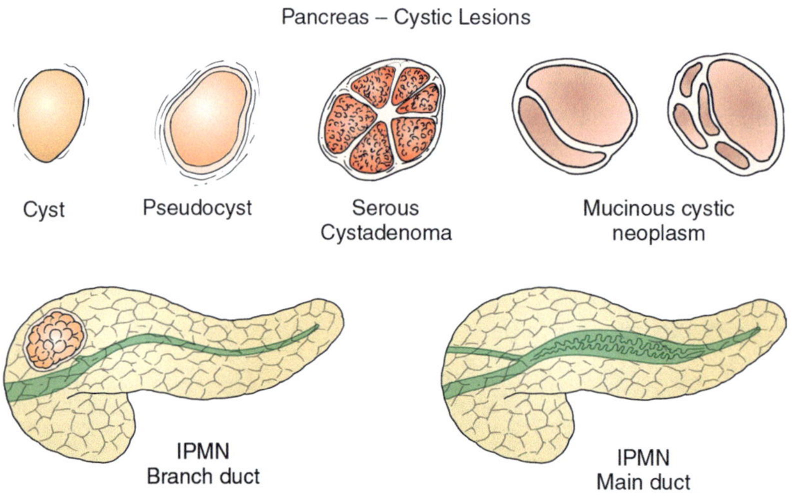

Figure 5.1. Cystic pancreatic lesions.

Source: https://radiologykey.com/wp-content/uploads/2021/06/f14-01-9780323680615.jpg.

Definition and Classification of Pancreatic Cystic Neoplasms

The understanding of pancreatic cystic neoplasms is of critical significance to clinical practice and research given the malignancy potential for their transformation. These can be largely divided into serous cystic neoplasms (SCN) and mucinous cystic neoplasms (MCN), with IPMN being a prominent subgroup of the mucinous type. SCNs are generally benign with a cystic morphology that is filled with clear fluid, but MCNs contain a mucin-secreting epithelium and can have the potential for malignant change. They should be identified because they have very different cancerous potential. Thus, an adequate understanding of their definitions and classifications assists in guiding clinical decisions and patient outcomes, specifically in surveillance and intervention strategies (Fischer & Wood, 2018). Recently, IPMN's role has drawn a great deal of attention due to its high incidence and risk of malignancy. IPMNs are classified based on their location in the pancreatic ductal system: main duct, branch duct, and mixed type. The majority duct type is most sinister due to its frequent relationship with invasive cancer, whereas branch duct IPMNs are generally associated with a lower short-term risk of malignancy. This dichotomy enables clinicians not only to risk-stratify these lesions but also to decide on monitoring and intervention protocols. The 2013 European consensus statement and subsequent guidelines suggest a balanced management of IPMNs according to symptoms, cyst size, and the presence of high-risk features such as solid components or main pancreatic duct dilation (Ateeb, 2023). Additionally, advances in diagnostic techniques such as radiologic imaging and metabolic profiling have further refined the classification and management of pancreatic cystic neoplasms. Precise imaging methods can uncover key features distinguishing between benign and potentially malignant lesions, directing surgical treatment when indicated. Studies involving the metabolic patterns of IPMNs and SCNs indicate encouraging directions for their differentiation and prediction of behavior. The detection of particular metabolites in cyst fluid, for example, has correlated with histological grading, providing a potential non-invasive diagnostic test. As knowledge of pancreatic cystic neoplasms increases, surveillance and refinement of classification systems are important in order to maximize patient outcomes and avoid risk from these problem lesions (Fischer & Wood, 2018; Ateeb, 2023) (Figure 5.2).

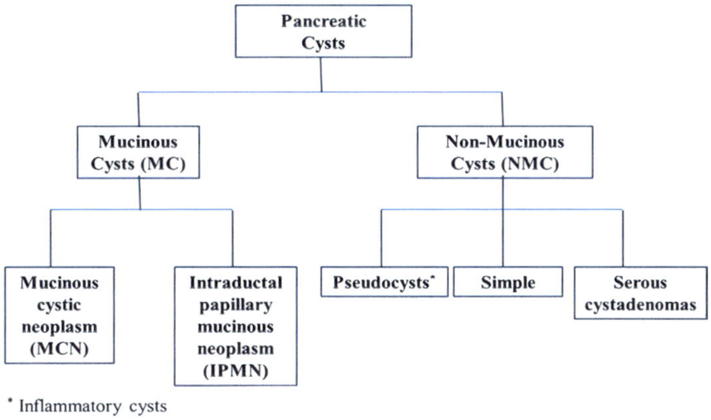

Figure 5.2. Classification of pancreatic cystic neoplasms.

Source: https://www.researchgate.net/profile/Aiman-Abu-Ammar/publication/315739129/figure/fig1/AS:478597510111232@1491117946779/Classification-of-pancreatic-cysts.png.

Importance of Understanding Different Types

Understanding the distinction among various types of cystic neoplasms of the pancreas is important for a number of reasons, primarily for the development of effective management strategies. Of these neoplasms, mucinous cystic neoplasms and serous cystadenomas exhibit drastically differing biological behaviors, clinical characteristics, and malignant potential. Serous cystadenomas, for instance, are typically benign and almost never develop into malignancies, and therefore clinicians can adopt a more conservative approach to monitoring and intervention. In contrast, mucinous cystic neoplasms possess high malignant potential and necessitate more aggressive diagnostic and therapeutic measures. The delineation between such neoplasms thus finally enhances outcomes by guiding individualized surveillance protocols and treatment modalities required for appropriate risk stratification. IPMNs once again demonstrate the requirement for differential types of pancreatic neoplasms since they possess unique characteristics and varying malignant potentials. IPMNs are also graded depending on how associated they are with pancreatic ducts and their grades of dysplasia, which determines clinical management. With increasing evidence suggesting a link between IPMNs and pancreatic cancer, being familiar with their individual behavior becomes highly crucial. There has been recent work documenting significant genetic alterations in IPMNs, which suggests that they need to be detected early and treated curatively if they can be detected in the pre-cancerous stage (Fischer et al., 2018). As surveillance protocols become more distinct, detection of heterogeneity of IPMNs will yield more precise follow-up and potential surgery recommendations, ultimately aiming to reduce pancreatic cancer-related morbidity. In addition, the greater amount of data on the molecular underpinnings of pancreatic cystic neoplasms confirms the requirement for differential understanding. Molecular characterization technologies have revealed key genomic alterations contributing to tumorigenesis that expose the pathways to initiating and developing such lesions (Löhr et al., 2017). Scientific studies provide valuable information that directs clinical interventions to provide early detection and prevention that can stop malignant conversions. Because each neoplasm category may present with varying clinical presentations, diagnostic pitfalls, and therapy, clinicians need important knowledge. Emphasizing the importance of subclassifying and knowing these entities not only gives a stronger academic presence to what the literature has to say about pancreatic pathology but also results in improved patient care and survival.

5.1. Serous Neoplasms

Serous neoplasms are a special category of pancreatic cystic neoplasms characterized by their benign nature and comparatively low malignant potential. Serous neoplasms are characterized by their predominance of serous fluid and histological picture of tiny cystic spaces lined by a single layer of bland epithelial cells. Unlike mucinous neoplasms, serous neoplasms do not possess any aggressive risk factors for malignant transformation. Subsequently, they are often handled with caution unless there are symptoms or other complications. Surveillance methods are primarily through routine imaging to evaluate tumor size and the development of new symptoms, in line with the overall goal of providing patient safety without unnecessary surgery in the majority of cases where tumors are asymptomatic and stable (Fischer & Wood, 2018). A total understanding of serous cystic neoplasms also involves knowledge of the diagnostic challenges they present. The need to differentiate these benign tumors from other more malignant forms of pancreatic neoplasms cannot be overly emphasized, as misdiagnosis would lead to overtreatment or under-treatment. Radiological imaging, especially via the intermediacy of computed tomography (CT) and magnetic resonance imaging (MRI), plays a critical role in assisting clinicians to visualize the appearance of these tumors. However, certain diagnosis in the majority of instances requires cytological study of cyst fluid, as imaging is not always specific for ruling out other cystic neoplasms such as mucinous cystic neoplasms or intraductal papillary mucinous neoplasms (Kwon & Simeone, 2011). With ongoing research, using of novel biomarkers from proteomics is likely to become more precise for diagnosis and distinction, ultimately rationalizing the management of these neoplasms. Given the benign course of serous neoplasms, contemporary medicine prefers conservative management techniques and reserves surgery only for a subset of cases. European evidence-based guidelines for pancreatic cystic neoplasms suggest that asymptomatic serous cystic neoplasms should, in most cases, not undergo surgical resection since this is now becoming increasingly frequent and individualized therapy is being employed. Ongoing surveillance and patient counseling are key components of this approach, with the psychosocial effects of having a pancreatic cyst addressed by it. This paradigm change functions to underscore careful monitoring being weighed against quality-of-life considerations and acceptance that prematurity is sometimes inevitable for lesions with unusual appearance or concerning symptoms (Fischer & Wood, 2018). Therefore, a meticulous appreciation of serous neoplasms is required for optimal patient outcomes in the big picture of pancreatic cystic neoplasm management (Figure 5.3).

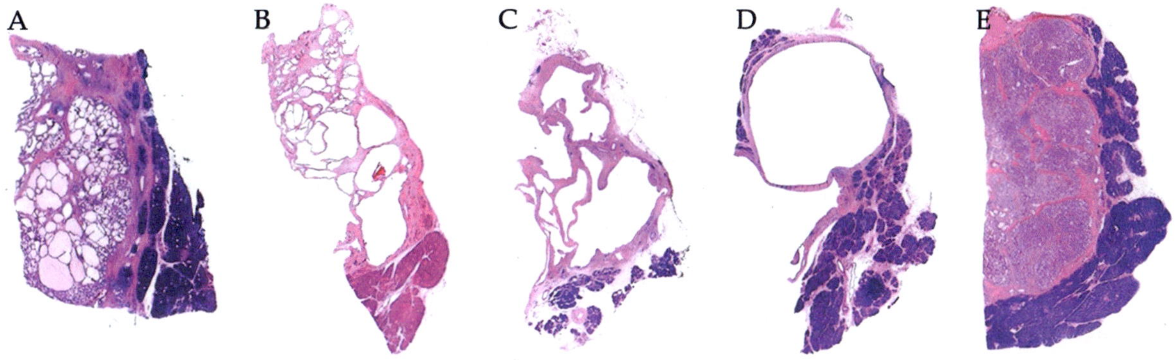

Figure 5.3. Serous neoplasms of the pancreas.

Source: https://images.journals.lww.com/ajsp/SocialThumb.00000478-201512000-00002.F1-2.jpeg.

5.1.1. Characteristics and Histological Features

Cystic pancreatic neoplasms exhibit a broad range of characteristics and histologic patterns that are important for classification. Serous cystadenomas are best characterized by their distinctive multilocular cystic appearance filled with clear, serous fluid and lined with a thin membrane of cuboidal or flat epithelial cells. Histologically, these lesions are characterized by a fibrous stroma, with disorganized capillaries and little cellular atypia, reflecting low malignant potential. Mucinous cystic neoplasms, however, which are often seen in women, contain more mucus and can have more complex cystic configurations. Histologically, they are characterized by a dense stroma and neoplastic epithelium, the latter of which may have various degrees of atypia, thus reflecting their malignant potential. This histological distinction is significant for the planning of management strategies for these pancreatic lesions, particularly in their individual malignancy risk (Azzopardi et al., 2014). Intraductal papillary mucinous neoplasms (IPMNs) complicate their presentation and histology, as they are often a ductal source within the pancreas. They are classified as main duct, branch duct, and mixed types, and each has variable implications for clinical behavior. Histologically, IPMNs are characterized by papillary projections and abundant mucin production, leading to ductal system dilation. The neoplastic cells covering the papillae may range from low-grade to high-grade dysplasia, emphasizing the potential to evolve into invasive carcinoma. These differences need careful monitoring and, in some cases, urgent surgical treatment, particularly for high-risk lesions with suspicious characteristics such as mural nodular enhancement or main pancreatic duct dilatation (Fischer & Wood, 2018). Awareness of these features guides additional clinical decision-making about management regimens. The neoplastic character of cystic neoplasms is inseparably linked with their histological presentation, and utmost care is needed for optimal surveillance regimens. Serous cystadenomas are primarily benign with little risk of malignant transformation, while mucinous cystic neoplasms and IPMNs warrant a more guarded strategy due to their intrinsic risk profiles. Recommendations are for surgical resection of mucinous neoplasms and certain IPMNs, specifically those with high-risk stigmata like size or excessive cytological atypia, to prevent the evolution of invasive disease. For asymptomatic branch duct IPMNs without worrisome features, a conservative surveillance approach can be recommended. This risk stratification based on histological examination is crucial in the planning of the management approaches since it greatly affects patient outcomes in the context of cystic pancreatic neoplasms (Azzopardi et al., 2014; Fischer & Wood, 2018).

5.1.2. Common Types and Their Clinical Presentations

The pancreatic cystic neoplasm classification is pivotal in appreciating their clinical manifestations and patient management implications. The most common types of such neoplasms include serous cystic neoplasms (SCNs) and mucinous cystic neoplasms (MCNs), both of which have unique morphological and clinical characteristics. SCNs are typically benign with low malignant potential, and they normally appear as well-circumscribed cysts with a central scar on imaging. On the other hand, MCNs, found predominantly in women, might carry malignant potential, particularly if atypical presentations, such as wall thickness of the cyst or solid components, are present. Their clinical presentation can be non-specific, e.g., abdominal pain, or they can remain asymptomatic for many years, presenting challenges to an early diagnosis and surveillance strategy. IPMNs are another significant form of pancreatic cystic lesions with variable clinical presentation and the potential for malignant transformation.

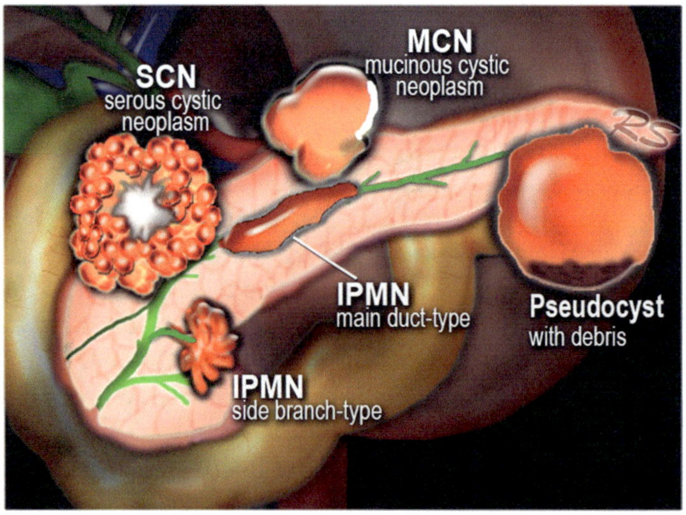

Figure 5.4. Mucinous cystic neoplasm pancreas causes.

Source: https://external-content.duckduckgo.com/iu/?u=https%3A%2F%2Fhealthjade.net%2Fwp-content%2Fuploads%2F2019%2F12%2Fmucinous-cystic-neoplasm.jpg&f=1&nofb=1&ipt=de1abc4f3cea928d8eac871ffdb1e0975a5a03313e45bb1504a704c9b4c5d941.

IPMNs arise from the pancreatic ducts and are further classified into main-duct, branch-duct, and mixed types. Main-duct types and the mixed types are at much higher risk of developing invasive cancer compared to the branch-duct types, and their management is therefore very challenging. Patients may be diagnosed with nonspecific abdominal pain, weight loss, or jaundice, but the majority are asymptomatic and discovered incidentally upon imaging for unrelated purposes. Such presentations require careful clinical evaluation and follow-up, given that early management is found to have a significant effect on patient outcomes (Shaikh, 2021). The management of IPMNs is dictated by their cystic nature and malignancy risk. Whereas resection for main-duct and mixed IPMNs is usually justified by their higher risk of malignancy, branch-duct IPMNs can be safely monitored if not for the presence of specific high-risk features, such as cyst growth or mural nodule formation. The preponderance of asymptomatic IPMNs also renders surveillance difficult, which requires repeated imaging to assess for changes in size or morphology. Advances in imaging, such as MRI with breath-hold magnetic resonance cholangiopancreatography, have improved the assessment of such neoplasms to better delineate potentially malignant features such as intramural nodules and communication with the ducts, thus improving stratification of risk and choice for surgical treatment (Pollini et al., 2019) (Figure 5.4).

5.1.3. Diagnostic Imaging Techniques Used

Diagnosis of cystic neoplasms of the pancreas is dependent on a range of diagnostic imaging modalities, which play a crucial role in the accurate identification and characterization of such lesions. Of all such commonly employed modalities, CT and MRI offer broad images of the pancreas and adjacent organs. CT scanning is capable of providing high-resolution images that can highlight cystic lesions, particularly in suspected malignancies. Parallel to this, MRI in the guise of magnetic resonance cholangiopancreatography (MRCP) is very helpful in the imaging of the pancreatic duct and demarcation of how cystic neoplasms are related to the main pancreatic duct. This ability is critical in differentiating between serous and mucinous neoplasms, a distinction pertinent to the subsequent management and potential surgeries, as encapsulated by existing guidelines (Azzopardi et al., 2014). Endoscopic ultrasound (EUS) is also a part of the diagnostic workup of pancreatic cystic lesions. EUS offers more proximal visualization of the pancreas, making more accurate evaluation of small lesions not seen on CT or MRI possible. Apart from high-resolution imaging of cystic lesions, EUS permits fine-needle aspiration (FNA) cytological assessment, which aids in distinguishing neoplasm types. The ability to sample cyst fluid obtains critical information on tumor markers and cytology that has a central impact on the assessment of the malignant potential of cystic neoplasms. For instance, the identification of certain markers may indicate a higher potential for malignancy, thus informing surveillance behaviors and surgical procedures (Fischer & Wood, 2018). Integration of EUS findings with imaging results presents an improved overall diagnostic accuracy and management of pancreatic cystic neoplasms. Recent advances in imaging modalities have significantly improved the monitoring and surveillance of cystic pancreatic lesions. In patients with IPMN and other cystic neoplasms, adherence to evidence-based surveillance guidelines is essential to monitor for size and morphological evolution that signals malignant change. This includes periodic imaging assessments with either CT or MRI, depending on the patient's specific clinical profile and risk factors. Most recent European guidelines favor conservative treatment in asymptomatic lesions but also indicate surgery when there are high-risk features, such as an enhancing mural nodule or marked dilation of the pancreatic duct (Marc et al., 2018). The new guidelines emphasize the use of diagnostic imaging not only at initial diagnosis but also on follow-up to avoid complications of pancreatic cancer occurrence.

5.2. Mucinous Neoplasms

Classification of pancreatic cystic neoplasms is important to the management and monitoring in practice, particularly for mucinous neoplasms that carry a significant risk of malignancy. MCNs are identified by the production of mucin and can be presented as either malignant or benign lesions. In comparison to serous cystadenomas, which are not of significant concern with the possibility of developing into cancer, MCNs will often need to be resected due to premalignant characteristics. Special diagnostic criteria, like imaging and histological examinations, are essential to differentiate such lesions from other cystic lesions, like IPMNs.

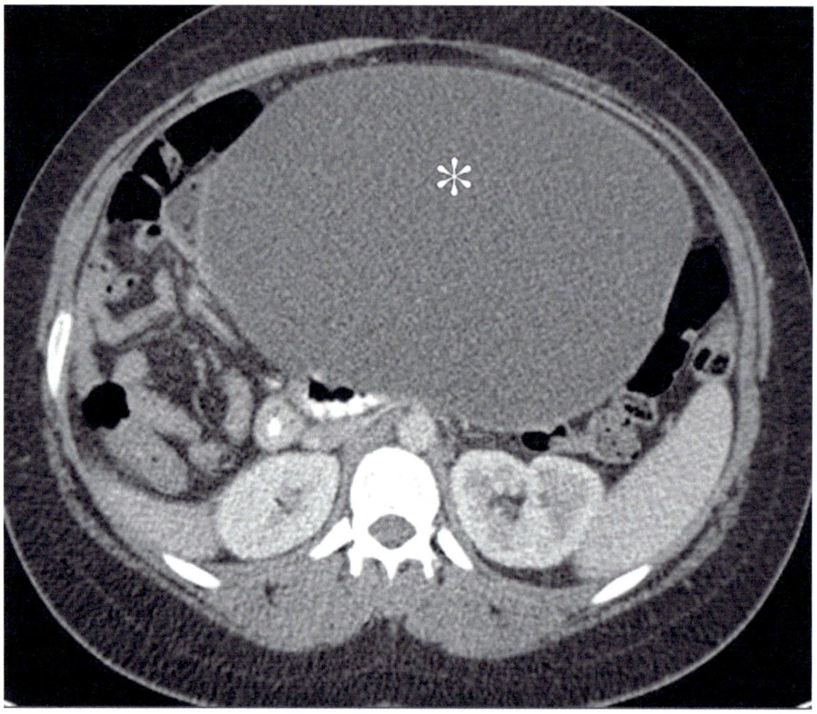

Figure 5.5. Mucinous neoplasms of the ovary.

Source: https://pubs.rsna.org/cms/10.1148/rg.2019180221/asset/images/large/rg.2019180221.fig1a.jpeg.

The need for proper differentiation is appreciated when employing surveillance protocols, emphasizing the vital role of proper diagnosis in patient outcomes. Lack of proper assessment of such lesions can result in a loss of potential for early intervention on malignant transformation. In the clinical setting, the treatment of mucinous neoplasms is guided by practice guidelines that include risk stratification based on imaging studies and clinical findings. The international consensus guidelines, or the Fukuoka criteria, are a set of criteria used to identify patients with IPMNs who are at risk for pancreatic cancer. Based on Lawson et al. (2015), these criteria define "high-risk stigmata" and "worrisome features" that would trigger intensified intervention upon them, such as surgical resection. The findings point out that patients with these criteria have a significantly increased cumulative incidence of pancreatic cancer, with a 28% seven-year risk for those in the highest-risk category. These publications emphasize the value of guideline compliance in clinical practice in the prompt surgical resection of mucinous neoplasms to avoid the threat of progression to invasive cancer. Besides surgical treatment, long-term surveillance of mucinous neoplasms following first diagnosis could also be warranted, particularly in those with branch duct IPMNs that do not have high-risk features. Recent practice has included suggestions that asymptomatic patients with minor lesions can safely be kept under close observation, but any change of findings or development of symptoms should be reassessed for management. In the opinion of Azzopardi et al. (2014), such practice strikes a balance between the risk associated with surgical therapy versus malignant change in such commonly indolent neoplasms. Continuous monitoring allows the physician to adjust management as indicated by the progression of the neoplasms or the clinical condition of the patient, finally improving outcomes and survival in these complex pancreatic lesions. A complete understanding and monitoring of mucinous neoplasms are still the most important aspect in contemporary pancreatic therapy (Figure 5.5).

5.2.1. Distinction Between Mucinous Cystic Neoplasms (MCNs) and Serous Neoplasms

The MCNs and SCNs need to be differentiated from each other in the treatment and diagnosis of pancreatic cystic neoplasms. MCNs appear in middle-aged women with mucin-producing epithelial cells are typically ensconced in a thick fibrous stroma. MCNs have a high potential for malignant transformation and hence need close monitoring and treatment. In contrast, SCNs predominantly occur in older women and are more benign in nature, the histological content consisting of a network of cystic spaces lined by cuboidal epithelial cells. Due to their reduced malignant potential, SCNs are likely to need less aggressive treatment protocols than MCNs. It is therefore important to understand these distinctions to customize surveillance strategies and treatment protocols for patients with pancreatic cystic lesions. In clinical practice, MCNs and SCNs are distinguishable through an examination of their imaging characteristics and histopathological presentation. Radiologically, MCNs present as unilocular or multilocular cystic masses with peripheral enhancement, while SCNs are generally well-defined microcystic lesions that can present with a "honeycomb" appearance on imaging examinations. The differential can also be validated through the cytologic study of the cyst fluid, where mucin presence in MCNs is paralleled to the lesion's malignant nature. Additionally, based on guideline-suggested criteria, e.g., Fukuoka criteria, clinicians are able to stratify patients into high-risk and low-risk categories for pancreatic cancer based on certain imaging features, thereby informing their treatment strategy. The effective implementation of these criteria is supplemented by data stratifying malignancy risk in branch duct IPMN patients, emphasizing the utility of differentiation of types of pancreatic cystic lesions (Lawson et al., 2015). Long-term follow-up is important in the case of patients with MCN-diagnosed, owing to the possibility of malignant transformation. The current guidelines for practice recommend surgery for symptomatic or large MCNs, particularly those greater than 4 cm, due to their potential for pancreatic cancer development. SCN monitoring is usually conservative since they are benign in behavior with a low malignancy rate. This is also reflected by the latest evidence-based European guidelines on pancreatic cystic neoplasms that advocate for conservative management except in the presence of absolute indications for surgery. Appropriate risk stratification and surveillance measures play a crucial role in optimizing patient outcomes, as evident from the contrasting management approaches of MCNs and SCNs in clinical practice (Fischer & Wood, 2018). Lastly, comprehension of the variations enhances a clinician's ability to individualize management strategies and prognosis for patients who have pancreatic cystic neoplasms (Figure 5.6).

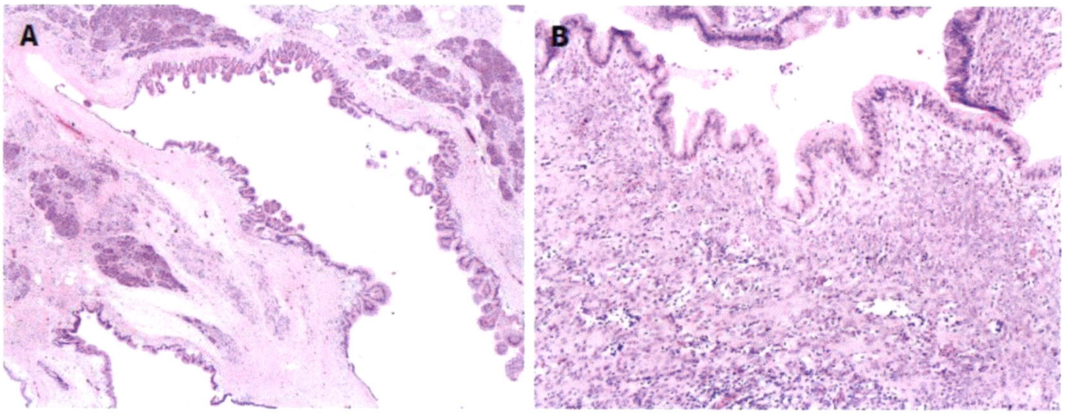

Figure 5.6. Pathological features and diagnosis of intraductal papillary mucinous.

Source: https://external-content.duckduckgo.com/iu/?u=https%3A%2F%2Ff6publishing.blob.core.windows.net%2F106d5768-5694-4b06-8052-770013bc0b06%2FWJGO-6-311-g010.jpg&f=1&nofb=1&ipt=fe621bb2c1600941b585e86534dfdac1bb072fb7f16dfcc3a60e0eac07392c8e.

5.2.2. Clinical Implications and Symptoms

Clinical relevance of pancreas cystic neoplasms also varies widely depending on the type of neoplasm and its potential to be cancerous. SCNs follow a benign course with mild clinical presentation and low progression to malignancy. MCNs and IPMNs, on the other hand, have features that indicate higher malignant potential. MCNs are usually found in women, with incongruous degrees of presentation of symptoms like abdominal pain and weight loss, which may raise suspicion for malignancy. IPMNs, grouped based on their association with the pancreatic duct, can produce obstructions and jaundice, particularly if they are noted with high-risk stigmata. Clinical follow-up is important for such neoplasms to detect any initial indication of progression to provide maximum management and outcome for the patient. Symptoms attributed to pancreatic cystic neoplasms can help in early diagnosis and treatment. IPMN patients may present with barely noticeable symptoms of gastrointestinal change or abdominal pain, but some cases are also asymptomatic. Significantly, the presence of some clinical features indicates urinary obstruction or distal bile duct involvement that requires emergent imaging or surgical evaluation. Stratification of risk based on the Fukuoka criteria plays a pivotal role in assessing the risk of malignant transformation. The general cancer risk in high-risk groups remains understandably elevated, with studies providing evidence of a seven-year cancer incidence in 28% of individuals who meet high-risk stigmata (Lawson et al., 2015). It is thus important to value these clinical observations and their implications for implementing the appropriate diagnostic sequences and treatments. The changing paradigm of recommendations for the management of pancreatic cystic neoplasms emphasizes the need for a more nuanced approach to clinical implications and follow-up. Plans for surveillance are recommended based on the type, size, and symptomatology of the neoplasm, based on the latest European consensus guidelines (Fischer & Wood, 2018). For instance, IPMN patients with absolute indications for surgery, such as an extreme dilatation of the main pancreatic duct or with enhancing mural nodules, should be closely monitored or assessed for surgery. Conservative therapy can be advised in asymptomatic lesions, but careful follow-up is mandatory to avoid malignant transformation. Ultimately, personalized management approaches taking into account both clinical significance and patient uniqueness will facilitate results and ensure interventions are warranted when needed.

5.2.3. Pathological Features and Diagnosis

The pathological features of pancreatic cystic neoplasms are significant in making the right diagnosis and subsequent management. Pancreatic cystic neoplasms can broadly be classified as serous and mucinous, both having distinct histological features. Serous cystadenomas consist of profuse small cysts lined by cuboidal cells with clear cytoplasm and central content containing glycogen. On the other hand, mucinous cystic neoplasms are characterized by mucin-secreting epithelial cells and a covering ovarian-type stroma. IPMNs have a higher degree of complexity, and possibly extend into the main pancreatic duct or its branches, and show a range of unusual cellular features corresponding to different malignant potentials. Correct discrimination between these neoplasms requires an understanding of both imaging and histopathological features since their treatment relies on it (Azzopardi et al., 2014).

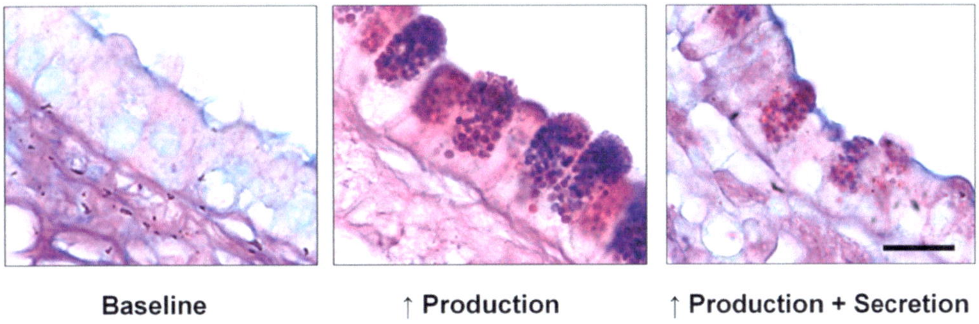

Figure 5.7. Regulated mucin secretion from airway epithelial cells.

Source: Adler KB, Tuvim MJ and Dickey BF (2013) Regulated mucin secretion from airway epithelial cells. Front. Endocrinol. 4:129. doi: 10.3389/fendo.2013.00129.

Imaging modalities such as CT and MRI provide the basis for the diagnosis of cystic neoplasms. Imaging is useful in the determination of the size, morphology, and some features of the cystic lesions that indicate their malignant potential. One such example is the indication of enhancing mural nodules or ductal architectural changes, which can be indicative of higher probabilities of malignancy. Practice today focuses on the importance of risk-stratified classification; therefore, for example, main duct IPMN with associated malignancy risk should be treated, while asymptomatic branch duct IPMN in the absence of worrisome features can be followed conservatively. It is consequently critical that there is integration of diagnostic imaging and careful clinical assessment for effective management of patients (Fischer & Wood, 2018). Beyond imaging and pathologic examination, surveillance guidelines for vigilant monitoring of neoplasms are also an essential component of patient management. Mucinous cystic neoplasms and IPMNs, particularly those with high-risk features such as increasing size or mural nodules, need careful follow-up and early treatment. Surveillance practices are likely to suggest regular imaging assessment, typically between one and two years depending on the primary findings, in order to catch any malignant change at an earlier time. Conversely, serous cystadenomas with their low propensity for malignancy may be observed at less frequent intervals, with heterogeneity of malignant potential among the range of cystic neoplasms. The development and enforcement of evidence-based guidelines assist in standardizing treatment and improving patient outcomes for those who are evaluated for pancreatic cystic lesions (Azzopardi et al., 2014) (Figure 5.7).

5.3. Intraductal Papillary Mucinous Neoplasms (IPMNs)

IPMNs are a significant subtype of pancreatic cystic neoplasms where mucin-secreting cells grow abnormally in the pancreatic ducts. These lesions are significant due to their potential for malignant transformation and thus their early detection and treatment are necessary. IPMNs are classified into three broad categories: main duct, branch duct, and mixed-type, the riskiest of them being the main duct type with the highest potential for the development of pancreatic ductal adenocarcinoma (PDAC). Surveillance of IPMNs is essential since patients typically present symptomatically, and detection is difficult until advanced stages. The transformation rate for branch duct IPMNs is estimated to be quite diverse, even more so, highlighting the importance of close surveillance and risk stratification in the management of individuals with such neoplasms. Practitioners must be aware of the distinctive characteristics and malignant potential of each group to properly guide treatment schemes. The malignant potential of IPMNs varies greatly based on their subtype, which affects the management and follow-up plan. Main duct IPMNs are very concerning, with a reported malignancy rate of 35% to 75%, suggesting surgical resection upon diagnosis. Branch duct IPMNs, although still risky, have lower rates of transformation, thereby supporting a more conservative monitoring approach. The decision-making process is one in which surgical risk must be balanced against the potential benefits of early intervention. New guidelines identify characteristics such as cyst diameter, mural nodules, and ductal dilation as important predictors for determining the necessity of surgical resection. Therefore, accurate IPMN characterization, in addition to a judiciously planned surveillance regimen, is critical to optimizing patient outcomes while avoiding unnecessary interventions. Awareness of these nuances consolidates the platform upon which clinicians make a diagnosis and treat IPMNs, considering that such lesions have special challenges in the clinical setting. For proper management to be enabled, careful knowledge of the imaging modalities and fluid cytology of IPMNs is required. Cross-sectional imaging, particularly MRI and CT, are essential instruments for initial diagnosis and characterization of cystic lesions. EUS with FNA also allows for fluid evaluation from cysts, which can be of critical significance, for instance, identification of the presence of cancer cells or mutation markers. A number of studies emphasize that an accurate diagnostic method not only maximizes surveillance results but also informs the decision regarding interventions. For instance, identification of increased carcinoembryonic antigen (CEA) concentration in cyst fluid can indicate mucinous character and arouse suspicion of cancer. The integration of aggressive imaging modalities with accurate fluid considerations delineates a broad plan for the observation of IPMNs. With incremental advances in technology and clinical practice, the management landscape for IPMNs becomes progressively complex, necessitating an interdisciplinary model that tunes patient safety to optimally effective anticancer therapy (Figure 5.8).

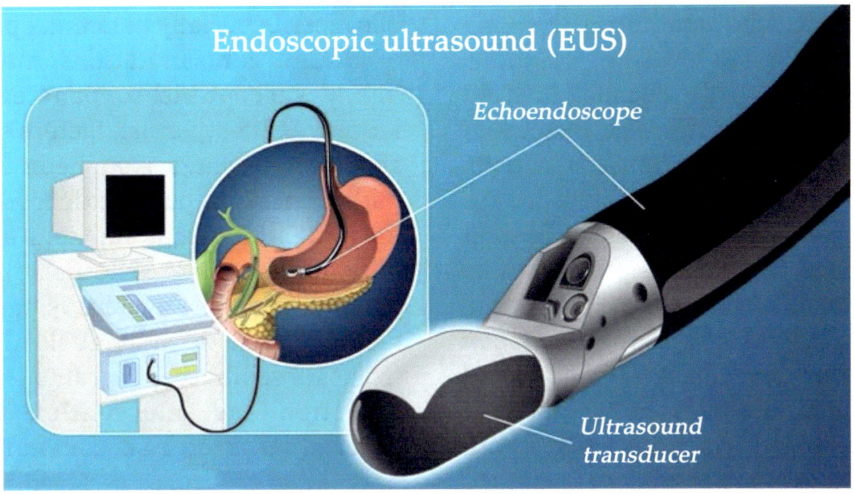

Figure 5.8. Endoscopic ultrasound (EUS).

Source: https://external-content.duckduckgo.com/iu/?u=https%3A%2F%2Fi.ytimg.com%2Fvi%2F0A4FNAQpeRc%2Fmaxresdefault.jpg&f=1&nofb=1&ipt=4929eec72a8ed8ea21fa464a4a342677ff81c44be3747e46e833d30f3fcaef82.

5.3.1. Definition and Classification of Intraductal Papillary Mucinous Neoplasms (IPMNs)

Classification of IPMNs holds the greatest significance in assessing their malignant potential and their management planning. IPMNs are primarily classified based on their site of origin and it is usually either the main pancreatic duct (MPD) or the side branches. There are three types of IPMNs identified by the World Health Organization, which include main duct IPMN, branch duct IPMN, and mixed type IPMN. They help to determine prognostic results and treatment interventions. For instance, main duct IPMNs have a higher risk of malignancy compared to their branch duct counterparts, and as such, varied surveillance measures and surgical intervention would be appropriate. These variations support the significance of accurate classification in the clinic based on its capability to inform effective intervention of management that can avoid potential malignant types in those affected (Fischer & Wood, 2018). Diagnosis and recognition of IPMN rely on sophisticated imaging techniques, which are necessary to differentiate the neoplasms from other pancreatic cystic lesions. Endoscopic ultrasonography, magnetic resonance imaging, and computed tomography have been useful in assessing the character of these neoplasms, such as their size, cystic character, and ductal involvement. High-resolution imaging will also detect the presence of suspicious findings such as mural nodules or main duct dilation, both of which are important indicators of a high risk for malignancy. In fact, studies have confirmed that MPD dilation of more than 5 mm typically indicates high-grade dysplasia or even invasive cancer (Ateeb, 2023). Thus, diligent imaging evaluation is not only vital for diagnosis but also for establishing the degree of urgency for therapeutic intervention, underlining the significance of radiologic information to clinical IPMN treatment. IPMNs are clinically managed based on a diligent assessment of their classification in terms of surveillance as well as possible surgical intervention. Since IPMNs may exhibit a broad range of histological characteristics, ranging from low-grade dysplasia to invasive carcinoma, monitoring mechanisms need to be individualized according to the nature and risk factors of each neoplasm. Active surveillance is usually suggested in guidelines for branch duct IPMNs measuring less than 4 cm, whereas main duct IPMNs, particularly if they are symptomatic, like jaundice or in case of an obvious MPD dilation, may require surgical resection. The European consensus on PCNs demonstrates the critical importance of multidisciplinary collaboration in developing guidelines for management, where every IPMN is considered according to its unique characteristics, thereby optimizing outcomes in patients at risk for pancreatic cancer (Fischer & Wood, 2018).

5.3.2. Risk Factors and Epidemiology

The epidemiology of pancreatic cystic neoplasms (PCNs) has become more prominent in recent years, particularly with advances in imaging technologies such as CT and MRI. These imaging technologies enable incidental detection of cystic lesions, and hence, an increased awareness of their prevalence has been established. PCNs are generally divided into a number of categories: serous cystic neoplasms, mucinous cystic neoplasms, and IPMN, each with its distinct risk factors and potential for malignancy. Notably, IPMN is recognized to be a premalignant condition with an unpredictable risk profile, and thus, management and surveillance strategies need to be taken into account in a complex way. As systematic reviews give ever-stronger evidence, early diagnosis is related to improved outcomes, underlining the need for additional research to perfect our understanding of the epidemiological patterns on which these lesions arise and how they may go on to develop into malignancy (Fischer & Wood, 2018). Risk factors for the development and progression of PCNs are multifactorial and can be influenced by genetic predisposition along with environmental conditions. A first-degree relative with a history of cancer, especially in familial pancreatic cancer or BRCA2 gene mutations, makes the patient highly susceptible to pancreatic neoplasms. Moreover, lifestyle risk factors such as smoking and obesity have also been involved in the pathogenesis of pancreatic lesions, and studies have identified that smokers have more cases of IPMN compared to non-smokers. A thorough grasp of such risk factors is paramount for the identification of individuals who will benefit from surveillance programs in favor of early detection and intervention. Tackling these determinants of risk can not only optimize preventive measures but also help to decrease overall morbidity and mortality from malignant change in pancreatic cystic neoplasms (Minelli et al., 2023).

As regards surveillance, the patients with IPMN present particular challenges because of its unpredictable risk for malignant transformation. New guidelines favor a selective approach with regard to cyst characteristics and associated risk factors. For instance, asymptomatic branch-duct IPMNs less than 4 cm in size may be treated conservatively, but those with suspicious features like enhancing mural nodules or main pancreatic duct dilatation require surgical resection. This strategic discrimination in the management is vital, as it avoids undertreatment of low-risk individuals while facilitating individualized intervention. Current research and clinical utilization of novel risk stratification scores with regard to contemporary imaging modalities will further shape surveillance policies to progressively follow patients with pancreatic cystic neoplasms more effectively. These measures aim to reduce the impending danger of malignancy while promoting enhanced patient outcomes (Fischer & Wood, 2018) (Figure 5.9).

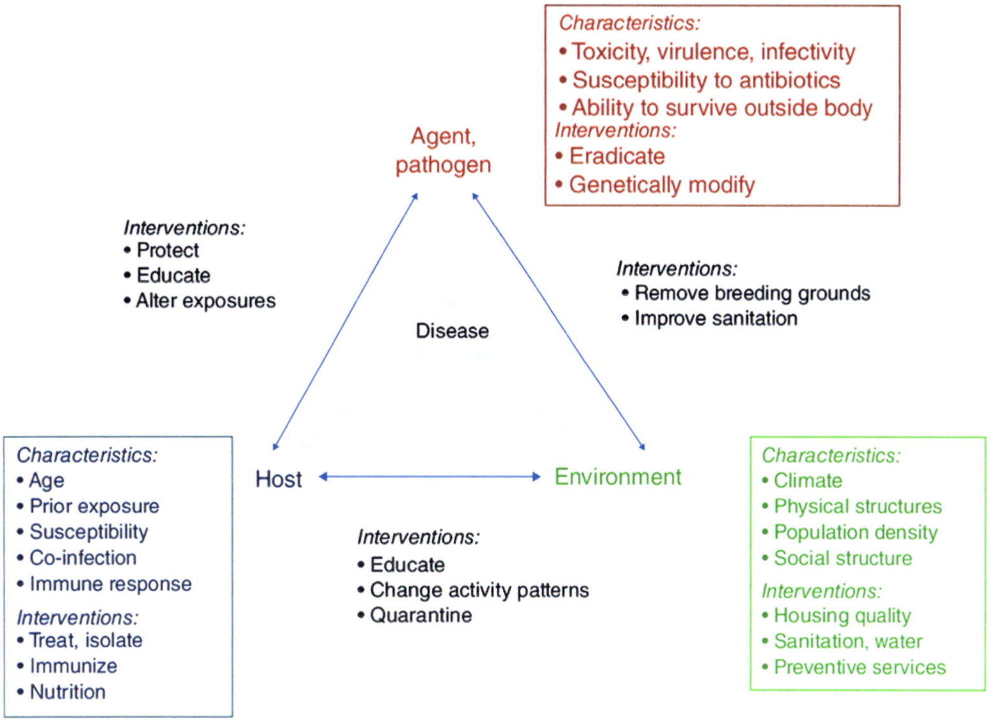

Figure 5.9. The "epidemiologic triad" of infectious disease.

Source: https://www.researchgate.net/profile/Yvette-Johnson-3/publication/323678367/figure/fig1/AS:659686567194624@1534292942583/The-epidemiologic-triad-of-infectious-disease-summarizes-the-factors-that-influence-an.png.

5.3.3. Diagnostic Criteria and Imaging Modalities

Diagnosis of cystic pancreatic neoplasms needs an extremely cautious approach with an amalgamation of diagnostic features and appropriate imaging modalities. Deciphering imaging modalities such as CT, MRI, and EUS is extremely crucial in identifying the nature of pancreatic cysts. These modalities are extremely helpful in discriminating serous cystadenomas, tending to have a characteristic pattern of numerous microcysts, from mucinous cystic neoplasms, with a recognized malignant transformation potential. Their effectiveness is also enhanced by the fact that these imaging techniques are able to provide detailed anatomical information, including the interaction between cysts and pancreatic ducts and adjacent vascular structures. As stressed in recent reviews, the rising detection rates for pancreatic cystic lesions highlight the necessity for accurate imaging to direct subsequent management and potential surgery (Azzopardi et al., 2014). Diagnostic features used for the diagnosis of pancreatic cystic neoplasms closely mirror their morphological characteristics and the clinical context in which they present. IPMNs, for instance, are categorized based on the involvement of the main pancreatic duct versus branch ducts, and this dictates the surveillance or surgical resection approach. Evidence-based recommendations support resection in the setting of IPMN with high-risk stigmata such as jaundice or an enhancing mural nodule (Fischer & Wood, 2018). Cyst size, symptom change, and imaging findings all play a role in assessing malignant potential. This stratification not only helps clinicians in formulating patient-specific treatment strategies but also highlights the importance of regular surveillance, particularly in asymptomatic patients falling within certain criteria. Multidisciplinary input fortifies the diagnosis and management of pancreatic cystic neoplasms. Experts in radiology, gastroenterology, and surgical oncology collaborate to review imaging reports with a consensus approach to separate benign disease from high-risk malignancy. Asymptomatic branch duct IPMN of less than 30 mm is recommended to be managed conservatively with appropriate caution so that patients with suggestive features are surgically assessed promptly (Azzopardi et al., 2014). This collaborative paradigm is critical to optimizing patient outcomes since the management of cystic lesions relies significantly on personal risk assessment and evolving knowledge about these complex structures. This degree of diagnostic intensity and imaging modality highlights the need for ongoing research and guideline revision in this rapidly changing body of research.

5.4. Malignant Potential of Cystic Neoplasms

The prognostic potential for malignancy of pancreatic cystic neoplasms is a significant consideration in both diagnosis and treatment. The difference between various types of neoplasms, particularly serous and mucinous neoplasms, is significant due to their varied prognoses. Mucinous cystic neoplasms, previously classified in most instances as potentially malignant, have had a greater risk of malignant transformation than their serous counterparts, which tend to be benign. High-risk features, including size and cyst wall characteristics, play a pivotal role in clinical management. Based on current guidelines, invasive interventions can be recommended for suspicious features of cysts because they can possess a greater rate of cancer. This high appreciation of cystic neoplasms not only guides treatment interventions but also indicates the importance of surveillance strategies in monitoring changes over time.

IPMNs are a unique group with deep significance regarding malignancy. This subtype is frequently separated into high-risk and low-risk groups according to criteria established, most importantly the Fukuoka criteria. Studies have shown that patients in the high-risk group, with features such as main duct involvement or mural nodules, have significantly greater rates of pancreatic cancer compared with patients with features in the low-risk group. Specifically, the cumulative incidence of pancreatic cancer can be as high as 28% during a seven-year follow-up in high-risk patients, whereas it is a meager 1.2% in their low-risk counterparts. The grim reality is brought out by these figures, and it underscores the importance of meticulous follow-up and early surgical intervention when necessary, as early diagnosis and treatment can actually enhance the prognosis of such patients (Lawson et al., 2015). Management strategies for pancreatic cystic neoplasms have been guided to a significant extent by the understanding of malignancy potential. Suggestions support resection in solid pseudopapillary tumors and mucinous neoplasms if there are observed malignancy risk factors. Branch duct IPMNs with nonsuspicious features, however, can be monitored with follow-up, provided they are asymptomatic and less than predetermined size limits. The challenge lies in properly choosing those lesions that require urgent surgical intervention and those that can be safely observed. As emphasized in recent literature, it is persistent attention to the nature of such neoplasms that is central to quality clinical practice. The continued evolution of imaging techniques and improved knowledge of cancer risk factors will certainly further simplify these management strategies, allowing for more individualized and effective patient treatment (Azzopardi et al., 2014) (Figure 5.10).

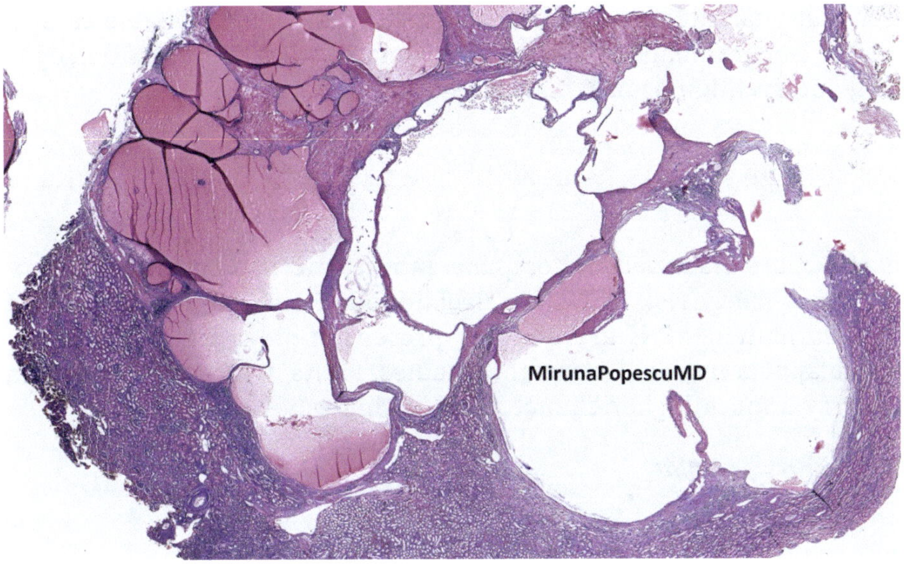

Figure 5.10. Multilocular cystic renal neoplasm of low malignant potential.

Source: https://objektyv-production.s3.amazonaws.com/media/13186/thumbnails/1670771000MCRNLMP%20kiko%201.jpg.

5.4.1. Factors Influencing Malignant Transformation

The likelihood of malignancy of pancreatic cystic neoplasms, particularly mucinous and IPMNs, is highly influenced by several factors including type of cyst, presenting features, and radiological features. Mucinous cystic neoplasms have shown a high propensity towards malignant change, hence the need for intense monitoring and optimal management. Recommendations are for resection of high-risk lesions showing features such as main duct involvement or mural nodules, while asymptomatic branch duct IPMNs without such features may be watched conservatively (Azzopardi et al., 2014). Diagnostic imaging technology has advanced to the extent that these lesions can increasingly be detected, which allows medical practitioners to better assess their risk of malignancy and make the best surveillance options. Fukuoka criteria, which apply symptomatic and imaging features to classify cysts, have an influence that cannot be overstated in the context of malignant transformation. Dividing patients into highest-risk and lowest-risk groups significantly directs clinical management decisions about BD-IPMNs. Studies have found that cumulative pancreatic cancer incidence is much higher in patients who were in the highest-risk group, with 7-year cancer incidence being 28% compared with 1.2% in those who were in the lowest-risk group (Lawson et al., 2015). Such stratification not only calls attention to the importance of early recognition of concerning features but also emphasizes the need for ongoing monitoring and early intervention, in an effort to improve patient outcomes by focusing on those with the highest risk. Finally, patient populations and clinical histories also play crucial roles in interpreting the variables involved in the malignant transformation of pancreatic cystic neoplasms. Age, gender, family background, and the presence of underlying pancreatic diseases or conditions affect the likelihood of neoplasias becoming malignancies. Additionally, recent studies show that genetic markers may also prove to be useful predictors of malignant conversion. It is the comprehension of such dynamic factors that plays a central role in the creation of a tailored surveillance program compatible with the risk profiles identified, but guaranteeing that patients receive the best available care. Taken together, these results inform a more nuanced strategy to manage pancreatic cystic neoplasms, weighing prudence for early intervention against unnecessary intervention.

5.4.2. Comparison of Serous and Mucinous Neoplasms in Terms of Malignancy

Both SCNs and MCNs are classified under pancreatic cystic neoplasms, but they are not alike when it comes to malignancy risk. SCNs are usually found as benign tumors with minimal risk for malignant transformation. SCNs are typically present in older females and are characterized by their honeycomb appearance under imaging studies. MCNs, which also predominantly occur in female patients, carry a much higher chance of becoming cancerous.

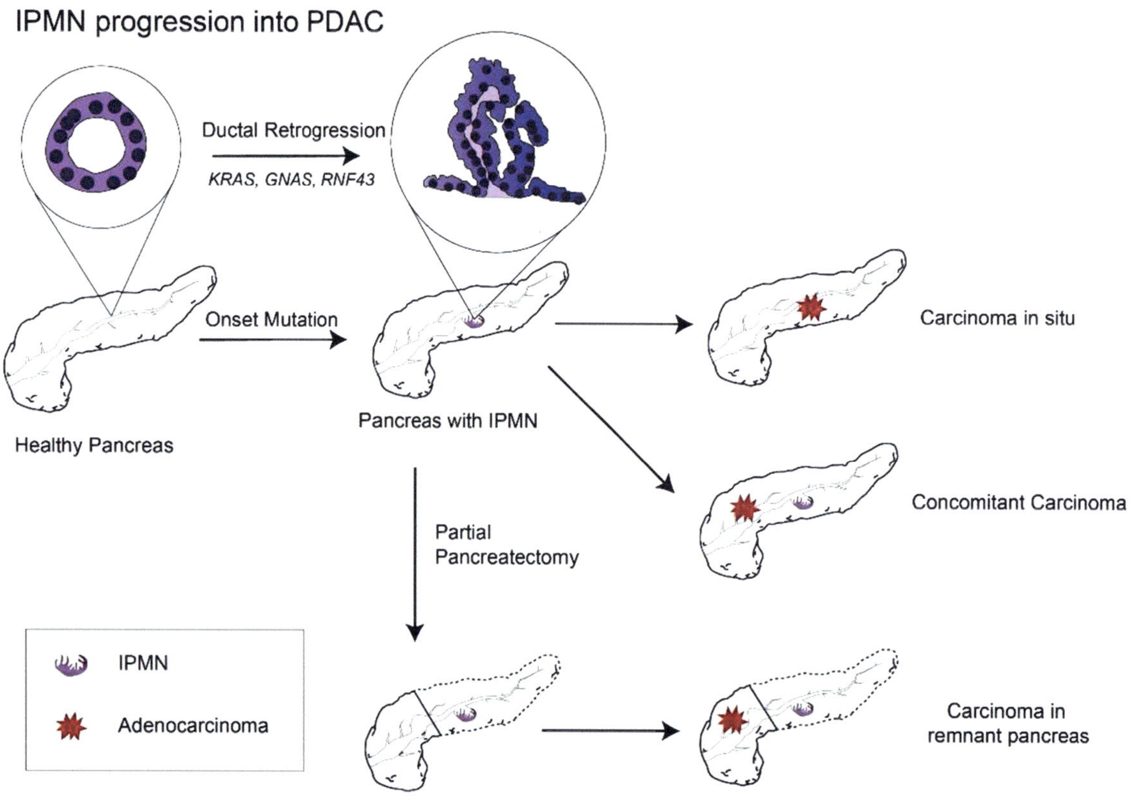

Figure 5.11. IPMN progression into PDAC.

Source: Li J, Wei T, Zhang J, Liang T. Intraductal Papillary Mucinous Neoplasms of the Pancreas: A Review of Their Genetic Characteristics and Mouse Models. *Cancers*. 2021; 13(21):5296. https://doi.org/10.3390/cancers13215296

The malignant potential of MCNs is exacerbated by the presence of certain histologic features, such as atypical cells or invasive components, which need close follow-up and, in the vast majority, surgical resection to avoid the development of invasive pancreatic cancer. Recognition of these fundamental differences is essential in guiding management and treatment decisions in patients with these distinct neoplastic lesions. The intracystic dynamics of IPMNs further contribute to the intricacy of pancreatic cystic neoplasms. Unlike SCNs and MCNs, IPMNs carry a recognized predisposition towards malignant transformation, which is stratified by various clinical and imaging determinants. High-risk stigmata according to the Fukuoka criteria are associated with a significantly elevated risk of malignancy and are predicted to be present in up to 28% of cases with cancer on a seven-year follow-up after diagnosis. Unlike for serous neoplasms, the malignant potential of IPMNs is highly variable according to morphologic and cytologic features. This heterogeneity emphasizes the need to implement stringent surveillance guidelines and stratify patients based on known risk factors to allow early intervention when malignant transformation happens (Lawson et al., 2015), thus optimizing patient outcomes for pancreatic neoplasms. The management strategy for serous versus mucinous neoplasms is actually determined by their different malignancy patterns. In SCNs, the conservative method is normally sufficient because the lesions never need to be treated surgically unless symptomatic or questionable diagnosis. In MCNs, particularly those with challenging appearances or large dimensions, surgical excision is advocated because of their intrinsic potential to undergo malignant change (Fischer & Wood, 2018). This therapeutic paradigm disparity reflects the need for distinct approaches based on the specific cystic neoplasm and the direct involvement of imaging and histopathologic assessment in decision-making. In addition, lifelong surveillance policies are now highlighted more strongly for patients with MCNs and IPMNs to alert them to any malignant transformation early on, further establishing the importance of an educated and proactive strategy to the treatment of pancreatic cystic neoplasms (Figure 5.11).

5.4.3. Role of Genetic Mutations in Malignancy Risk

Knowledge of the genetic mutation's involvement in pancreatic cystic neoplasms is key in identifying the risk of malignancy. IPMNs, in particular, are significant markers of susceptibility to pancreatic cancer because they can develop neoplasms. The key oncogenic drivers of such lesions are KRAS and GNAS mutations, which are present in low-grade dysplastic lesions that have a propensity to progress to high-grade or invasive carcinoma. The stability of the mutations underscores the importance of vigilant monitoring to pre-empt the diagnosis of malignant transformation. Emerging evidence in molecular pathology suggests that additional genes participating in the tumorigenesis of IPMNs have been identified through whole exome sequencing, confirming the multifactorial nature of the contribution of genetics to the malignancy risk of pancreatic neoplasms (Hu et al., 2024). Moreover, the molecular character of pancreatic cystic lesions has become increasingly complicated with the discoveries of genetic heterogeneity. IPMNs tend to have multiclonal and multifocal morphology, each with a distinct genetic signature that renders risk stratification and management difficult. The genetic heterogeneity necessitates building elaborate surveillance protocols based on individual patient profiles. With further studies, the focus on genetic mutations will be an absolute determinant in the identification of high-risk lesions and the selection of appropriate intervention modalities. The merger of genetic studies with advanced imaging techniques can complement new algorithms, allowing personalized monitoring and therapeutic plans in high-risk patients for the onset of pancreatic cancer (Mormul et al., 2023). Pancreatic cystic neoplasms, particularly IPMNs, require long-term follow-up based on the understanding of the involved genetic mutations leading to malignant transformation. With the risk that low-grade lesions have of progressing to high-grade dysplasia or invasive carcinoma, clinicians must adopt an in-depth risk-stratification plan. The recent identification of new genes implicated in IPMN pathogenesis has broadened the framework for following malignancy risk. Especially, this molecular information not only dictates disease pathology insight but also actionable data to enhance patient outcomes with tailored surveillance plans. With an emphasis on genetic markers, healthcare practitioners are then well-placed to address the complexities that come with cystic neoplasms and extend intervention promptly, thus avoiding malignancy in groups at high risk (Mormul et al., 2023; Hu et al., 2024).

5.5. Surveillance Strategies

Effective surveillance strategies for pancreatic cystic neoplasms are instrumental in the prompt detection and treatment of the possible malignancies. The need for systematic surveillance is largely because of the various malignant potential of various types of cysts. SCNs, for instance, are largely benign and often do not require intense surveillance. IPMNs, however, are very challenging because of their heterogeneity and varying risk of progression into pancreatic cancer. Research advises a careful and considered assessment of cyst characteristics and patient history in order to risk-stratify patients according to their individual risk profiles, necessitating a more tailored approach to imaging and clinical assessment at follow-up periods, particularly for larger mural nodules or ductal dilatation (Fischer & Wood, 2018).

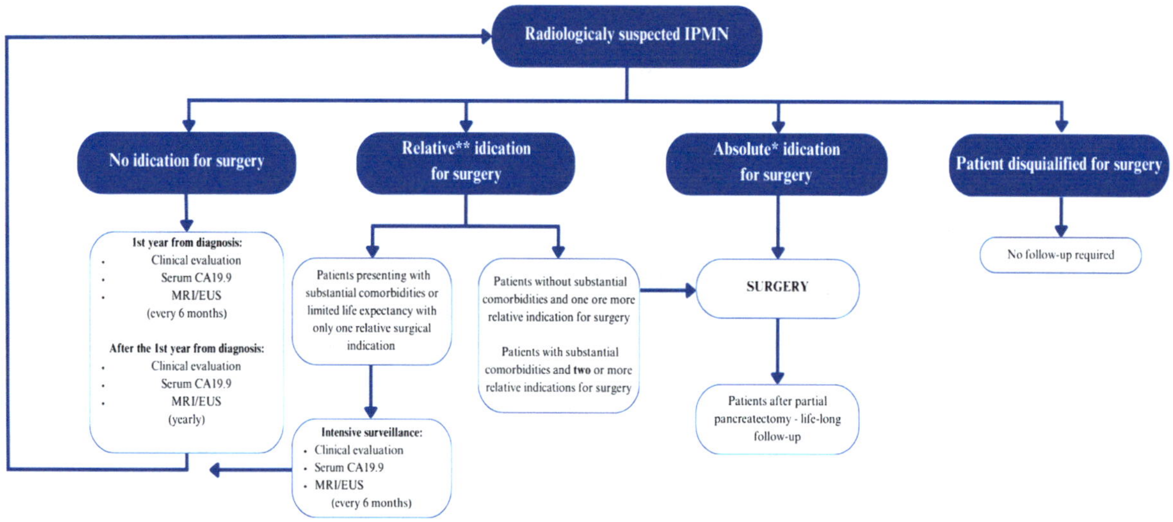

Figure 5.12. Diagnostics and management of pancreatic cystic lesions.

Source: Rogowska J, Semeradt J, Durko Ł, Małecka-Wojciesko E. Diagnostics and Management of Pancreatic Cystic Lesions—New Techniques and Guidelines. *Journal of Clinical Medicine*. 2024; 13(16):4644. https://doi.org/10.3390/jcm13164644

The deployment of next-generation imaging modalities plays a fundamental role in optimal surveillance of pancreatic cysts. Imaging studies such as MRI and EUS are absolutely vital in the follow-up of cystic lesions, providing typical information regarding cyst morphology and, potentially, evolution over time. The integration of these imaging technologies allows clinicians to detect subtle alterations that indicate malignant transformation. Furthermore, the detection of biomarkers through cyst fluid analysis can enhance the specificity of surveillance regimens. While cytological examinations have been generally indeterminate in the past, recent proteomic research offers promising avenues for the discovery of protein markers of malignancy in cystic neoplasms (Kwon

& Simeone, 2011). This novel paradigm for surveillance emphasizes the importance of periodic reevaluation in the treatment of clinical decisions. Follow-up long-term is particularly emphasized in the treatment of patients with diagnosed IPMNs due to the high risk of malignant transformation associated with such lesions. Recommendations in the current era promote conservative management of asymptomatic IPMNs, particularly lesions less than 4 cm in diameter. Yet, symptomatic or larger lesions or lesions with high-risk features should be treated surgically. According to the guidelines, continuous monitoring should be performed for the patients, with the interval determined depending on the presence and development of suspicious features like mural nodules or main pancreatic duct dilatation. Central, however, to such evidence-based recommendations is their aim to minimize the risk of progression while not diminishing the effectiveness of related overtreatment morbidity (Fischer & Wood, 2018). With ongoing research and the development of new biomarkers, the sensitivity of surveillance paradigms will play a key role in maximizing outcomes in individuals with various types of pancreatic cystic neoplasms (Figure 5.12).

5.5.1. Guidelines for Monitoring Cystic Neoplasms

Pancreatic cystic neoplasms, particularly IPMNs and SCNs, need regular follow-up since they possess varying malignant potential. The guidelines emphasize the detection of high-risk and low-risk cysts, particularly since the former may have the potential to become pancreatic cancer if not treated in a manner appropriate. Current guidelines suggest following patients with IPMNs who possess particular high-risk features, such as MPD dilatation and increased serum CA 19-9, with periodic imaging to facilitate early malignant transformation diagnosis. The high-risk features play a crucial role in determining whether intervention through surgery or observation is necessary, highlighting the importance of establishing individualized surveillance strategies to promote optimal patient outcomes. Monitoring practices are, therefore, crucial in a bid to counteract the dire morbidity and mortality of pancreatic cancers at advanced stages of presentation (Ateeb, 2023).

The incorporation of systematic imaging protocols, particularly through EUS, has been highlighted in the guidelines as a key step towards monitoring cystic neoplasms. EUS facilitates the accurate characterization of cystic lesions and improves the likelihood of achieving cyst fluid for further evaluation. The current focus on metabolomics and biomarker studies, as evident from the literature, promises to enhance diagnostic sensitivity and malignant risk stratification of pancreatic cysts. For instance, studies have been able to prove that it is possible to differentiate benign and malignant lesions with high accuracy through the use of metabolomic profiling and, hence implement it in the clinical setting. Furthermore, the integration of cytological examination of cyst fluid with EUS also guides management further by identifying markers of aggressiveness in the lesion so that unnecessary surgery is avoided in benign cysts, while high-risk patients are treated early (Antunes., 2020). Follow-up and surveillance in patients with cystic neoplasms are also extremely crucial, particularly in those patients with a history of high-grade dysplasia or known IPMNs. The guidelines propose an approach based on early results, such that patients with low-grade dysplasia are imaged less often and patients with signs of concern imaged in accordance with more aggressive monitoring regimens. Most importantly, new evidence shows that small changes in the features of the cysts, even a slight enlargement of MPD diameter, can presage a change in the risk profile of a cyst. Thus, there needs to be an active and responsive management of cystic neoplasms. This addresses not only the individualized cancer risk of the patient but also broad goals of early treatment and diagnosis, thereby culminating in survival improvement and improving the quality of life of the patient affected by pancreatic neoplasms (Ateeb, 2023) (Figure 5.13).

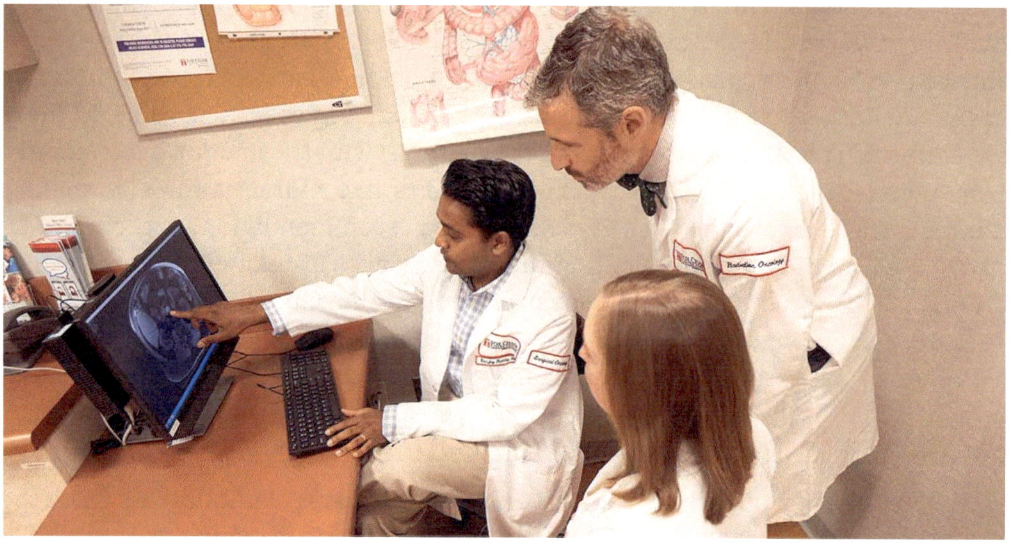

Figure 5.13. Pancreatic cyst treatment option.

Source: https://www.foxchase.org/sites/default/files/assets/Multidisciplinary-Care-Pancreatic-Reddy-Meyers_1200x630.jpg.

5.5.2. Role of Imaging in Surveillance

Imaging is central to the monitoring of cystic neoplasms of the pancreas, especially the discrimination between cyst types, including serous and mucinous neoplasms, and their subtypes, including IPMNs. Ultrasound, CT, and MRI are some of the techniques that yield valuable information about cyst morphology, size, and the presence of malignancy markers. Effective surveillance requires a particular imaging approach so that clinicians are able to monitor changes in cyst appearance over time, as indicated by the risk of malignant transformation. Because certain features recorded on imaging—wall irregularity and solid components, are signs of the risk of malignancy, careful evaluation is important in guiding management decisions as well as in determining the need for surgical intervention (Fischer & Wood, 2018). The European evidence-based guidelines for pancreatic cystic neoplasms emphasize the utility of multimodal imaging in combination with clinical assessments in an effort to obtain optimal patient outcomes. An example is that follow-up imaging should be recommended for asymptomatic mucinous neoplasms and IPMNs less than 40 mm in size to allow observation non-invasively rather than their removal surgically immediately (Marc et al., 2018). Given that the malignant risk of such neoplasms varies, awareness of the typical appearance of these lesions is essential in establishing surveillance policies. Radiographic findings, i.e., interval change in cyst size or new development of features, are components of identifying the need for more aggressive investigation, such as endoscopic ultrasonography or biopsy for cyst fluid aspiration and additional diagnostic evaluation. The addition of new imaging modalities can further enhance the accuracy of diagnosis of cystic neoplasms, particularly between benign and malignant. Coupling proteomics and new biomarker analysis with new imaging can enable layered treatment of patients. By using liquid biopsies and protein profiling within cyst fluid, clinicians may obtain useful information beyond imaging alone. As evidence continues to validate the utility of such new biomarkers, there is real hope to incorporate protein-based diagnostic testing into routine surveillance protocols and ultimately decomplicate risk stratification of patients with pancreatic cystic neoplasms. Such multiparametric surveillance can significantly improve patient management by enabling appropriate timely intervention in some cases and reassurance for those at lower risk (Figure 5.14).

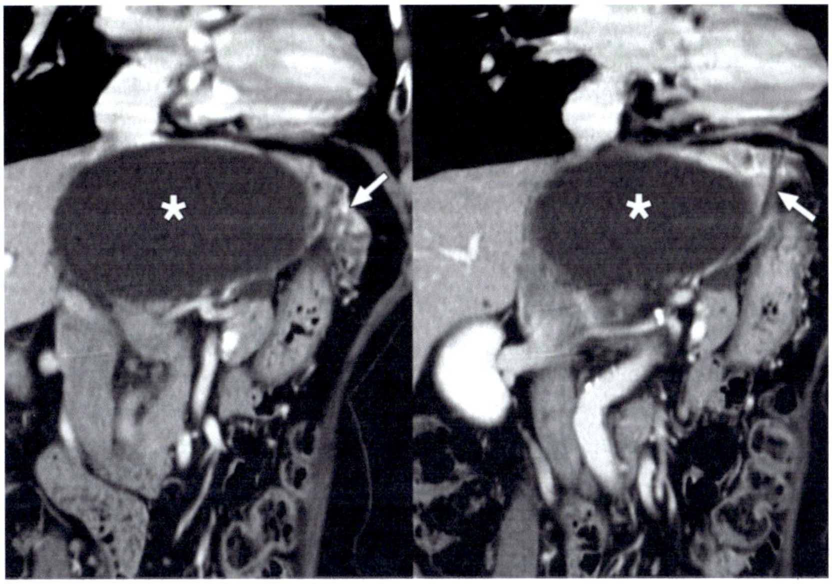

Figure 5.14. Differentiation between biliary cystic neoplasms.

Source: https://www.ajronline.org/cms/10.2214/AJR.09.4026/asset/images/11_09_4026_01b.jpeg.

5.5.3. Importance of Multidisciplinary Approach in Management

The management of pancreatic cystic neoplasms, particularly the differentiation between mucinous and serous types, underlines the utmost significance of a multidisciplinary strategy. This strategy includes the integration of diverse expertise, including surgeons, radiologists, pathologists, and gastroenterologists, each with their unique special knowledge and data required for accurate diagnosis and planning of therapy. For instance, standardized and evidence-based recommendations, as elaborated in European consensus statements, emphasize the imperative of cooperative care in the decision-making for the appropriate management strategy for various cystic neoplasms, especially IPMN. The coordination among experts not only directs surveillance and surgical decisions but also facilitates overall evaluation of the unique risk factors of each patient, enhancing patient outcomes overall (Fischer & Wood, 2018). In the management of asymptomatic pancreatic cysts, a multidisciplinary strategy becomes more applicable. Research illustrates that outcomes may range substantially based on complete assessments in which the analysis of cyst fluid and imaging studies is incorporated. By bringing together specialists who can analyze and interpret these results collectively, healthcare providers are able to devise forward-looking and individualized management strategies. More specifically, recommendations advise follow-up of asymptomatic mucinous cystic neoplasms less than 1.5 cm in size as larger neoplasms are more likely to develop into malignancy. This nuanced finding is based on shared experience and expertise across specialties, attesting to the value of comprehensive patient assessment in practice (Morris-Stiff et al., 2013). In addition, the multidisciplinary approach ensures constant sharing in the discussion of the dynamic evolution of pancreatic cystic lesions. With advancements in imaging modalities and increased insight into the malignant character of numerous neoplasms, collaboration allows continued refinement of management algorithms. Continuous case discussion and joint assessment make revisions of treatment guidelines feasible with the emergence of new evidence, allowing evidence-based care responsive to the heterogeneity of pancreatic pathologies. Lastly, adopting a multidisciplinary approach to practice not only ensures all aspects of patient care are addressed but also fosters a culture of collaborative learning and adaptation required by the challenges associated with managing pancreatic cystic neoplasms.

5.6. Current Research and Advances

Recent research endeavors towards cystic neoplasms of the pancreas have highlighted significant improvements in diagnostic strategies and therapeutic modalities. Particular emphasis has been laid on the differentiation between the various subtypes of PCNs, i.e., SCN, MCN, and IPMN. The problem of dependable differential diagnosis of these lesions before intervention is still of prime importance in light of their diversified malignant potentials. Present studies employing newer imaging modalities, such as CT and MRI, aim to maximize diagnostic performance. Further, the integration of clinical-radiologic parameters with newer radiomics analysis has also been promising and has given rise to models with the ability to distinguish these neoplasms and improve prognostication. The validation of effective diagnostic tools is thus critical to direct therapy and enable personalized care (Vargas et al., 2024). With advancements in diagnostic methods, ablative thermo therapies, particularly EUS-guided ablation, are also emerging as significant alternatives to traditional surgery for managing precancerous pancreatic cysts.

The EUS-guided ablation allows minimal access to therapy methods with different modalities such as alcohol, chemotherapy drugs, and radiofrequency ablation. Studies have shown that these techniques can achieve cyst resolution in a significant proportion of treated patients, making EUS-guided ablation an option for patients who cannot undergo surgical resection. This new technique is not only used to treat cystic neoplasms but is also showing effectiveness in the initial therapy of pancreatic cancer. With more research, the safety and effectiveness of EUS-guided ablation are being increasingly clarified, promising improved management for these challenging conditions (Vargas et al., 2024). The rapidly expanding field of pancreatic cystic neoplasm research also underscores the importance of regular follow-up, particularly in those patients who have been diagnosed with low-risk cysts such as SCN. Although MCN and IPMN both require surgical intervention due to their malignant potential, SCN merely requires serial surveillance to determine any change in size or characteristics. Future studies suggest standardized surveillance protocols to better define patients who may need intensified follow-up or intervention. The addition of radiomics to surveillance protocols may also further refine risk stratification to better enhance patient outcomes. With improving comprehension of the biology and behavior of numerous cystic neoplasms, the aspiration is to optimize management strategy based on the individual patient profile—the risk of malignancy versus avoiding invasive therapy (Zhang et al., 2023) (Figure 5.15).

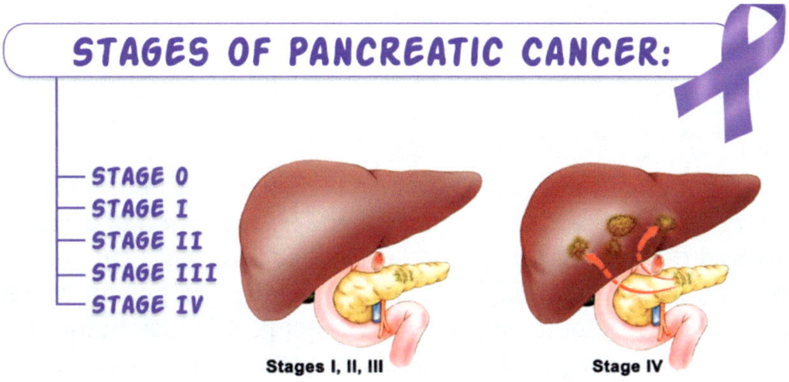

Figure 5.15. Stages-of-pancreatic-cancer.

Source: https://drkapendra.com.np/wp-content/uploads/2023/03/stages-of-Pancreatic-Cancer-1024x576.png.

5.6.1. Emerging Therapies and Treatment Options

New therapies and treatment strategies for pancreatic cystic neoplasms are essential in their ability to solve the complex nature of malignancies because they are at the juncture of the challenge of diagnosis and the challenge of treatment. One novel solution is the utilization of targeted molecular therapies, which aim to take advantage of certain genetic mutations prevalent in pancreatic neoplasms. Current research has identified gene mutations such as KRAS that are commonly mutated in the serous and mucinous neoplasms. Such targeted therapies have been encouraging in initial clinical trials, and this implies that a genetic profiling-driven personalized treatment regimen can optimize the therapeutic result. Further, advances in immunotherapy have raised hopes, especially among IPMN patients, since such treatment is likely to activate the patient's immune system against cancer cells, with a potential effect on the overall survival rate in heavily pretreated individuals (Tonini et al., 2021). Further, novel imaging modalities are transforming pancreatic cystic neoplasm surveillance and early detection. As emphasized by recent reviews, the integration of advanced imaging modalities such as MRI with contrast-enhanced techniques and EUS is important in differentiating benign versus malignant cysts. Enhanced imaging strategies aid clinicians in arriving at more precise decisions for treatment strategy and surveillance protocols, particularly for high-risk patients, including patients with mucinous pancreatic cysts and family histories of pancreatic cancer (Singhi et al., 2019). The ability to adequately characterize cystic neoplasms reduces the risk of unnecessary surgical interventions while enabling early diagnosis of malignant change, thereby optimizing patient results. Finally, tailored surveillance programs are becoming the most important principle in the management of pancreatic cystic neoplasms, particularly in patients classified as high-risk. These programs are often multidisciplinary in scope and involve genetic counseling and meticulous design of overarching management plans based on patient-specific profiles. By utilizing advanced genetic screening and risk stratification techniques, medical professionals can selectively recall patients with a higher risk of malignant evolution based on criteria such as germline mutations or repeated histories of pancreatitis. Along with advancing protocols, fine-tuning of indications for surgical treatment based on radiographic findings as well as biomarker evaluation will be critical to the improvement of prognosis in patients of these challenging neoplasms, ultimately leading to a paradigm in the management of pancreatic disease (Singhi et al., 2019; Tonini et al., 2021).

5.6.2. Recent Findings in Genetic Research

Recent developments in genetic studies have greatly contributed to our knowledge of pancreatic cystic neoplasms. Of particular interest among these is the investigation of certain genetic mutations associated with IPMNs and their malignant potential. Studies show that mutational changes in genes like KRAS, GNAS, and TP53 are commonly detected in IPMNs, proposing a mechanistic route to malignant transformation. These genetic markers not only provide insight into the pathophysiology of cystic neoplasms, but they also provide a basis for the development of targeted molecular therapies. By being able to isolate these mutations through high-level genomic sequencing, clinicians can better stratify patients based on their risk for progression so that individualized treatment decisions can be made that better enhance patient outcomes.

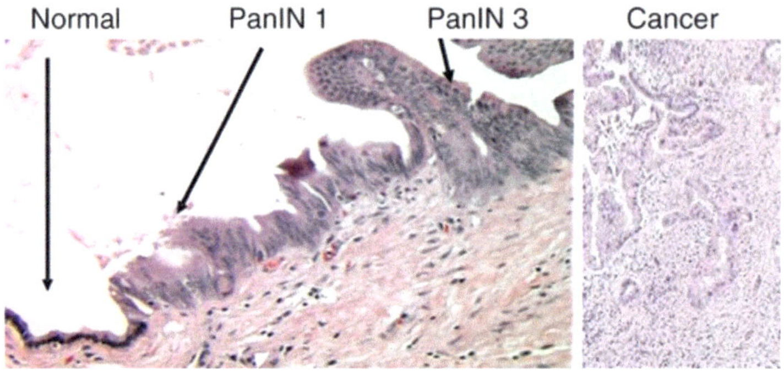

Figure 5.16. Desmoplasia of pancreatic ductal adenocarcinoma (PDAC).

Source: By Palladin_expression_neoplasia.png: see abovederivative work: Nephron T|C - This is a retouched picture, which means that it has been digitally altered from its original version. Modifications: removed reference to 'palladin' -- the micrograph are nice on their own. The original can be viewed here: Palladin expression neoplasia.png: . Modifications made by Nephron., CC BY 1.0, https://commons.wikimedia.org/w/index.php?curid=10486641

In addition, biomarker utility in pancreatic cyst management has been brought into the spotlight, providing insight into significant implications for surveillance and treatment approaches. For instance, the use of carbohydrate antigen 19-9 (CA 19-9) is a key marker in assessing pancreatic lesion behavior, PDAC. Its current application highlights utility beyond diagnostic deficiencies; elevated levels of CA 19-9 can be applied to signify malignancy despite benign pancreatic disease. As in existing literature, the use of glycoproteins is extended to the larger gastrointestinal and even beyond the gastrointestinal context, which suggests that CA 19-9 might play a pivotal role in managing patients in different therapeutic contexts, including potential therapeutic targeting in pancreatic disease (Lee et al., 2020). The integration of genetic biomarkers and advanced machine learning techniques also assists further in streamlining the management of pancreatic cysts. The development of tools like CompCyst is an example of this disciplined process that leverages clinical, imaging, and cyst fluid analysis to facilitate more efficient decision-making processes. From using patient cohort data to train algorithms, researchers have discovered unique profiles that have been found to characterize cysts according to their malignant potential more accurately than traditional criteria. CompCyst not only shows the ability to limit undue procedures but also highlights the evolving role of genetic investigations in optimizing the monitoring of these neoplasms. Ultimately, these developments portend a paradigm shift in the management of pancreatic cysts by practitioners with solutions that optimize the reduction of patient morbidity with minimal healthcare costs (Springer et al., 2019) (Figure 5.16).

5.6.3. Future Directions in the Study of Pancreatic Cystic Neoplasms

Emerging research into pancreatic cystic neoplasms is becoming increasingly interested in developing more precise diagnostic accuracy and therapeutic methods. More recent advances in metabolomics and genomics analysis have opened up promising research paths to distinguishing between serous and mucinous neoplasms, particularly IPMNs. The integration of metabolomic profiling, with the ability to detect small biochemical variations in cystic fluid, adds predictive value to the degree of dysplasia found in these lesions. As postulated in recent studies, some metabolites could potentially act as biomarkers to differentiate between low-risk and high-risk cysts and thereby inform clinical management and surveillance policy. This is an important step towards precision pancreatic oncology for early and precise detection of pre-malignant lesions, especially because advanced pancreatic cancer is associated with a dismal prognosis (Ateeb, 2023). Future advances also encompass the application of newer imaging modalities, including Endoscopic Ultrasound with Fine-needle Aspiration (EUS-FNA), which have been demonstrated to be highly effective in obtaining useful cytological and biochemical information. Recent research indicates that EUS-FNA not only raises the diagnostic yield for cystic neoplasms but also has the potential to detect individual alterations that can potentially be used to predict malignancy. Moreover, the addition of molecular marker analysis of mutations in KRAS and GNAS to routine assessments would further improve diagnostic accuracy to allow more tailored management practices. This proactive stance underscores the need for the adoption of a multi-disciplinary model to optimize patient outcomes by balancing the need to intervene surgically with the risks of over-treatment of benign lesions (Antunes., 2020). Lastly, the future of pancreatic cystic neoplasm research will probably be marked by a focus on thorough surveillance regimens after resection. Results indicate that even low-grade dysplastic lesion patients have a significant rate of recurrence, and thus, stringent follow-up becomes critical. Subsequent studies must clarify the exact risk factors that lead to recurrence and malignant degeneration in these individuals. They should also explore the clinical utility and cost-effectiveness of intensified monitoring approaches under the guidance of established biomarkers and imaging modalities. Evidence-based monitoring protocols empowerment of patients with IPMNs will not only improve early detection of malignancy transformation but might also maximize therapy approaches, ultimately improving patient outcomes against this challenging disease (Ateeb, 2023).

A CLOSER LOOK

PREVALENCE, DIAGNOSIS, AND MANAGEMENT OF PANCREATIC CYSTIC NEOPLASMS (PCNS)

PCNs are increasingly found with the widespread application of high-resolution imaging modalities such as CT and MRI. Their frequency in the general population is 2%–13 %, which rises with age, particularly above the age of 60 years. There are multiple subtypes of cystic tumors with varying malignant potential, of which the most common include SCNs, MCNs, IPMNs, and SPNs. SCNs are typically benign with little follow-up, while MCNs and IPMNs are mucinous and highly malignant when transformed, especially the main duct type IPMN. PCN diagnosis relies on imaging tests coupled with fluid analysis. Cross-sectional imaging, such as MRI with MRCP, is best suited to assess cyst communication with the pancreatic duct and internal structure evaluation, such as septations and mural nodules. EUS with FNA plays a crucial role in cyst fluid sampling for analysis of levels of CEA, amylase content, cytology, and molecular markers such as KRAS and GNAS mutations that differentiate mucinous from non-mucinous cysts. Treatment of PCNs depends on the type, size, and risk factors of the cyst. Low-risk cysts, particularly small branch-duct IPMNs without worrisome features, can typically be managed with follow-up on serial imaging, while high-risk cysts—those with mural nodules, dilatation of the main pancreatic duct, or positive cytology—typically require surgical resection. Surgical approaches include pancreaticoduodenectomy (Whipple procedure) for lesions in the head and distal pancreatectomy for body or tail lesions. Enucleation is appropriate in some cases for low-risk lesions. Postoperative follow-up is tailored based on final pathology, especially if there is high-grade dysplasia or invasive carcinoma. Biomarkers and newer imaging technologies like radiomics and artificial intelligence are going to improve diagnostic accuracy and individualized management plans for pancreatic cystic neoplasms in future research.

SUMMARY

The complex nature of pancreatic cystic neoplasms, particularly the distinction between serous and mucinous types, underscores the need for meticulous diagnosis and planning for therapy. Serous neoplasms are typically benign, while mucinous types, particularly IPMNs, have a high risk of malignant transformation. The Mayo Clinic and other institutions have highlighted the utility of imaging modalities, such as MRI, in identifying potentially malignant features of these lesions. As outlined, branch-duct IPMNs illustrate the challenge in management, with a need for an individualized approach to each patient based on individual risk factors and imaging characteristics, which underlines the necessity for an interdisciplinary clinical approach to making treatment decisions (Minelli et al., 2023). The new recognition of IPMNs' malignant potential emphasizes the pressing need for early diagnosis and surveillance measures. As pancreatic cancer is increasingly becoming recognized as a major cause of cancer death, strategies for the detection of precursor lesions like IPMN have become of utmost importance. It has been reported that MPD dilation and elevated levels of CA 19-9 are related to higher risks of advanced histological outcomes and malignancy (Ateeb, 2023). Therefore, IPMNs, especially those with suggestive features, should be closely followed so that intervention may be initiated at the proper time. The capability of imaging and metabolic profiling to provide information about the nature of such neoplasms is a sophisticated step in clinical practice. Moreover, follow-up after surgery in patients with previously resected IPMN is indicated because surveillance reveals a strong risk of recurrence. Research has indicated that the grade of dysplasia at initial diagnosis affects malignant transformation risk significantly, especially among those with low-grade or high-grade dysplasia without correlated PDAC (Ateeb, 2023). What this indicates is that patients must be extremely vigilant following resection, and it illustrates the need for further research regarding dynamic surveillance protocols capable of addressing patient-specific pathways. Ongoing investigation into the metabolic profiles may continue to enhance diagnostic accuracy, and therapeutic interventions are feasible, with better outcomes for patients with pancreatic cystic neoplasms.

The literature on cystic neoplasms of the pancreas highlights a significant distinction between serous and mucinous neoplasms, significantly placing IPMN into focus due to their malignant nature. Widespread use of advanced imaging modalities has led to an increase in the incidental detection of these tumors, requiring accuracy in diagnosis and risk stratification. Some radiologic features, such as MPD dilatation, have been shown by research to be important indicators of risk for malignancy in IPMN. For instance, MPD dilatation of more than 5 mm suggests high likelihood of high-grade dysplasia or carcinoma and provides additional support for clinical vigilance within surveillance protocols to detect early malignant change, according to Ateeb (2023). In addition to radiological features, new technologies in metabolomics and biomarker analysis also promise to increase diagnostic accuracy in the distinction between cystic malignancy and benign cystic lesions. Cyst fluid and plasma metabolomic profiling is a significant development in clinical practice. Not only does this research unlock the application of non-invasive diagnostic tests, but it also the determination of typical metabolic profiles that are linked to the histological grade of dysplasia. For instance, studies have indicated that certain metabolite levels can be used to predict the severity of dysplasia in IPMNs, which points towards a potential future where management would be guided by metabolomic analysis and unnecessary surgeries would be avoided, as well as being debated in Antunes. (2020). Moreover, the need for regular surveillance and follow-up in IPMN patients cannot be overestimated. Studies have indicated a high recurrence rate of these lesions following surgery, with clinical management strategies still under development. There is evidence to indicate that patients with low-grade dysplasia (LGD) or high-grade dysplasia (HGD) are at high risk for malignant transformation, and strict follow-up regimens are required. Notably, age is an important predictor of recurrence risk, which requires personalized surveillance regimens in elderly patients or those with baseline IPMN. Thus, an integrated strategy combining radiological, metabolic, and clinical assessments is needed to maximize patient results and minimize the economic impact of this rapidly expanding disease, summarizing the key points offered in this comprehensive review of pancreatic cystic neoplasms.

KEY TERMS FROM THIS CHAPTER

- Abundant mucin production
- Carcinoembryonic antigen (CEA)
- Clinical lesions
- Intraductal papillary mucinous neoplasms
- Microcystic lesions
- Neoplastic cells
- Pancreatic cancer
- Serous cystic neoplasms (SCN)
- Tiny cystic spaces
- Biological behaviors
- Chemotherapy drugs
- Cystic morphology
- Main pancreatic duct (MPD)
- Neoplasms
- Neoplastic character
- Serous cystadenomas
- Surgical treatment

References

1. Antunes, S. de J. R. F. (2020). *Biomarkers for Classification and Risk Assessment of Pancreatic Cystic Neoplasms* [Doctoral dissertation]. https://core.ac.uk/download/401085509.pdf (accessed on 26 May 2025).
2. Ateeb, Zeeshan (2022). Improvement of the diagnosis and management of cystic tumors of the pancreas. Karolinska Institutet. Thesis. https://hdl.handle.net/10616/48416 (accessed on 26 May 2025).
3. Azzopardi, N. (2014). *Cystic Lesions of the Pancreas* [Doctoral dissertation]. https://core.ac.uk/download/46602499.pdf (accessed on 26 May 2025).
4. Minelli, C., Balducci, F., Cavalleri, C., Milanetto, A. C., Ferrara, F., Crimì, F., Quaia, E., & Vernuccio, F. (2023). Intraductal papillary mucinous neoplasms of the pancreas: Uncommon imaging presentation, evolution and comparison of guidelines. *European journal of radiology open*, *11*, 100531. https://doi.org/10.1016/j.ejro.2023.100531 (accessed on 26 May 2025).
5. Besselink, M. B., Bruno, M. J., Cahen, D. L., Cunningham, D., Del Chiaro, M., Gress, T. M., et al. (2018). European evidence-based guidelines on pancreatic cystic neoplasms. https://core.ac.uk/download/575949730.pdf (accessed on 26 May 2025).
6. . Morris-Stiff, G., Falk, G. A., Chalikonda, S., & Walsh, R. M. (2013). Natural history of asymptomatic pancreatic cystic neoplasms. *HPB : the official journal of the International Hepato Pancreato Biliary Association*, *15*(3), 175–181. https://doi.org/10.1111/j.1477-2574.2012.00522.x
7. Lawson, R. D., Hunt, G. C., Giap, A. Q., Krinsky, M. L., Slezak, J., Tang, R. S., Gonzalez, I., Kwong, W. T., Fehmi, S. A., & Savides, T. J. (2015). Pancreatic cysts suspected to be branch duct intraductal papillary mucinous neoplasm without concerning features have low risk for development of pancreatic cancer. *Annals of gastroenterology*, *28*(4), 487–494.
8. Fischer, C. G., & Wood, L. D. (2018). From somatic mutation to early detection: Insights from molecular characterization of pancreatic cancer precursor lesions. *The Journal of Pathology, 246*, 395–404. https://doi.org/10.1002/path.5154.
9. Hu, Y., Jones, D., Esnakula, A., Krishna, S. G., & Chen, W. (2024). Molecular pathology of pancreatic cystic lesions with a focus on malignant progression. *Cancers, 16*. https://www.semanticscholar.org/paper/78e9dfb2e0ba765f0fd8fa05192d2755e7183972 (accessed on 26 May 2025).
10. Kwon, R. S., & Simeone, D. M. (2011). The use of protein-based biomarkers for the diagnosis of cystic tumors of the pancreas. *International journal of proteomics*, *2011*, 413646. https://doi.org/10.1155/2011/413646
11. Lee, T., Teng, T. Z. J., & Shelat, V. G. (2020). Carbohydrate antigen 19-9—tumor marker: Past, present, and future. *World Journal of Gastrointestinal Surgery, 12*, 468–490. https://doi.org/10.4240/wjgs.v12.i12.468.
12. Löhr, M., Domínguez-Muñoz, J. E., Rosendahl, J., Besselink, M. G., Mayerle, J., Lerch, M. M., Haas, S., et al. (2017). United European Gastroenterology evidence-based guidelines for the diagnosis and therapy of chronic pancreatitis (HaPanEU). *United European Gastroenterology Journal, 5*, 153–199. https://doi.org/10.1177/2050640616684695.

13. Mormul, A., Włoszek, E., Nowoszewska, J., Fudalej, M., Budzik, M., Badowska-Kozakiewicz, A., & Deptała, A. (2023). Rare non-neuroendocrine pancreatic tumours. *Cancers, 15*. https://www.semanticscholar.org/paper/d28b4e8fb443349ef0cb082e8ead14a1841f64da (accessed on 26 May 2025).
14. Pollini, T., Andrianello, S., Caravati, A., Perri, G., Malleo, G., Paiella, S., Marchegiani, G., et al. (2019). The management of intraductal papillary mucinous neoplasms of the pancreas. *Minerva Chirurgica, 74*(5), 414–421. https://www.semanticscholar.org/paper/46fa6c15fc7d64b6ef90c958f7264aee10ba1e3d (accessed on 26 May 2025).
15. Shaikh, S. (2021). Editorial for "Abbreviated magnetic resonance imaging with breath-hold 3-dimensional magnetic resonance cholangiopancreatography: Assessment of malignant risks of pancreatic intraductal papillary mucinous neoplasms". *Journal of Magnetic Resonance Imaging, 54*. https://www.semanticscholar.org/paper/5a8a4219e6dbb86860df394c467d0b845db1b35c (accessed on 26 May 2025).
16. Singhi, A. D., Koay, E. J., Chari, S. T., & Maitra, A. (2019). Early detection of pancreatic cancer: Opportunities and challenges. *Gastroenterology, 156*, 2024–2040. https://doi.org/10.1053/j.gastro.2019.01.259.
17. Søreide, K., & Marchegiani, G. (2021). Clinical management of pancreatic premalignant lesions. *Gastroenterology, 162*, 379–384. https://doi.org/10.1053/j.gastro.2021.09.073.
18. Springer, S., Masica, D. L., Dal Molin, M., Douville, C., Thoburn, C., Afsari, B., Li, L., et al. (2019). A multimodality test to guide the management of patients with a pancreatic cyst. *Science Translational Medicine, 11*. https://doi.org/10.1126/scitranslmed.aav4772.
19. Tonini, V., & Zanni, M. (2021). Pancreatic cancer in 2021: What you need to know to win. *World Journal of Gastroenterology, 27*, 5851–5889. https://doi.org/10.3748/wjg.v27.i35.5851.
20. Vargas, A., Dutta, P., Carpenter, E. S., & Machicado, J. D. (2024). Endoscopic ultrasound-guided ablation of premalignant pancreatic cysts and pancreatic cancer. *Diagnostics, 14*, 564. https://doi.org/10.3390/diagnostics14050564.
21. Zhang, Y., Wu, J., He, J., & Xu, S. (2023). Preoperative differentiation of pancreatic cystic neoplasm subtypes on computed tomography radiomics. *Quantitative Imaging in Medicine and Surgery, 13*, 6395–6411. https://doi.org/10.21037/qims-22-1192.

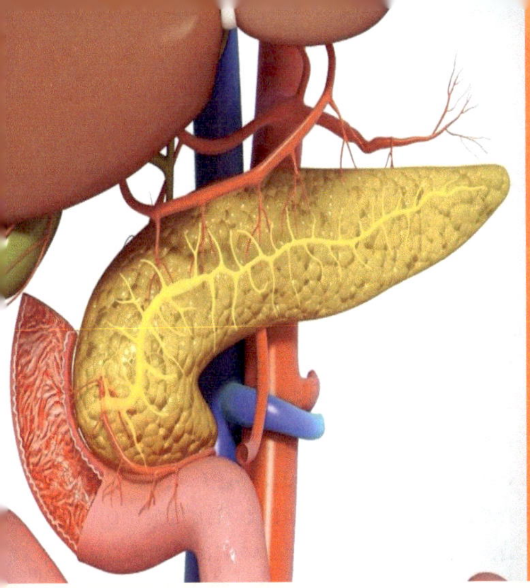

Chapter 6

PANCREATIC CYSTS

Contents

Introduction

The pancreas plays a crucial role in the endocrine and digestive system, but there can be certain abnormalities in this organ, one of which is most commonly pancreatic cysts. These fluid-filled sacs are etiologically and clinically variable and occur as incidental findings on imaging studies or are symptomatic depending upon type and size. Increased imaging modalities, particularly cross-sectional imaging modalities such as computed tomography (CT) and magnetic resonance imaging (MRI), have immensely enhanced the detection of pancreatic cysts and solid tumors. As more information is gained regarding these cysts, differentiation between benign and malignant lesions is important to provide proper intervention and management (Scialpi et al., 2016). Consequently, a solid foundation on the characterization of pancreatic cysts is par for the course in order to improve patient outcomes and inform therapeutic interventions best. Among various pancreatic cysts, Intraductal Papillary Mucinous Neoplasms (IPMNs) stand out for potentially leading to pancreatic cancer. IPMNs are hard to diagnose because they do not show overt symptoms in advance. Therefore, early detection and risk assessment become a function of greater concern. Evidence is in support that the use of advanced imaging technology, including multi-modal MRI, significantly enhances the accuracy of diagnosis in IPMNs (Bagci et al., 2018). Moreover, the integration of artificial intelligence algorithmic approaches, including Convolutional Neural Networks (CNNs), has opened new means to the analysis of imaging data with the view to optimizing diagnostic accuracy. Recognition of the nuances of cystic lesions is not only of value for clinical decision-making, but also highlights the value of ongoing research into optimal diagnostic practices in pancreatic cysts. The worth of separating out pancreatic cysts is not merely in their clinical management, but also in the recognition of their significance regarding pancreatic well-being and associated risks. With the poor outcome of pancreatic cancer, particularly from undetected or inappropriately treated cysts, an interdisciplinary diagnostic and treatment approach cannot be stressed more. Proper evaluation with multimodal imaging modalities like ultrasound, CT, and MRI plays a pivotal role in the management of cystic pancreatic lesions to ensure a better success rate through early detection and treatment (Scialpi et al., 2016). Accordingly, a thorough review of the nature, characteristics, and management of pancreatic cysts forms the foundation of this essay, leading to an in-depth discussion of their clinical significance and advanced trends in the diagnostic process (Figure 6.1).

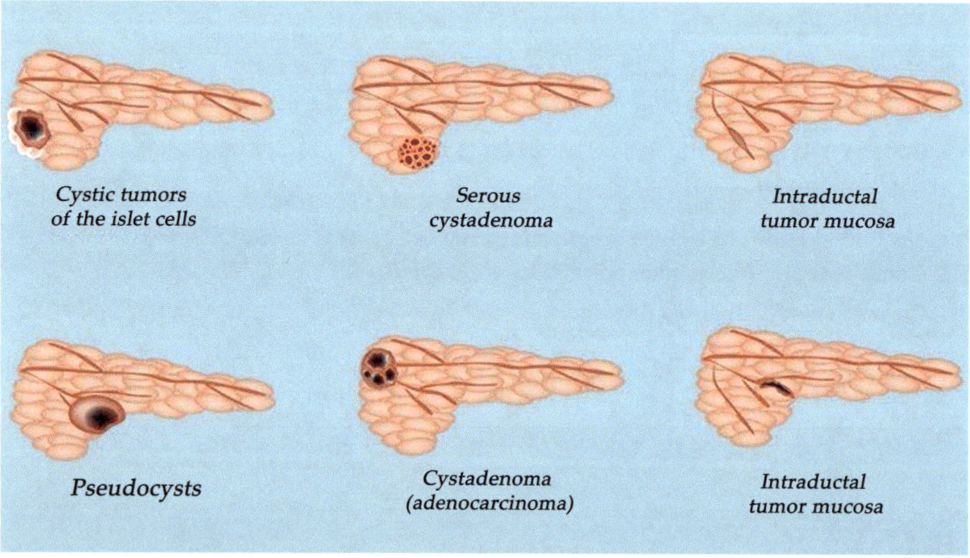

Figure 6.1. Pancreatic cyst.

Source: https://images.everydayhealth.com/images/digestive-health/pancreatitis/what-is-a-pancreatic-cyst-722x406.jpg?sfvrsn=fa1bab39_0.

Definition of Pancreatic Cysts

Pancreatic cysts are fluid-filled cystic spaces that develop in or on the surface of the pancreas, an organ involved in digestion and metabolism. Cysts come in a range of sizes, contents, and potential malignancies. Serous cystadenomas, mucinous cystadenomas, and IPMNs are the most frequent types. Benign cysts are most frequently asymptomatic and are discovered incidentally as part of unconnected imaging exams. However, certain cystic lesions are at a high risk of developing pancreatic cancer, such as mucinous cysts, which need careful monitoring and assessment. These variations highlight the necessity of accurate diagnosis in order to determine the best clinical management strategy for patients found to harbor such cysts (Moyer et al., 2019). The clinical importance of pancreatic cysts extends beyond detection because the potential for malignancy is a dangerous health threat. With increasingly frequent and sensitive cross-sectional imaging modalities, pancreatic cyst detection has risen, which is increasingly becoming a public health problem. It is impossible to distinguish between benign and potentially malignant cysts, and therefore, surveillance and intervention strategies are critical components of patient management.

Redo surgery may be feasible, but with the risk of morbidity, and therefore an exquisite balance between advantage and potential complications must be weighed (Moyer et al., 2019). Accordingly, endoscopic ultrasound-guided chemoablation is a significant departure from modes of treatment, which aim to minimize the risks of such lesions but improve patient safety and overall outcomes.

Pathology of pancreatic cysts also encompasses a variety of differential diagnoses that must be considered during clinical evaluation. While predominantly benign, pancreatic cysts can mimic more dangerous entities, such as gastrointestinal stromal tumors (GISTs), which themselves can be present as cystic abdominal masses. In some cases, these pathologies also involve cystic degeneration, which also complicates diagnosis. Accurate imaging and histological analysis are the way to make the correct diagnosis because they also affect the management approach. Therefore, clinicians are advised to be vigilant in regard to cyst behavior and long-term changes since altered clinical management can become necessary to balance the dynamic nature of such cysts and their potential influence on patient health (Figure 6.2).

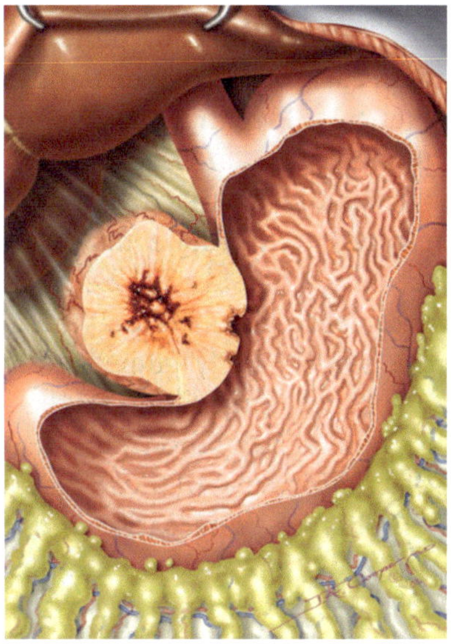

Figure 6.2. Gastrointestinal stromal tumor.

Source: https://external-content.duckduckgo.com/iu/?u=https%3A%2F%2Fpubs.rsna.org%2Fcms%2F10.1148%2Frg.232035901%2Fasset%2Fimages%2Fmedium%2Fg03mr25c1x.jpeg&f=1&nofb=1&ipt=ed43172170a61ba35e00946b75d35e7a276ff20549b79beaafc8a9ffe0780dfe.

Importance of Studying Pancreatic Cysts

Pancreatic cyst investigation is highly necessary due to its potential association with pancreatic cancer, particularly pancreatic ductal adenocarcinoma (PDAC). The cystic neoplasms could be significant indicators of underlying malignancy, and certain of them have intermediate malignant potential. Awareness of the pathophysiology of different pancreatic cysts can lead to early detection and treatment, thereby improving patient outcomes. There is evidence that some patients with benign cystic tumors are at increased risk for the development of PDAC in later years, and therefore, it is imperative to be able to differentiate benign from possible pre-malignant cystic lesions.

Identification of consistent biomarkers for these lesions might enhance early diagnosis and enable the establishment of individualized surveillance plans for individuals at increased risk. Heeding these issues underscores the importance of studying pancreatic cysts as a means to modulate the unpredictable nature of pancreatic malignancies. Furthermore, examination of microRNA (miRNA) expression profiles in pancreatic cysts is capable of offering insights into the first steps of carcinogenesis. Investigation of how specific miRNAs are managed as pancreatic cysts evolve into malignant states can clarify the underlying biological pathways involved in the development of PDAC. For instance, down-regulation of miRNA has been shown on a large scale in PDAC compared to benign cysts, with single miRNAs controlling directly oncogenes that have a major role in transformation (Jiao et al., 2012). By identifying these molecular changes, researchers are not only able to make more accurate diagnostic criteria but can even potentially find therapeutic targets for the treatment of early pancreatic cancer. The inherent diversity of pancreatic cysts calls for a reflective approach, underlined by the value of ongoing research in this field. In addition, pancreatic cyst research brings together multidisciplinary methods, such as genetics, radiology, and molecular biology. The combination of these disciplines allows for an integrated understanding of cystic lesions and their impact on pancreatic function. Characterization of pancreatic cysts can be better done by utilizing newer imaging techniques and genetic markers, allowing for clinical decision-making regarding management and follow-up. By characterizing the biological behavior of the cyst types, the clinician can determine whether surgical treatment is indicated or whether monitoring alone is sufficient. This common platform emphasizes the necessity for constant research to yield data that can impact clinical guidelines and, ultimately, improve patient care in the context of pancreatic illness. In general, the importance of researching pancreatic cysts extends beyond basic diagnosis to encompass a broad spectrum of patient management and therapeutic interventions.

6.1. Types of Pancreatic Cysts

Information regarding the various forms of pancreatic cysts is essential for accurate diagnosis and treatment of pancreatic illness. Intraductal papillary mucinous neoplasm or IPMN is perhaps one of the most significant categories because it carries the potential for transformation into pancreatic cancer. IPMN occurs primarily in two types: main duct and branch duct. The main duct IPMN is characterized by the marked dilation of the main pancreatic duct, whereas the branch duct IPMN depicts the dilatation of the secondary branches resembling a bunch of grapes. Studies indicate IPMN is usually detected in older adults, with a higher incidence in men, approximately age 65. Their anatomical location, frequently in the head of the pancreas, contributes to their clinical relevance, especially considering the risk factors for cancer progression. Another fascinating type of pancreatic cyst is the choledochal cyst, a congenital lesion often diagnosed with inhomogeneous widening of extrahepatic bile ducts. The pathology occurs because of an abnormal common bile and pancreatic duct junction near the sphincter of Oddi, which has led to several different diagnostic classifications, such as the Todani and Komi classifications. These categorizations bring to the forefront the differences in anatomy and provide data regarding the correct surgical and therapeutic interventions. Descriptive imaging techniques like magnetic resonance cholangiopancreatography (MRCP) and endoscopic retrograde cholangiography (ERCP) are critical in visualizing and studying choledochal cysts so that increased anatomical accuracy is achieved for assessment (Lee et al., 2009). The implications of these cysts extend beyond diagnosis; they can be associated with significant complications, and the treatment must be individualized. Pseudocysts are also a common type of pancreatic cyst, and they typically present due to acute pancreatitis or pancreatic injury. Unlike other cystic formations, pseudocysts lack an epithelial lining but instead have fibrous tissue and an inflammatory debris wall. The development of pseudocysts typically follows the extent of interstitial damage to the pancreas and is more common in those with an alcoholic or gallstone history. Symptomatic cysts can present with abdominal pain, nausea, or indeed with complications like infection and rupture and can require surgery. Thus, recognition of the typical characteristics of pseudocysts is crucial for the clinician, as early diagnosis and intervention will ultimately decide patient outcome in relation to the underlying pancreatic pathology (Figure 6.3).

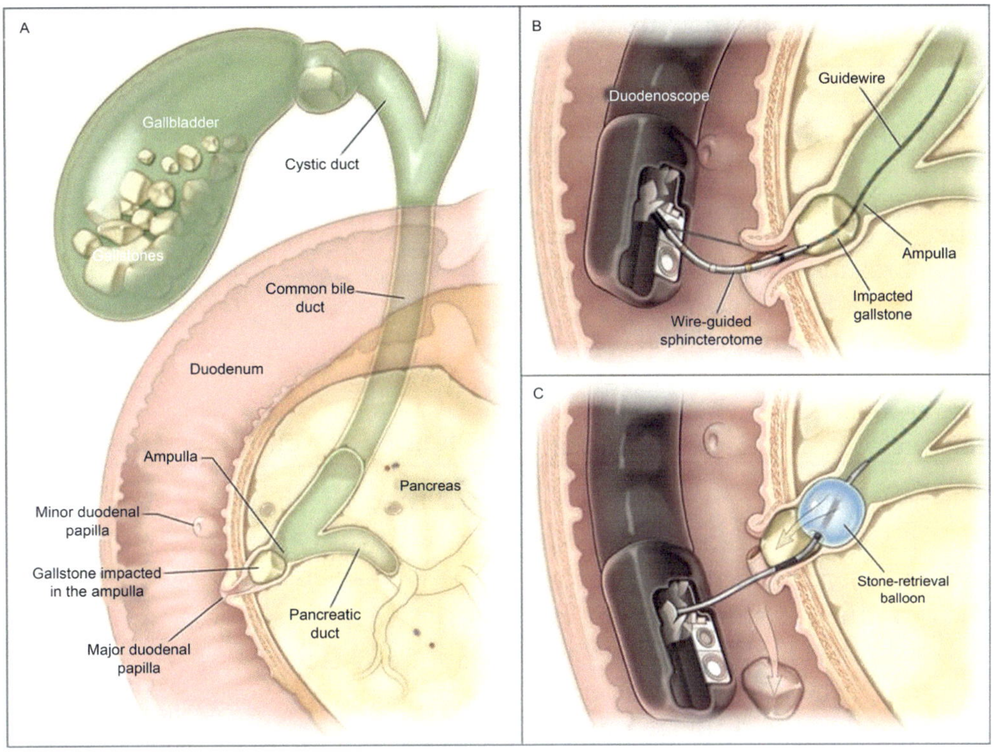

Figure 6.3. Endoscopic retrograde cholangiopancreatography.

Source: https://tebmedtourism.com/wp-content/uploads/2020/05/nejmct1208450_f1.jpeg.jpg.

6.1.1. Serous Cystadenomas

The group of pancreatic cysts contains various neoplastic and non-neoplastic states among which serous cystadenomas are particularly benign in nature. With their contents as serous fluid and honeycomb type, they are typically identified as a distinct group due to their rarity and predictable behavior. Typically occurring in the body or tail of the pancreas, serous cystadenomas occur predominantly in women in the age group of 60-70 years. Their diagnosis is also made easier by imaging modalities such as computed tomography (CT) and magnetic resonance imaging (MRI), which allow visualization of characteristic features such as numerous small cysts with intracystic septations. Unlike other cystic lesions, serous cystadenomas are typically not symptomatic; thus, treatment is primarily reserved for circumstances where there is diagnostic uncertainty or when they are complicated, e.g., abdominal pain or discomfort. The link between serous cystadenomas and genetic predispositions informs us of the complexity of pancreatic cysts. While they mostly arise sporadically, there is also a reported instance of von Hippel-Lindau syndrome (VHL), an autosomal-dominant inherited disease that predisposes patients to numerous tumors, including pancreatic cystadenomas (Ganeshan et al., 2018). This genetic correlation suggests that caution should be exercised in patients with serous cystadenomas, as their treatment may be of a diverse nature based on genetics. Moreover, knowledge of molecular biology and pathogenesis of serous cystadenomas should be good to be able to achieve the best result for the patient. With the development of genetic testing and diagnostics, there is heightened interest in studying the broader effects of hereditary factors on the presentation and management of pancreatic cysts. Management of serous cystadenomas is primarily observation and management for operation when indicated, distinguishing them from possibly malignant lesions.

From clinical experience, serous cystadenomas are characterized by a benign course, which influences the decision to intervene (Mosimann et al., 1990). While operative resection in most cases is reserved for symptomatic or those with indeterminate diagnoses, close monitoring in asymptomatic individuals is warranted. Intervals of imaging follow-up can be useful to track patterns of growth and potential complications. This conservative attitude is reflective of the desire to avoid unnecessary operations while aggressively treating any alterations that can signal malignancy. With advancing research in the area of pancreatic cysts, a well-balanced comprehension of serous cystadenomas will support clinical practice such that patients undergo personalized and evidence-based management for these distinctive pancreatic lesions (Figure 6.4).

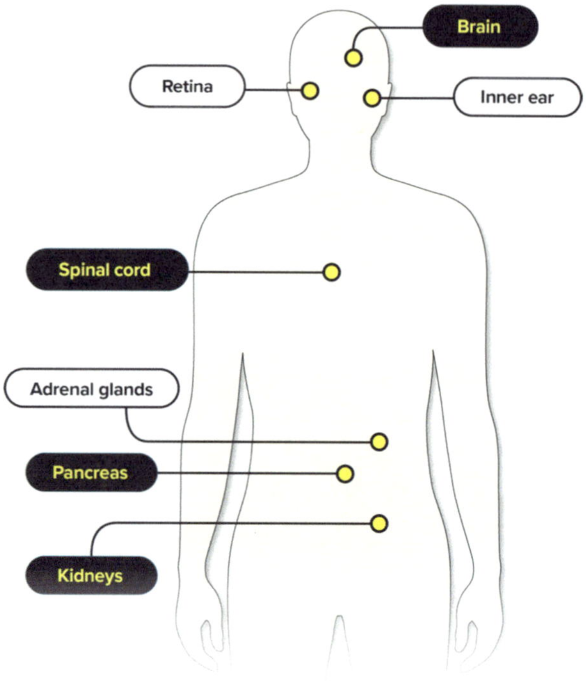

Figure 6.4. Von Hippel-Lindau (VHL) disease.

Source: https://www.welireghcp.com/static/img-person-unbranded-ce2ba66a464e6fb7f956297ca813526d.png.

6.1.2. Mucinous Cystic Neoplasms (MCNs)

MCNs are an important subgroup of cystic lesions of the pancreas, characterized by the presence of mucin-producing epithelial cells and a characteristic stroma, such as ovarian-type stroma. MCNs most frequently occur in the body or tail of the pancreas and, more often than not, occur in females and present in middle-aged patients. The clinical challenge is their potential for malignancy; hence, accurate diagnosis and management are critical. Imaging modalities such as CT and MRI are focal points for the diagnosis of these cysts, with some features, such as cyst size and the presence of solid components, serving as predictors for intervention. This necessitates addressing the risk assessment and treatment planning in a multidisciplinary fashion since some MCNs have the potential to become invasive adenocarcinomas if they are not treated. Previous studies have also emphasized the critical role of standard guidelines in determining high-risk mucinous cystic neoplasms. The Fukuoka criteria, for instance, help clinicians stratify patients by the degree of risk of malignant transformation by taking into account specific features such as cyst size and mural nodules. One retrospective study showed that there was a wide variation in the risk of cancer by these traits, showing the cumulative incidence of high-risk stigmata patients for the development of pancreatic cancer within seven years to be 28%, compared to just 1.2% for the absence of these traits (Lawson et al., 2015). This underscores the necessity of applying rigid criteria in clinical decision-making, as early intervention can be paramount in reducing the risk of cancer progression. The occurrence and possible severity of mucinous cystic neoplasms are also depicted in the overall scenario of asymptomatic pancreatic cysts. Yet another study had faulted the 2015 American Gastroenterological Association (AGA), 2012 Fukuoka, and the 2010 American College of Radiology (ACR) guidelines and discovered variations in their sensitivity in malignancy prediction. Crucially, 92.6% of the cancer or high-grade dysplastic patients would have been excluded using AGA guidelines alone, compared to the wider criteria employed by Fukuoka guidelines (Xu et al., 2017). This finding places the focus on employing detailed guidelines in clinical practice in order to avoid mismanagement and improve patient outcomes. Jointly, the understanding of MCNs addresses the critical need for early detection, rigorous evaluation, and purposeful intervention in pancreatic cysts.

6.1.3. Intraductal Papillary Mucinous Neoplasms (IPMNs)

IPMNs are an important subtype of pancreatic cysts that are characterized by the development of mucin-producing epithelial cells within the ductal system of the pancreas. IPMNs can be further classified as branch-duct IPMNs and main-duct IPMNs, and both of them are of varied clinical significance and management. Branch-duct IPMNs are often known to have a benign outcome, but must be watched very carefully because some will progress to high-grade dysplasia or invasive carcinoma. Conversely, main-duct IPMNs possess a more sinister character and are prone to necessitate surgical intervention due to their greater association with malignancy. Understanding the pathophysiology and heterogeneous character of these neoplasms is a vital component in the provision of clinical judgment and improving patient outcomes. The clinical presentation of IPMNs is largely asymptomatic, which hinders timely diagnosis and management. With advancements in imaging modalities, these cystic lesions are increasingly found incidentally on regular abdominal scans, and therefore, there is a need for rigorous evaluation protocols. Different guidelines exist to calculate the risk of malignancy in pancreatic cysts, yet their validity varies. For example, it was assessed how accurately the 2015 AGA, Fukuoka, and ACR guidelines predicted the risk of high-grade dysplasia or cancer in resected cysts. Findings indicated that the AGA criteria may exclude a considerable number of patients who would require treatment, and hence there is a requirement for greater diagnostic accuracy to effectively treat IPMNs and lower the risk of pancreatic cancer, bearing in mind that 15.2% of asymptomatic branch duct IPMNs had heterogeneity on histopathological examination (Xu et al., 2017). Increased imaging capacity in recent years has allowed improved detection and characterization of intraductal papillary mucinous neoplasms to fundamentally change management practices. Imaging modalities, including MRI and endoscopic ultrasound (EUS), have become critical in differentiating IPMNs from other cystic neoplasms and assessing risk for malignancy. Moreover, evolving knowledge of the biological behavior of these neoplasms has influenced clinical practices and promoted surveillance approaches. Thus, interdisciplinary collaboration among gastroenterologists, radiologists, and pathologists is essential for optimal patient outcomes. With improvement in the management of IPMN over time, the health practitioners have the role of keeping up with such advancements to prevent delay in timely intervention, as well as effects of over-treatment, with due respect for acceptable false-positive rates (Neri, 2017) (Figure 6.5).

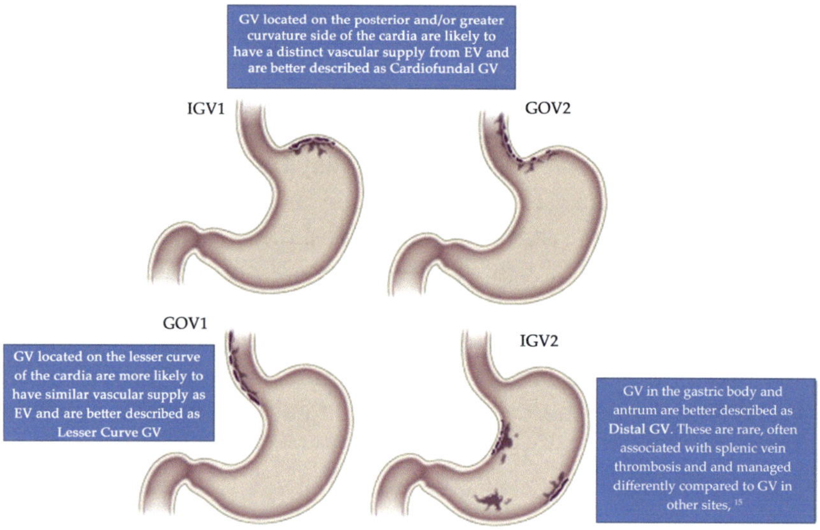

Figure 6.5. Management of bleeding gastric varices.

Source: https://gastro.org/wp-content/uploads/2022/03/gr1-2-1.jpg.

6.2. Causes and Risk Factors

Pancreatic cyst formation may be secondary to a variety of intrinsic and extrinsic causes that are primarily responsible for its development. The predominant etiologies are usually underlying diseases and genetic predispositions. Patients with a previous history of pancreatic or familial syndromes such as Peutz-Jeghers syndrome or von Hippel-Lindau syndrome are at a higher risk of experiencing pancreatic lesions such as cystic structures. In addition, alcoholic, smoking, and metabolic disease-induced chronic pancreatitis have been suspected to play a role in the pathogenesis of cysts in the context of ongoing pancreatic inflammation and injury. The chronic inflammatory environment within the pancreas enhances neoplastic activity, thereby creating a fertile soil for cyst formation. Besides genetic problems and chronic inflammation, age and gender are also determining factors for the prevalence of pancreatic cysts. Epidemiological literature states that the frequency of cystic lesions rises remarkably with increasing age, primarily in patients over the age of 50 years. Besides, a gender imbalance has been documented wherein most cases occur among women, particularly in the scenario of serous cystadenomas. Research points out that serous cystic neoplasms (SCNs) are common among older women and typically are symptom-free for many years. However, because of their ability to produce abdominal pain or other symptoms, their timely diagnosis and follow-up are crucial, especially considering that SCNs, as mostly benign, deserve precise management approaches towards their yet uncertain malignancy (Garcete et al., 2015). Increased use of sophisticated imaging modalities is yet another factor in the risk for pancreatic cyst development. The wide use of abdominal imaging, particularly in the elderly, has led to an increase in the detection of cystic pancreatic lesions that would have otherwise remained asymptomatic. While most of these cysts are likely to be benign, certain types, such as mucinous cystic neoplasms and intraductal papillary mucinous neoplasms, are recognized to have high malignant potential (Azzopardi et al., 2014). This has spurred healthcare recommendations to advise surveillance and step-wise management on a series of criteria, reserving surgery for high-risk cysts but conservatively managing asymptomatic cysts. Thus, the interplay of these causes and risk factors warrants the necessity of stringent monitoring and assessment of pancreatic cysts in clinical practice (Figure 6.6).

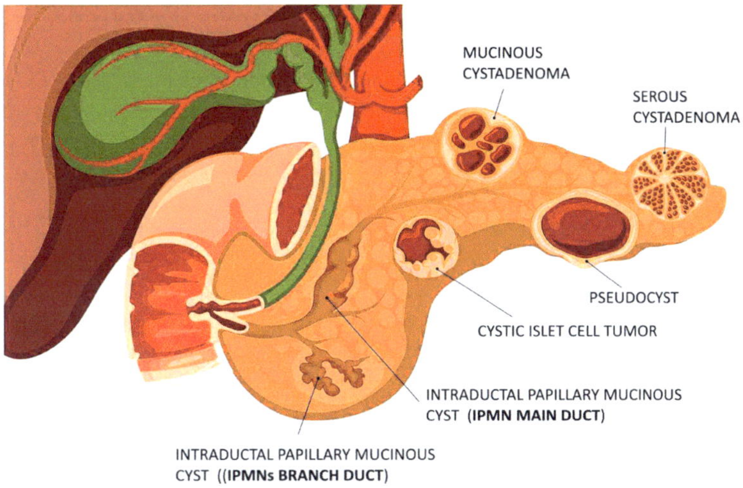

Figure 6.6. Causes and risk factors of pancreatic cysts.

Source: https://stgaccinwbsdevlrs01.blob.core.windows.net/newcorporatewbsite/blogs/october2023/Lymphoepithelial-Cysts.jpg.

6.2.1. Genetic Predispositions

Genetic predispositions are relevant in identifying the etiology of pancreatic cyst formation, particularly in high-risk families or individuals. Heredity is significant in the etiology of many pancreatic diseases, including cystic lesions. Peutz-Jeghers syndrome, familial pancreatic cancer (FPC), and mutations in BRCA1/2 have been associated with increased risk of pancreatic cyst formation. These genetic markers may induce disordered cell growth, manifested as cystic lesions that may require further investigation and follow-up. Recognition of these inherited associations puts the spotlight on genetic counseling and periodic screening protocols for susceptible patients so that early identification of potentially harmful lesions can be done, thereby improving clinical outcomes. The Italian multicenter program illustrates how efficiently surveillance programs were instituted in individuals with known genetic predispositions. This research has included asymptomatic high-risk patients for routine MRCP or EUS to detect pre-malignant lesions or early pancreatic cancer. Quite interestingly, the findings indicated a high prevalence of cystic lesions among the participants, with diagnostic yield for MRCP and EUS determining the importance of targeted screening interventions. Indeed, the findings indicated that individuals with a family history of pancreatic cancer were more likely to show significant cystic lesions. Thus, not only is the genetic susceptibility a risk factor for the development of pancreatic cysts, but also a basis for designing strong surveillance programs, which can help promote enhanced early detection (Signoretti, 2019). Furthermore, recent studies reveal that some genetic mutations can influence the type and aggressiveness of the pancreatic cysts. Individuals with certain genetic predispositions have been shown to have more complex cystic development or an increased frequency of associated malignancies. This kind of association points towards individualized management based on certain genetic backgrounds. Furthermore, understanding such genetic markers will also dictate clinical management regarding the timing of surgery and the need for long-term surveillance for high-risk groups. In general, defining the contribution of genetic predispositions to pancreatic cyst formation is important for maximizing patient outcomes and better understanding pancreatic pathology overall (Scott et al., 2003).

6.2.2. Environmental Factors

Pancreatic cyst formation, similar to pancreatic ductal adenocarcinoma (PDAC), is strongly influenced by environmental factors. The confluence of external environmental exposures and intrinsic genetic susceptibilities cannot be overlooked. Pancreatic injury after chronic exposure to harmful agents such as alcohol and other chemicals has been implicated, a process before cyst formation and the potential evolution to its more sinister equivalents like cancer. For instance, alcohol's toxic effect on pancreatic tissue is known to trigger a state of chronic pancreatitis, which is regarded as a major risk factor for PDAC. Natural environmental influences, such as diet or exposure to endocrine disruptors, also are able to modify pancreatic function further to complicate the landscape around cyst formation and the risks of malignancy that accompany chronic pancreas insult (Toma, 2017). In addition to chemical exposures, lifestyle is also central to determining a person's risk of developing pancreatic cysts and associated diseases. Physical inactivity in combination with poor dietary habits is increasingly recognized as a central environmental component that predisposes towards obesity and diabetes mellitus. These provide a background that provokes a metabolic environment to encourage pancreatic failure and cyst development. The link between obesity and pancreatic disease includes inflammatory pathways destabilizing pancreatic cell architecture, thereby inducing cyst growth and ultimately the conversion to malignancy. Excess weight has, in particular, been observed to exacerbate chronic pancreatitis in the pancreas, thereby accelerating the injury-repair cycle that most typically results in cyst formation (Blackburn et al., 2021). Also, the presence of primary cilia on pancreatic cells emerges as a critical environmental factor implicated in cyst regulation and pancreatic function. These cellular organelles are involved in various signaling pathways that impact cellular growth and differentiation, and alterations affecting their development may lead to abnormal pancreatic physiology. The primary cilia of pancreatic β-cells are critical in insulin secretion and cellular signaling, and any defect in them leads to diseases referred to as ciliopathies. As evidence shows, such impairment not only distorts insulin synthesis but also directly takes part in the development of pancreatic cysts by modifying the structural integrity of the tissues. Therefore, realizing the intricate relationship between environmental factors, cellular response, and their combined impact on pancreatic health becomes imperative for the establishment of prophylactic measures and therapeutic regimens for disorders like pancreatic cysts (Blackburn et al., 2021) (Figure 6.7).

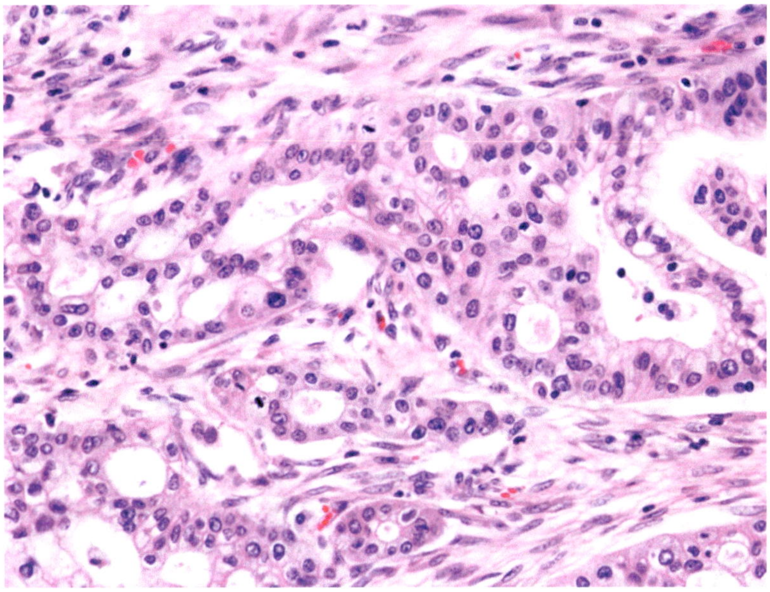

Figure 6.7. Pancreatic ductal adenocarcinoma (PDCA).

Source: By user:KGH - Own work, CC BY-SA 3.0, https://commons.wikimedia.org/w/index.php?curid=552903

6.2.3. Lifestyle Choices and Their Impact

The correlation between lifestyle behaviors and the pathogenesis of pancreatic cysts is better appreciated in the current medical literature. While the pathophysiology of pancreatic cysts is multifactorial, certain lifestyle factors such as alcohol consumption, diet, and obesity play major roles in their development and growth. Studies have proven that diets rich in fats and sugars are proven to lead to obesity and insulin resistance, two of the risk factors for pancreatic disease. In addition, alcoholism has also been linked to inflammation of the pancreas and cysts. If these risk factors could be understood, then patients would be taking necessary precautions to reduce their potential for developing such a condition, stressing the value of a balanced lifestyle regarding nutrition and moderation. Further, exercise and physical activity are integral components of a healthy way of life and will have significant impacts on the individual health implications of pancreatic health. Regularly engaging in physical activity has the ability to contribute to weight management and increased insulin sensitivity, factors that play an important role in pancreas cyst prevention. A systematic review that examines lifestyle patterns and eating habits points out that the interventions prove to be effective in managing related health issues, specifically illnesses such as obesity and type 2 diabetes that can cause pancreatic dysfunction (Namoosi and Reyhaneh, 2024). Adding exercise at intervals and higher quality food to one's diet not only enhances one's overall health but also can decrease the chances of the formation of pancreatic cysts. In addition, psychological problems concerning lifestyle habits, such as stress management and sleep patterns, also contribute to the health of the pancreas. Stress, if it is chronic, can lead to hormonal imbalance and metabolic disorders, which are likely to enhance the possibility of forming pancreatic cysts. Adequate stress management through mindfulness practices and adequate sleep can provide a positive environment for the health of the pancreas (Mann, 2021). As science continues to advance, it is clear that controlling the risk of pancreatic cysts must include an integrated process encompassing diet, physical activity, and psychological well-being. By prioritizing these habits of lifestyle, individuals can enhance health outcomes and be better able to deal with the complexities associated with pancreatic health conditions.

6.3. Symptoms and Diagnosis

The presentation of pancreatic cysts is usually a diagnostic challenge because they are nonspecific. A significant majority of individuals with pancreatic cysts remain asymptomatic and hence delays in diagnosis. When symptoms have developed, these can be presented in the form of abdominal pain, reported in about 27% of cases, in association with pancreaticobiliary complications in the form of jaundice or pancreatitis in 9% of the patients. In addition, some cases may have diabetes mellitus, which is found in roughly 5% of the cases. The variability of symptomatology is proof of the importance of careful evaluation in patients who come in with atypical abdominal complaints, particularly those who are at risk for developing pancreatic cysts, such as those with inherited syndromes like von Hippel–Lindau disease (Ganeshan et al., 2018).

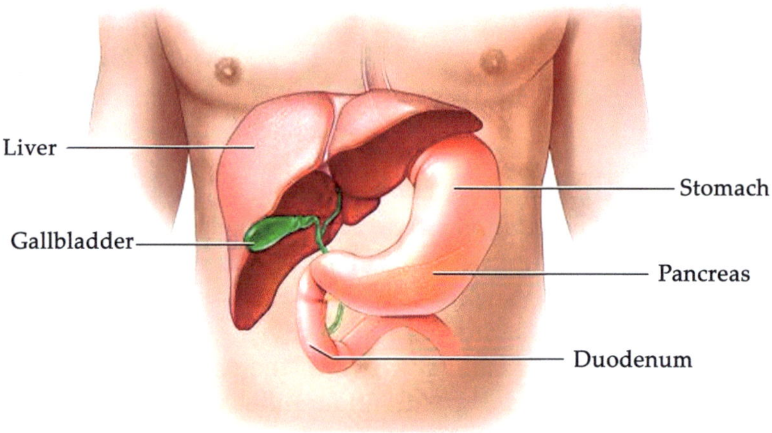

Figure 6.8. Symptoms associated with pancreatic cysts.

Source: https://assets.mayoclinic.org/content/dam/media/en/images/2023/02/10/pancreas.jpg.

Recognition of these potential clinical presentations can facilitate early diagnosis and treatment, which minimizes the risk of complications of such conditions. Diagnosis of pancreatic cysts would typically be a multi-modal procedure that employs imaging modalities such as ultrasound, CT, and MRI. These are invaluable in identifying the nature, size, and location of the cysts, relevant in the determination of their nature and potential need for intervention. A large percentage of symptomatic patients are treated within a year of diagnosis, increasingly due to uncertain diagnoses at presentation, characterized by cyst growth and size patterns. In fact, indications for surgery may arise from symptoms or complications, resulting in diagnostic necessity. A study showed that 39% of serous cystic neoplasm patients did not have any surgery over a period of three years, reflecting the role of surgical evaluation in different cases (Garcete et al., 2015). This extensive diagnostic process is important in differentiating benign and malignant cystic masses. Diagnosis of pancreatic cysts requires a complete investigation of patient history, symptoms, and imaging findings. Genetic testing would also be warranted in patients who are suspected of having such conditions as von Hippel–Lindau syndrome, which makes one susceptible to pancreatic cysts among other cancers (Ganeshan et al., 2018). That the cysts are in the context of VHL underscores the role of monitoring and surveillance imaging to track any change in cyst characteristics. The management plan must be tailored to the patient's unique risk profile, cyst size, and cyst behavior, balancing the thoroughness of the investigations with the need to avoid excessive exposure to invasive interventions. Also, an understanding of the natural history of the different types of cysts, like serous cystic neoplasms, informs clinical decision-making because the majority are non-progressive over the years and must be dealt with conservatively rather than surgically (Garcete et al., 2015) (Figure 6.8).

6.3.1. Common Symptoms Associated with Pancreatic Cysts

The symptom presentation associated with pancreatic cysts varies considerably in every patient, at times leading to misdiagnosis or delayed treatment. Asymptomatic patients are present in the majority of cases, particularly when the cysts are small and benign. When symptoms do occur, they may be as subtle as intense abdominal pain, which manifests as upper abdominal or back pain. This pain is caused by the pressure exerted on surrounding organs or tissue by the cysts. Also, when cysts develop, they may block the pancreatic duct or become inflamed, leading to other associated issues such as pancreatitis, defined by intense abdominal pain and gastrointestinal disturbances (Scialpi et al., 2016). The second most common symptom of pancreatic cysts is changes in appetite and, therefore, weight loss. Patients may complain of experiencing nausea and satiety in the initial stages, as the presence of a cyst may hamper normal digestive function. In the more severe cases, when there is an infected or ruptured cyst, patients may have a more serious presentation with fever, chills, and jaundice, which are manifestations of underlying complications such as infection or bile duct obstruction. These symptoms necessitate immediate medical treatment, as without it, there will be serious consequences for pancreatic function and overall health (Carlo et al., 2018). Observing carefully and early action are paramount to prevent exacerbation. In addition to gastrointestinal symptoms, systemic symptoms such as fatigue or nonspecific malaise can occur in some patients with pancreatic cysts. These may be due to the chronic nature of the disease, but the body may also be in a state of constant battle with inflammation or infection. Laboratory tests and radiologic imaging like CT or MRI, are significant for the proper diagnosis and treatment of pancreatic cysts. Given that asymptomatic cases are often discovered incidentally on imaging workup for other reasons, awareness of these common symptoms will likely promote proactive follow-up and therapeutic planning (Scialpi et al., 2016). In summary, awareness of the symptomatology of pancreatic cysts is crucial for timely diagnosis and optimal management of this often neglected condition.

6.3.2. Diagnostic Imaging Techniques

Diagnosis of pancreatic cysts largely relies on advanced diagnostic imaging techniques, which have become the cornerstone of their identification and characterization. The growing access and technical advancement of cross-sectional imaging modalities such as CT and MRI have significantly raised the detection rate of pancreatic cysts. These imaging methods enable physicians to visualize the pancreas more effectively, which makes it easy to differentiate between benign and potentially malignant cystic tumors. The potential to detect cysts at earlier stages contributes to better decision-making in management, illustrative of the critical role that diagnostic imaging has in achieving successful patient care for patients with pancreatic disease (Kocjan, 2010). Amongst the imaging modalities used, EUS with fine needle aspiration (FNA) offers a unique advantage in pancreatic cyst diagnosis. EUS, due to its proximity to the pancreas, provides higher sensitivity to small cystic lesions that easily slip by on routine imaging. EUS FNA also permits the collection of cyst fluid for cytopathological and molecular analyses. This allows for a finer classification of cysts between mucinous and non-mucinous tumors and, on occasion, malignancy. The ability to be capable of performing EUS and FNA within one procedure both boosts the diagnostic yield and subsequent management options and illustrates the invaluable place of this technique within the total evaluation of pancreatic cysts (Kocjan, 2010). Despite imaging techniques, management of pancreatic cysts remains problematic due to the lesions' heterogeneity. Because imaging can accurately define the presence and nature of the cysts, this information, coupled with clinical assessment and cytology, is necessary to provide optimal care to the patient. Various guidelines are being formulated to optimize the diagnostic algorithms, but presently, there is no single integrated approach that adequately directs the practitioners. Ongoing assessment of cystic lesions by imaging must be supplemented by multidisciplinary strategies so that benign and malignant cysts are accurately identified and treated. Thus, in the complex context of pancreatic cysts, imaging diagnostic modalities continue to be key determinants of clinical decision-making and ultimately the outcome of care (Meziani et al., 2012) (Figure 6.9).

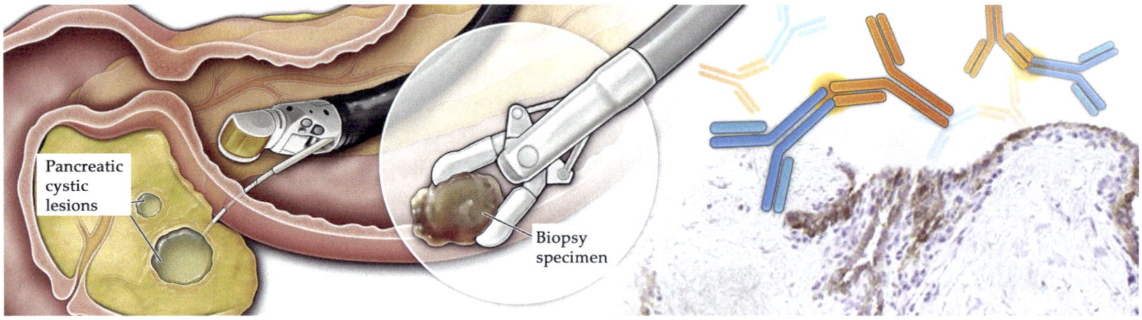

Figure 6.9. EUS-guided through-the-needle biopsy sampling of pancreatic cystic lesions.

Source: https://www.giejournal.org/cms/10.1016/j.gie.2020.04.040/asset/9ad17cb9-eb12-4396-83db-cf6f18eb5785/main.assets/fx1_lrg.jpg.

6.3.3. Role of Laboratory Tests in Diagnosis

Diagnostic workup in the lab is crucial in differentiating between malignant and benign lesions in pancreatic cysts. Serum markers, such as CA 19-9, aid doctors in establishing the likelihood of malignancy in cysts of the pancreas. A raised level of CA 19-9 in conjunction with radiological workup may heighten suspicion for a cystic neoplasm over an incidental cyst. While laboratory testing alone cannot provide a definitive diagnosis, it contributes to the overall diagnostic picture. For instance, the correlation of certain laboratory findings with the clinical presentation has a significant bearing on management, for instance, the requirement for surgery or follow-up. Laboratory testing thus becomes an important adjunct to imaging techniques, leading clinicians toward a heightened consciousness of pancreatic cysts and their complications, which in turn influence patient outcomes.

In addition to serum markers, cytologic examination obtained with FNA assists in diagnosing pancreatic cysts, particularly when imaging results are inconclusive. This biochemical examination allows for the evaluation of the cystic fluid, providing crucial information as to the nature of the cyst. For instance, the identification of atypical cells or specific cytologic findings may indicate a premalignant lesion or malignancy. Rapid on-site assessment (ROSE) plays an important role in this environment, allowing pathologists to inspect the cyst fluid in real-time during the FNA. This real-time feedback allows clinicians to make rational patient management decisions, often deciding whether or not surgical treatment is required. Using laboratory tests such as cytological examination, physicians can optimize the diagnostic process for pancreatic cysts and limit the risks associated with unneeded procedures, a testament to the test's essential role in clinical practice (Carico et al., 2015). Regular laboratory checks are also important in monitoring pancreatic cysts in the long term, particularly for those with low-risk characteristics. The laboratory studies have a utilitarian function beyond the primary diagnosis; they form an integral component in sustained observation of cyst expansion and symptom progression. For example, a conservative therapy may involve serial imaging and baseline serum studies to evaluate any change in cyst characteristics. For SCN, natural history and slow growth behavior, as evidenced in studies, justify the foundation for conservative follow-up rather than immediate surgery (Garcete et al., 2015). The results emphasize the importance of laboratory results in initial diagnosis and long-term management, providing useful information to optimize patient outcomes while minimizing unnecessary treatments.

6.4. Treatment Options

Treatment of pancreatic cysts involves a variety of treatments that vary with the type of cyst, the size, and the malignant potential. For asymptomatic incidentally discovered cysts, a policy of watchful waiting with regular follow-up is typically employed, particularly in serous cystadenomas, which are typically benign and do not require emergent treatment. However, in the case of mucinous cysts, which have a significant risk for the development of pancreatic cancer, more aggressive treatment is needed. Surgical resection may be able to eliminate the malignancy risk from the body, but this is very morbid and thus, stringent patient selection and assessment are crucial in the avoidance of complications of such aggressive therapy. The new techniques employed in the treatment of pancreatic cysts demonstrate the evolution of less invasive treatments. The recent advancements in EUS-guided chemoablation have also been encouraging, especially for neoplastic cysts. The technique allows for direct infusion of therapeutic agents into the cystic lesions, which could minimize the need for more invasive surgical interventions. The efficacy of these ablation techniques has also improved as non-alcoholic chemoablation cocktails have developed with a good safety profile, which is minimal in terms of causing complications such as post-procedure pancreatitis. Thus, EUS-guided chemoablation is a potentially game-changing component of the treatment algorithm in individual patients to achieve maximum effect with minimum risk to the patient (Moyer et al., 2019). Even though new developments in therapeutic possibilities have created new doors for the treatment of pancreatic cysts, the genetic and clinical histories also play significant roles in defining therapy. In hereditary diseases such as VHL, in which patients are at risk of having multiple pancreatic lesions, an individualized approach is necessary. In VHL patients with cystic pancreas, individual surveillance regimens might be necessary, together with balancing the indications for surgery according to lesion characteristics. Genetic counseling and genetic testing are useful in managing risk stratification and identification of complications.

Enhanced detection of VHL-associated tumor expression through diagnostic imaging is crucial for early treatments, thus better patient outcomes as well as affecting the treatment of pancreatic cysts (Ganeshan et al., 2018) (Figure 6.10).

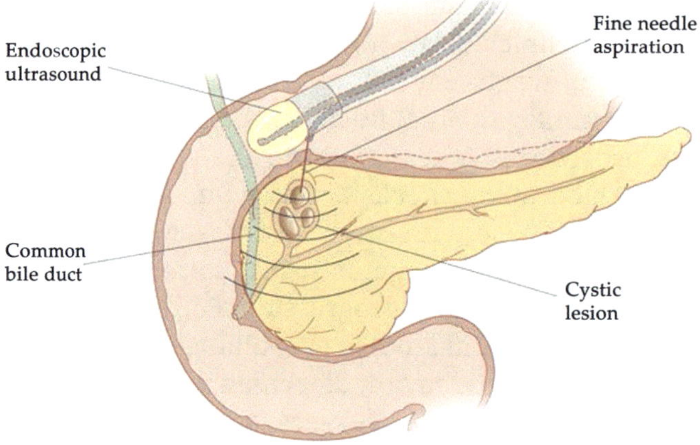

Figure 6.10. Treatment of pancreatic cystic tumors.

Source: https://stanfordhealthcare.org/medical-treatments/t/therapeutic-endoscopy/procedures/treatment-pancreatic-cystic-tumors/_jcr_content/tab-nav-component/tab-nav-parsys/imagewithcaption/image.img.full.high.jpg/1474756098885.jpg.

6.4.1. Observation and Monitoring

The process of monitoring and observation plays a key role in the management of pancreatic cysts, particularly in SCNs. With the continuous improvement of imaging technology and diagnostic criteria, watchful waiting is increasingly being utilized for asymptomatic patients with SCNs by clinicians. The approach provides the opportunity to avoid unnecessary surgery, which can carry significant risks and morbidity. Specifically, as has been reported in observational accounts, the majority of patients with SCNs can safely be managed without expedited resection, particularly if predictive variables such as age, pain, and imaging solid components are considered. This strategy toward observation is indicative of a refined understanding of benign cystic neoplasms and emphasizes the importance of individualized patient management strategies to optimize outcomes and reduce health burdens (Gomatos et al., 2016). Observation also involves continued surveillance of the cysts' characteristics over time through serial imaging examinations. Radiologic follow-up, typically through high-resolution imaging modalities such as MRI or CT scans, enables the clinician to follow up with cyst size, morphology, and status of complications. The decision between observation and intervention rests on guidelines that suggest standard time intervals of follow-up imaging based on cyst size and history of symptoms. Continued advancements in imaging techniques reaffirm the value of observation protocols to avoid overtreatment while allowing for early intervention in case such changes characterizing malignancy arise. Educating patients and incorporating them in their management through awareness of the significance of these observation protocols fosters trust, counteracting concern over risk of delayed treatment (Gomatos et al., 2016). Further, microbiological analysis of pancreatic cyst fluid is an interesting field to explore and follow up. Recent data have indicated a unique bacterial community in the pancreatic cysts, implying that the local microbiome may play a role in the pathophysiology of the lesion. Microbiological data may provide additional insight into the cyst's behavior and potential malignancy evolution. Detection of specific bacterial genera associated with pancreatic cysts, as indicated by comprehensive studies, can inform surveillance strategies and enhance predictive models of cyst enlargement or disappearance. By integrating this new data into typical observation routines, clinicians may optimize monitoring strategies and tailor interventions based on the evolving clinical setting of pancreatic cysts.

6.4.2. Surgical Interventions

Surgical interventions play a critical role in the treatment of pancreatic cysts, particularly if the lesions exhibit malignant suggestive features or show significant symptoms. Advances in imaging techniques have significantly enhanced the diagnostic accuracy of cystic neoplasms, hence the evaluation and monitoring strategies.

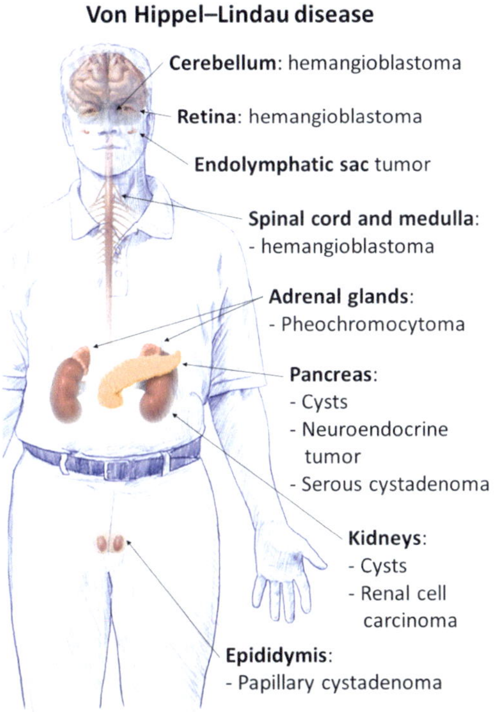

Figure 6.11. Von hippel-lindau disease (VHL).

Source: By Mikael Häggström, M.D. Author info- Reusing images- Conflicts of interest:NoneMikael Häggström, M.D.The figure is using an image by Schunemann V, Huntoon K, and Lonser RR - Image source:Figure 1, from: Schunemann V, Huntoon K, Lonser RR (2016). "Personalized Medicine for Nervous System Manifestations of von Hippel-Lindau Disease.". Front Surg 3: 39. DOI:10.3389/fsurg.2016.00039. PMID 27446927. PMC: 4928600.- "Available via license: Creative Commons Attribution 4.0 International"Source for diseasesLeung RS, Biswas SV, Duncan M, Rankin S (2008). "Imaging features of von Hippel-Lindau disease.". Radiographics 28 (1): 65-79; quiz 323. DOI:10.1148/rg.281075052. PMID 18203931., CC BY 4.0, https://commons.wikimedia.org/w/index.php?curid=126783017

As has been suggested, the reliance on routine and advanced imaging procedures is the foundation on which the diagnosis of pancreatic cysts is made, and this influences the decision to perform or not perform surgical intervention (Neri, 2017). The synchronization between accurate diagnosis and the timing of surgery is needed; patients with cysts with uncharacteristic features or with symptoms are typically candidates for surgical excision. It is a proactive effort that attempts to diminish the risk of developing into pancreatic cancer and, in the process, maximizes the patient outcome. Surgical therapy of pancreatic cysts is largely a series of surgical procedures, such as cystogastrostomy, pancreaticoduodenectomy, or distal pancreatectomy, based on the nature of the cyst and the site. Surgical therapy gains significance, especially with IPMNs and MCNs, which carry the threat of malignant transformation. Systematic evaluation of the characteristics of the cysts, including size, cytology, and symptoms, helps direct surgical treatment. Also, clinical guidelines, especially in diseases like VHL, imbue individualized surgery with seriousness in high-risk groups. Directed surgery, not only for addressing immediate health problems but also offering a site for long-term follow-up of complications, is ultimately supported. Decision-making for the surgical treatment of pancreatic cysts is typically multifactorial, with the risk versus benefit of surgery. While the indication to resect potentially malignant cysts is of utmost concern, surgery-related risk such as postoperative complication in the form of pancreatic fistula or delayed gastric emptying must be considered with careful deliberation. Patient condition, age, and comorbidities are also central to decision-making for surgery. A patient-centered approach is the implementation of intensive conversations with regard to the result of delayed operation versus the hazard of intervention. In the end, the formulation of personalized surgical plans emphasizes the need to balance efficacy with safety in the treatment of pancreatic cysts to optimize patient care and improve overall prognoses (Figure 6.11).

6.4.3. Endoscopic Procedures

Endoscopic procedures have become indispensable instruments in managing pancreatic cysts, particularly in the diagnosis and management of cystic lesions with malignant potential. With the advent of EUS, it is possible to obtain precise imaging and aspiration of aspirate and histological material from the cysts, hence making an accurate diagnosis possible. With the rising prevalence of pancreatic cystic lesions in a changing population, effective surveillance and treatment are more important. Endoscopic guidance not only enhances the quality of diagnosis but also provides a platform for therapeutic applications such as drainage of cysts and thereby prevents intervention by more invasive surgical techniques with increased risk of morbidity. Thus, EUS is an important component of the contemporary clinical assessment of pancreatic cysts, helping in the unambiguous distinction of benign from potentially malignant lesions that need more invasive therapeutic modalities. The advances in endoscopic technology highlight the promise of endoscopic ultrasound-guided chemoablation as a viable therapy for neoplastic pancreatic cysts. This minimally invasive procedure involves the delivery of the chemotherapeutic agents directly into the cyst cavity, thereby targeting and reducing the size of the cyst as well as lowering the risk of complications of traditional surgical procedures. The effectiveness of this procedure has been variably reported in studies, which has spurred ongoing work to optimize the protocol and enhance the outcome for patients. Of special note is the departure from alcohol-based chemoablation due to the safety concerns associated with alcohol-induced pancreatitis. The potential has been realized through the administration of a non-alcohol chemoablation cocktail that is accompanied by positive adverse event reporting alongside maximal therapeutic effectiveness. Thus, the integration of this technology within the treatment pathway for pancreatic cysts represents a significant step forward in gastroenterological intervention (Moyer et al., 2019). Also, the implications of endoscopic practice take precedence over short-term therapeutic outcomes, such as longer-term concerns of patient quality of life and usage of health resources. Implementing minimally invasive techniques like EUS-guided chemoablation, healthcare providers are able to decrease the mental stress and bodily morbidity generally described with more aggressive surgery methods. This technique has also been shown to decrease post-operative recovery and hospital stay, a factor of utmost importance in the treatment of elderly or comorbid patients. Ongoing investigation and clinical trials are essential to refine these techniques further and establish comprehensive treatment programs tailored to a patient's requirements and nature of the cyst. In general, advances in endoscopic interventions remain to establish their pivotal position in the therapy of pancreatic cysts, maximizing efficacy and safety while remaining in agreement with the prevailing trend towards patient-focussed care (Al-Haddad et al., 2014) (Figure 6.12).

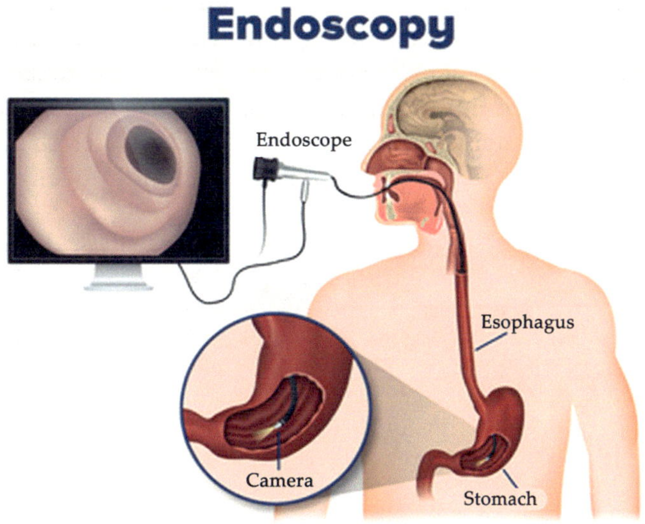

Figure 6.12. Endoscopic procedures.

Source: https://medstarhealth-delivery.sitecorecontenthub.cloud/api/public/content/services%2Fendoscopy-illustration?v=4ff38de2.

6.5. Complications Associated with Pancreatic Cysts

The presence of pancreatic cysts can cause a variety of complications that vary in severity. With the progression of the cysts, compression or obstruction of the organs in the surrounding abdominal cavity can occur, leading to painful or gastrointestinal symptoms. More concretely, pancreatitisobiliary symptoms such as jaundice or cholangitis can occur due to bile duct obstruction, thus normally necessitating urgent intervention. The risk for such complications makes a need for caution and investigation of cyst enlargement. Indeed, surgical interventions are usually considered not just in symptomatic patients but even in situations where concerns are triggered by the suspicious nature of the cyst, particularly in cases presenting with significant enlargement or suspicious findings on imaging tests (Garcete et al., 2015). The second critical characteristic of complications with pancreatic cysts is the risk of malignant transformation, especially in the case of mucinous cystic neoplasms. While serous cysts are deemed benign, the risk in some mucinous cysts is high for their progression to pancreatic cancer, which continues to have an extremely poor prognosis. The challenge is in discriminating between cystic lesions that need to be operated on because they could be cancerous. Due to this, surveillance measures must be put into action cautiously, balancing the danger of the surgical process with that of malignancy. These evaluations cannot be overstated, as early detection and resection of malignant cysts can contribute significantly to influencing patient outcomes and survival (Moyer et al., 2019). Patients may also experience complications from surgical interventions after pancreatic cyst management. With advancements in surgical techniques, they too carry their own risks associated with them, such as postoperative infections, hemorrhage, and leakage of pancreatic enzymes, leading to additional morbidity. Pancreatic surgery has long-term complications as well, such as exocrine or endocrine deficiency, particularly when a significant portion of the pancreas is excised. Patients with complications of pancreatic surgery after surgery have different survival rates, which makes it necessary for individualized postoperative care and follow-up. Moreover, newer advancements in minimally invasive methods, such as endoscopic ultrasound-guided chemoablation, demonstrate favorable alternatives to surgery, reducing rates of complications with ongoing effective neoplastic cyst management (Moyer et al., 2019) (Figure 6.13).

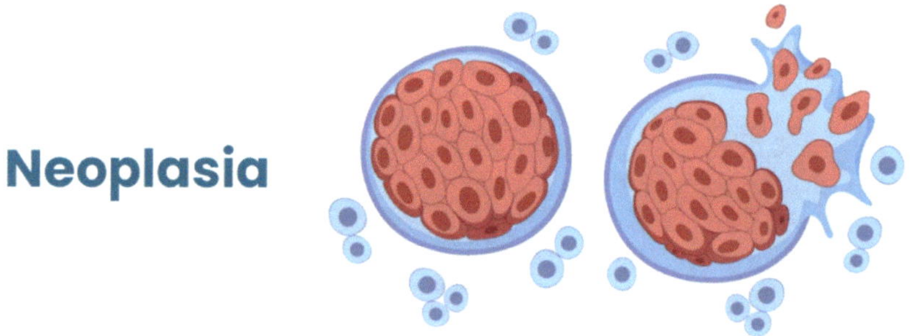

Figure 6.13. Neoplasia.

Source: https://www.medicoverhospitals.in/images/articles/neoplasia.webp.

6.5.1. Risk of Infection

The presence of pancreatic cysts also raises severe issues of risk of infection, which is possible, particularly when cysts are complicated by co-morbid diseases such as acute pancreatitis or choledochal cysts. Infection becomes a prevalent condition when there is a disruption of the integrity of the pancreatic tissue, leading to circumstances under which bacteria can invade the cystic spaces. As has been discussed in the review of choledochal cysts, embryogenic infection may produce biliary and pancreatic system complications and hence is a very essential differential diagnosis to be added while diagnosing pancreatic cysts. Prompt clinical evaluation is subsequently required to minimize the risk of the infection complications, such as ascending cholangitis or pancreatitis, which may exacerbate morbidity and even increase the risk of lethal outcomes in patients with pancreatic cysts (Koncoro et al., 2012). Aside from the short-term impact on the pancreas's functioning, the risk resulting from infection also encompasses long-term health outcomes. For instance, infected pancreatic cysts can lead to abscess formation that necessitates drainage or surgery. The risk of untreated infections developing into systemic complications is a testament to the gravity with which health professionals must approach cases of pancreatic cysts. Treatment calls for a multi-disciplinary approach based on radiological assessment to identify continuing complications and laboratory investigations that yield evidence of infection or inflammation. Also, complete knowledge of the infection etiology, such as possible modes of transmission and the importance of co-morbid conditions, is crucial in the creation of treatment regimens (Crocetti et al., 2015). Lastly, preventive measures and early intervention are critical in decreasing infection risk in pancreatic cyst patients. Close observation, good imaging studies, and immediate therapeutic interventions can significantly reduce complications. In addition, the clinician's role is not just in direct treatment; patient education of infection-suggestive symptoms is of the highest priority. A multidisciplinary team of primary care, gastroenterology, and surgical teams provides a solid foundation where all aspects of patient care are addressed. Finally, detection of the polyvalent risk of infection in the setting of pancreatic cysts enhances early detection and integrated treatment strategies, ultimately bettering patient outcomes and reducing the expense of complications resulting from it (Figure 6.14).

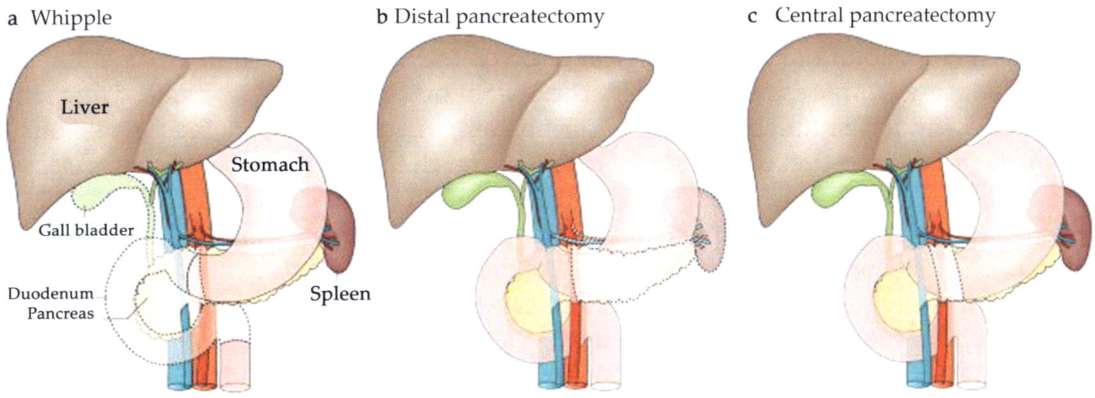

Figure 6.14. Diagnosis and management of pancreatic cystic neoplasms.

Source: https://media.springernature.com/lw685/springer-static/image/art%3A10.1038%2Fs41575-019-0195-x/MediaObjects/41575_2019_195_Fig3_HTML.png.

6.5.2. Potential for Malignant Transformation

The risk of malignant transformation of pancreatic cysts is an area of great clinical interest due to the influence it exerts on patient management and outcome. Pancreatic cysts, found incidentally on imaging investigations, may have varying levels of premalignant potential. Some lesions, such as mucinous cystic neoplasms and solid pseudopapillary neoplasms, carry a high risk of malignant transformation, with the consequent need for careful evaluation. Guidelines recommend surgery for the treatment of certain high-risk cystic lesions, particularly when criteria for malignancy have been suggested. In contrast, lesions like serous cystadenomas are very unlikely to undergo malignant change, pointing to the significance of proper diagnosis to guide clinical practice and avoid the risk of overtreatment of benign conditions (Azzopardi et al., 2014). Asymptomatic pancreatic cysts present a difficult situation, as the majority are benign but bear an intrinsic risk of malignant development. It has been demonstrated that while the majority of pancreatic cysts are stable, some may present with signs indicative of high-grade dysplasia or invasive carcinoma. Data show that less than a quarter, around 15.2%, of cysts that are resected in asymptomatic individuals reveal high-grade dysplasia or malignancy (Xu et al., 2017). Risk factors in such changes are patient age and cyst size, and clinical practice in the management of asymptomatic cysts is weighted by predetermined practice patterns, as these try to balance the risks of operation against malignant potential not yet identified by present techniques. Evolving guidelines for the evaluation of pancreatic cysts highlight the challenge and the advancement of identifying malignant potential. For example, the sensitivity and specificity variability of established protocols such as the AGA and Fukuoka guidelines appears to arise from their relative ability to detect high-grade lesions. Importantly, application of AGA criteria can result in substantial numbers of false-negative instances of malignancy, so single usage of these guidelines would be at the expense of patient safety. Continued refinement in the imaging and diagnostic criteria is required to better stratify risk in pancreatic cysts so that informed interventions can be made, resulting in improved outcomes for patients (Xu et al., 2017).

6.5.3. Impact on Pancreatic Function

The growth of pancreatic cysts may have significant effects on pancreatic function by disrupting the organs normal structure and physiological activity. Cystic formations of this nature have the potential to induce a compressive effect on the surrounding pancreatic tissue, which disrupts the exocrine and endocrine functions. The exocrine component of the pancreas is responsible for digestion through the excretion of digestive enzymes, and the endocrine component is responsible for the maintenance of glucose homeostasis by the secretion of hormones like insulin. When cysts develop, they can block the pancreatic ducts, trapping the enzymes and leading to additional inflammation, further complicating the overall condition of the pancreas. This obstruction also precludes insulin release, creating a scenario that can cause insulin resistance or diabetes related to deranged glucose metabolism, thus illustrating the widespread influence of cyst growth on pancreatic function. Interestingly, cyst formation mechanisms and effects on pancreatic islet beta-cell function illustrate the interconnectedness of developmental signal transduction events and metabolic outcomes. Signaling pathway dysregulation, such as that of the canonical Wnt pathway, has been implicated in causing hypoplasia of the pancreas, proposing the importance of stringent regulation mechanisms for the maintenance of pancreatic structure and function (Cano et al., 2016). Abnormal activation of such pathways during cystogenesis may trigger abnormal cell fate decisions within the pancreatic epithelium.

This diversion results in the formation of gut-like tissue rather than typical pancreatic architecture. These consequent changes affect not only the structural make-up of the pancreas but also hinder its effectiveness in insulin production and secretion, thereby exacerbating metabolic imbalances potentially seen in individuals with pancreatic cysts. Moreover, the Vhlh gene function in pancreatic function underscores the delicate balance that has to be achieved to maintain glucose homeostasis. Disruption of the VHL protein in pancreatic beta-cells has been shown in studies to lead to profound glucose intolerance caused primarily by impaired insulin secretion in response to increased glucose levels. While insulin production continues to be nominal, mechanisms of secretion become faulty, causing major dysregulation of metabolic function (Puri et al., 2009). This observation highlights that even though structural deformation caused by cyst formation greatly impacts the pancreas, genetics also has a significant influence. Thus, the interface between cyst-driven morphological alterations and internal genetic vulnerabilities underscores the complexity of pancreatic nature and the necessity for integrative therapeutic modalities to act on these poly-faceted pathologies.

6.6. Current Research and Advances

Recent advancements in the management and comprehension of pancreatic cysts have rendered endoscopic ultrasound-guided chemoablation a promising option. It is a lesser-invasive procedure for the treatment of neoplastic cysts, taking advantage of the possibility to directly administer therapy into the cystic lesion. The efficacy of an alcohol-free chemoablation cocktail that prevents the risks of pancreatitis usually caused by alcohol-based cocktails is highlighted in recent studies. With a less toxic side effect profile, this technique is a significant step towards safer alternatives to treat potentially malignant cysts.

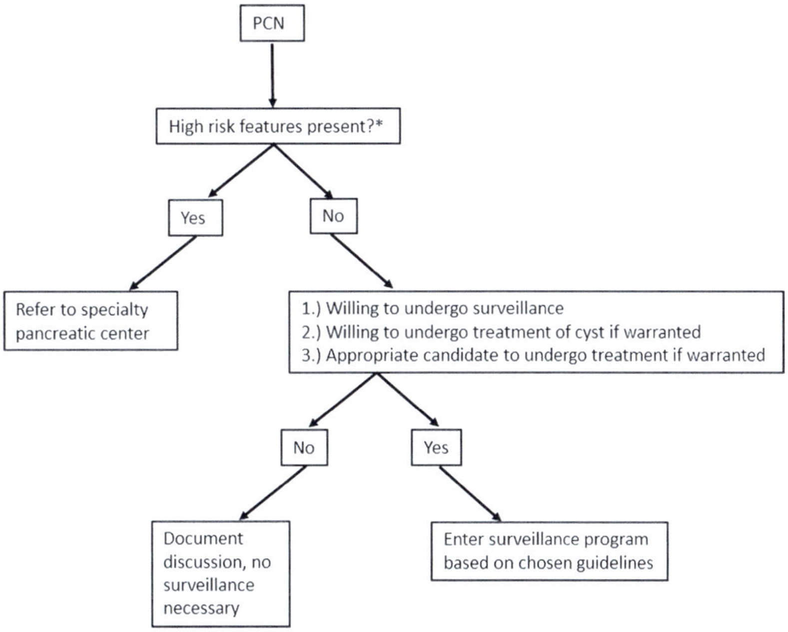

Figure 6.15. Management of pancreatic cysts and guidelines.

Source: https://journals.sagepub.com/cms/10.1177/26317745211045769/asset/10215ba3-646f-4e15-948b-183c28d561b4/assets/images/large/10.1177_26317745211045769-fig11.jpg.

The efficacy of chemoablation makes it a strong candidate to be a standard component of the treatment regimen, thereby addressing an important public health problem of the mismanagement of cystic lesions with the potential for cancerous development of the pancreas (Moyer et al., 2019). Pancreatic cyst type differentiation and identification are critical to establishing the best intervention strategy. The available guidelines, such as the 2015 AGA and the 2012 International Consensus/Fukuoka guidelines, provide an algorithmic methodology for assessing the risk of malignancy within the cysts. More recent data, however, have shown the limitations of these guidelines, particularly with the observation of a low sensitivity rate of AGA criteria in detecting high-grade dysplasia or cancer. In a study of resected cyst patients, the AGA guidelines would have excluded 92.6% of patients with high-grade dysplasia or cancer, while the Fukuoka and ACR guidelines were more sensitive but at the expense of specificity (Xu et al., 2017). The findings again point towards ongoing optimization of guidelines to enhance diagnostic performance and patient outcome. Besides, additional studies are needed to further clarify the risk factors for the malignant transformation of pancreatic cysts. Notably, patient age and cyst diameter were major predictors; the risk for high-grade dysplasia or cancer was higher with cyst diameter > 3 cm and higher year of age. This has to be handled with cautious management in the patient, in a way that individualized surveillance and treatment approaches can be provided. With increasing progress in the area, the integration of predictive factors with advances in imaging modality and treatment approaches will further lead to improved stratification of patients and personalized clinical decision-making. All these advances point towards a significant change in pancreatic cyst management, reaffirming the central role of good research in refining diagnostic and treatment modalities (Xu et al., 2017) (Figure 6.15).

6.6.1. Innovations in Diagnostic Techniques

Subsequent technological advancements in pancreatic cyst diagnostic techniques have significantly enhanced clinician performance in the detection and characterization of such lesions. One such development is increased use of EUS, which allows real-time visualization of the pancreas, thereby facilitating greater accuracy in the diagnosis of cystic formations. Not only does EUS facilitate differentiation of malignant and benign cysts but also provides an avenue for FNA to obtain cytologic samples. This minimally invasive method has turned out to be vital, particularly in high-risk patients who may harbor precursors of pancreatic cancer. By making it available to detect early lesions and precursors, EUS allows physicians to stage prompt interventions, thus leading to better outcomes for patients. The refinement of EUS methods and the development of new equipment have made diagnostic examinations faster and easier in both simple and difficult cases in pancreatic pathology. At the same time, developments in imaging techniques have greatly contributed to the early detection and management of pancreatic cysts. MRI and CT scans have been developed to provide improved images and more accurate anatomical detail. The imaging tests can allow for accurate measurements of the size, shape, and potential for malignancy of pancreatic cysts to facilitate informed clinical decisions. In addition, pancreas MRI has become increasingly popular since it is non-ionizing, and thus a safer option for serial imaging, particularly in children or in those requiring long-term follow-up. , The integration of radiomics into advanced imaging modalities has tremendous promise for the molecular diagnosis of pancreatic lesions, and in so doing may revolutionize risk stratification and surveillance paradigms for individuals at high risk of pancreatic cancer. Furthermore, the advent of biomarker research points to a pivotal shift in the model of diagnosis for pancreatic cysts. A number of studies have examined the potential of serum and cyst fluid biomarkers to be used as adjuncts to traditional imaging approaches. Molecular markers derived from cystic fluid, for instance, can help elucidate the biological behavior of pancreatic cysts and thereby assist in determining their nature—malignant or benign. As highlighted in recent National Institute of Diabetes and Digestive and Kidney Diseases-sponsored workshops, there are ongoing attempts to harmonize diagnostic criteria derived from these biomarkers, which will ultimately find more personalized methods of managing patients (Lee et al., 2017). This new paradigm not only offers better diagnoses but also informs treatment pathways, harmonizing clinical care with contemporary research aimed at improving surveillance and outcomes in patients with pancreatic cysts (Meziani et al., 2024) (Figure 6.16).

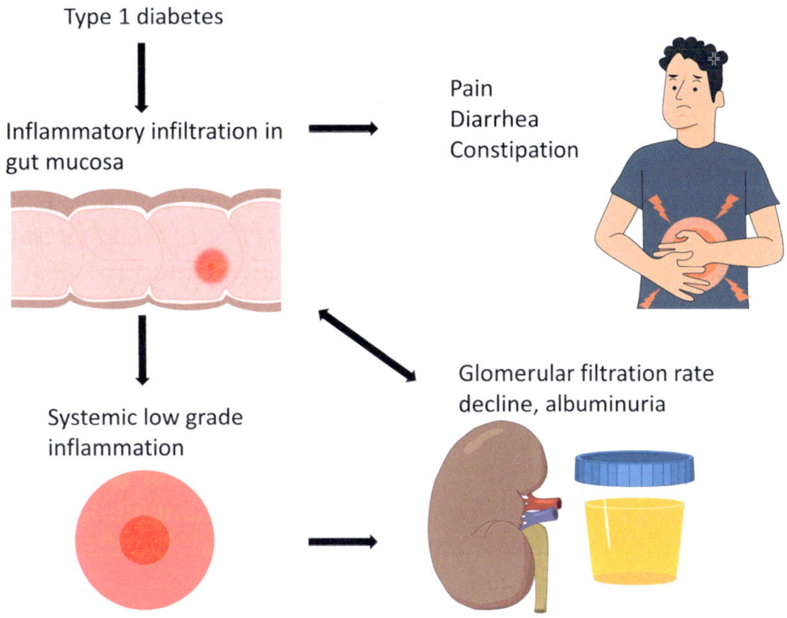

Figure 6.16. Progression of diabetic kidney disease and gastrointestinal symptoms in patients with type I.

Source: Fedulovs A, Tzivian L, Zalizko P, Ivanova S, Bumane R, Janeviča J, Krūzmane L, Krustins E, Sokolovska J. Progression of Diabetic Kidney Disease and Gastrointestinal Symptoms in Patients with Type I Diabetes. *Biomedicines*. 2023; 11(10):2679. https://doi.org/10.3390/biomedicines11102679

6.6.2. Emerging Treatment Modalities

The management of pancreatic cysts is evolving as new approaches are incorporated into clinical practice to improve patient outcomes with less risk of surgery. The tradition has been resection or observation, particularly in cysts with high malignant potential, such as MCNs and IPMNs (Jani et al., 2025). The advent of minimally invasive techniques, such as laparoscopic and endoscopic ultrasound-guided procedures, provides a paradigm shift in the treatment of these cysts. Increasing evidence suggests that these techniques can identify cystic lesions more accurately with fewer complications from open surgery. Moreover, as imaging modalities improve, the doctors can currently identify an individual type of cyst, hence more individualized and effective treatment protocols (Jani et al., 2025). Apart from minimally invasive procedures, adjunct therapies such as ethanol ablation are also gaining traction, particularly among well-chosen patients with cystic lesions that pose a significant diagnostic challenges. Ethanol ablation may be employed to reduce the size of cysts and allow for the treatment of patients without requiring further radical surgery (Jani et al., 2025). This modality is of interest where cystic masses are found to be benign after thorough evaluation. Furthermore, novel biomarkers are redescribing the diagnostic landscape, as evidenced by the identification of vascular endothelial growth factor A (VEGF-A) as an emerging pancreatic fluid biomarker for differentiating between serous cystic neoplasms and more sinister lesions. The incorporation of these biomarkers into standard clinical practice could enhance diagnostic accuracy, potentially avoiding unnecessary surgeries for benign cystic lesions while allowing timely treatment of those necessitating intervention. The interaction of advanced diagnostic techniques and emerging treatment modalities is setting a new standard of care for pancreatic cyst management. As more research comes to light, the biological foundation of these pancreatic lesions is being increasingly revealed, which could render the future of management ever more dependent on the use of personalized medicine approaches. For instance, further investigation of the synergistic effect of combination therapy, e.g., the simultaneous measurement of CEA and VEGF-A levels during cyst fluid analysis, would justify treatment planning. This paradigm change emphasizes the need for multidimensional assessment involving both biochemical parameters and imaging techniques. With evolving clinicians to these advances, the final goal stands: optimizing therapeutic effects while minimizing risks from traditional therapies for pancreatic cysts.

6.6.3. Future Directions in Pancreatic Cyst Research

The future of pancreatic cyst research is poised to make significant advances, particularly in diagnostic techniques and risk stratification. Current techniques for evaluating pancreatic cysts are largely imaging modalities such as MRI and CT scans, providing an insight into cystic nature and potential malignancy, but with intrinsic limitations, particularly in discriminating benign from malignant lesions. Against this background, ongoing studies are aimed at designing biomarker-based protocols that would enhance diagnostic accuracy and thereby define improved management protocols for patients with pancreatic cysts. For instance, identifying specific molecular profiles for each of the types of cysts would aid in providing a more personalized treatment approach. In the future, also, awareness of preoperative predictors of malignancy in mucinous cystic neoplasms—a subject characterized by the scarcity of meaningful data—will be critical in planning clinical decision-making within a few years (Postlewait et al., 2017). As pancreatic cysts are increasingly becoming an expansive arena in medicine, the push is to include genetic and epigenetic data in upcoming research studies. Early detection of pancreatic cancer remains a challenge, with the majority of patients being diagnosed at advanced stages when the treatment is limited and the prognosis is poorer (Meziani et al., 2024). Research with the goal of genetic predisposition in patients with pancreatic cysts can potentially bridge this gap. Identification of high-risk groups, most notably those with familial lifetime risk of developing pancreatic cancer, is central to the start of successful surveillance programs. Furthermore, such schemes must determine which are the best subjects to screen and the optimum time intervals to follow cysts. This will result in improved patient outcomes and possibly allow for earlier intervention in the higher-risk group. In addition, upcoming studies on pancreatic cysts will likely include a multi-faceted process where not only clinical and genetic considerations will be included, but also such advancements in treatment approaches. Minimally invasive surgeries are more and more being preferred for the management of pancreatic cysts, and they provide a platform to study their outcome compared to standard surgery. In addition, research in newer pharmacologic treatments against cystic growth and potential malignant change can offer less invasive alternatives to patients. This exploration of these less invasive methods is consistent with the greater goal of reducing morbidity from pancreatic resection. Generally, as scientists work towards understanding the intricacies of pancreatic cysts, these collective efforts could lead to numerous advances in diagnosis, management, and patient care practices and potentially alter the direction of pancreatic cyst research in the future (Postlewait et al., 2017; Meziani et al., 2024).

A CLOSER LOOK

PANCREATIC CYST SURVEILLANCE CLINIC

A Pancreatic Cyst Surveillance Clinic is a multidisciplinary clinical center that is set up to follow and treat patients with pancreatic cystic lesions, particularly those who have a potential for malignant transformation. As incidental pancreatic cysts are usually incidentally discovered by imaging for unrelated disease, a specialty clinic has a critical function in risk stratification, avoiding unnecessary resections and allowing early detection of pancreatic cancer.

The main role of a pancreatic cyst surveillance clinic is to deliver evidence-based, guideline-concordant care. Patients are assessed with high-resolution imaging—primarily MRI with MRCP—and occasionally EUS, especially in the setting of worrisome features (e.g., mural nodules, main pancreatic duct dilation, or cyst growth). The provider panel of the clinic may consist of gastroenterologists, pancreatic surgeons, radiologists, pathologists, and genetic counselors, with comprehensive assessment enabled. Cytology and molecular markers (e.g., KRAS and GNAS mutations) and CEA levels and amylase analysis of fluid on EUS-FNA (fine-needle aspiration) assist in the determination of the cyst subtype and evaluation of cancer risk.

Surveillance intervals are determined based on international consensus guidelines (e.g., Fukuoka, AGA, or European guidelines), with more frequent imaging in high-risk cysts and longer intervals for stable, low-risk lesions. Branch-duct IPMNs <3 cm with no high-risk features are typically monitored by imaging at 6–12 monthly intervals, and those with main duct involvement or suspicious features can be offered surgery or more intensive monitoring. Pointedly, the clinic also promotes patient education and shared decision-making, ensuring that patients get information about the risk, benefit, and justification for intervention or surveillance.

High-volume cyst clinics also use new technology like radiomics, machine learning-based image interpretation, and genomic cyst fluid profiling, which might offer better risk stratification. Databases for follow-up observation of cyst growth and outcome are maintained in some centers, which aid in research in pancreatic disease. Ultimately, a pancreatic cyst surveillance clinic works towards maintaining an equilibrium avoidance of overtreatment and with early detection of malignancy, with individualized care for a growing number of patients with pancreatic cystic neoplasms (Northrup et al., 2021).

SUMMARY

In a case of pancreatic cysts, sure that the significance of accurate diagnosis and appropriate management choices should not be overstated. With improvements in imaging technologies, cystic pancreatic lesions are increasingly being diagnosed. This phenomenon is a necessity for medical practitioners to be knowledgeable about the various types of pancreatic cysts, such as mucinous cystic neoplasms and IPMNs. According to new guidelines, the differentiation between benign and potentially malignant lesions is most important since diseases like IPMNs represent known precursors of pancreatic cancer with the poorest prognosis among all malignancies (Azzopardi et al., 2014). The treatment of such lesions needs to be tailored to their characteristics, which emphasizes the need for a proper understanding of their pathophysiology and natural history. The implications of the identification of the cystic lesions of the pancreas reach far beyond mere diagnosis; they highlight the need for follow-up and management strategies in patients. As an example, asymptomatic branch duct-origin IPMNs without features of high risk can often be followed rather than receiving immediate surgery. Yet mucinous cystic neoplasms and other high-risk ones need urgent surgical excision to prevent potential malignancy (Azzopardi et al., 2014). Thus, the conclusion reached in the management of pancreatic cysts reiterates once again the imperative of individualized patient care interventions not only based on imaging findings but on the broader context of the patient's clinical situation. This is in line with ongoing efforts toward better comprehension of neoplasms of the pancreas and their intrinsic risks. Ultimately, the diagnosis and treatment of pancreatic cysts are evolving, particularly with the emergence of advanced diagnostics such as Convolutional Neural Networks (CNNs) for the assessment of IPMNs. These systems enhance the accuracy of risk stratification, which is paramount in setting the necessary clinical interventions (Bagci et al., 2018). With increasing medical technology advancements, the application of artificial intelligence in diagnostics is set to revolutionize the industry through heightened accuracy that can help lead to enhanced patient outcomes. In conclusion, a wide-angle approach to managing pancreatic cysts entails the combination of clinical expertise, technological advancements, and patient results. The importance of recognition of the neoplastic potential of some cysts and the hope of new diagnostic techniques will play a central role in establishing paradigms of management of these demanding lesions in the future.

The pathophysiology of pancreatic cysts tells us a great deal about their formation, classification, and potential impact on the health of the patient. Most importantly, the cysts are classified into various types, including serous cystadenomas, mucinous cystic neoplasms, and intraductal papillary mucinous neoplasms. Each of these has distinct clinical manifestations and varying outcomes for the formation of malignancies. To illustrate, mucinous cystic neoplasms are of particular interest because they present a risk of pancreatic cancer. It is important to recognize these differences for the purpose of guiding proper measures of management and intervening when warranted. Furthermore, advances in imaging modalities, such as MRI and CT scans, facilitate accurate diagnosis and evaluation of pancreatic cysts, ultimately towards better patient care. The biological processes of pancreatic cyst formation are a field of ongoing research interest. Recent evidence suggests that cellular signaling-related and microenvironmental interaction-related factors are central determinants in the pathogenesis of such lesions. In greater specificity, studies show that the growth and differentiation abnormalities of cells, especially epithelial tissues, underlie cystic changes. For example, the role of the extracellular matrix (ECM) in regulating epithelial cell polarity is essential for normal acinar morphogenesis, as discussed in a study showcasing paracrine signaling pathways in cell organization (Bryant et al., 2017). Such findings may open doors to targeted therapies by targeting these dysregulated cellular pathways in patients with pancreatic cysts. Secondly, the implications of pancreatic cyst management transcend the diagnosis and treatment; they encompass extension to patient education and follow-up. Patients with pancreatic cysts should be informed of their status in an open manner, sensitive to the risk of having presenting symptoms progressing from benign to malignant. Imaging follow-up at regular intervals and monitoring cyst characteristics are central elements in effective management so that immediate interventions may be done if transformation hints are noted. In addition, patient symptom awareness, such as abdominal discomfort or a change in appetite may facilitate earlier detection of complications or related conditions. Treatment of both medical and educational aspects of pancreatic cysts is an overarching patient care approach, generally leading to improved outcomes for patients with these lesions (Puri et al., 2009).

KEY TERMS FROM THIS CHAPTER

- Abnormal activation
- Anatomical location
- Back pain
- Baseline serum
- Close observation
- Contemporary clinical assessment
- Cytology
- Diets
- Epithelial cells
- Epithelial lining
- Familial pancreatic cancer (FPC)
- Fine needle aspiration (FNA)

References

1. Postlewait, L. M., Ethun, C. G., McInnis, M. R., Merchant, N., Parikh, A., Idrees, K., Isom, C. A., Hawkins, W., Fields, R. C., Strand, M., Weber, S. M., Cho, C. S., Salem, A., Martin, R. C., Scoggins, C., Bentrem, D., Kim, H. J., Carr, J., Ahmad, S., Abbott, D. E., ... Maithel, S. K. (2017). Association of Preoperative Risk Factors With Malignancy in Pancreatic Mucinous Cystic Neoplasms: A Multicenter Study. *JAMA surgery*, *152*(1), 19–25. https://doi.org/10.1001/jamasurg.2016.3598 (accessed on 26 May 2025).
2. Aguero Garcete, G., Angiolini, M. R., Araujo Acuna, I., Arcidiacono, P., et al. (2015). Serous cystic neoplasm of the pancreas: A multinational study of 2622 patients under the auspices of the International Association of Pancreatology and European Pancreatic Club. https://core.ac.uk/download/53527604.pdf (accessed on 26 May 2025).
3. Al-Haddad, M., Anand, B. S., Baron, T. H., Berg, D. E., Bhutani, M. S., Bottrell, C. B., Boyle, M., et al. (2014). Clinical evaluation, imaging studies, and cytologic study recommendations for pancreatic and biliary cytology. https://deepblue.lib.umich.edu/bitstream/2027.42/106723/1/dc23095.pdf (accessed on 26 May 2025).
4. Lee, L. S., Andersen, D. K., Ashida, R., Brugge, W. R., Canto, M. I., Chang, K. J., Chari, S. T., DeWitt, J., Hwang, J. H., Khashab, M. A., Kim, K., Levy, M. J., McGrath, K., Park, W. G., Singhi, A., Stevens, T., Thompson, C. C., Topazian, M. D., Wallace, M. B., Wani, S., ... Singh, V. K. (2017). Endoscopic Ultrasound and Related Technologies for the Diagnosis and Treatment of Pancreatic Disease - Research Gaps and Opportunities: Summary of a National Institute of Diabetes and Digestive and Kidney Diseases Workshop. *Pancreas*, *46*(10), 1242–1250. https://doi.org/10.1097/MPA.0000000000000936(accessed on 26 May 2025).
5. Northrup, H., Aronow, M. E., Bebin, E. M., Bissler, J., Darling, T. N., de Vries, P. J., Frost, M. D., Fuchs, Z., Gosnell, E. S., Gupta, N., Jansen, A. C., Jóźwiak, S., Kingswood, J. C., Knilans, T. K., McCormack, F. X., Pounders, A., Roberds, S. L., Rodriguez-Buritica, D. F., Roth, J., Sampson, J. R., ... International Tuberous Sclerosis Complex Consensus Group (2021). Updated International Tuberous Sclerosis Complex Diagnostic Criteria and Surveillance and Management Recommendations. *Pediatric neurology*, *123*, 50–66. https://doi.org/10.1016/j.pediatrneurol.2021.07.011 (accessed on 26 May 2025).
6. Xu, M. M., Yin, S., Siddiqui, A. A., Salem, R. R., Schrope, B., Sethi, A., Poneros, J. M., Gress, F. G., Genkinger, J. M., Do, C., Brooks, C. A., Chabot, J. A., Kluger, M. D., Kowalski, T., Loren, D. E., Aslanian, H., Farrell, J. J., & Gonda, T. A. (2017). Comparison of the diagnostic accuracy of three current guidelines for the evaluation of asymptomatic pancreatic cystic neoplasms. *Medicine*, *96*(35), e7900. https://doi.org/10.1097/MD.0000000000007900 (accessed on 26 May 2025).
7. Azzopardi, N. (2014). Cystic lesions of the pancreas. https://core.ac.uk/download/46602499.pdf (accessed on 26 May 2025).
8. Scialpi, M., Reginelli, A., D'Andrea, A., Gravante, S., Falcone, G., Baccari, P., Manganaro, L., Palumbo, B., & Cappabianca, S. (2016). Pancreatic tumors imaging: An update. *International journal of surgery (London, England)*, *28 Suppl 1*, S142–S155. https://doi.org/10.1016/j.ijsu.2015.12.053 (accessed on 26 May 2025).
9. Bagci, U., Bolan, C. W., Corral, J. E., Hussein, S., et al. (2018). Deep multi-modal classification of intraductal papillary mucinous neoplasms (IPMN) with canonical correlation analysis. *arXiv Preprint*. http://arxiv.org/abs/1710.09779 (accessed on 26 May 2025).

10. Jani, N., Bani Hani, M., Schulick, R. D., Hruban, R. H., & Cunningham, S. C. (2011). Diagnosis and management of cystic lesions of the pancreas. *Diagnostic and therapeutic endoscopy*, *2011*, 478913. https://doi.org/10.1155/2011/478913

11. Ganeshan, D., Menias, C. O., Pickhardt, P. J., Sandrasegaran, K., Lubner, M. G., Ramalingam, P., & Bhalla, S. (2018). Tumors in von Hippel-Lindau Syndrome: From Head to Toe-Comprehensive State-of-the-Art Review. *Radiographics : a review publication of the Radiological Society of North America, Inc*, *38*(3), 849–866. https://doi.org/10.1148/rg.2018170156 (accessed on 26 May 2025).

12. Blackburn, E. (2021). The emerging role of pancreatic β-cell primary cilia in diabetes mellitus. https://core.ac.uk/download/482673598.pdf.

13. BN, N., Bruno, M. J., Fuhler, G. M., Jose, J., et al. (2017). Pancreatic cyst fluid harbors a unique microbiome. https://core.ac.uk/download/154410540.pdf (accessed on 26 May 2025).

14. Popivanov, G., Tabakov, M., Mantese, G., Cirocchi, R., Piccinini, I., D'Andrea, V., Covarelli, P., Boselli, C., Barberini, F., Tabola, R., Pietro, U., & Cavaliere, D. (2018). Surgical treatment of gastrointestinal stromal tumors of the duodenum: a literature review. *Translational gastroenterology and hepatology*, *3*, 71. https://doi.org/10.21037/tgh.2018.09.04 (accessed on 26 May 2025).

15. Meziani, J., Fuhler, G. M., Bruno, M. J., Cahen, D. L., & Overbeek, K. A. (2024). Pancreatic Cancer Screening: A Narrative Review. *Techniques and Innovations in Gastrointestinal Endoscopy*, *26*(4), 323-334. https://doi.org/10.1016/j.tige.2024.08.001 (accessed on 26 May 2025).

16. Bruno, M. J., de Jong, K., & Fockens, P. (2012). Epidemiology, diagnosis, and management of cystic lesions of the pancreas. https://core.ac.uk/download/pdf/8627672.pdf.

17. Bryant, D. M., Datta, A., Mostov, K. E., Sandilands, E., et al. (2017). Fibroblast-derived HGF drives acinar lung cancer cell polarization through integrin-dependent RhoA-ROCK1 inhibition. https://core.ac.uk/download/96883587.pdf (accessed on 26 May 2025).

18. Gomatos, I. P., Halloran, C., Ghaneh, P., Raraty, M., Polydoros, F., Campbell, F., Evans, J., Sutton, R., Garry, J., Whelan, P., & Neoptolemos, J. P. (2016). Management and Outcome of 64 Patients with Pancreatic Serous Cystic Neoplasms. *Digestive surgery*, *33*(3), 203–212. https://doi.org/10.1159/000442094 (accessed on 26 May 2025).

19. Cano, D. A., Flores Martínez, Á., Hebrok, M., et al. (2016). Loss of pancreas upon activated Wnt signaling is concomitant with emergence of gastrointestinal identity. https://core.ac.uk/download/186618050.pdf (accessed on 26 May 2025).

20. Cano, D. A., Hebrok, M., & Puri, S. (2009). A role for von Hippel-Lindau protein in pancreatic beta-cell function. https://core.ac.uk/download/323072356.pdf. Puri, S., Cano, D. A., & Hebrok, M. (2009). A role for von Hippel-Lindau protein in pancreatic beta-cell function. *Diabetes*, *58*(2), 433–441. https://doi.org/10.2337/db08-0749

21. Carico, E., Carnuccio, A., Di Giulio, E., et al. (2015). Rapid on-site evaluation (ROSE) in pancreatic cancer diagnosis: Doing more with less. https://core.ac.uk/download/54521845.pdf (accessed on 26 May 2025).

22. Carr, R. A., Dolejs, S., Hancock, B. A., et al. (2017). Pancreatic cyst fluid vascular endothelial growth factor A and carcinoembryonic antigen: A highly accurate test for the diagnosis of serous cystic neoplasm. https://core.ac.uk/download/159342255.pdf (accessed on 26 May 2025).

23. Morris-Stiff, G., Falk, G. A., Chalikonda, S., & Walsh, R. M. (2013). Natural history of asymptomatic pancreatic cystic neoplasms. *HPB : the official journal of the International Hepato Pancreato Biliary Association*, *15*(3), 175–181. https://doi.org/10.1111/j.1477-2574.2012.00522.x. Jiao, L. R., Frampton, A. E., Jacob, J., Pellegrino, L., Krell, J., Giamas, G., Tsim, N., Vlavianos, P., Cohen, P., Ahmad, R., Keller, A., Habib, N. A., Stebbing, J., & Castellano, L. (2012). MicroRNAs targeting oncogenes are down-regulated in pancreatic malignant transformation from benign tumors. *PloS one*, *7*(2), e32068. https://doi.org/10.1371/journal.pone.0032068

24. Crocetti, D., D'Orazi, V., Grazi, G. L., et al. (2015). Peliosis hepatis: Personal experience and literature review. https://core.ac.uk/download/54526950.pdf (accessed on 26 May 2025).

25. Moyer, M. T., Maranki, J. L., & DeWitt, J. M. (2019). EUS-Guided Pancreatic Cyst Ablation: a Clinical and Technical Review. *Current gastroenterology reports*, *21*(5), 19. https://doi.org/10.1007/s11894-019-0686-5 (accessed on 26 May 2025).

26. Lawson, R. D., Hunt, G. C., Giap, A. Q., Krinsky, M. L., Slezak, J., Tang, R. S., Gonzalez, I., Kwong, W. T., Fehmi, S. A., & Savides, T. J. (2015). Pancreatic cysts suspected to be branch duct intraductal papillary mucinous neoplasm without concerning features have low risk for development of pancreatic cancer. *Annals of gastroenterology*, *28*(4), 487–494.Hoorens, A., Id, A., Frederik, V., Delvaux, G., De Vogelaere, K., & Meert, V. (2012). Unusual appearance of a pendulated gastric tumor: Always think of GIST. https://core.ac.uk/download/84041173.pdf (accessed on 26 May 2025).

27. Kocjan, G. (2010). Fine needle aspiration cytology of the pancreas: A guide to the diagnostic approach. https://core.ac.uk/download/14426738.pdf (accessed on 26 May 2025).

28. Koncoro, H., & Wibawa, I. D. (2012). Acute pancreatitis as a complication of choledochal cyst. https://media.neliti.com/media/publications/63839-EN-acute-pancreatitis-as-a-complication-of.pdf (accessed on 26 May 2025).

29. Lee, H. K., Park, S. J., Yi, B. H., Lee, A. L., Moon, J. H., & Chang, Y. W. (2009). Imaging features of adult choledochal cysts: a pictorial review. *Korean journal of radiology*, *10*(1), 71–80. https://doi.org/10.3348/kjr.2009.10.1.71Mann, S. (2021). Polycystic ovarian syndrome and insulin resistance: An evaluation of treatment modalities and complication prevention. https://core.ac.uk/download/427713199.pdf (accessed on 26 May 2025).

30. Mosimann, F., Ribaux, C., & Schnyder, P. (1990). Cystic neoplasms of the exocrine pancreas. *HPB surgery : a world journal of hepatic, pancreatic and biliary surgery*, *2*(3), 165–175. https://doi.org/10.1155/1990/24762Namoosi, R. (2024). Study of food patterns among patients with polycystic ovarian syndrome. https://core.ac.uk/download/620847719.pdf (accessed on 26 May 2025).

31. Neri, V. (2017). Management of Pancreatic Cystic Lesions. InTech. doi: 10.5772/65117(accessed on 26 May 2025).

32. Scott, R. J. (2003). Familial adenomatous polyposis (FAP) and other polyposis syndromes. https://core.ac.uk/download/pdf/8390115.pdf.

33. Signoretti, M. (2019). Screening for pancreatic cancer in high-risk individuals. https://core.ac.uk/download/188831832.pdf (accessed on 26 May 2025).

34. Toma, Jelena, "Contribution of Activating Transcription Factor 3 to development of acinar-to-ductal cell metaplasia" (2017). *Electronic Thesis and Dissertation Repository*. 4719. https://ir.lib.uwo.ca/etd/4719 (accessed on 26 May 2025).

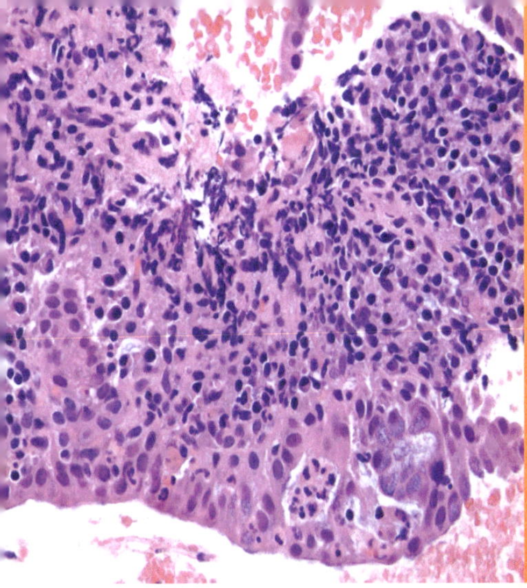

Chapter 7

AUTOIMMUNE PANCREATITIS

Contents

Introduction

Autoimmune pancreatitis (AIP) is a newly recognized manifestation of pancreatitis with an autoimmune-mediated inflammatory process around the pancreas. It's a complex condition and generally categorized into two types: Type 1 which exists along with IgG4-related disease, and Type 2 which is characterized by specific histopathological features. Type 1 AIP typically has elevated serum IgG4 levels and is most commonly linked to systemic manifestations, while Type 2 is more localized and occurs in younger patients without concomitant elevation of IgG4. Differentiation between the two types is important as it determines prognosis and management, guiding clinicians toward a more favorable therapeutic approach based on individual patients' needs. Treatment of autoimmune pancreatitis is important in view of the risk of progression from acute attack to chronic pancreatitis, with significant morbidity in terms of reducing the quality of life of the patients. The treatment approach is based on the use of corticosteroids that are well reported to exert a rapid response in the modulation of inflammation and relief of symptoms. Recent studies have indicated that corticosteroids are able to stop autoimmune pancreatitis from advancing to chronic stages, and thus their importance in clinical practice (González et al., 2013). However, the heterogeneity of response towards corticosteroid therapy among patients, on the basis mainly of the distinct pathophysiological processes of Type 1 and Type 2 AIP, points out the complexities associated with successful therapy. Relapse prevention is also a critical component of autoimmune pancreatitis management because relapse can lead to poor outcomes, like irreversible pancreatic damage. Understanding the pathophysiologic mechanisms can give clinicians an idea of how they can develop targeted interventions to prevent relapse. Cognitive assessment of corticosteroid response and probability of prolonged remission are essential components in the realm of patient management (González et al., 2013). Secondly, heterogeneity of clinical presentation and treatment response among the involved individuals necessitates ongoing research to establish more precise diagnostic criteria and treatment modalities and, lastly, to improve long-term outcomes in patients with autoimmune pancreatitis (Figure 7.1).

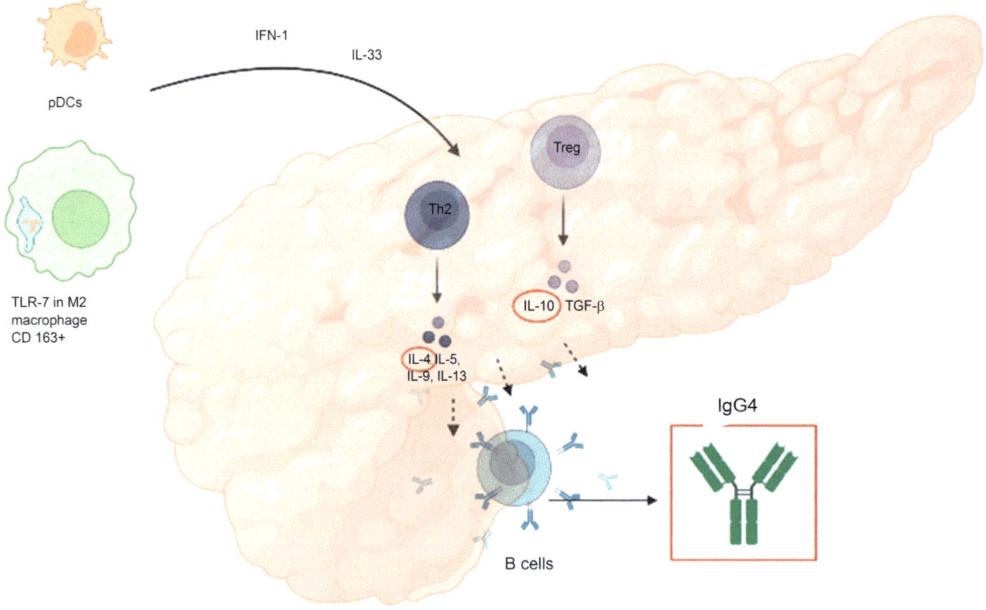

Figure 7.1. Autoimmune pancreatitis (AIP).

Source: Nista EC, De Lucia SS, Manilla V, Schepis T, Pellegrino A, Ojetti V, Pignataro G, Zileri dal Verme L, Franceschi F, Gasbarrini A, et al. Autoimmune Pancreatitis: From Pathogenesis to Treatment. *International Journal of Molecular Sciences*. 2022; 23(20):12667. https://doi.org/10.3390/ijms232012667

Definition of Autoimmune Pancreatitis (AIP)

The understanding of AIP mandates a clear definition of its complexity and clinical significance. Autoimmune pancreatitis is characterized by an inflammatory process in the pancreas that starts as a result of a dysregulated immune reaction against the tissue of the pancreas. It is further categorized into two broad forms: Type 1, which is usually associated with IgG4-related disease, and Type 2, which is not associated with the IgG4 subclass. Clinically, AIP is characterized by abdominal pain, jaundice, and weight loss and usually imitates pancreatic cancer. The complex nature of AIP makes diagnosis a challenge, as it involves differentiating from autoimmune and other causes of pancreatitis. There is an urgent need for early identification and precise diagnostic criteria since untreated conditions result in serious complications and influence patients' quality of life. Diagnosis of autoimmune pancreatitis is in itself problematic because the clinical presentation overlaps with other pancreatic disorders. For example, the presentation of AIP can be such that it imitates chronic pancreatitis, and this makes correct diagnosis difficult unless it is approached in a stringent and multidisciplinary manner. To guide clinicians, protocols have been established to harmonize the diagnostic procedures, which generally include serological examination for autoimmune markers, imaging methods such as MRI and EUS, and, in some cases, biopsy in order to confirm the inflammatory process. The Spanish Pancreatic Club, for example, has developed a consensus for managing chronic pancreatitis, which reflects the subtlety that clinicians face in diagnosis and management. These frameworks are crucial in the improvement of diagnostic sensitivity and patient care in autoimmune diseases like AIP (González et al., 2013). In the treatment of AIP, response patterns to corticosteroid therapy are significant in the prediction of treatment outcome and relapse prevention. The corticosteroids are still the mainstay of therapy, particularly for Type 1 AIP, which responds favorably to steroid therapy. Patients typically experience relief of symptoms and diminution in pancreatic inflammation following corticosteroid therapy. However, the outcome in Type 1 and Type 2 AIP varies, with Type 1 responding more to corticosteroid sensitivity than Type 2. The variation brings out the need for treatment regimens that are tailored to individual consideration of the disease pathology and patient response. Furthermore, ongoing research should concentrate on addressing relapse rates post-treatment and on optimizing long-term management plans for better outcomes in patients suffering from this complex autoimmune disease (Gleeson et al., 2025).

Importance of Distinguishing Between Type 1 And Type 2

Differentiation between Type 1 and Type 2 AIP is essential for accurate diagnosis, treatment, and management. Type 1 AIP is most frequently associated with IgG4-related disease, characterized by elevated serum levels of IgG4 and lymphoplasmacytic inflammation. This specific association not only teaches clinicians about the systemic nature of the disease but also allows for targeted therapies, such as corticosteroids, that have been found to be remarkable for their potential to reduce inflammation and improve patient outcomes. Type 2 AIP, on the other hand, lacks the IgG4 elevation and has distinct pathological features. Identification of such differences avoids misdiagnosis and ensures that patients are being treated appropriately because of their distinctive condition, thus eliminating the risks of complications arising from mismanagement and enhancing patient care and prognosis as a whole (Gleeson et al., 2025). Identification of differences in pathophysiology between Type 2 and Type 1 AIP is also important in making effective predictions regarding clinical behavior and response to treatment. Type 1 AIP is likely to present with more aggressive clinical manifestations, e.g., the involvement of the other organs like the biliary tree, salivary glands, and lymph nodes, and therefore, it becomes crucial to notice the indications of systemic illness. Type 2 AIP, on the other hand, typically presents as a focal process within the pancreas and can be treated successfully with medical therapy alone. Identification of these distinctions enables clinicians to utilize stricter monitoring regimens for Type 1 patients and consider alternative therapeutic options. This tailored treatment not only enhances the quality of care but also reduces the risk of mismanagement, which could complicate patient suffering (Chapman et al., 2019). From a relapse prevention standpoint, Type 1 and Type 2 AIP differentiation have important long-term treatment plan implications. Type 1 AIP is distinguished by its spontaneous remission and relapse tendency and can sometimes necessitate an active management regimen that can include persistent corticosteroid treatment or immunosuppressants. Type 2 AIP, on the other hand, has a lower propensity for recurrence and can most effectively be treated by more conservative therapy for the majority of patients. It is awareness of these patterns of relapsing disease that allows clinicians to develop patient-specific management strategies that consider the risks and benefits of long-term steroid treatment. This strategic distinction ultimately serves not only patients' physical well-being but also their mental well-being, as expectation management of disease behavior contributes to improved patient satisfaction and adherence (Gleeson et al., 2025) (Figure 7.2).

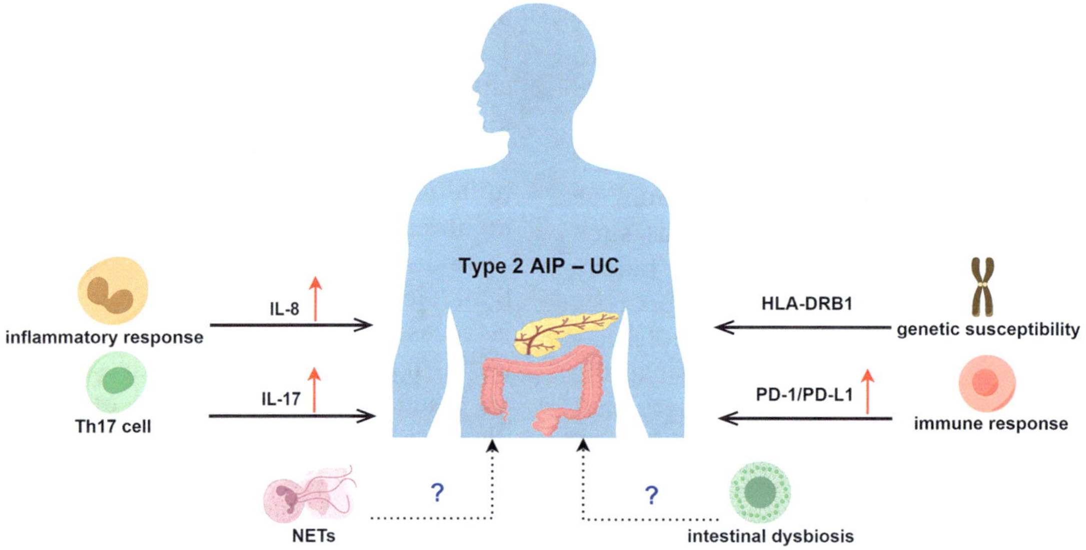

Figure 7.2. Type 2 autoimmune pancreatitis associated with ulcerative colitis.

Source: Nan N and Wang D (2023) Type 2 autoimmune pancreatitis associated with ulcerative colitis. Front. Immunol. 14:1288390. doi: 10.3389/fimmu.2023.1288390

7.1. Understanding Autoimmune Pancreatitis (AIP)

AIP investigation involves understanding its two distinct forms, Type 1 and Type 2, both with their unique pathological characteristics. Type 1 AIP would be associated with IgG4-related disease, demonstrated by elevated levels of serum IgG4 and tissue infiltration of IgG4-positive plasma cells. This subtype, originally identified by the presence of extraintestinal manifestations, has significant clinical overlap with other autoimmune conditions, and it is challenging to diagnose and manage. Conversely, Type 2 AIP, while less common, is distinguished from its relative based on its inability to induce elevation of IgG4 and clean histological characteristics. Symptomatology and organ involvement in both types are equally critical in the process of differentiation, as Type 1 has been discovered to have extra-systemic signs and symptoms that may either precede or accompany pancreatic signs in such a manner that diagnostic workup becomes extremely difficult (Gleeson et al., 2025). Treatment of AIP relies on the use of corticosteroids, which have been shown to be very effective in managing symptoms and achieving remission. Both types rely on corticosteroids not only as a treatment option but also as a diagnostic tool, since a response can be used to diagnose AIP. The routine corticosteroid regimen initiates high doses and tapers them afterward to prevent potential side effects. In Type 1 AIP, corticosteroid response is rapid, with significant improvement in clinical manifestations and inflammatory markers. Type 2 AIP, although responsive, will take a longer treatment duration to achieve similar results. Risk of relapse remains for both types, and thus regular follow-up and perhaps maintenance therapy become a must (Hibi et al., 2016). The challenge of preventing relapse in autoimmune pancreatitis is itself evidence of the complexity of long-term management. Given the nature of AIP, where relapses and spontaneous remissions are not uncommon, prevention of relapse is itself central to maximizing the results of patients. Evidence indicates that continuation of sustained corticosteroid therapy, combined with regular follow-up measurements, can be very effective in decreasing the occurrence of relapse. Additionally, changes in lifestyle, such as dietary modifications and alcohol avoidance, are also recommended to avoid triggers that may aggravate the condition. The patient must be educated by healthcare professionals about the risk of relapse and the necessity of adhering strictly to treatment protocols because an early intervention at the inception of the signs will radically alter the disease course (Gleeson et al., 2025). It is thus crucial to value the processes of autoimmune pancreatitis, including its types, corticosteroid sensitivity, and relapse prevention, to enhance the quality of treatment for the affected (Figure 7.3).

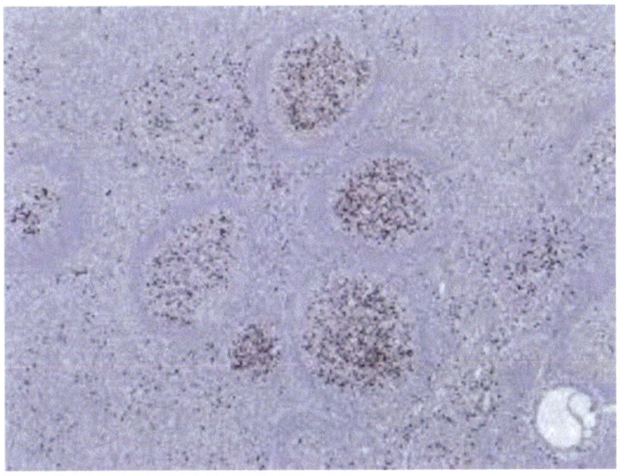

Figure 7.3. IgG4-positive plasma cells.

Source: https://encrypted-tbn0.gstatic.com/images?q=tbn:ANd9GcQPufosSVionRsZpTN71flkzTLtl XbYxM13pw&s.

7.1.1. Pathophysiology of Autoimmune Pancreatitis

The pathophysiology of autoimmune pancreatitis entails a complex interaction among immune mechanisms leading to inflammation and resultant injury in the pancreas. Autoimmune pancreatitis is generally classified as Type 1 or Type 2 autoimmune pancreatitis, and the two differ histopathologically. Type 1 is most often accompanied by IgG4-positive plasma cells and a systemic pattern of IgG4-

related disease, which points towards humoral immunity in pathogenesis. On the other hand, Type 2 has a lymphocytic infiltrate but does not typically present with IgG4 elevation. It is necessary to be aware of these diverse immune patterns because the treatment strategies are quite dissimilar. Genetic participation is another equally significant component of autoimmune pancreatitis pathophysiology, independent of the immune process. Quantitative trait loci (QTLs) recently discovered play a very crucial role in modulating the severity of disease. For example, five QTLs for autoimmune pancreatitis were located on chromosomes 2, 4, 5, and 6 in studies that have established a genetic predisposition to the condition in some mouse models. Discovery of these loci improves not only our understanding of the genetic etiology of autoimmune pancreatitis but also opens doors to novel therapeutic interventions to modify disease severity and potentially prevent progression of the disease to chronic pancreatitis. Corticosteroids remain the cornerstone of the treatment of autoimmune pancreatitis, particularly for Type 1 disease. Corticosteroids possess potent anti-inflammatory action, lessening the immune response responsible for pancreatic inflammation. Evidence suggests that corticosteroids can inhibit the progression of autoimmune pancreatitis into chronic pancreatitis, as outlined in the pertinent studies. This capability is important because chronic pancreatitis tends to cause irreversible damage and the development of complications such as diabetes and pancreatic cancer. Secondly, identifying the differential sensitivity of Type 1 and Type 2 autoimmune pancreatitis to corticosteroids will allow clinicians to treat each patient individually, enhancing overall treatment outcomes as well as reducing the risk of relapse.

7.1.2. Symptoms and Clinical Presentation

AIP's clinical presentation can often lead to diagnostic misgivings due to similar symptoms with other pancreatic diseases. It can typically arise in older patients, predominantly men, with an average age at diagnosis of around 63 years. Patients typically present with jaundice, which is due to obstructive lesions of the biliary tree secondary to the pancreatic swelling in AIP. In addition, presenting features such as significant weight loss and new-onset diabetes mellitus are also common presentations. The presentation of these, with diffuse or focal pancreatic enlargement, is a significant sign for health care providers when screening for potential cases of AIP, as the disease is responsible for 5%–6% of all chronic pancreatitis and can present similarly to pancreatic malignancies (Gleeson et al., 2025). In addition to the pancreatic manifestation, AIP can also manifest with systemic features that will complicate its clinical picture. The extrapancreatic manifestations can affect many organs, such as the biliary system, salivary glands, and kidneys. These extrapancreatic manifestations can lead to conditions such as sclerosing cholangitis and Sjögrens syndrome, which can obscure the true diagnosis of AIP. They may also develop retroperitoneal fibrosis or lymphadenopathy, which may occur with, if not preceding, the pancreatic symptoms. The heterogeneity in presentation warrants the application of wide-based imaging and serologic diagnostic workup, particularly the serum IgG4 level, which is elevated in a very high proportion of patients with type 1 AIP (Gleeson et al., 2025). The corticosteroid response is a major characteristic of autoimmune pancreatitis therapy because it significantly alters the clinical course of the disease. Patients typically respond rapidly to corticosteroids, which can enhance their clinical symptoms within a few weeks upon treatment initiation. Steroid effectiveness is not just a therapeutic standard but also an index of diagnosis, as a response to steroid treatment can confirm the autoimmune cause of the pancreatitis. Relapse afterwards is nonetheless a source of concern, with studies indicating that relapses after spontaneous remissions are common occurrences. Therefore, comprehension of the early signs of AIP and their systemic implications is crucial for prompt intervention and successful relapse prevention measures (Figure 7.4).

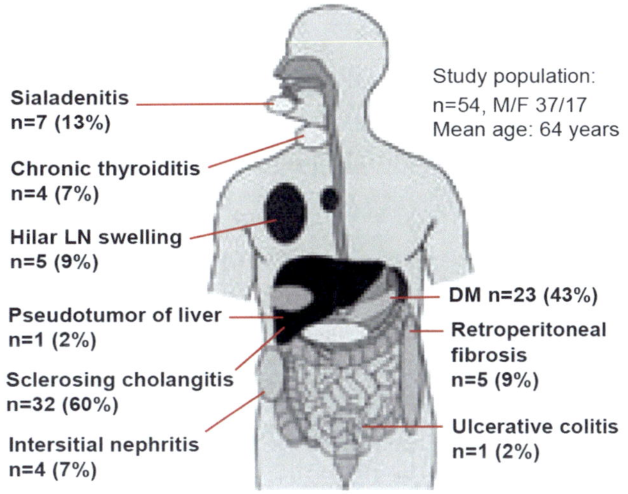

Figure 7.4. Extrapancreatic lesions.

Source: https://www.researchgate.net/profile/Toshiro_Fukui/publication/51636123/figure/fig1/AS:341283626340354@1458379765576/Extrapancreatic-lesions-of-which-sclerosing-cholangitis-is-the-most-commonly-observed.png.

7.1.3. Diagnostic Criteria and Methods

The diagnostic criteria of AIP are crucial in the differentiation between its types, particularly Type 1 and Type 2. The early diagnoses usually utilize clinical symptoms such as abdominal pain, jaundice, and weight loss that usually overlap with other pancreatic illnesses. Imaging tests, including magnetic resonance imaging (MRI) and endoscopic retrograde cholangiopancreatography (ERCP), are very important in the diagnosis, as they reveal characteristic lesions and narrowing of the pancreatic duct. Additionally, serological tests for the measurement of immunoglobulin G4 (IgG4) levels are also essential, particularly in Type 1 AIP, where increased IgG4 is typically present, with Type 2 AIP having normal values. These modalities emphasize the multi-modal strategy required for accurate diagnosis, combining clinical signs, imaging findings, and laboratory examinations to dramatically impact patient outcomes by facilitating early intervention. Compounding diagnosis is added by the heterogeneity of chronic pancreatitis (CP), which can appear early in the disease course of AIP. Absence of a widely utilized gold standard for diagnosis in the early stages of CP may lead to misdiagnosis if presentation is atypical. Diagnostic heterogeneity between operators and centers has been reported by the Spanish Pancreatic Club, highlighting the need for uniform protocols that improve consensus in the treatment of CP (González et al., 2013). Thus, practitioners need to keep their guard up in case of identification of AIP, since appropriate diagnosis not only prescribes treatment regimens but also determines prognosis. With specific diagnostic criteria, healthcare providers can identify AIP from other forms of pancreatitis and proceed with more accurate therapeutic interventions and better patient management. Upon diagnosis, treatment of AIP generally involves the use of corticosteroids, which have proven effective in managing inflammation and halting disease progression. A research work from Shinshu University highlights the observation that corticosteroids can halt the progression of autoimmune pancreatitis into chronic pancreatitis, a critical point in intervention for clinicians (González et al., 2013). Regular follow-up evaluations, such as imaging and serology, remain essential in monitoring response to treatment. A crucial realization is, in fact, the variation in response to corticosteroids between Type 1 and Type 2 AIP. With continued research informing treatment protocols, the use of strict diagnostic criteria and adaptive treatment approaches will provide enhanced outcomes and mitigate the risk of relapse, eventually optimizing autoimmune pancreatitis management as a whole.

7.2. Type 1 Autoimmune Pancreatitis (AIP)

Type 1 AIP is gradually being characterized as a unique form of pancreatitis according to its underlying immunological pathogenesis and clinical profile. Type 1 AIP is classically observed in middle-aged males, with abdominal pain, weight loss, and complications of pancreatitis among the presenting symptoms. Notably, type 1 AIP has been observed to be frequently linked with elevated concentrations of IgG4, an important factor in pathogenesis. The potential for ductal obstruction and thickening of the pancreatic duct is are classic feature of the disease, making type 1 AIP a compelling differential diagnosis consideration for pancreatitis. Its clinical relevance is additionally heightened by its association with other autoimmune diseases, and thus solid understanding is critical to guide effective management. Besides, the early intervention can prevent the progression of chronic pancreatitis, which indicates the urgency of proper identification and treatment of type 1 AIP (González et al., 2013). The management strategy in type 1 AIP primarily involves the use of corticosteroids, which are extremely efficacious in remitting and symptomatically enhancing the condition. Administration of corticosteroids here is of utmost relevance in that it has been established that corticosteroids have the ability to stop the process of becoming chronic pancreatitis, and in turn, optimize the outcome of the patient. Systematic review of clinical reaction to steroid therapy demonstrates an overwhelmingly high rate of remission in favor of corticosteroid treatment as a first-line treatment. Nevertheless, heterogeneity in response insists on an individualized treatment regimen in accordance with patient-specific factors. Type 1 AIP management also involves watching for potential side effects due to steroids, which can impact the successful long-term management of the disease. While corticosteroids are useful, keeping in mind that there is a risk of relapse after stopping treatment is especially significant given the multifactorial etiology of this autoimmune condition (González et al., 2013). Relapse prevention of type 1 AIP is a clinical conundrum, wherein the patient can experience recurrent attacks despite successful initial treatment with corticosteroids. Relapse risk needs to be addressed through continuous long-term management utilizing follow-ups and lifestyle modifications. Further, recent evidence suggests that combination treatments, except corticosteroids, can offer additional relapse protection. Such therapeutic interventions include immunomodulators, which have the potential to augment immune function and decrease inflammation. Current trials and research seek to further optimize such strategies, revealing the best treatment protocols. Lastly, a comprehensive understanding of the disease pathophysiology, coupled with advances in the therapeutic strategy, is essential in the achievement of sustained remission and the improvement of the quality of life of type 1 autoimmune pancreatitis patients (González et al., 2013) (Figure 7.5).

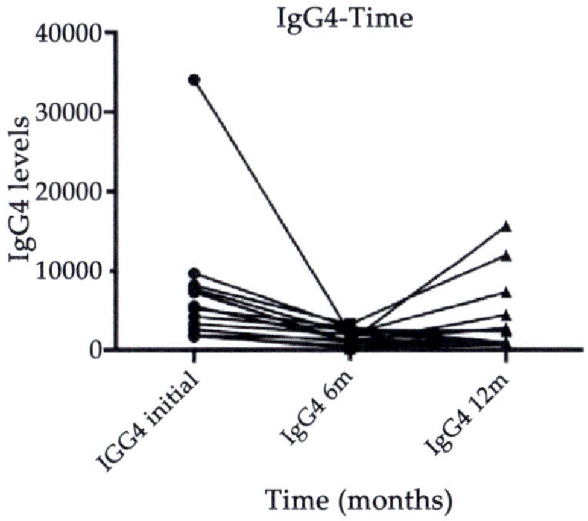

Figure 7.5. Immunoglobulin G4 (IgG4) levels.

Source: https://www.researchgate.net/publication/337819589/figure/fig1/AS:833512622022662@1575736303514/gG4-levels-and-IgG4-time.png.

7.2.1. Characteristics and Demographics

In characterizing the demographics and presentation of AIP, it is critical to draw a distinction between its two main forms: Type 1 and Type 2. Type 1 AIP, which is often associated with IgG4-related disease, predominantly occurs in older men, typically diagnosed in their 60s and 70s. This age group is significant in that its distribution is atypical from that of Type 2 AIP, with more frequent presentation in younger patients with no gender predilection. Its clinical presentation and treatment response may be significantly variable between these types, highlighting the importance of demographic factors in the management of the disease. Moreover, Type 1 AIP is also found to be linked with other autoimmune conditions as well as an elevated concentration of serum IgG4, which highlights its systemic nature beyond the pancreas. Demographic studies have shown that autoimmune pancreatitis expresses differential characteristics in geography and ethnicity. For instance, Type 1 AIP is more prevalent in Asia than in Europe and North America, with implications for genetic susceptibility or environmental influences on disease prevalence. This is of particular relevance to the broader understanding of AIP, where variation in presentation and course may become evident across populations. Rates of Type 2 AIP also appear to be more international in their consistency, although the exact pathophysiology is not as well defined. As the researchers monitor these population trends, the findings do justify the need for particular screening tests in high-risk groups, encouraging early diagnosis and treatment to reduce complications. Population dynamics of autoimmune pancreatitis overlap into treatment outcomes and relapse rates, particularly corticosteroid administration. Studies have shown that Type 1 and Type 2 AIP patients considerably have different corticosteroid responses with Type 1 tending to have an optimum positive response to corticosteroids, which is of crucial significance to modulate the disease. Type 2 AIP patients, however, do not always receive the same level of benefit from corticosteroids, which may imply that there are differing pathophysiologies. Demographic factors such as gender and age also have important implications for treatment and outcomes. It is crucial for healthcare professionals to know the nature of such populations so that they can devise personalized treatment plans. As novel treatments become available, population and disease characteristics observations will play a key role in maximizing patient care as well as predicting relapse capacities in autoimmune pancreatitis patients (Jones et al., 2016).

7.2.2. Association with Immunoglobulin G4-Related Disease (IgG4-RD)

The association between AIP and IgG4-related disease is a key area of research in understanding pancreatic disorders. AIP has been classified into two general categories, and Type 1 AIP is identified as strongly associated with IgG4-related systemic disease. The typical disorder includes several extrapancreatic manifestations, including salivary gland, kidney, and lymph node disorders. The presence of elevated serum IgG4 is a feature of this subtype, which is also featured by histological changes with a rich lymphoplasmacytic infiltrate.

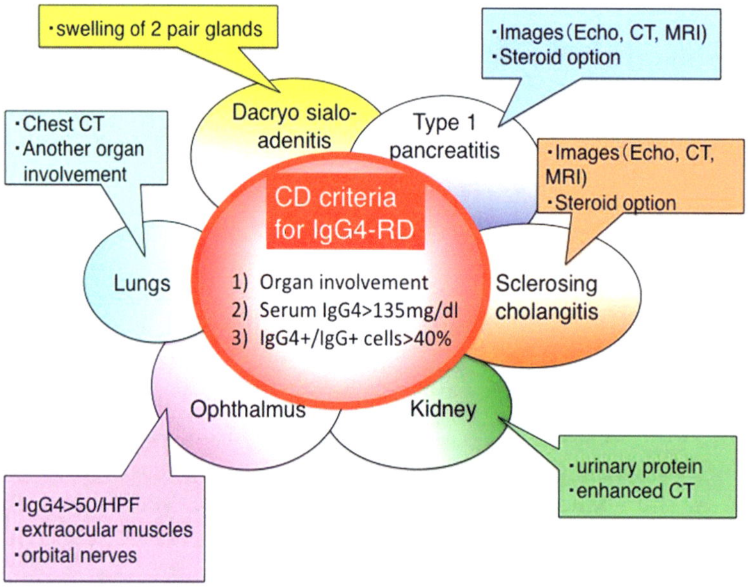

Figure 7.6. Diagnose IgG4-related disease (IgG4-RT).

Source: https://ard.bmj.com/content/annrheumdis/76/11/e46/F1.large.jpg.

These observations emphasize the utility of IgG4 as a marker in diagnosing Type 1 AIP, as opposed to Type 2 AIP, which is often lacking in such systemic associations and an increase in IgG4. Awareness of these distinctions is crucial for effective management and treatment strategies aimed at preventing complications of chronic disease. The clinical relevance of the association of IgG4-related disease and autoimmune pancreatitis also adds emphasis to the need for individually tailored therapy. Corticosteroid therapy has been reported to be a first-line treatment for both types of AIP, but it can react very differently in the two. In Type 1 AIP, corticosteroids can rapidly induce remission and decrease plasma IgG4, as indicated by resolution of pancreatic inflammation and associated systemic manifestations. The efficacy of Type 2 AIP is varied, typically demanding other immunosuppression modalities due to its distinct pathophysiological mechanisms. This difference indicates that even as corticosteroids play a vital role in Type 1 AIP treatment, more work must be done in studying optimal treatment options for Type 2 AIP patients to make sure that complete care is offered across the spectrum of autoimmune pancreatitis. Both types of autoimmune pancreatitis are at risk for relapse and require additional investigation of their relationship with IgG4-related disease. Evidence suggests IgG4-related diseases can recur after successful corticosteroid management, prompting research on long-term management strategies. Relying on research by González et al., 2013, the author describes the application of corticosteroids in preventing autoimmune pancreatitis from progressing to chronic pancreatitis and cites an urgent need for sustained surveillance and early intervention. In addition, the Spanish Pancreatic Club emphasizes that an interdisciplinary approach of managing complications due to chronic pancreatitis should be implemented, with an understanding of heterogeneity of therapeutic protocols between different centers (González et al., 2013). Identifying these associations will allow clinicians to better modify their therapeutic regimens, which will ultimately improve long-term outcomes of patients and prevent recurrence of autoimmune pancreatitis (Figure 7.6).

7.2.3. Treatment Options and Outcomes

AIP's treatment is very heterogeneous according to the illness subclassification—predominantly Type 1 and Type 2. Type 1 AIP, often associated with IgG4-related disease, generally responds well to corticosteroids, which are the first-line treatment. Clinical evidence suggests that steroids are effective in inducing remission and preventing progression of the disease, reducing the risk of complications such as chronic pancreatitis, which has a tremendous effect on quality of life in patients. Corticosteroids also have a key function in managing the acute inflammatory stage, and studies have evidenced their efficacy in symptom resolution as well as improvement of pancreatic function. Corticosteroid response in Type 2 AIP may be less predictable; therefore, treatment is generally more specifically individualized, reflecting the multifaceted nature of this illness. Consequently, a comprehensive understanding of these treatment regimens is necessary for optimal patient results. In addition to corticosteroids, other immunosuppressive therapies have been found to be central to the management of AIP, particularly in steroid non-responders or those with relapse on tapering. Azathioprine and mycophenolate mofetil have been effective in maintaining remission and preventing recrudescence. Such immunotherapies are essential addenda, particularly in preventing high corticosteroid doses in an attempt to minimize side effects. Moreover, multidisciplinary interaction between gastroenterologists, immunologists, and even hepatologists is required in the optimal treatment regimens based on patient-specific disease phenotypes and comorbidities (Chapman et al., 2019). Regular monitoring of treatment outcomes and quality of life assessments in the patients is important, optimizing management regimens with respect for long-term prognosis. Prevention of relapse is a significant problem in the management of Type 1 and Type 2 AIP, with the emphasis placed on long-term follow-up and monitoring. Relapse is high in rate, particularly in Type 1 disease, for whom therapy with corticosteroids may have to be continued to avoid relapses. There is growing evidence to recommend the use of maintenance immunosuppressive therapy as a preventive measure against flare-ups and overall pancreatic well-being. Serial monitoring of serum IgG4 concentrations and repeated imaging are also part of the continuous assessment of disease activity and treatment response. Such proactive monitoring and management reflects patient-centered care practices that allow for early interventions that prevent risks associated with chronicity and complications (v). Last but not least, knowledge of the dynamic treatment approaches at one's disposal and outcomes is critical to improving overall management of autoimmune pancreatitis.

7.3. Type 2 Autoimmune Pancreatitis (AIP)

Type 2 AIP represents an unusual type of autoimmune pancreatitis distinct from the IgG4-type. While Type 1 AIP is characterized by an increase in serum IgG4 and widespread fibrosis, Type 2 AIP is characterized mainly by a younger age group and is often found with an inflammatory cell predominance, with significantly neutrophils. This distinctive cellular composition leads to a heterogeneous clinical presentation, and in most instances, chronic recurrent abdominal pain and pancreatic exocrine deficiency with no diffuse damage and scarring characteristic of Type 1 disease. Type 2 AIP is also usually accompanied by corticosteroid resistance, thus rendering management approaches more challenging compared to its IgG4-related equivalent, which invariably demonstrates sensitivity to steroid treatment. One of the most important aspects of Type 2 AIP management is to understand its corticosteroid response and how it fits into preventing relapse.

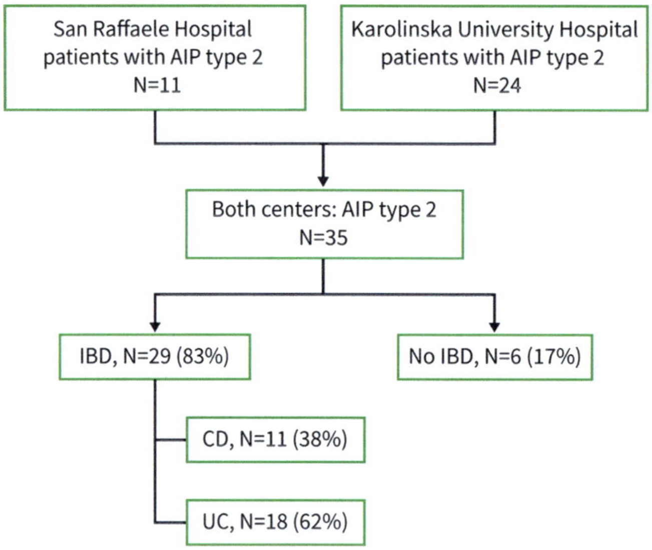

Figure 7.7. AIP-autoimmune pancreatitis.

Source: https://www.researchgate.net/publication/360458769/figure/fig1/AS:11431281180730493@1691703881180/AIP-autoimmune-pancreatitis-IBD-inflammatory-bowel-disease-CD-Crohns-disease.png.

Studies have established that while corticosteroids are able to alleviate symptoms, they are ineffective at inducing remission in patients with Type 2 AIP on a long-term basis. Unlike Type 1 AIP, where remission is associated with higher doses of corticosteroids, in Type 2 patients, there may be only transient improvement, making it challenging to keep the disease under control. In addition, the unique pathologic features of Type 2 AIP, not defined by elevated levels of IgG4 seen with Type 1 AIP, suggest that alternative therapeutic strategies may be required to better achieve treatment outcomes. Therefore, an approach to management that is multidimensional and individualized to the patient is critical in addressing the complexities inherent to Type 2 AIP. Efforts toward elucidating the pathophysiology of Type 2 AIP are critical, considering the clinical complexity of the disease. Identification of type-specific biomarkers for Type 2 AIP would significantly assist in the improvement of diagnostic criteria and prognosis, currently based mainly on clinical and radiologic manifestations. In addition, understanding the implicated inflammatory mechanisms may offer novel therapeutic windows aside from corticosteroids, such as immunomodulators or biologics. Better comprehension of the immunologic picture of the disease could improve the patients' prognosis by lowering relapse rates and increasing sustained remission. Overall, handling the complexity of Type 2 autoimmune pancreatitis requires the collaborative action of the medical community towards enhancing the diagnostic sensitivity and the effectiveness of treatment, establishing a platform for improved clinical guidelines (González et al., 2013) (Figure 7.7).

7.3.1. Distinct Features Compared to Type 1

The distinction between Type 1 and Type 2 AIP is critical to clinicians managing this complex illness. Type 1 AIP, in IgG4-associated disease, is observed with a systemic fibro-inflammatory process that involves not just the pancreas but also the multiple organ systems. This involves lymphoplasmacytic infiltration and marked fibrosis leading to significant morphological changes such as pancreatic enlargement or mass formation, often accompanied by jaundice and other systemic manifestations. The increased serum IgG4 levels are the hallmark of the condition, with studies demonstrating them to be increased in approximately 68%–95% of Type 1 AIP patients, suggesting an interesting immune response that differentiates it from Type 2 AIP, where such immunologic markers are typically absent. Conversely, Type 2 AIP demonstrates more localized pathology confined mostly to the pancreas itself without any systemic features as in Type 1. Type 2 patients also present with distinct histological features, e.g., an excess of neutrophilic infiltrate compared to lymphoplasmacytic cells of Type 1 disease. Such differentiation presents a clear clinical picture, in that Type 2 AIP is usually encountered in younger patients, typically less than 50 years of age, without the systemic IgG4 disease. This aspect significantly alters management strategies, as Type 2 AIP is less responsive to corticosteroid treatment than Type 1 and thus demands more tailored interventions. Furthermore, the prognosis and relapse rates are greatly different for the two varieties. Type 1 AIP shows corticosteroid responsiveness that not only alleviates symptoms but also plays an important part in preventing disease progression to chronic pancreatitis, as explained in new studies. In contrast, Type 2 AIP tends to have a more indolent presentation despite being an incomplete and less consistent response to corticosteroids, possibly with challenges in managing relapses. These differences are of paramount importance for practitioners to be able to devise effective treatment strategies and to be able to anticipate the clinical behavior of patients with these two types of autoimmune pancreatitis.

7.3.2. Clinical Implications and Patient Demographics

AIP, particularly its two types—Type 1 and Type 2—has a mixed clinical presentation and patient population. Type 1 AIP, with a tendency for IgG4-related disease, is predominantly found in older men and is associated with other systemic conditions. Type 2 AIP, however, involves younger individuals and females to a greater extent. All these differences in populations emphasize the need for gender- and age-stratified clinical management. Besides, the clinical usefulness of this classification is in the differing patterns of treatment as Type 1 may be corticosteroid-responsive while Type 2 is not responsive to corticosteroids. Thus, patient classification may permit better diagnostic returns and certain treatment regimens that limit the risk of disease worsening and better quality of life in the cohort. Clinical relevance of AIP exceeds the original diagnosis and treatment, extending to prevention of relapse and considerations for management. Type 1 AIP patients often experience relapses and may require constant treatment with corticosteroids to remain in remission, creating a need for long-term observation and strict management protocols. The relapses are potentially linked with underlying epigenetic changes that affect inflammatory responses, as demonstrated by longitudinal analysis of DNA methylation patterns in autoimmune illnesses such as ANCA-associated vasculitis (Jones et al., 2016). Adding surveillance of such epigenetic markers on a regular basis may further advance our understanding regarding patient-specific treatment outcomes and relapse susceptibility. Consequently, disease management approaches must be adapted to accommodate the findings to achieve the clinical goal of stable remission and minimize the relapse rate among AIP patients. Demographic characteristics and clinical significance of AIP also intersect with treatment approaches such as apheresis, whose popularity as an adjunct therapy to corticosteroids is on the rise for serious conditions. Apheresis is the technique of the removal of autoantibodies from the bloodstream and has proved useful in the management of a large number of autoimmune disorders. The effectiveness and utility of apheresis can vary significantly among various age groups. Young Type 2 AIP patients, for example, might respond differently to this therapy than elderly Type 1 AIP patients. Therefore, knowledge of these demographic nuances is vital not simply for the assessment of treatment efficacy but also to optimize therapeutic measures. In trying to enhance patient outcomes in autoimmune pancreatitis, consideration of data on clinical presentation and patient demographics will be significant in developing individualized treatment strategies, taking cognizance of the specific challenges presented by this complex disease (Figure 7.8).

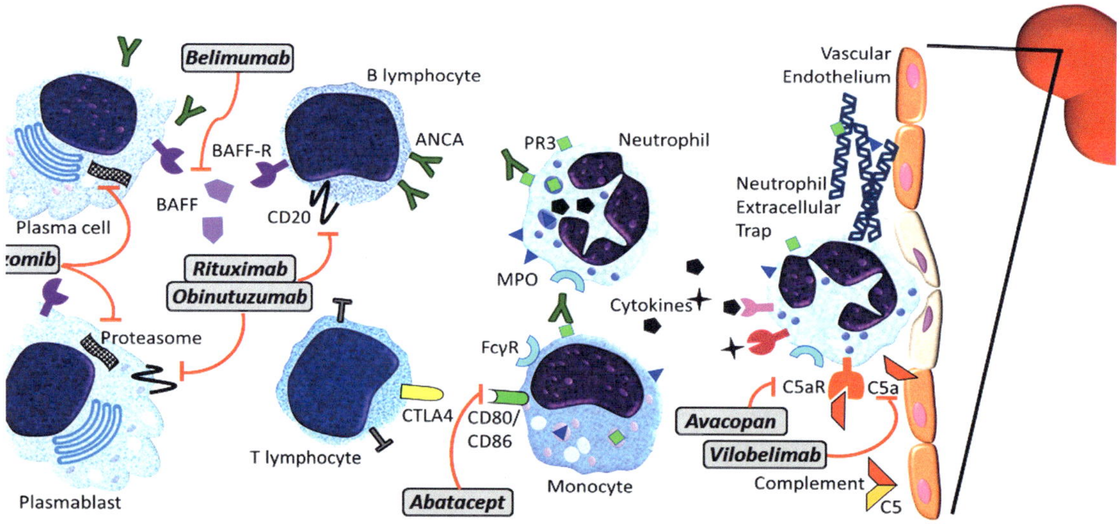

Figure 7.8. ANCA-associated vasculitis.

Source: Almaani S, Fussner LA, Brodsky S, Meara AS, Jayne D. ANCA-Associated Vasculitis: An Update. *Journal of Clinical Medicine.* 2021; 10(7):1446. https://doi.org/10.3390/jcm10071446

7.3.3. Treatment Strategies and Effectiveness

In evaluating the treatment for AIP, corticosteroids emerge as a cornerstone treatment due to their immunosuppressive property. AIP's exceptional sensitivity to corticosteroids is characterized by the fact that most of the patients show dramatic improvement in both clinical features and imaging at the time of initiation of treatment. Studies show that corticosteroids not only enhance symptoms such as jaundice and weight loss but also have great promise in the prevention of progression to chronic pancreatitis, as evidenced by a study by Gleeson et al., 2025, where it is discussed how corticosteroids can effectively prevent such a situation in patients. This extremely high efficacy of corticosteroids suggests that there is real potential for disease control from early intervention, so the importance of early diagnosis and treatment. The treatment strategy should also consider, however, the differing responses reported between Type 1 and Type 2 AIP. Type 1 AIP, which is frequently associated with IgG4-related disease, generally responds well to corticosteroid treatment given its inherent immunological character. Type 2 AIP, on the other hand, can be variable in its reaction, considering the distinctive pathological features of the disease that incline away from the paradigm of IgG4 involvement (Gleeson et al., 2025). Therapeutic regimens, therefore, must be addressed by practitioners keeping these differences in perspective and tailored based on the patient's individual AIP type and reaction. Identification of the nuances of these forms is paramount to maximizing treatment success and tailoring patient care. The risk of relapse, despite the effectiveness of corticosteroids in managing AIP, is a significant confounding factor that renders constant vigilant management of the patient of foremost concern. Relapse rates for AIP can be remarkably high, rendering spontaneous remission an additional confounding factor in clinical presentation. Therefore, maintaining a good follow-up schedule with adherence to medication and regular imaging follow-up is crucial to monitor for possible recurrences (Gleeson et al., 2025). In addition, research also demonstrated that in some patients, low-dose corticosteroids are capable of decreasing the risk of flare and sustaining the anti-inflammatory effect of the drugs. This prophylactic management not only maximizes the length of effective treatment but also enhances the aim of preventing acute exacerbations, in this instance, ensuring the quality of life of autoimmune pancreatitis patients as a top objective of their comprehensive treatment regimen.

7.4. IgG4-Related Disease (IgG4-RD)

The intricate relationship between IgG4-RD and autoimmune pancreatitis points to the challenges in diagnosing and treating pancreatic disease. Characterized by a rise in serum concentrations of IgG4, IgG4-RD occurs in various forms, with autoimmune pancreatitis being a common presentation. It has been mistaken for pancreatic malignancy based on shared imaging features. The clinical symptoms and laboratory findings similarity between type 1 autoimmune pancreatitis, commonly associated with IgG4-RD, and other pancreatitis types necessitates careful differentiation. The presence of a mass-forming pancreatitis and typical imaging characteristics can give rise to misinterpretations that make clinical management challenging, and therefore, clinicians need to keep in mind IgG4-RDs peculiarities and its therapeutic context in the future. Treatment with corticosteroids is an important part of IgG4-RD treatment, particularly in autoimmune pancreatitis associated with it. The available literature shows that corticosteroids are not only beneficial in relieving symptoms but also in inhibiting autoimmune pancreatitis from developing into chronic pancreatitis. The research emphasizes the importance of early use of corticosteroids to avoid complications resulting from untreated or poorly treated IgG4-RD. Chronic inflammation will lead to irreversible damage and chronic diseases such as chronic pancreatitis, which is challenging to treat in patients. Therefore, identification of the corticosteroid response in the case of IgG4-RD can direct the therapeutic intervention and enhance the quality of care for the patient, underlining the need for early detection and active treatment modalities. Moreover, prevention of relapse in IgG4-RD remains a topic of first concern after corticosteroid therapy. While the initial good response to corticosteroids, the relapse potential is great and necessitates ongoing monitoring and possible adjunctive therapies to preserve remission. The consensus of opinion is that simultaneous treatment with corticosteroids and immunosuppressants may produce a more long-term response with less frequency of relapse, harmonizing management strategies with the disease's complexities. Healthcare practitioners need to be vigilant, as the development of chronic pancreatitis, aided by recurrences, highlights the necessity of an integrative treatment process for this multifaceted condition. This highlights the importance of individualized treatment regimens as well as the use of newer therapies that may assist in long-term remission for IgG4-RD patients, further elucidated in work presented by González et al. (2013) (Figure 7.9).

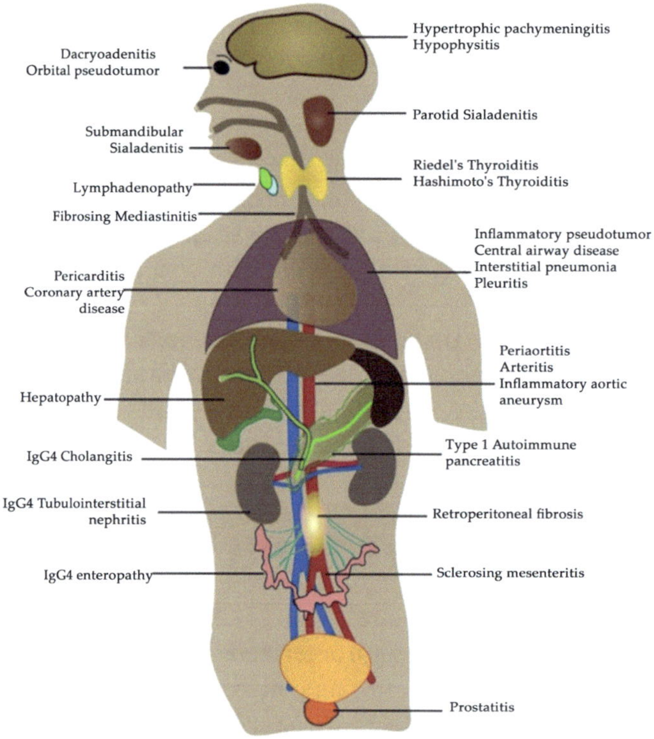

Figure 7.9. Immunoglobulin G4-related disease.

Source: https://els-jbs-prod-cdn.jbs.elsevierhealth.com/cms/attachment/db259aff-1e41-404a-a6e3-d27322c2c70e/gr1_lrg.jpg.

7.4.1. Role of Immunoglobulin G4 (IgG4) in Autoimmune Conditions

The role of IgG4 in autoimmune disorders has drawn great attention, especially among AIP. The disease falls into two categories, and Type 1 AIP is particularly associated with elevated levels of IgG4. Essentially, IgG4 serves as a biomarker for IgG4-associated illness, which comprises a chronic inflammatory process across several organs. In AIP, IgG4-positive plasma cell accumulation results in characteristic histopathological alterations, such as storiform fibrosis and lymphocytic infiltration. Understanding the immunologic mechanisms governing abnormal IgG4 production explains its bifunctional nature as a pro-inflammatory mediator and immune response regulator, rendering it challenging to define in autoimmune disease processes. This dualism poses questions regarding the therapeutic management of AIP and related conditions, particularly the determination of the most beneficial immune modulation and stabilization approaches. The treatment of autoimmune pancreatitis often includes corticosteroids, which successfully suppress inflammation and induce remission. Corticosteroids target specifically immune dysregulation, which is reinforced by the presence of IgG4-mediated responses.

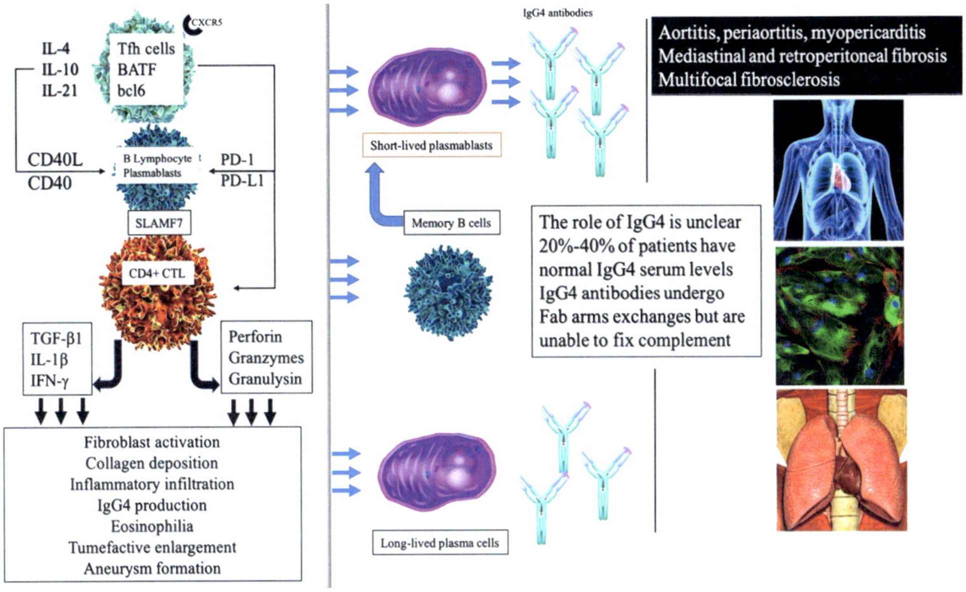

Figure 7.10. Role of IgG4 in autoimmune conditions.

Source: https://heart.bmj.com/content/heartjnl/107/10/790/F2.large.jpg.

Research has revealed that corticosteroids are effective in reducing levels of serum IgG4, resulting in symptomatic improvement and improved pancreatic function. Heterogeneity in the response of patients to corticosteroids necessitates the application of individualized therapeutic regimens. Complete remission can be achieved in some patients, while others may experience relapse despite similar treatment regimens. It has been pointed out in current research that the understanding of the complexities of corticosteroid responsiveness with reference to IgG4 dynamics will add importantly to the prognostication of patients and hence the follow-up management strategies, making patient stratification a very important component of treatment planning. Given the intricacies involved with IgG4-related disorders, the prevention of relapse becomes an important thrust area in autoimmune pancreatitis management. Evidence indicates that the maintenance of optimal levels of IgG4 following therapy is essential to minimize relapse and progression of the disease. An intensive follow-up regime involving regular monitoring of the serum level of IgG4 can identify those patients at higher risk of recurrent attack. Furthermore, a majority consensus is to use long-term immunosuppressive strategies in certain cases, especially in cases of aggressive disease. By the inclusion of insight into IgG4s role in pathophysiology and successful management, healthcare providers are able to foster better outcomes for patients with the challenge of autoimmune pancreatitis. Further studies need to be conducted to optimize these approaches to develop a holistic model for disease profile assessment and intervention planning (González et al., 2013) (Figure 7.10).

7.4.2. Diagnostic Challenges and Biomarkers

The diagnostic challenges of AIP are significant, primarily as a consequence of the overlapping clinical characteristics and the ubiquity of the symptoms in other biliary and pancreatic diseases. Diagnosis of Type 1 AIP, which often coexists with IgG4-related disease, is most challenging to differentiate from Type 2 AIP since both conditions feature overlapping symptoms like abdominal pain, weight loss, and jaundice. Furthermore, rising serum IgG4 levels is a likely biomarker but always lack specificity. The elevated IgG4 can occur in other conditions and, therefore, cannot be utilized for diagnosis alone. Effective diagnosis depends on a combination of imaging modalities, serological tests, and histologic confirmation, highlighting the complexity of accurate diagnosis in such circumstances (Wang et al., 2023). Biomarkers drive diagnosis and treatment of AIP but tend to be complex to interpret, requiring a sophisticated understanding of the pathophysiology that is being interrogated and subtle consideration of clinical context. IgG4 levels are usually measured to support the diagnosis of IgG4-related disorders, but in isolation, they are not specific, as up to 30% of patients with AIP will have normal levels of IgG4. In addition, temporal variation in biomarker levels could compromise interpretation and necessitate serial measurements in some instances. Detection of other biomarkers, including some autoantibodies, is in progress and potentially might enhance diagnostic sensitivity in subclassifying AIP and distinguishing AIP from other pancreatitis, e.g., malignancies and chronic pancreatitis. Research on novel biomarkers may ultimately give rise to more individualized therapeutic approaches (Chapman et al., 2019). In addition, diagnostic criteria tend to offer a template for clinicians but, in doing so, can create difficulties with individualized patient management. The British Society of Gastroenterology has set out management guidelines for primary sclerosing cholangitis, which can also have overlapping features of the presentation in AIP. These guidelines act as essential points of reference; however, the variability of patient presentations and responses to therapy mean that attention must be drawn beyond protocol-driven care. Individualization of the diagnostic approach allows for consideration of special situations, which can generally affect disease prognosis and treatment response. Therefore, awareness of the limitations of existing biomarkers and clinical practice guidelines is important, allowing practitioners to guide the diagnostic area of autoimmune pancreatitis to the best possible patient outcomes (Wang et al., 2023).

7.4.3. Treatment Approaches Specific to Immunoglobulin G4-Related Disease (IgG4-RD)

The treatment choices for IgG4-RD, particularly in autoimmune pancreatitis, are primarily corticosteroid therapy since the illnesses are highly responsive to glucocorticoids. Treatment is frequently initiated with high-dose corticosteroids, which have been observed to alleviate symptoms and reduce inflammation in affected organs, including the pancreas. Patients tend to have a pronounced clinical and radiological responses along with significant clinical improvement within weeks of initiation of therapy. This aggressive treatment highlights the diagnostic utility of corticosteroids in that marked relief of symptoms may aid the diagnosis of IgG4-RD. Secondly, tapering the steroid dose is a common practice for maximizing the therapeutic effect with due regard paid to the adverse effects of prolonged corticosteroid treatment, and thus the monitoring of symptoms and laboratory parameters needs to be done cautiously during the course of therapy (Gleeson et al., 2025). In addition to corticosteroids, other immunosuppressive agents can be tried in IgG4-RD patients, particularly corticosteroid-resistant or relapsing patients. Azathioprine, mycophenolate mofetil, and rituximab are currently being explored as add-ons or steroid alternatives. Azathioprine and mycophenolate mofetil are beneficial in terms of remission maintenance and reducing corticosteroid use; however, they are somewhat constrained by side effects and inconsistent efficacy. Rituximab, a CD20-positive B-cell-targeted monoclonal antibody, has proved extremely effective in reducing IgG4-related symptoms in refractory disease and has the potential to be a key relapse preventing factor. Thus, a multidisciplinary treatment approach is often required to tailor the treatment protocols for each patient according to the response and presentation, and therefore, optimum management of this multifactorial disorder (Gleeson et al., 2025). Relapse prevention is a key part of IgG4-RD management, given the spontaneous remission tendency and subsequent relapses that characterize the disease. Follow-up and serum IgG4 measurement are key elements in monitoring for disease activity and in changing treatment. Few reports suggest that patients on a low-dose corticosteroid regimen can reduce relapse and maintain remission, albeit at the cost of potential long-term steroid side effects. There is new evidence that supports the use of alternative immunosuppressive therapy in maintenance therapy, particularly in patients with widespread organ involvement or multiple relapses. Further investigation is necessary to create standardized protocols and guidelines for IgG4-related disease treatment, the delineation of the roles of newer agents, such as rituximab, to further enhance outcomes and diminish the severity of this refractory autoimmune disease (Figure 7.11).

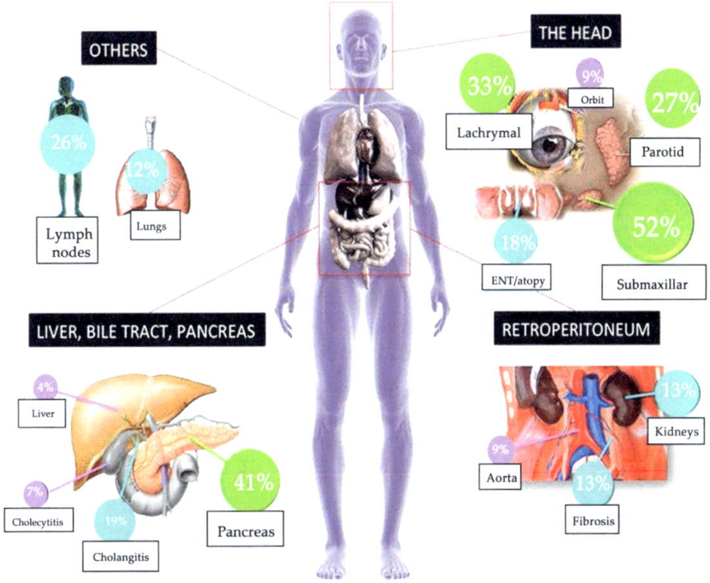

Figure 7.11. IgG4-related disease (IgG4-RD) of autoimmune pancreatitis.

Source: https://i.pinimg.com/736x/06/b0/18/06b0181f8b02165f0ce538f783961c20--autoimmune-arthritis.jpg.

7.5. Corticosteroid Response

The corticosteroid sensitivity of AIP is a significant parameter for managing it, particularly in Type 1 AIP with an IgG4-associated inflammatory process. Corticosteroids possess a very strong immunosuppressive action and bring about prompt clinical resolution with immediate relief of symptoms such as jaundice, abdominal pain, and loss of weight. This therapeutic responsiveness not only aids in the relief of the acute disease burden but also helps establish AIP distinct from malignancies, where this kind of quick response is less frequent.

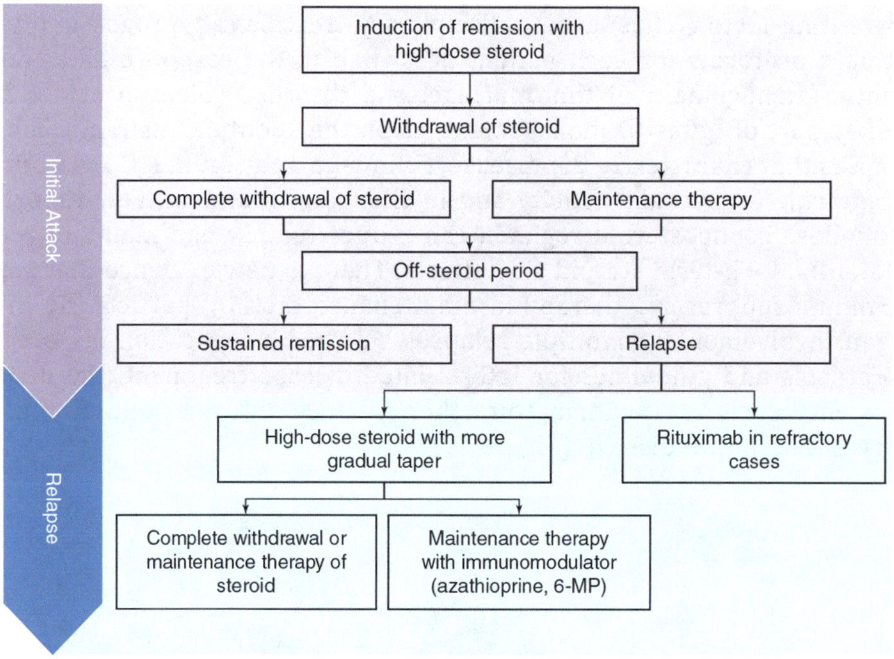

Figure 7.12. Steroid therapy for autoimmune pancreatitis (AIP).

Source: https://i0.wp.com/basicmedicalkey.com/wp-content/uploads/2017/06/A323555_1_En_22_Fig2_HTML.jpg?w=960.

It is apparent that even a brief course of corticosteroids can cause significant reductions in swelling of the pancreas and associated complications, attesting to their utility as both diagnostic and therapeutic agents in suspecting AIP. Therefore, an understanding of the mechanisms of corticosteroid responsiveness is essential to optimize patient management in various forms of this complex disease. Corticosteroids are not only therapeutic in controlling symptoms of autoimmune pancreatitis but also critical to prevent the progression and chronicity of the disease. Research indicates that early treatment with corticosteroids can abort conversion from AIP to chronic pancreatitis and hence prevent late complications such as pancreatic insufficiency and diabetes. This preventive aspect emphasizes the need for early intervention following diagnosis due to the fact that procrastination will lead to significant morbidity. Furthermore, prevention with corticosteroids remains an active area of research. Observations reveal that while a few patients experience spontaneous remissions, many of them can experience relapses of the disease; hence, the need to establish an individualized long-term regimen of corticosteroids, considering the ratio between effectiveness and potential side effects, particularly in recurrent AIP attacks. Even the treatment of corticosteroid response in autoimmune pancreatitis encompasses the subject of long-term prognosis of patients. Even though early responsiveness, relapses can impact life quality and necessitate re-evaluation of long-term plans. Experiments reveal that long-term corticosteroid treatment has numerous side effects, including osteoporosis and metabolic syndrome, and doctors have had to weigh other immunosuppressive drugs or adjunctive medications that could minimize these risks without diminishing control over the disease (Gleeson et al., 2025). Close monitoring and a well-planned corticosteroid tapering program are crucial in avoiding complications from prolonged use so that the patients can achieve an equilibrium state. Thus, knowing corticosteroid response in depth is critical in formulating proper management programs that balance short-term curative actions and long-term welfare of autoimmune pancreatitis patients (Figure 7.12).

7.5.1. Mechanism of Action of Corticosteroids

Corticosteroids are at the forefront of immune response modulation in the treatment of autoimmune disorders, particularly in the case of Type 1 and Type 2 IgG4-related diseases. Corticosteroids act primarily by binding and activating glucocorticoid receptors (GRs), transcription factors that modulate the expression of numerous genes that manage Pancreatitis inflammation and immune modulation. Upon binding, the corticosteroid-GR complex moves into the nucleus, there to act on anti-inflammatory genes for transcription and at the same time suppress pro-inflammatory cytokines. This functions both to reverse the inflammatory activity of autoimmune pancreatitis and to reverse tissue damage from autoimmune attack. Notably, the disease-modulating effect of corticosteroids in IgG4-related disease, characterized by widespread plasma cell infiltration, identifies their central role in disease management and emphasizes the need for gentle therapy to maximize patient benefit (Kersten et al., 2024). Corticosteroid action on immune functions also involves suppression of inflammatory cell proliferation and activation. Corticosteroids block the synthesis of key pro-inflammatory mediators, such as tumor necrosis factor-alpha (TNF-α) and interleukin-6 (IL-6), thereby downregulating the overall inflammatory environment. The blockade even extends to the level of the targeted blocking of antigen presentation, as corticosteroids interfere with the function of dendritic cells and macrophages, which play a central role in initiating immune responses. Besides, by suppressing the expression of major histocompatibility complex (MHC) class II molecules on antigen-presenting cells, corticosteroids suppress T-cell activation, a crucial step in the autoimmune cascade of diseases such as Type 1 autoimmune pancreatitis. This total immunosuppression is one of the significant reasons for the immediate clinical and biochemical response to corticosteroid therapy (Kersten et al., 2024). While corticosteroids are effectively proven in the treatment of autoimmune pancreatitis, prevention of relapse remains a constant challenge. While initial treatment can produce remission, long-term use of corticosteroids can result in complications such as increased vulnerability to infections, osteoporosis, and metabolic syndromes that require close monitoring and steroid-sparing strategies. In the context of IgG4-related disease, understanding the mechanisms of relapse is essential to optimize treatment regimens. How to maintain remission is unknown and potentially will necessitate switching to other immunosuppressive medications following steroids or the application of adjunct therapy to preserve long-term benefits. Hence, understanding the intricate activities of corticosteroids not only maximizes short-term therapeutic outcomes but also forms the basis to devise beneficial protocols to impede the relapse of disease with time (Wang et al., 2023).

7.5.2. Efficacy in Treating Autoimmune Pancreatitis (AIP)

The efficacy of corticosteroids in managing AIP has been well-established, particularly their capacity for immediate symptom relief and attainment of remission. Corticosteroids act through the eradication of disease inflammation, effectively managing clinical symptoms like jaundice and abdominal pain. Research indicates that patients with AIP tend to respond favorably to corticosteroid treatment, with most improving quite significantly within weeks of the therapy. Early corticosteroid therapy has been observed to arrest the development of autoimmune pancreatitis into chronic pancreatitis and hence prevent potential long-term sequels such as pancreatic insufficiency and the formation of complications such as diabetes mellitus. Consequently, the role of corticosteroids is not only therapeutic but also preventive, a point that contributes to their importance in the management of this complex disease.

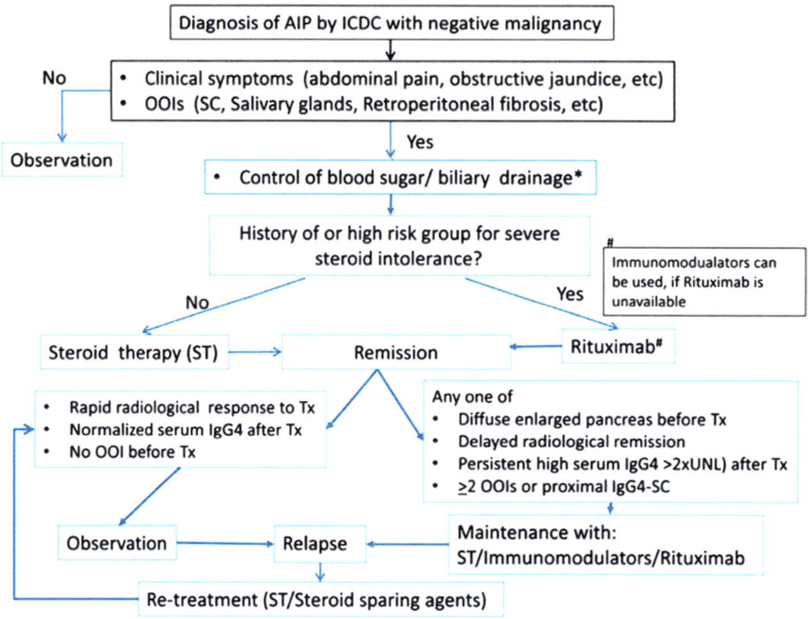

Figure 7.13. International consensus for the treatment of autoimmune pancreatitis.

Source: https://ars.els-cdn.com/content/image/1-s2.0-S1424390316312509-gr1.jpg.

Further, the distinction between Type 1 and Type 2 autoimmune pancreatitis reinforces differences in treatment response and patient outcome. Type 1 AIP, typically linked with IgG4-related disease, typically responds well to corticosteroids as a result of underlying pathophysiologic mechanisms of IgG4-positive plasma cell infiltration and severe fibrosis (Gleeson et al., 2025). Patients in this category may need prolonged corticosteroid treatment to stay in remission, and close surveillance is required to control any adverse effects of prolonged therapy. Type 2 AIP, in which there is lymphoplasmacytic infiltration without substantial IgG4, might not show as consistent a response to corticosteroids. The variation in treatment strategy as a result of this makes it adjustable to the specific type of autoimmune pancreatitis, emphasizing the complexity of effective management in the clinic. Relapse prevention is a significant concern in the management of autoimmune pancreatitis, particularly with the disease's propensity for spontaneous remissions followed by potential recurrences later. Following initial corticosteroid treatment, the relapse rate is a significant consideration that needs to be addressed by doctors. Tapering corticosteroids is a strategy for reducing this risk, with observation of serum levels of IgG4 as a potential relapse biomarker (Gleeson et al., 2025). Some studies suggest that certain patients will go into sustained remission following a successful taper, whereas others will need intermittent treatment with corticosteroids to proactively treat relapsing symptoms. Moreover, new treatments and combination therapy regimens are also being investigated to encourage better long-term control of AIP and reduce corticosteroid usage, which has several side effects. The present research is attempting to maximize these approaches for better patient outcomes and establish a more formalized methodology for relapse prevention (Figure 7.13).

7.5.3. Potential Side Effects and Management

The management of AIP, particularly in Type 1 IgG4-related disease patients, is generally centered on corticosteroid treatment. Corticosteroids are useful for inducing remission, but they also have the potential to produce certain side effects. The most frequent side effects are weight gain, hyperglycemia, osteoporosis, and susceptibility to infections. For example, long-term corticosteroid use leads to the development of steroid-induced hyperglycemia that complicates the clinical situation in AIP patients (Griebel et al., 2023). Because of the significant short- and long-term side effects of corticosteroid therapy, such risks should be handled with caution. Measurement of blood glucose and the use of lifestyle interventions, including diet and exercise, can reduce some side effects, thus improving patient outcomes with the treatment. In patients who experience relapse after corticosteroid tapering, alternative management may be sought. The use of other immunosuppressive agents, such as azathioprine or mycophenolate mofetil has been controversial for remission induction in a few situations, especially when corticosteroid side effects become unacceptable (Gleeson et al., 2025). But even those have their adverse effect profiles, such as risk of infection and hepatotoxicity, necessitating ongoing monitoring for potential side effects. Clinical decision-making must be done with a full discussion regarding the risks versus benefits of continued corticosteroid therapy versus alternative treatments. Several disciplines, including a gastroenterologist, endocrinologist, and on occasion an immunologist, can optimize the success of patient-specific management plans. The exploration of more recent therapy in the form of biologics can provide a brighter prognosis for AIP management with reduced risk compared to the current therapy of corticosteroids. Vedolizumab, for instance, has worked well for refractory AIP, with remission induction and maintenance achievable without the harsh side effects that often accompany long-term corticosteroid therapy (Griebel et al., 2023). This is particularly important for patients who experience difficulty with side effects from systemic corticosteroids or patients with recurrent relapses. Additionally, understanding the pathophysiological mechanisms behind AIP can help in personalized treatment strategies. Future research into detecting certain biomarkers specific to individual therapy responses would enable a more individualized treatment protocol, ultimately improving the quality of life for patients with this frustrating disease.

7.6. Relapse Prevention Strategies

Relapse prevention in AIP is essential for optimal management of both type 1 and type 2 presentations. Because of the pathophysiology of AIP, characterized by lymphoplasmacytic cell invasion with resultant fibrosis, biomarker identification is imperative for assessing disease activity. Elevated serum IgG4 is a significant marker for type 1 AIP, which strongly correlates with IgG4-related disease. Routine follow-up of such biomarkers can yield information regarding patient response to corticosteroid treatment, which is crucial for the early detection and management of potential relapses. Early diagnosis enables clinicians to adjust treatment regimens promptly and thus prevent the development of chronic pancreatitis, which can complicate patient prognoses significantly as detailed by Heerde et al. (2013). This strategic plan emphasizes the importance of personalized medicine in the treatment of AIP, particularly the balance between efficacy and potential side effects of prolonged steroid therapy. The integration of lifestyle modification, such as diet adjustment and stress management, is likewise important in the prevention of relapse of AIP. Patients must eat a healthy balanced diet with a high antioxidant content and low fat content to improve overall pancreatic health. Research has shown that dietary intervention can help suppress inflammatory responses, thus playing a supplementary role to drug therapy, with the former primarily tackling symptoms on the autoimmune axis. Coping strategies against stress like relaxation and mindfulness are also encouraged to help suppress exacerbations. Patient education is also important in informing patients of potential relapse-inducing factors so they can proactively manage themselves.

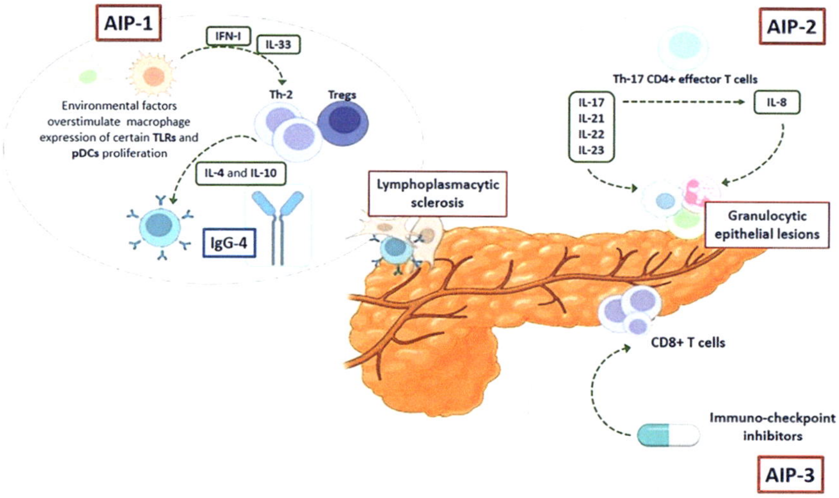

Figure 7.14. Autoimmune pancreatitis: Cornerstones and future perspectives.

Source: https://external-content.duckduckgo.com/iu/?u=https%3A%2F%2Ff6publishing.blob.core.windows.net%2F34ebc8d1-970e-4d88-b0d9-dcb0699d9ad4%2FWJG-30-817-g001.png&f=1&nofb=1&ipt=c7646c6cf57d614a0c552466837dee980977bca24efa4efd01745ff9085d0e9f.

This multi-faceted relapse prevention model is singular in that it addresses not only disease course determinants that are key factors of biology and psychosociality but also emphasizes the necessity of an integrated treatment plan. Finally, corticosteroid maintenance therapy in both AIP types is pivotal. Corticosteroids are very potent, with a tendency to cause spontaneous remission in most cases; long-term use must, however, be exercised very carefully because of potential adverse effects. Regular testing of steroid responsiveness in the patient is necessary, as it dictates the management schedule as well as tapering and maintenance doses. Significantly, studies have indicated that some patients benefit from the employment of adjunct therapy, such as immunosuppressants, to improve relapse rates without augmenting steroid dependency. Corticosteroids not only control inflammation but are also applied as a diagnostic tool when a good response to therapy is seen and signifies AIP. Relapse prevention must then involve a coordinated effort to weigh the effectiveness of treatment against the risk factor involved in the application of corticosteroids, as seen in studies (Figure 7.14).

7.6.1. Importance of Monitoring and Follow-Up

Monitoring and follow-up are both crucial to the treatment of autoimmune pancreatitis, with a direct influence on the prognosis of the patient. Due to the inherent complications associated with both Type 1 and Type 2 autoimmune pancreatitis, vigilant monitoring enables medical specialists to assess response to treatment as well as detect complications at an early stage. Given the unpredictability of this condition, where symptoms range from pain to potential pancreatic insufficiency, monitoring regularly becomes a critical necessity to modify treatment modalities accordingly. Clinicians should be aware of a thorough understanding of the differential features pertaining to different types of autoimmune pancreatitis because its heterogeneity might necessitate divergent management plans and follow-up duration in a bid to prevent complications and disease progression. The success of corticosteroid therapy in autoimmune pancreatitis also underscores the need for long-term follow-up. Though corticosteroids can achieve remission in the majority of patients, relapse may develop if the disease itself is not well controlled. Close monitoring enables appropriate changes in treatment regimens and may reduce the risks of flare or complications due to prolonged corticosteroid therapy. By evaluating patient response to corticosteroid therapy in a systematic way, clinicians can individualize treatment regimens to enhance efficacy and decrease adverse effects, thereby improving the overall quality of life of the patients. Moreover, the establishment of general guidelines and consensus statements, such as those devised by expert panels, serves to emphasize the role of monitoring and follow-up in treating autoimmune pancreatitis. These interventions standardize care across different healthcare settings and offer patients evidence-based treatments uniquely tailored to their specific disease parameters. For example, guidelines set by multidisciplinary panels consider not only clinical presentations but also require regular assessment of inflammatory markers and imaging modalities for monitoring disease activity. These systematic strategies promote a more effective healthcare environment, ultimately resulting in better patient outcomes and alleviating the long-term burden of autoimmune pancreatitis (Gleeson et al., 2025; González et al., 2013).

7.6.2. Long-Term Management Options

Long-term management of AIP relies on constant monitoring and adjustment to effectively address the distinct pathophysiological presentations of Type 1 and Type 2 diseases. Corticosteroids are the cornerstone of therapy due to their powerful anti-inflammatory properties, reducing pancreatic inflammation and the progression of disease to chronic pancreatitis. Studies have established that corticosteroids can be employed to cause remission, but extended application of the drugs is likely to lead to complications, one of them being steroid-induced hyperglycemia. Physicians must weigh the benefits of treatment with corticosteroids against the risks present, especially among patients who are not able to tolerate long courses of steroids. Ongoing evaluation of the patient is required for readjusting treatment plans and choosing the best management techniques that enhance the quality of life at the lowest risk of recurrent disease, hence prioritizing individualized management in both variants of autoimmune pancreatitis. In cases where corticosteroids fail or have harmful side effects, alternative immunosuppressive treatment options can be explored. For instance, drugs like azathioprine and mycophenolate mofetil can help maintain remission with fewer complications. However, studies on these alternative options are still limited, pointing to the need for good clinical trials to establish firm guidelines. Recent case reports describing vedolizumab, an integrin inhibitor, have shown promise in treating refractory cases of autoimmune pancreatitis. In fact, these cases indicate that vedolizumab can produce and sustain remission while posing less risk for harmful side effects compared to traditional steroid therapies. Continued studies on such biological agents are still key to enabling greater long-term treatment opportunities and relief for patients who experience relapse or side effects from traditional regimens (Griebel et al., 2023). Relapse prevention remains a serious problem in the long-term care of autoimmune pancreatitis, arguing for continued follow-up and customized approaches to treatment. The tapering schedule and dosage of corticosteroids need to be carefully monitored to prevent an escalation of symptom recurrence with abrupt reductions leading to rebound effects. Maintenance therapy regimens, including low-dose corticosteroids or other immunosuppressants, must be evaluated carefully based on response and side effect profile for individual patients. Therapeutic drugs such as biologics or target therapies should be included in long-term treatment regimens as increasing evidence supports their efficacy and safety. Lastly, multidisciplinary management by gastroenterologists, endocrinologists, and nutritionists can optimize integrated care so patients with autoimmune pancreatitis can lead productive lives with effective management of the disease (Figure 7.15).

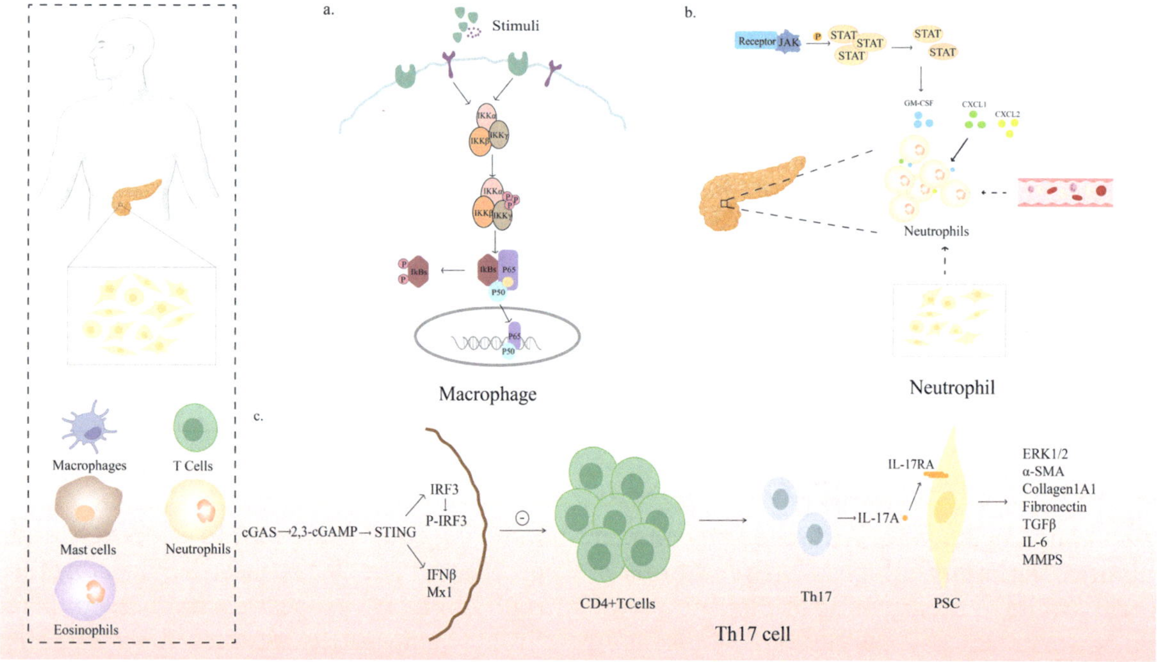

Figure 7.15. Immune cells and immune cell-targeted therapy in chronic pancreatitis.

Source: Zhang Y, Zhang W-Q, Liu X-Y, Zhang Q, Mao T and Li X-Y (2023) Immune cells and immune cell-targeted therapy in chronic pancreatitis. Front. Oncol. 13:1151103. doi: 10.3389/fonc.2023.1151103

7.6.3. Lifestyle Modifications and Patient Education

Lifestyle modification and patient education are also significant aspects of the management of autoimmune pancreatitis, particularly in terms of relapse prevention and the general well-being of the patient. Given the chronic nature of the disease, adopting a holistic strategy using diet, exercise, and stress management becomes imperative. For example, a healthy diet with antioxidants and minimal inflammatory foods can reduce symptoms and correct nutritional deficiencies, which typically exist in patients with pancreatic diseases. In addition, getting the patient to exercise regularly at moderate levels can improve overall physical health as well as reduce stress, both of which are crucial for proper immune functioning and recovery. Ultimately, encouraging patient-centered care with a focus on these lifestyle changes, and also continued education around the disease itself, can significantly improve patient results and level of life. Patient education is the foundation of effective management schemes for autoimmune pancreatitis and is at the heart of fighting against the complexities of the disease. Apart from being aware of the character of the disease, patients should also be informed about potential precipitating factors and the need to adhere to treatment, such as corticosteroids. Through educational interventions, patients can be empowered by their attending physicians with the needed information for the identification of early stages of relapse, allowing timely medical interventions. In addition, patients must be empowered in their own care through the open discussion of symptom management and treatment plans with their health professionals. Patient education materials that maximize patient comprehension, such as clear guidelines and visual descriptions, can play a significant role in enhanced compliance and self-care behaviors and, consequently, decrease the risk of disease progression or recurrence. Also, gut microbiota and autoimmune disease interaction have been in the limelight over the past few years, indicating the potential for dietary modification and patient counseling with respect to microbiome status. Mounting evidence indicates that dysbiosis, or imbalance in gut microorganisms, is involved in inflammation and autoimmune activity in a variety of diseases, including those of the pancreas. Consequently, patient education regarding the role of prebiotics, probiotics, and fibers in the re-establishment of gut health is becoming more prevalent. Making food choices that promote a healthy microbiome not only improves pancreatic function but also maximizes body inflammatory reserves to treat and prevent recurrence. As noted in literature, lifestyle intervention in modulating the gut microbiota has a significant therapeutic effect on autoimmune pancreatitis and ought to be a major component of patient education and management plans.

A CLOSER LOOK

MANAGEMENT AND TREATMENT OF AUTOIMMUNE PANCREATITIS (AIP)

Management and treatment for AIP must be approached in the context of a nuanced recognition of its various subtypes, particularly Type 1 and Type 2. Type 1 AIP is characterized by its association with IgG4-related disease, which typically necessitates thorough evaluation for extrapancreatic manifestations. Type 2 AIP is primarily characterized by its idiopathic nature and is most often seen in younger patients. Because of the etiological variations, management approaches include the application of corticosteroid therapies in both types with established effectiveness. Nevertheless, management recommendations vary across clinical practices, which has been a need for combined guidelines focusing on optimizing treatment.

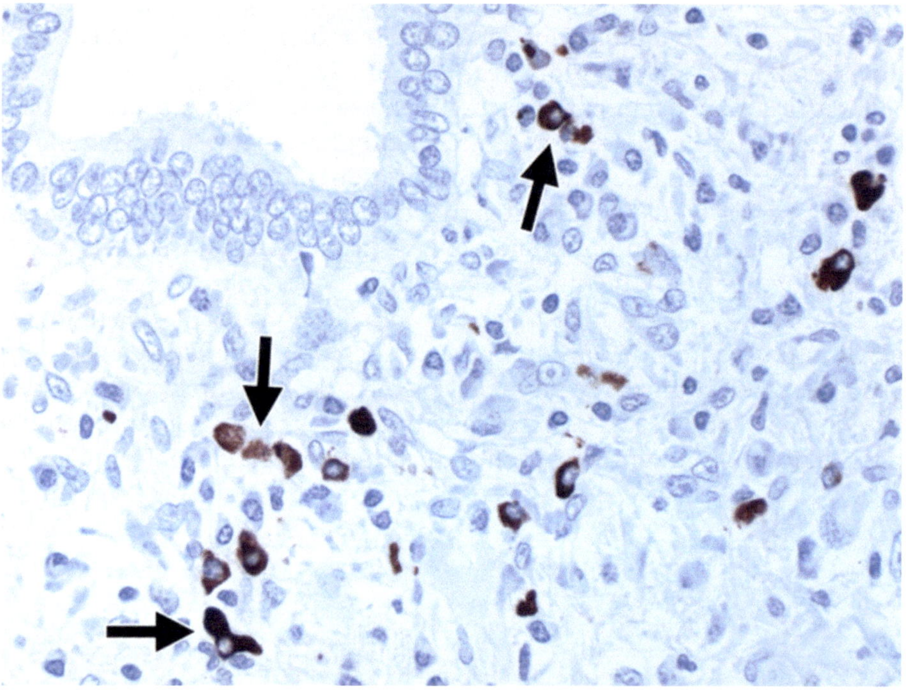

Source: https://pubs.rsna.org/cms/10.1148/rg.315105735/asset/images/large/105735fig02c.jpeg.

This practice variability renders case handling cumbersome and imposes the necessity of individualized patient care approaches considering both the biochemical and clinical characteristics of the disease. Corticosteroid use in preventing the progression of autoimmune pancreatitis to chronic pancreatitis is essential. Studies establish that early initiation of treatment with corticosteroids can significantly lower the risk of chronic complications like awful pain and loss of pancreatic function characteristic of chronic pancreatitis. The evidence establishes that corticosteroids not only relieve the symptoms but also cause resolution of the inflammatory activity associated with AIP when used in treating AIP. It is critical, therefore, for clinicians to initiate corticosteroid therapy cautiously, modulating the dose and duration of treatment based on patients individual response. Ongoing monitoring of the success of treatment and adverse effects is necessary to further tailor management approaches and give patients appropriate care for AIP. Relapse prevention is a critical challenge in autoimmune pancreatitis management as repeated episodes and exacerbations can significantly decrease patients quality of life. Variable relapse rates are evidenced, and corticosteroid tapering schedules are a matter of serious concern in the clinic. Long-term follow-up studies demonstrate that some patients are long-term remitters, but others develop recurrent exacerbations after successful initial treatment. This heterogeneity makes formalized monitoring regimens with patient education essential to identify early relapse characteristics. Also, interprofessional collaboration with gastroenterologists and endocrinologists has the potential to facilitate more collaborative styles of care management, enabling timely interventions that can reduce the likelihood of relapse and improve long-term outcomes for patients suffering from this complex condition (Figure 7.16).

SUMMARY

Assessment of AIP according to type and treatment response, it is evident that the differentiation of Type 1 and Type 2 AIP is crucial so that it can be well controlled. Type 1 AIP, most frequently seen with IgG4-related disease, has typical features such as elevated serum levels of IgG4 and a systemic type with fibro-inflammatory characteristics, while Type 2 AIP possesses typical pathological features with little resemblance to systemic disease. Distinguishing between these two types is important because it will determine treatment and enable prediction of disease progression. Additional research will be needed to elucidate the nuances of each type so clinicians can tailor interventions to optimize patient benefit and avoid complications of chronic pancreatitis. The role of corticosteroids in the management of AIP cannot be overstated. These medications are known to have excellent efficacy in relief of symptoms and inflammation decrease of the pancreas, particularly in Type 1 AIP, where very high response rates are typically seen. Early treatment with corticosteroids not only prevents the progression of AIP to chronic pancreatitis but also renders them a valuable diagnostic tool. An understanding of the steroid responsiveness of AIP has implications for maintaining remission because spontaneous remissions and relapses are common with this entity. A standardized corticosteroid therapy regimen, along with appropriate monitoring and follow-up, is necessary to effectively manage such relapses and enhance the quality of the patients' lives with AIP. Along with this, AIP must be addressed using multidisciplinary management approach with respect to the management of potential complications and concomitant conditions. Because of the systemic character of IgG4-related disease, recognition of other organ involvement is necessary for the comprehensive treatment of patients (Gleeson et al., 2025). Multidisciplinary collaboration among gastroenterologists, endocrinologists, and other experts guarantees meticulous monitoring and management of the pancreatic manifestations as well as any associated symptoms such as jaundice or diabetes. In the long run, advances toward defining the immunological underpinnings of AIP will yield innovative treatments, possibly leading to enhanced long-term outcome and reduced relapse and therefore maximal patient outcomes and minimal disease burden.

The studies of AIP have revealed that significant differences between Type 1 and Type 2 forms are seen in their pathophysiological characteristics and associated systemic features. Type 1 AIP is usually seen in association with IgG4-related disease, which is expressed by elevated serum levels of IgG4 in 68%–95% of the cases. This relationship highlights the complexity of AIP as a pancreatic and systemic fibro-inflammatory condition characterized by lymphoplasmacytic infiltration and pancreatic fibrosis. These changes are responsible for notable morphological alterations, including pancreatic enlargement, and the potential for organ dysfunction. Type 2 AIP, with comparable clinical manifestations, differs in its histopathological characteristics and implies the employment of distinct therapeutic approaches. It is of most significance to determine these differences in an effort to develop precise treatment and diagnostic plans for affected individuals (Gleeson et al., 2025). Moreover, the epidemiology of AIP is primarily based on Japan, which shows differences in rate of prevalence and incidence in different populations. Estimated prevalence in the Japanese population is 2.2 per 100,000, and the annual incidence rate is 0.9 per 100,000. Because AIP is a significant proportion of chronic pancreatitis (approximately 5%–6%), its epidemiology has important implications for public health policy and planning. AIP affects older men, with manifestations of jaundice, weight loss, and new onset of diabetes. Interestingly, extra-pancreatic organ involvement, including the biliary tree and kidneys, typically happens at the same time as pancreatic symptoms, contributing to complexity of clinical management. This multifaceted clinical presentation of the disease necessitates an integrated diagnostic and therapeutic approach, enhancing patient outcome through a directed therapeutic strategy (Gleeson et al., 2025). Investigations into the genetic etiology of AIP have provided crucial insights into its pathogenesis. With the help of powerful intercross mouse models, five QTLs determining the severity of AIP were localized on different chromosomes. This new approach paves the way towards a broader understanding of the genetic factors for susceptibility and disease severity. The implication of these findings is tremendous, as it suggests predisposition to guide individualized treatment strategies and possible measures for relapse prevention. With further studies unfolding the intricacies of autoimmune disorders, the concordance of clinical findings with genetic information will be pivotal in optimizing the individualized treatment regimens in AIP. Besides, understanding the response to corticosteroid therapy and awareness of relapses will prove necessary for boosting the long-term care of this disease.

KEY TERMS FROM THIS CHAPTER

- Age-stratified clinical management
- Complex condition
- Corticosteroid sensitivity
- Diabetes mellitus
- Glucocorticoid receptors (GRs)
- Inflammatory cell predominance
- Augmenting steroid dependency
- Complex disease
- Devise effective treatment
- Disease management
- Glucocorticoids
- Kidney

References

1. Abad González, A., Aparicio, J. R., Aparisi, L., Boadas, et al. (2013). The Spanish Pancreatic Club recommendations for the diagnosis and treatment of chronic pancreatitis: Part 1 (diagnosis). https://core.ac.uk/download/599238294.pdf (accessed on 26 May 2025).
2. Akyuz, F., Algül, H., Arlt, A., et al. (2024). Type 1 autoimmune pancreatitis in Europe: Clinical profile and response to treatment. https://core.ac.uk/download/610638482.pdf (accessed on 26 May 2025).
3. Chapman, M. H., Thorburn, D., Hirschfield, G. M., Webster, G. G. J., Rushbrook, S. M., Alexander, G., Collier, J., Dyson, J. K., Jones, D. E., Patanwala, I., Thain, C., Walmsley, M., & Pereira, S. P. (2019). British Society of Gastroenterology and UK-PSC guidelines for the diagnosis and management of primary sclerosing cholangitis. *Gut*, *68*(8), 1356–1378. https://doi.org/10.1136/gutjnl-2018-317993 (accessed on 26 May 2025).
4. Asghari, F. (2025). Molecular, immunological and genetic studies on murine autoimmune pancreatitis. https://core.ac.uk/download/198099004.pdf (accessed on 26 May 2025).
5. Gleeson, D., Bornand, R., Brownlee, A., Dhaliwal, H., Dyson, J. K., Hails, J., Henderson, P., Kelly, D., Mells, G. F., Miquel, R., Oo, Y. H., Sutton, A., Yeoman, A., & Heneghan, M. A. (2025). British Society of Gastroenterology guidelines for diagnosis and management of autoimmune hepatitis. *Gut*, gutjnl-2024-333171. Advance online publication. https://doi.org/10.1136/gutjnl-2024-333171 (accessed on 26 May 2025).
6. Hibi, T., Hirata, I., Hokari, R., et al. (2016). Endoscopic and clinical evaluation of treatment and prognosis of Cronkhite-Canada syndrome: A Japanese nationwide survey. https://core.ac.uk/download/323078062.pdf.
7. Jones, B. E., Yang, J., Muthigi, A., Hogan, S. L., Hu, Y., Starmer, J., Henderson, C. D., Poulton, C. J., Brant, E. J., Pendergraft, W. F., 3rd, Jennette, J. C., Falk, R. J., & Ciavatta, D. J. (2017). Gene-Specific DNA Methylation Changes Predict Remission in Patients with ANCA-Associated Vasculitis. *Journal of the American Society of Nephrology : JASN*, *28*(4), 1175–1187. https://doi.org/10.1681/ASN.2016050548(accessed on 26 May 2025).
8. Kersten, R. H. J. (2024). Cholangiocellular defense mechanisms in IgG4-related cholangitis: Role of autoantigens and autoantibodies. https://core.ac.uk/download/604744591.pdf (accessed on 26 May 2025).
9. Griebel, P., Tran, F., Luehring, J., & Schreiber, S. (2023). Case report: Induction and maintenance of steroid-free remission with vedolizumab in a case of steroid-dependent autoimmune pancreatitis. *Frontiers in immunology*, *14*, 1201363. https://doi.org/10.3389/fimmu.2023.1201363 (accessed on 26 May 2025).
10. Wang, H., & Wu, S. (2023). IgG4-related digestive diseases: Diagnosis and treatment. https://core.ac.uk/download/587878803.pdf (accessed on 26 May 2025).

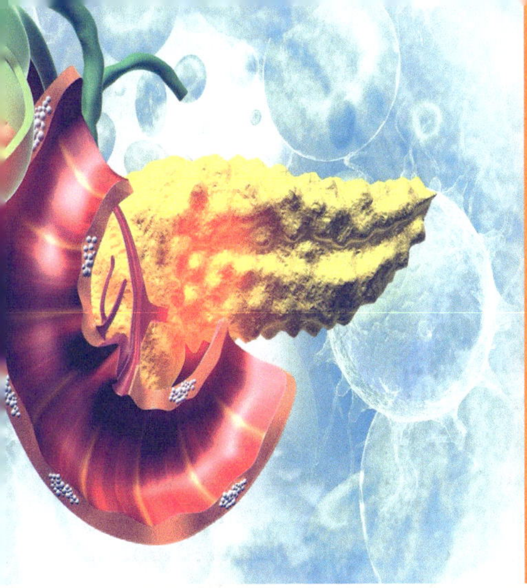

Chapter 8

PANCREATIC INFECTIONS AND ABSCESSES

Contents

Introduction

Amongst gastrointestinal pathology, pancreatic infections and abscesses constitute a seminal intersection of pathology that demands profound comprehension and best care. The pancreas plays a critical role in digestion and metabolism; however, its susceptibility to infection, particularly following acute pancreatitis, can lead to severe systemic complications. Infected necrosis falls under this category and is a significant problem because necrotic pancreas tissue can be a reservoir of bacteria to result in secondary infections. Besides the immediate threats to the health of the infected individuals, such infections make treatment interventions employed to cure pancreatic diseases more complicated. With growing understanding of microbial etiology, identification of each pathogen responsible for such infections is now a matter of utmost concern for targeted therapeutic measures that enhance recovery in patients with this life-threatening disease. Etiology of pancreatic infections is especially diverse and involves a multitude of microbial causes that make treatment more challenging. Understanding this microbial environment is important, particularly because infection can be endogenous or exogenous. Polymicrobial infection, as with deep tissue infection, can be frustrating in their capacity to make the clinical scenario more complicated by having a resistant pattern to the antibiotic. Prior surgical intervention and the presence of underlying pathology increase the complexity of the infectious environment surrounding the pancreas. The increasing rates of resistant organisms, particularly in developing infection within the healthcare environment, call for strict measures in antimicrobial stewardship to halt the proliferation of treatment-resistant strains. Tackling such underlying microbial dynamics is key to designing effective drainage regimens and antibiotic therapies that can facilitate recuperation at the cost of reduced recurrence of pancreatic abscesses. Therapeutic intervention of pancreatic infection has shifted significantly, with emphasis being laid on the early drainage and appropriate antibiotic management. The initial management is generally decompression of infected tissue, which is highly critical in alleviating symptoms and preventing system complications. Drainage procedures, ranging from percutaneous to surgery, are selected based on the clinical presentation of the patients and the severity. Following the early management phase, the choice of antibiotic therapy must be judiciously modified based on the isolated pathogens and resistance patterns. Additionally, adding supportive care interventions such as fluid and electrolyte replacement fortifies the overall therapeutic strategy, promoting recovery in the patient. As ongoing advances are being made in the understanding of the pathophysiology underlying pancreatic infections, it is hoped that more effective management paradigms will result in improved outcomes for patients while surmounting the difficulties of infected necrosis and microbiological sequelae (Figure 8.1).

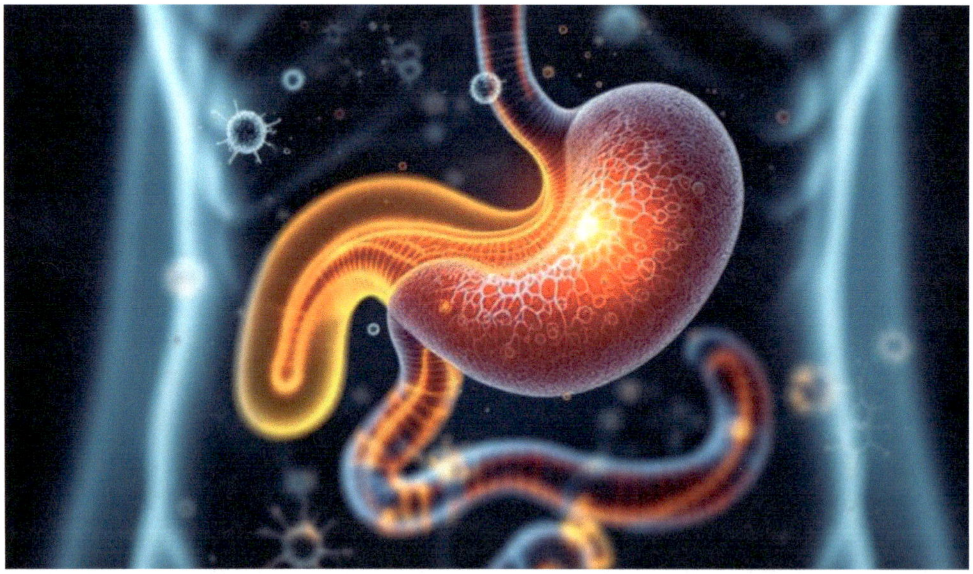

Figure 8.1. Pancreatic abscess.

Source: https://mdsearchlight.com/wp-content/uploads/2024/12/26573-1733788961998-728x420.jpg.

Definition of Pancreatic Infections and Abscesses

Pancreatic infections and abscesses are most frequently found as a complication of acute pancreatitis with necrotizing inflammation of the pancreas. Such a condition can lead to the formation of infected necrosis — an infected local collection of pancreatic tissue with overlying normal tissue. Pancreatic injury results in an inflammatory response that leads to the formation of necrotic tissue, which is an ideal location for bacterial colonization. The microbial pathogenesis typically involves mixed flora and the existence of specific pathogens, including Enterobacteriaceae and, less commonly, fungi, making their overall treatment more challenging. Knowledge of the infection dynamics is important; once pancreatic necrosis develops, risk for secondary complications is increased, and treatment needs to be addressed promptly to minimize morbidity and prevent the evolution to systemic infection. Pancreatic abscesses, in the clinical setting, are classified based on etiology and presentation timing. The development of early abscesses can occur shortly after the onset of pancreatitis, whereas late abscesses occur weeks to months later. The clinical presentation can present as recurring pain in the abdomen, fever, and signs of systemic infection, underlining the need for early diagnosis and treatment. Diagnostic imaging in the shape of abdominal ultrasound or computed tomography is crucial in the proper assessment of the presence, location, and size of these infections. Prompt diagnosis is crucial, as treatment delay can be succeeded by severe complications, including sepsis, multi-organ failure, or even death in high-risk patients (Herrera et al., 2014). Effective treatment of pancreatic infections demands a multidisciplinary approach, with incorporation of surgical and medical interventions. Drainage of the abscess forms the primary therapeutic method, which can be performed percutaneously or surgically, depending on severity and the general condition of the patients. In addition to drainage, antibiotic treatment is also essential in the management of the underlying microbial pathogenesis and prevention of further infection. Suggestions are that empirical antibiotic treatment should be started on the basis of local resistance patterns and the patient's clinical status. This combined strategy—both drainage and directed antimicrobial treatment, is effective in the improvement of patient outcome. However, ongoing re-evaluation of the treatment plan is necessary as the condition evolves and infection resolves (Herrera et al., 2014) (Figure 8.2).

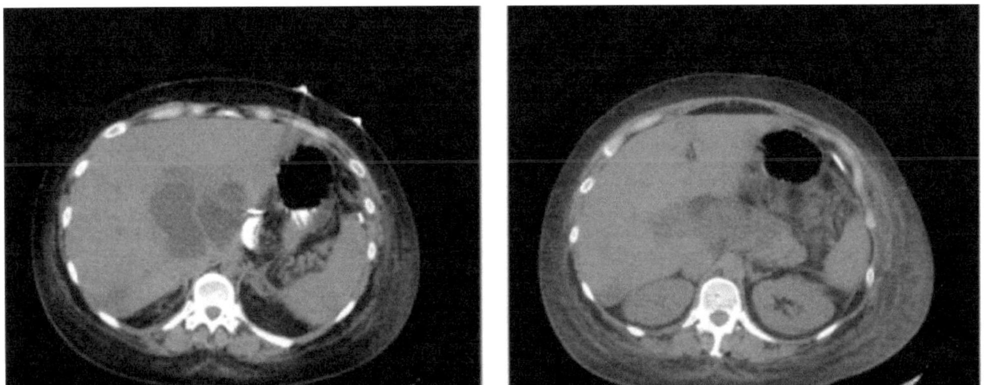

Figure 8.2. A case of recurrent pancreatitis complicated by liver abscesses.

Source: https://external-content.duckduckgo.com/iu/?u=https%3A%2F%2Fsymbiosisonlinepublishing.com%2Fgastroenterology-pancreatology-liverdisorders%2Fimages%2Fgastroenterology-pancreatology-liverdisorders64-g001.gif&f=1&nofb=1&ipt=27f0c82ec523e73dcea5fc8bbbd858f773034966a3f5cef3c2344dc607477802.

Importance of Understanding the Condition

A good understanding of pancreatic abscesses and infections is pivotal in successful clinical management and improved patient outcomes. Awareness of the condition enables clinicians to diagnose infected necrosis, which is a complication of acute pancreatitis, in time. Once aware of the signs and symptoms that define this condition, clinicians are capable of initiating proper drainage intervention to reduce the complications that are associated with fluid collections and necrotic tissue. The most important insight that follows from the understanding of microbial pathogenesis of these infections allows clinicians to more accurately individualize antibiotic treatment, and ultimately reduce the morbidity of pancreatic infections. As is stated, Complicated intra-abdominal infections are a serious cause of morbidity and typically result in an unfavorable outcome, particularly in high-risk patients (Sartelli, 2010). Hence, complete knowledge of the disease is evidently tied to the ability to perform timely interventions, whose impact has considerable implications on clinical outcomes. Moreover, knowledge about the consequences of pancreatic infection calls for special insight into involved risk factors that contribute to poor prognosis. Evidence has highlighted a direct correlation between certain factors such as age and localized peritonitis and high mortality rates among patients suffering from pancreatic infections (Antonelli et al., 2024). AbSeS classification is an important measure of the severity of the condition and stratifying risk within the intensive care unit (ICU) population. By using this classification, patients' needs can be better predicted and resources are more effectively managed by clinicians. Lastly, awareness of persistent inflammation and late intervention as indicators of bad prognosis emphasizes the need for continuous monitoring and reassessment of therapy strategies. This awareness ultimately enhances the capacity of healthcare providers to prevent potential complications and thereby improve survival rates. Finally, awareness of pancreatic infections and abscesses facilitates interdisciplinary health team interaction, a key element of modern patient care. Experts like gastroenterologists, surgeons, radiologists, and infectious diseases physicians must be in close communication with each other in order to deal with the intricate issues presented by such conditions. Through a shared understanding of the underlying pathology and the intricacies of patient management, teams can minimize diagnostic maneuvers and coordinate treatment regimes. Multidisciplinary approaches also facilitate the timely deployment of new treatments, potentially with better results. The gravity of managing such infections is evident in data that total mortality to date was 35.2%, and this significantly highlights the urgent need for a unified effort towards enhanced care delivery (Antonelli et al., 2024). Collective knowledge is therefore not only advisable but actually necessary in further optimizing treatment efficacy and enhancing patient outcomes in the context of the pancreatic infections.

8.1. Anatomy and Physiology of the Pancreas

The pancreas is an organ within the abdominal cavity which possesses a multiple-functioning role in both the digestive and the endocrine system. The anatomy of the pancreas can be compartmentalized into various areas: head, body, and tail. The head of the pancreas is situated within the duodenal curve, while the tail extends towards the spleen. Composed of endocrine tissues and exocrine tissue, the pancreas also secretes enzymes needed for digestion, such as proteases, amylase, and lipase—and hormones that are critical for glucose control, such as insulin and glucagon. The exocrine component of pancreas constitutes the majority of pancreatic tissue and releases digestive enzymes into the small intestine via the pancreatic duct. Such a complex anatomy is essential to understand the physiological function and susceptibility to diseases of the organ, particularly pancreatic infections and abscesses that commonly arise as a result of disrupted digestive process. In the pancreas, secretion of enzymes and regulation of hormones are under strict control for efficient digestive function. The acinar cells of the exocrine pancreas are responsible for synthesis of digestive enzymes secreted in an inactive form to avoid autodigestion. These enzymes are later activated in the small intestine. The endocrine pancreas, which is structured predominantly into clusters known as islets of Langerhans, regulates blood glucose levels by releasing glucagon and insulin. Disrupting the balance may lead to metabolic disorders, pointing to the organs double function. With the pancreatic complex vascular supply provided by the celiac artery and inferior mesenteric artery, any pathological disruption—like that due to infections—can lead to systemic complications, including sepsis. The changes in normal anatomy and physiology are most significant factors in inducing conditions like pancreatic infection and secondary abscess development. Pancreatic infections are most often secondary to underlying acute or chronic pancreatitis, usually due to gallstones or alcohol. Pancreatitis causes inflammation that leads to patches of necrosis within the pancreatic tissue, creating a rich environment for bacterial growth. As infected necrotic tissue accrues, abscesses can develop and complicate treatment and healing. The microbial pathogenesis of such infections is usually polymicrobial flora with aerobic as well as anaerobic bacteria causing the disease process. Drainage and appropriate antibiotic therapy are crucial in the treatment of such abscesses and in the recovery of pancreatic function. With growing depth of insight into the anatomy and physiology of the pancreas also comes the depth of treatment for complications arising from infection, and the significance of the in-depth academic study of this organ's disease and health process (Saarinen et al., 2012) (Figure 8.3).

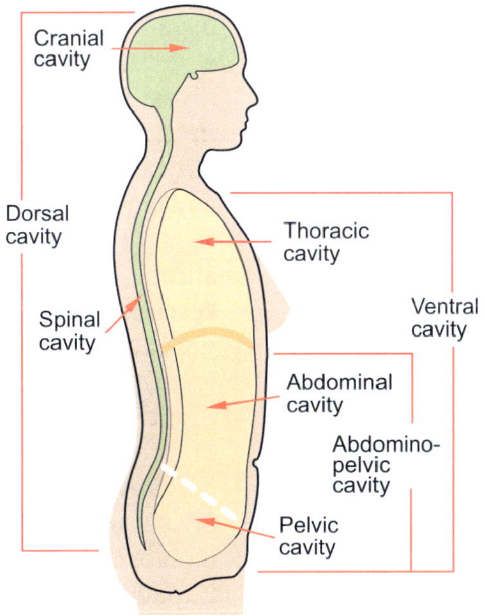

Figure 8.3. Abdominal cavity.

Source: By Vectorization: Mysid in Inkscape, based on http://training.seer.cancer.gov/module_anatomy/unit1_3_terminology3_cavities.html. Image renamed from File:Body cavities.svg (SVG), Public Domain, https://commons.wikimedia.org/w/index.php?curid=5678872

8.1.1. Structure of the Pancreas

The pancreas, being a critical organ in the abdominal cavity, has both endocrine and exocrine functions. It is a narrow, elongated gland situated behind the stomach, stretching transversely from the spleen to the duodenum. It consists of four anatomically separate regions: the head, body, tail, and uncinate process. The head of the pancreas is located in the duodenal curve, which is beneficial to its exocrine function of secreting digestive enzymes which drain into the gastrointestinal tract. The body and the tail are located towards the spleen and are in contact with several blood vessels, such as the splenic artery and vein, which supply it with blood. It is essential to recognize this organization since it forms a foundation for understanding how infectious processes such as the formation of an abscess can disrupt these intricate anatomical relationships and lead to widespread clinical effects. In addition to its organization, the pancreatic parenchyma is composed of acinar cells that secrete digestive enzymes and islets of Langerhans that secrete hormones such as insulin and glucagon. The pancreatic ducts, particularly the main pancreatic duct, are passages for these digestive enzymes to the duodenum, highlighting the role of the organ in both metabolism and digestion. Any compromise of these ductal systems, either by mechanical blockage or inflammation, can make an individual susceptible to pancreatic infections. These infections most often arise from disorders such as acute pancreatitis, where necrotic material becomes colonized by bacteria to develop infected necrosis. This dynamic interaction between pancreatic structure and susceptibility to infections points to the complexities in managing pancreatic abscesses,a formidable challenge that often calls for considerable drainage and antibiotic therapy to facilitate healing (Rolston, 2017). And the structural anatomy of the pancreas is also essential in understanding the complications in pancreatic infections and abscesses. Infections that lead to infected necrosis are usually polymicrobial infections, which complicate diagnosis and therapeutic intervention. The anatomy of the pancreas, with its ductal and vascular system, offers hints about the pathways through which infections can disseminate, tending to manifest serious complications, particularly in critically ill patients. Such complications can be in the form of complicated intra-abdominal infections whose influence on morbidity and mortality rates is considerable (Sartelli, 2010). Therefore, a profound knowledge about the anatomy of the pancreas is required not only for the diagnosis of infections but also for the practice of correct drainage techniques and antibiotic therapy in managing such life-threatening infections optimally.

8.1.2. Functions of the Pancreas in Digestion

Pancreas plays a critical role in digestion, basically through its exocrine activities. The organ releases pancreatic juice containing a potent mixture of enzymes critical in the digestion of carbohydrates, proteins, and fats in the small intestine. These enzymes are amylase, lipase, and proteases such as trypsin and chymotrypsin. Secretion of these enzymes is tightly controlled and is called upon by hormonal stimuli, particularly cholecystokinin (CCK) and secretin, released from the duodenum with the onset of food in the gut. Such enzymatic activity is responsible for nutrient absorption, and it illustrates the pancreas structural function of providing energy homeostasis and overall digestive health. Interference with synthesis or secretion of such enzymes can lead to malabsorption syndromes and have profound impacts on health and nutritional status. In addition to its exocrine functions, the pancreas also possesses important endocrine functions that contribute indirectly to digestion. The pancreas secretes insulin and glucagon hormones that are essential to glucose metabolism. Insulin stimulates the uptake of glucose by tissues, while glucagon increases blood glucose when necessary. These hormones maintain blood sugar balance following meals, thereby ensuring digested food-derived energy is put into operation or stored accordingly. Such homeostasis is important given the impact of pancreatic activities on digestive illness and disease. For instance, pancreatic infections and abscesses, discussed in the case of pancreatic pathology, may lead to profound endocrine impairment and cause an increase in metabolic complications like diabetes. It is important to comprehend such interactions to know how pancreas health influences digestion as a whole and metabolic equilibrium (Canadian Medical Association, 1990). In addition, the clinical significance of pancreatic function is particularly urgent when translated into pathological contexts such as acute pancreatitis that can cause serious complications such as infected necrosis and pancreatic abscess. The inflammatory process disrupts exocrine and endocrine pancreatic functions and typically follows gallstone disease or chronic alcoholism. The necrotic tissue resulting from the extreme inflammation puts the patient at risk for infection, bringing microbial etiology into the picture (Luiten et al., 1998). The interplay between infection and impaired pancreatic function reinforces the importance of early diagnosis and interventions, like drainage and antibiotic therapy, to manage these complications effectively. Such management is not only crucial in the alleviation of short-term symptoms but also in the prevention of long-term damage to pancreatic function and gastrointestinal health. The realization of the two roles of the pancreas serves to underscore the requirement for a holistic approach to the management of pancreatic disease and thus constitutes a clinical topic of relevance (Figure 8.4).

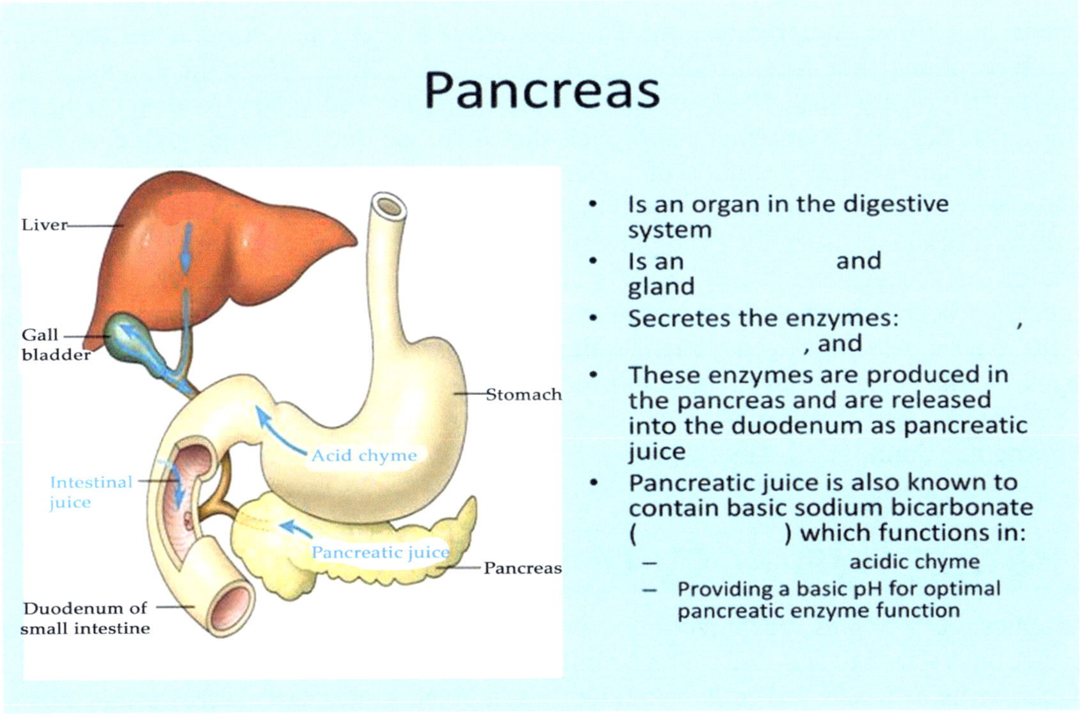

Figure 8.4. Functions of the pancreas in digestion.

Source: https://i.pinimg.com/736x/16/2a/94/162a94403995b1de5328ed2f496fb6b6.jpg.

8.1.3. Role Of The Pancreas in Metabolic Processes

The pancreas plays a significant role in metabolism, primarily through its exocrine and endocrine function. The pancreas, when functioning as an exocrine organ, secretes digestive enzymes such as amylase, lipase, and proteases that facilitate the breakdown of carbohydrate, fats, and proteins in the small intestine. This enzymatic activity facilitates the absorption and utilization of nutrients and thereby provides a foundation for metabolic health. In evaluating the consequences of pancreatic insufficiency, particularly when there are abscesses and infections, metabolic derangement can be made possible. For instance, pancreatitis, or inflammation of the pancreas, can impair enzyme secretion to result in malabsorption and secondary metabolic disturbances. The pathological character of such processes illustrates the way that systemic infections, which have a tendency to cause pancreatic abscesses, increase metabolic disorders further and influence general health outcomes, as illustrated in discussions of sepsis syndromes (Gonik et al., 1994). In addition to its exocrine functions, the pancreas also has a vital endocrine role in regulating blood glucose levels through the secretion of hormones such as insulin and glucagon. Insulin, which is secreted from the beta cells, facilitates glucose entry into tissue and thus decreases blood glucose concentration, whereas glucagon, secreted from the alpha cells, brings about mobilization of stored glucose in the liver in the case of fasting. Should pancreatic abscesses or infections have been developed, then these hormonal controls are lost and lead to conditions such as hyperglycemia or, in cases very severe indeed, diabetic ketoacidosis. The interaction between metabolic control and microbial infection is also most important, particularly as disrupted endocrine function can lead to heightened physiological stress and impaired healing. The interactive process also emphasizes the importance of early interventions that take into account infectious as well as metabolic concerns in clinical management (Herrera et al., 2014). Metabolic derangements secondary to pancreatic infections require a multidisciplinary treatment approach that includes both microbiological and metabolic control. Early drainage and drainage of pancreatic abscesses not only eliminate the infectious burden but also recover pancreatic function, essential for metabolic equilibrium. In addition, antimicrobial treatment directed by the patient's microbial etiology of the infection is essential for resolution of the abscess and avoidance of systemic sequelae like septic shock. As highlighted in contemporary research, management of the causative infection alongside monitoring of metabolic parameters can lead to improved patient outcomes. Therefore, understanding the multifactorial role played by the pancreas in metabolic processes is crucial for healthcare providers because it provides insight into the outcomes of infection on overall metabolic and endocrine health of infected patients (Gonik et al., 1994).

8.2. Pathophysiology of Pancreatic Infections

The pathophysiology of pancreas infection is a complex interaction between the necrotic pancreas tissue, infections related to site, and systemic inflammatory responses. Necrotizing pancreatitis from acute pancreatitis can lead to the development of infected pancreatic necrosis that significantly complicates patient outcome. When the pancreas is inflamed, enzymes are prematurely activated, causing tissue damage that is a fertile ground for infection. This necrotic tissue is a medium for bacterial culture, which infects the compromised tissue and causes local and systemic inflammatory reactions. This resultant accumulation of inflammatory mediators may cause promotion of organ dysfunction, and consequently, there is an innate need for early intervention to achieve effective management of such infections (Farooq et al., 2017). Microbial etiology plays an important role in the progression of pancreatic infection, with aerobic and anaerobic organisms being commonly involved. Bacteriology has identified *Escherichia coli*, *Klebsiella pneumoniae*, and Enterococcus as frequent in infected pancreatic necrosis with anaerobes such as Bacteroides potentially contributing to the pattern of infection. Polymicrobial infection complicates treatment since the antibiotic cover must be sufficiently broad-spectrum to act against numerous pathogens simultaneously. The emergence of resistant bacteria makes it difficult, necessitating an individualized culture sensitivity-based approach to antibiotic therapy. Information on the microbial pancreate infection profile is essential to design efficient therapeutic strategies and optimize outcomes. Treatment of pancreatic infection usually involves both drainage and antibiotic therapy to deal with both the local infection and systemic disease efficiently. Percutaneous catheter drainage (PCD) has proven to be a groundbreaking intervention in infected pancreatic necrosis, providing an alternative less invasive method to drain infected fluid collections and necrotic debris. It not only assists in infection control but also stabilizes the patient's status, enabling recovery without emergent surgery. The integration of PCD with judiciously selected antibiotics significantly improves survival and reduces the incidence of severe complications from infected necrosis. Lastly, thorough understanding of pancreatic infection pathophysiology steers these therapeutic modalities towards improved prognosis in affected patients (Farooq et al., 2017) (Figure 8.5).

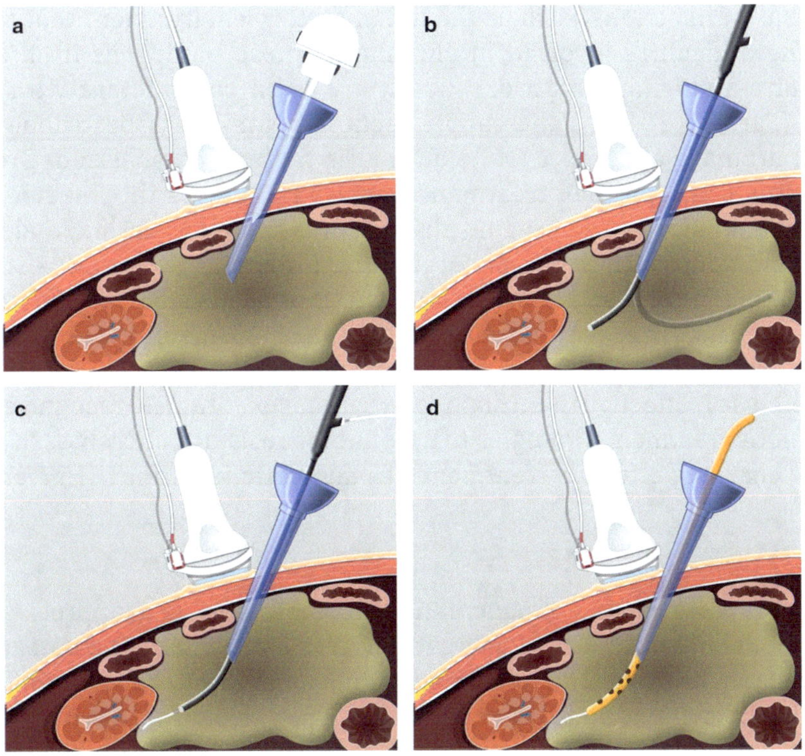

Figure 8.5. Percutaneous catheter drainage (PCD).

Source: https://commons.wikimedia.org/wiki/File:Schematic_of_the_modified_percutaneous_catheter_drainage_procedure_under_the_triple_guidance_of_choledochoscopy,_ultrasonography_%28US%29,_and_computed_tomography_%28CT%29.webp

8.2.1. Mechanisms Leading to Pancreatic Infections

The evolution of pancreatic infections is often a multifold process initiated by acute pancreatitis, whose etiology can be multiple such as gallstones, alcoholism, or metabolic disease. The inflammatory process involved in acute pancreatitis can lead to necrosis of the pancreatic tissue to create a permissive setting for microbial colonization. Since necrotic tissue contains plenty of nutrients and inflammatory mediators, it is also a fertile ground for bacterial growth, typically from the gut. This dysbiosis and loss of local immune suppression as a result of tissue destruction significantly increase the risk of infectious complications in the form of infected pancreatic necrosis. Understanding these mechanisms is crucial, as they identify the underlying infection pathophysiology of the infections that frequently complicate pancreatitis and render interventions more targeted and effective in clinical practice. Infected pancreatic necrosis typically results from bacterial colonization of necrotic tissue, which indicates an imperative for timely identification and treatment. Microbial etiology can be polymicrobial, being a mixture of enteric flora such as *Escherichia coli*, *Klebsiella pneumoniae*, and Enterococcus species. The remarkable point is that the role of these microbes is not mere colonization; they can also produce toxins and induce further inflammation, hastening necrotic changes. Additionally, factors such as host immune response and biofilm formation can make the course of infection multifaceted, so much so that treatment with antibiotics alone becomes challenging to bring about successfully. This changing paradigm highlights the need to learn the mechanisms of infections, such as the inflammatory environment that promotes bacterial colonization and the difficulties involved in eliminating these pathogens from a necrotic bed, as seen in complex intra-abdominal infections which are often concomitant with bad prognosis in high-risk patients (Sartelli, 2010). Pancreatic infection treatment is best done by an integrated method, with both drainage and appropriate antibiotic therapy emphasized. Drainage of infected collections is often the centerpiece of treatment because it removes the infected necrotic material and reduces the inflammatory process. But physical treatment by drainage alone is usually not sufficient without the concomitant use of targeted antimicrobial therapy. Also, the outcome in clinical terms is contingent on early therapy since in case of delayed therapy there is significant morbidity, which is an indicator of bacterial adaptive mechanisms of evading immune responses. So even though control of necrosis and infection is the first step, a proper comprehension of the processes is required for effective treatment of such cases. Studies recognize the necessity of reconfiguring antibiotic treatment strategies to account for resistant microbial strains, a challenging but critical field of ensuring effective treatment of pancreatic infections (Herrera et al., 2014).

8.2.2. Types of Pancreatic Necrosis

It is worth knowing the various types of pancreatic necrosis to be able to appreciate the complexities of pancreatic infections and abscesses. Pancreatic necrosis can simply be categorized into sterile necrosis and infected necrosis. Sterile necrosis occurs due to injury to pancreatic tissue by enzymatic damage, typically in the context of acute pancreatitis. The infected tissue may remain unchanged in microbial invasion, which provides a very critical phase where risks for secondary infections must be closely monitored. Infected necrosis, however, provides the presence and proliferation of infectious microbes in necrotic pancreas tissue and manifests a much more catastrophic clinical presentation. The pathogenesis of the two forms can disrupt management strategies, necessitating an understanding of the underlying microbial etiology and its resultant therapeutic implications, including the potential for surgical intervention or aggressive antimicrobial treatment. Microbial etiology of pancreatic necrosis is a central factor governing the course of the disease. Various studies have confirmed that infected necrosis is most often associated with a variety of bacterial pathogens, most commonly from the gastrointestinal system. Mostly, Gram-negative bacilli such as *Escherichia coli* and *Klebsiella pneumoniae* are commonly implicated in these infections. Their presence increases the inflammation response, which may lead to abscess formation and systemic effects such as sepsis. Sterile and infected necrosis distinction is relevant since management is quite distinct; infected necrosis usually needs prompt drainage, either percutaneously or surgically, along with antibiotic therapy. Such customized treatment is significant not only to prevent infection but also to alleviate co-morbidities so that patient outcome during an acute episode of pancreatic illness can be optimized. Control and prevention strategies are significant as instruments to handle pancreatic necrosis effectively.

Adequate drainage of infected pancreatic necrosis is required since it facilitates infectious material removal with the added benefit of not placing too much burden on the immune system. Performed percutaneously, the procedure is nowadays a favorite in the majority of clinical settings, commonly under imaging examinations to identify areas and areas of involvement of necrotic tissue. The procedure tends to be less invasive compared to traditional surgical techniques, with more beneficial shorter recovery times. In addition, systemic antibiotic therapy is generally tailored based on microbial culture results, indicating the necessity of definite identification of infecting pathogens in the process of infection. Consistent with this, management of these infections through adequate drainage and antimicrobial therapy is not only necessary for relief of acute patient distress but also to prevent further complication of infection of the pancreas and their consequential risk, demonstrating the dynamic character of this clinical dilemma (Figure 8.6).

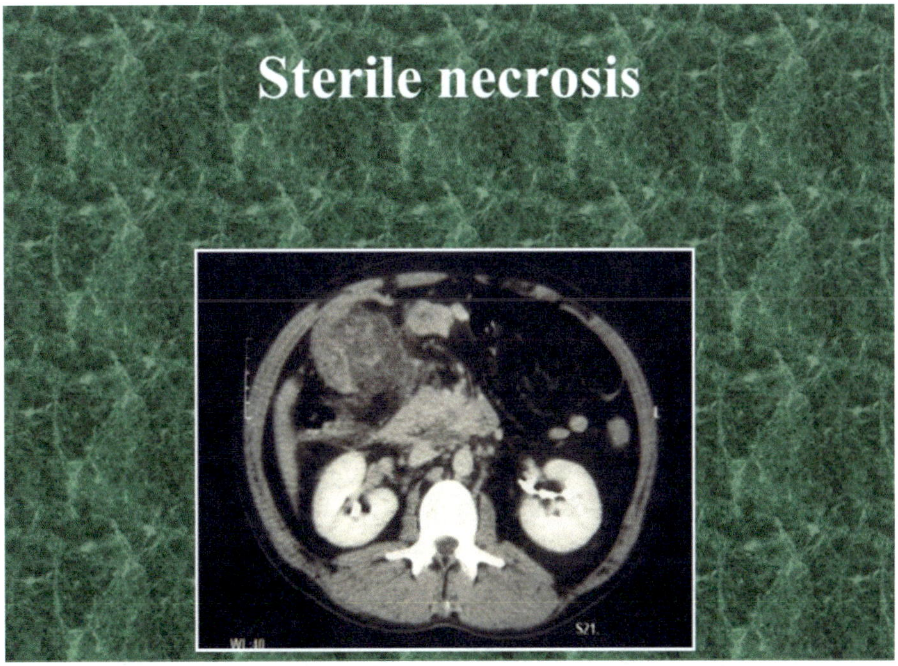

Figure 8.6. Sterile and infected necrosis.

Source: https://slideplayer.com/slide/5304601/17/images/12/Sterile+necrosis.jpg.

8.2.3. Consequences of Untreated Infections

The consequences of untreated infections, particularly in pancreatic infections and abscesses, are deadly and widespread. With increased development of the infection without intervention, bacterial proliferation can lead to the formation of pus-filled cavities, or abscesses. The abscess is a critical challenge to treatment in the clinic because it can exert pressure on the surrounding organs, causing functional impairment and exacerbation of pain. Early identification and drainage of such collections are essential to preventing further complications.

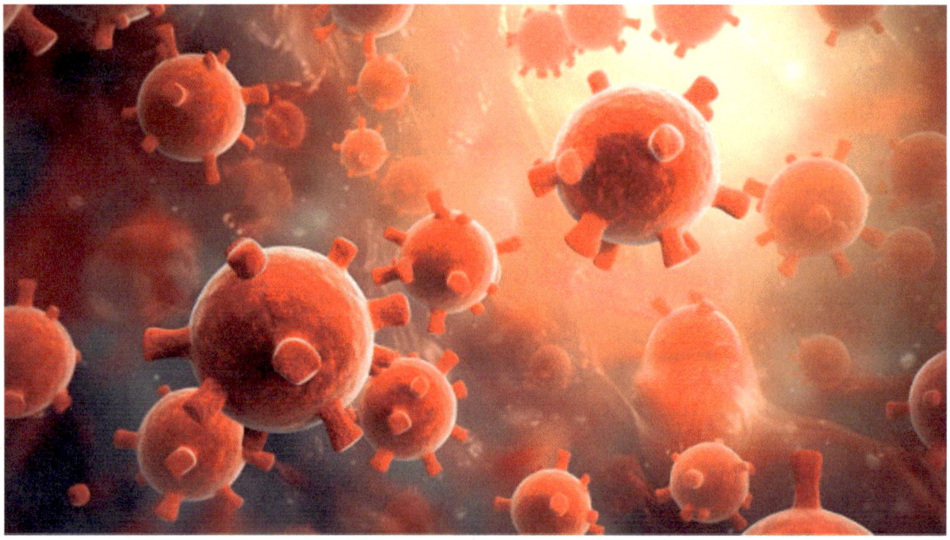

Figure 8.7. Untreated yeast infections: risks and effects.

Source: https://external-content.duckduckgo.com/iu/?u=https%3A%2F%2Fcdn.shortpixel.ai%2Fspai3%2Fq_lossy%2Bret_img%2Bto_auto%2Fsponauglewellness.com%2Fwp-content%2Fuploads%2Fwhat-happens-to-untreated-yeast-infections.jpg&f=1&nofb=1&ipt=1903ff4de0e2e75e049d4b1f79a606183785780e0f8873f0b467d860044c4b71.

Moreover, if left untreated, the infections lead to septicemia, which is described as the introduction of pathogens into systemic circulation, producing systemic inflammatory response syndrome (SIRS) and even leading to multi-organ failure. Thus, understanding and effectively managing the risk of untreated infections is vital to improving patient outcomes and streamlining healthcare system loads (Herrera et al., 2014). Looking at pancreatic infections in particular, the consequence of forgoing early treatment can be terminal. Acute pancreatitis, for instance, presents with severe abdominal pain but rapidly progresses to include complications such as infected pancreatic necrosis. Infected necrosis is linked to mortality risks, with studies establishing mortality rates of various pancreatitis complications like infected pancreatic necrosis to reach up to 80% (Herrera et al., 2014). Infections, if not treated, may disrupt the normal physiological mechanisms of the pancreas and lead to severe tissue damage. Furthermore, the development of systemic infections also contributes to clinical management complexity since it typically entails intensive care measures like surgical drainage and antimicrobial treatment. Therefore, such awareness of severe consequences underscores the necessity for immediate and effective infection treatments in infected patients. The long-term effect of untreated infection extends beyond the direct harm to health by potentially evolving into chronic conditions affecting quality of life. For instance, patients who survive severe infections may remain with such effects as chronic pain, gastrointestinal derangements, and psychological derangements. In the case of pancreatic infection, complications of pseudocyst formation may generate additional morbidity that necessitates further medical care. Moreover, undetected infections may burden the healthcare system in the form of enhanced courses of treatment, such as extended hospitalization or rehabilitation. The intradepartmental resolution for the management of pancreatic infections and their sequelae thus becomes more applicable, going beyond the acute care period to encompass consideration of long-term management (Herrera et al., 2014). This wider understanding of the complication of untreated infection highlights the need for effective medical treatments in averting both short-term and long-term threats to health (Figure 8.7).

8.3. Microbial Etiology of Pancreatic Infections

Microbial causality of pancreatic infections is polyfactorial and often dominated by multidrug-resistant pathogens, which pose tremendous challenges to the management of patients. Among patients with acute pancreatitis, *Klebsiella pneumoniae*, *Pseudomonas aeruginosa*, and *Acinetobacter baumannii* were the most frequent isolates in a study to determine the distribution of pathogens. Specifically, multidrug-resistant organisms (MDROs) was abnormally high at 87.57%, with 87.57% of infected pancreatic samples having resistance patterns that complicate treatment regimens (Farooq et al., 2017). The incidence of these organisms reflects an emergent shift of the microbial environment due to factors such as antibiotic overuse and the impaired immune status of patients with severe acute pancreatitis. This calls for ongoing surveillance of the microbial patterns in order to guide effective therapeutic interventions and improve patient outcomes. Prolonged hospital stay and severe presentation in the form of septic shock and acute kidney injury are associated with MDRO infections in pancreatic pathology. The implications of these infections transcend acute management because they play a critical role in determining the long-term prognosis of the affected patients. The association of infected pancreatic necrosis with the occurrence of organ dysfunction further underscores the paramount significance of early detection and treatment. With changing treatment paradigms, not only does the management of these infections include antibiotic therapy but also the appreciation of the fine line between the timing and modality of intervention, i.e., percutaneous catheter drainage and surgical necrosectomy, which may prove pivotal to control of septic process and prevention of morbidity (Farooq et al., 2017). Empirical antibiotic therapy of pancreatic infection continues to be bedeviled with difficulty due to the extensive spread of resistant strains. Antibiotic choice must consider regional microbial ecology and resistance patterns, which underscores the necessity of microbiological investigations before treatment is started. The multiplicity of microbial inhabitants complicates therapy, and it has been suggested that individualized approaches, such as adjustments of antibiotics based on culture reports, could enhance patient recovery rates. Moreover, with modern treatment regimens increasingly tending towards a conservative "step-up" approach, including effective drainage practices becomes pivotal within the management of infected necrosis. Within such settings, the antimicrobial therapy can be personalized based on direct inoculation results, which can potentially improve clinical outcomes and reduce the burden of life-threatening infections among patients with acute pancreatitis (Chen et al., 2025) (Figure 8.8).

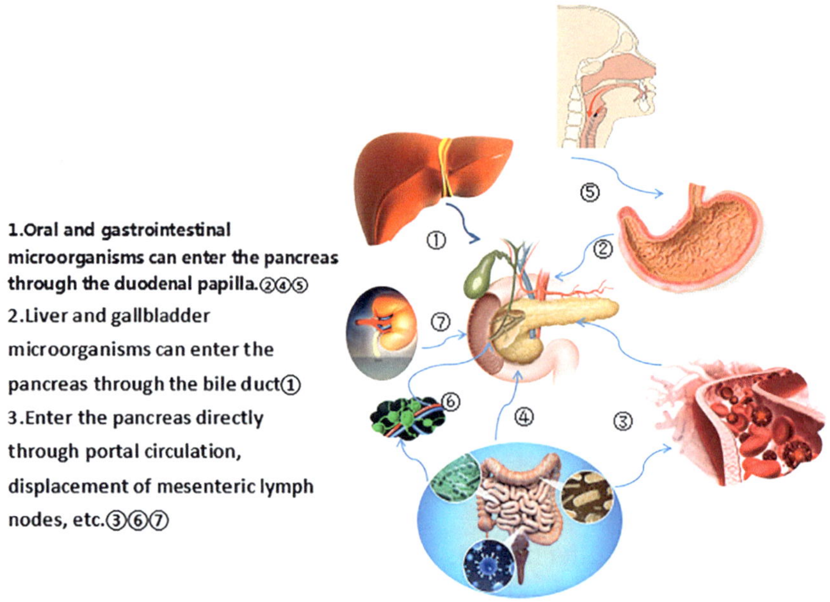

Figure 8.8. Progress of pancreas-related microorganisms and pancreatic cancer.

Source: Zhang W, Zhang K, Zhang P, Zheng J, Min C and Li X (2021) Research Progress of Pancreas-Related Microorganisms and Pancreatic Cancer. Front. Oncol. 10:604531. doi: 10.3389/fonc.2020.604531

8.3.1. Common Pathogens Involved in Infections

Infections that accompany pancreatic abscess are most frequently caused by specific bacterial pathogens that vary in prevalence depending on geographic and demographic factors. Of these pathogens, *Klebsiella pneumoniae*, especially carbapenemase-producing species, is the most well-known and renders them resistant to standard antibiotic therapy. Two such cases of infected pancreatic lesions where *K. pneumoniae* was isolated as a sole pathogen were reported in one study to influence treatment planning (Di Carlo et al., 2011). The emergence of multidrug-resistant pathogens like *K. pneumoniae* requires understanding these pathogens not only to treat them but also to devise adequate prevention strategies for avoiding potential surgical complications. Hence, early microbiological diagnosis is of prime importance in providing optimal therapeutic results to patients with pancreatic infection, as seen in the referenced cases where combined antibiotic therapy was responsible for recovery. Apart from *Klebsiella pneumoniae*, some other pathogens that are most frequently implicated in pancreatic infection include *Escherichia coli* and the Enterobacter species. Polymicrobial infection poses a specific challenge to clinicians because the existence of more than one organism complicates treatment programs and necessitates broad-spectrum antibiotics as an initial measure until specific pathogens are identified (Rolston, 2017). Furthermore, patient histories are important to review, as the conditions of chronic pancreatitis and neoplasms can provide conditions for bacterial colonization and subsequent infection. Understanding these associations further provides an argument for aggressive diagnostic work-ups considering not only the usual pathogens but also predisposing conditions that allow for more virulent infections. This integration of data is critical to both acute therapy and long-term planning in the treatment of pancreatic infections. Finally, antibiotic therapy of pancreatic abscesses must be tailored to the etiologic pathogens and their corresponding antibiotic susceptibility. As rates of antibiotic-resistant organisms continue to escalate, particularly among patients with risk factors such as solid tumors or with invasive procedures, selection of the antibiotic drugs requires diligent analysis. The frequency of resistant pathogens like MRSA and extended-spectrum beta-lactamase (ESBL)-producing organisms necessitates close monitoring and an adaptable treatment plan (Rolston, 2017). In addition, innovative approaches like combination antibiotic therapy and source control, i.e., abscess drainage, are increasingly becoming critical to treat the complexities of infected pancreatic necrosis. This evolving scenario of microbial etiology highlights the need for ongoing research and clinical vigilance in tackling infections in relation to pancreatic pathology.

8.3.2. Risk Factors for Microbial Colonization

The risk factors for microbial colonization in pancreatic infections and abscesses are complex and sometimes interdependent. One of the important factors is chronic pancreatitis, which may give rise to pancreatic necrosis. The compromised pancreatic tissue provides a favorable site for bacterial invasion. As has been noted in more recent literature, emergence of multidrug-resistant organisms like the *Klebsiella pneumoniae* carbapenemase producers has posed a question regarding how well these patients can be treated (Di Carlo et al., 2011). Further, among patients with background diseases like diabetes or compromised immunity, there is increased vulnerability to infection with lowered immune function. All of these put together create a perfect storm for microbial colonisation, one that poses difficulties both for diagnosis and treatment. In clinical cases, interventions spanning anatomical barriers significantly enhance microbial colonization risk. Surgical procedures, particularly procedures related to resection or drainage of the pancreas, can intentionally bring in infection or enable the spread of infection. Infection development associated with numerous medical devices, such as drainage catheters, has been substantiated; occlusion and breakdown of natural barriers commonly lead to infection (Rolston, 2017).

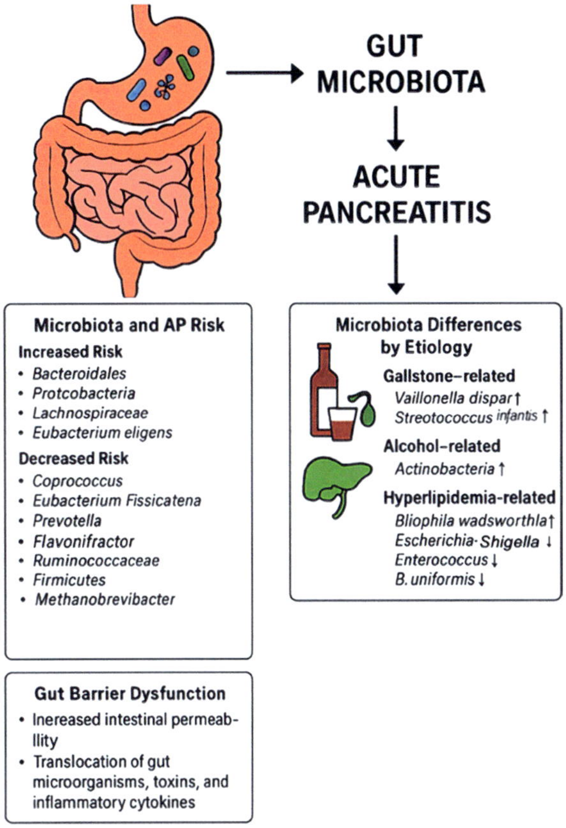

Figure 8.9. Exploring the role of gut microbiota and probiotics in acute pancreatitis.

Source: Nista EC, Parello S, Brigida M, Amadei G, Saviano A, De Lucia SS, Petruzziello C, Migneco A, Ojetti V. Exploring the Role of Gut Microbiota and Probiotics in Acute Pancreatitis: A Comprehensive Review. *International Journal of Molecular Sciences*. 2025; 26(7):3433. https://doi.org/10.3390/ijms26073433

Also, the existence of other factors, such as longer hospital stay and the administration of antibiotics, promotes the development of resistant pathogens and increases the intricacy of management methods. Therefore, identifying and restraining these risks is crucial to the success of the therapeutic treatment of pancreatic infections. In addition, lifestyle and general systemic health factors also cannot be excluded while identifying microbial colonization risks. Solid cancer patients, particularly those undergoing immunosuppression due to treatment, are prone to infections from numerous conditions because opportunistic pathogens tend to engage with malignant conditions more often (Rolston, 2017). As researchers continue to witness novel colonization practices, such as predisposition to deep tissue polymicrobial infections, it is essential for health professionals to implement rigorous infection control measures. Ensuring nutrition, optimizing glycemic control in diabetic patients, and offering immediate surgical treatment can significantly reduce the risk of microbial colonization and subsequent pancreatic infections and abscess (Figure 8.9).

8.3.3. Diagnostic Methods for Identifying Pathogens

Identification of the pathogen in pancreatic abscesses and infections is crucial in guiding therapy. Blood cultures, a tried and established diagnostic method, have provided insights into microbial etiology of such infections for a long time. In one such study on pyogenic liver abscesses, positive blood cultures strongly correlated with increased 30-day mortality, emphasizing the importance of early and accurate pathogen recognition (Wendt et al., 2024). While blood cultures are still a mainstay, they are not infallible, particularly in polymicrobial infections that are prevalent in pancreatic abscesses, where multiple pathogens make diagnosis more complicated. Thus, a battery of diagnostic instruments is generally needed to achieve a composite microbial profile, which will enable clinicians to tailor antibiotic therapy in an effective manner. Recent advances in molecular diagnostics have also further improved our capability to identify pathogenetic microbes related to pancreatic infection. The use of techniques such as polymerase chain reaction (PCR) makes it possible to detect specific bacterial DNA quickly, particularly valuable in cases where conventional culture methods can be unsuccessful because of prior antibiotic treatment or usage of organisms that are difficult to culture. Additionally, 16S rRNA targeted next-generation sequencing (TNGS) has been a strong methodology, allowing more precise description of complex bacterial communities than with traditional methodologies (Dyrhovden et al., 2023). This approach is priceless in the detection of low-abundance organisms that have the potential to play an important role in infection dynamics, thus contributing to improved clinical decision-making. In combination, these new methods highlight the dynamic evolution of pathogen detection in pancreatic abscess treatment. In the clinic, the integration of diagnostic modalities is important for the optimization of patient outcomes in pancreatic infections. Techniques such as Abdominal ultrasound and computed tomography (CT) imaging provide critical structural data, allowing localization of abscess formation and guiding the planning for subsequent drainage. Besides, combining imaging techniques with microbiological analysis enhances the specificity of pathogen identification. For instance, the reverse analysis of pyogenic liver abscesses in one study demonstrated that enterobacterales were the most frequent recognized pathogens, further confirming the significance of an extensive microbiological diagnosis to attain appropriate management (Wendt et al., 2024). Therefore, an extensive diagnostic process encompassing imaging, regular culture, molecular techniques, and metabolic profiling is required to address the complications associated with pancreatic infection and pave the way for improved intervention outcomes.

8.4. Clinical Presentation of Pancreatic Abscesses

The clinical presentation of pancreatic abscesses is generally multifactorial and may be quite variable depending on causes and the nature of the illness. The patients typically present with persistent abdominal pain that may be localized to the epigastrium and may radiate to the back, occasionally pointing towards complications of acute pancreatitis or pancreatectomy. Fever, tachycardia, and leukocytosis are common systemic responses that may accompany the abdominal symptoms, indicating an infectious process. These presentations require early investigation since delayed diagnosis can lead to severe complications such as sepsis or multi-organ failure.

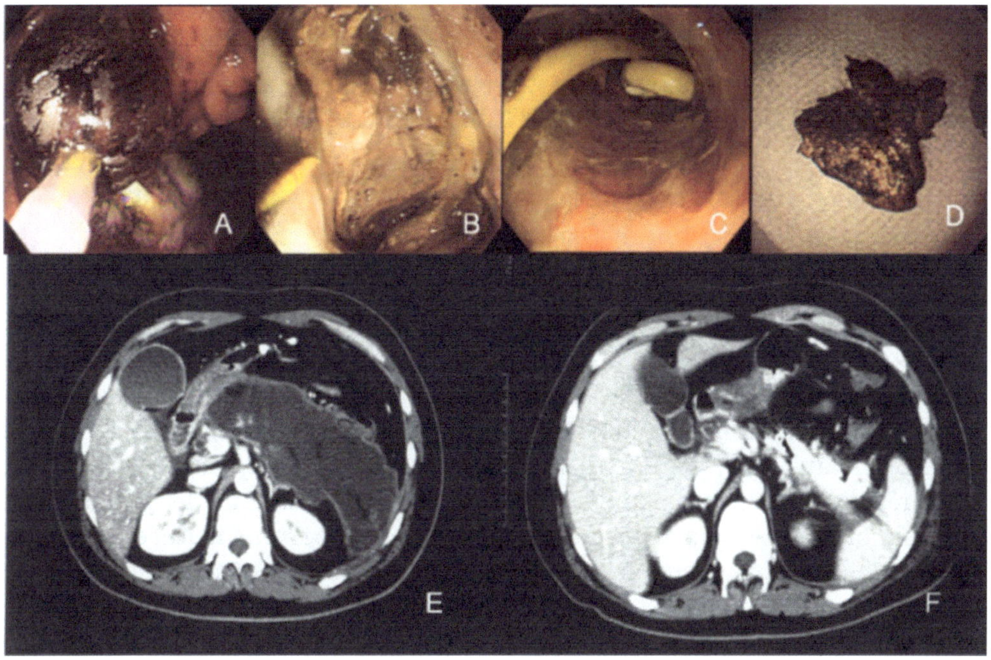

Figure 8.10. Necrosectomy for pancreatic abscess.

Source: https://www.researchgate.net/profile/Hiroshi-Imaizumi/publication/265532947/figure/fig2/AS:295805970862081@1447537047324/Necrosectomy-for-pancreatic-abscess-with-GF-Q260J.png.

The classic presentation of abdominal tenderness or rigidity usually results in imaging studies that can further define the nature and extent of any abscess formation (Di Carlo et al., 2011). Thus, accurate detection of such symptoms plays a crucial role in deciding the subsequent diagnostic and therapeutic interventions. Imaging modalities also play a significant role in clinical evaluation of pancreatic abscesses and provide useful information on the size, site, and type of abscess. CT scans are also considered to be the gold standard for diagnosis since they are capable of delineating fluid collection and pancreatic necrosis with ultra-high precision. Magnetic resonance imaging (MRI) may also be used, particularly in patients with CT contraindications. Imaging may also distinguish between sterile pancreatic necrosis and infected necrotic tissue beyond anatomical assessment, which is critical for determining treatment modalities. Anti-entity microbiological testing is facilitated by these imaging modalities, which assist in elucidating the microbial etiology of the infection. Amplified evidence has shown that some pathogens, such as carbapenemase-producing organisms, have been increasingly implicated in pancreatic infections that may necessitate tailor-made therapeutic approaches according to culture (Herrera et al., 2014). Pancreatic abscess treatment is typically a multidisciplinary intervention that includes surgical intervention, drainage technique, and appropriate antibiotic therapy. Percutaneous drainage is most often utilized in the treatment of symptomatic abscesses, especially well-encapsulated ones. Drainage is facilitated with the help of ultrasound or CT guidance so that it is targeted therapy with minimal damage to the surrounding tissues. Concurrently, broad-spectrum antibiotics are initiated to cover the bacterial infection, with a change based on reports of culture sensitivity. It should be noted that clinical success largely depends on the appropriateness and timing of these interventions. Chronic infection abscesses may need more invasive surgical procedures, including laparotomy or necrosectomy, to allow for adequate drainage and debridement. Hence, recognition of the clinical picture and early treatment are important in an attempt to restrict morbidity and encourage recovery in patients with pancreatic abscesses (Di Carlo et al., 2011) (Figure 8.10).

8.4.1. Symptoms Associated with Pancreatic Infections

The symptoms of pancreatic infections are multifaceted and typically evolve as the condition progresses. The patients first present with severe stomach pain, typically in the upper abdomen, that extends to the back. The pain typically accompanies nausea and vomiting because the inflamed pancreas disrupts normal digestive functions. As the infection progresses, additional symptoms of fever, chills, and abdominal distension develop, which are indicative of the possibility of infected necrosis. They are manifestations of a more severe state of pancreatitis, in which infected necrotic material is capable of causing systemic inflammatory processes. Early identification of these early predictors is therefore critical in preventing subsequent complications, as patients will go on to develop septicemia or multi-organ failure if untreated. An important feature of the management of pancreatic infections is recognizing some infection symptoms over sterile inflammation. Worth mentioning, infections can be characterized by the presentation of purulent fluid accumulation within the abdominal cavity that can be detected by imaging studies. Sustained hyperthermia, white blood cell elevation, and inflammatory markers are indicators of an underlying infectious process. Additionally, patients may exhibit symptoms of cardiovascular instability or respiratory distress as the infection progresses. Because of the complexities involved in making a diagnosis for infected pancreatitis, clinical assessment as well as imaging tests such as ultrasound or CT scan is necessary for differentiating between sterile necrosis and infected collections to facilitate appropriate and timely treatment (Farooq et al., 2017).

The treatment of pancreatic infections is dependent upon the identification of these symptoms and the application of appropriate therapeutic measures. With infected necrosis, drainage procedures such as percutaneous catheter drainage become important in symptom relief and treatment of the infection source. Improvement in fever and abdominal pain after drainage can be a sign of clinical improvement. However, continuous monitoring is required since residual infectious process may still be present, thus continuous antibiotic therapy becomes a necessity (Rolston, 2017). Furthermore, surgery can also be attempted in more severe cases where a response to non-operative management is not observed. Ultimately, clinical results for pancreatic infections patients are greatly determined by early detection and effective symptomatic management, thus it is evident that a multidisciplinary treatment strategy is imperative.

8.4.2. Diagnostic Imaging Techniques

Diagnosis using imaging techniques is at the core of diagnosing and managing pancreatic infection and abscess. A variety of modalities, including ultrasound, CT, and MRI, yield critical information about the anatomical and pathologic changes in the pancreas. Ultrasound, often the first modality of choice, can readily identify fluid collections and guide further intervention. However, CT has now become the standard of reference for pancreatic complication diagnosis due to its high accuracy and specificity for the detection of necrotizing pancreatitis and abscess. Accurate cross-sectional imaging acquired through CT not only delineates the scope of illness but also assists in differentiating between solid and fluid collections, which is important in the decision on the appropriate drainage procedures (Rolston, 2017). Last but not least, choice of imaging modality must be tailored to the individual patient situation so as to permit optimal possible treatment outcomes. In complicated intra-abdominal infections, imaging is more than just simple diagnostic work-up; it is fundamental to therapeutic treatment. CT imaging, for example, has radically transformed the management of pancreatic abscess by enabling accurate measurement of abscess size and location and thereby influencing drainage techniques.

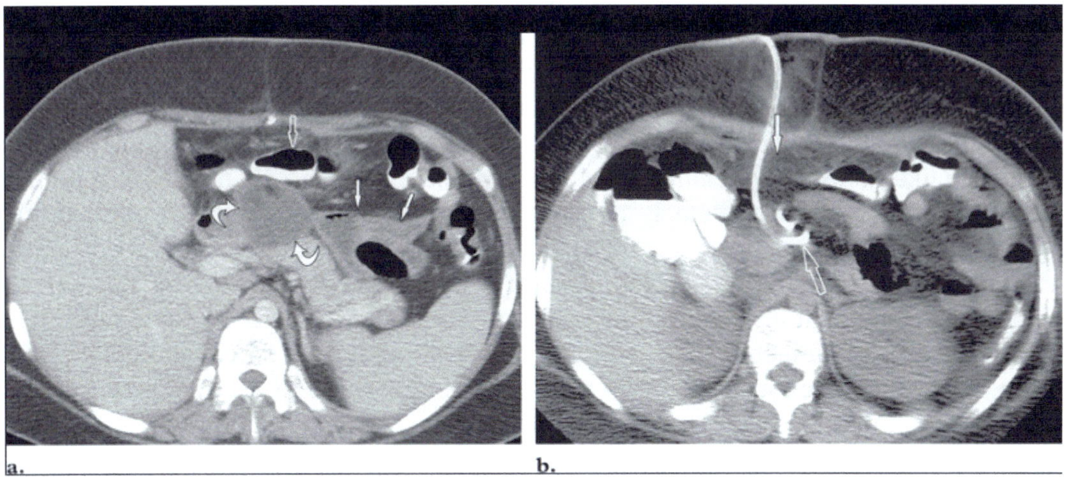

Figure 8.11. Imaging-guided drainage of a pancreatic abscess in a 16-year-old male.

Source: https://www.researchgate.net/profile/Mukesh-Harisinghani/publication/8563278/figure/fig8/AS:341053136752648@1458324812784/maging-guided-drainage-of-a-pancreatic-abscess-in-a-16-year-old-male-patient-a-Axial.png.

Pre-procedural imaging facilitates interventions being safe and effective and reduces the risk of complications associated with drainage procedures (Sartelli, 2010). Imaging techniques also play an important role in monitoring the result of the treatment so that clinicians can monitor changes in abscess shape or resolution over time. Prompt imaging follow-ups can lead to changes in clinical management, such as altering antibiotic therapy or ordering repeat drainage, illustrating the importance of dynamic imaging in patient care. In addition, with the advancement of newer imaging modalities, such as endoscopic ultrasound (EUS), diagnostic accuracy and therapeutic intervention have significantly increased in the treatment of pancreatic infection. EUS, with real-time imaging of the pancreas and surrounding structures, not only aids diagnosis but also allows direct interventions like drainage and aspiration of pancreatic fluid collections. Combination with fine-needle aspiration can provide cytological material further elucidating microbial cause and guiding targeted antibiotic therapy. As infections are similar to solid tumors and pose diagnostic challenges, the standard imaging findings enabled by such techniques are useful in early and precise diagnosis of pancreatic complications (Rolston, 2017). Continuous technological advancements are likely to further optimize management strategies and improve patient outcomes in the complex setting of pancreatic infections and abscesses (Figure 8.11).

8.4.3. Laboratory Findings in Infected Patients

In the diagnosis of pancreatic infections and abscesses, laboratory findings play a significant role in diagnosing and treating the conditions. A routine examination frequently includes complete blood counts, which reveal leukocytosis, a sign of an ongoing infectious process. Elevated C-reactive protein (CRP) levels may also be revealed, indicating that there is inflammation within the body. In addition, there may be liver function test abnormalities in these instances, particularly when infection has prolonged to cause an abscess. These abnormalities are important for the clinicians to detect because they identify the severity of infection and complications. Early intra-laboratory detection of such markers can guide interventions and result in appropriate surgical or medical interventions, which are critical in the optimization of patient outcomes in pancreatic infections and abscesses, where early treatment is essential. Microbiological analysis is a foundation in the management of infected pancreatic necrosis, with culture and sensitivity being crucial in the determination of microbial etiology. Common pathogens encountered in such cases are enteric Gram-negative bacteria like *Klebsiella pneumoniae*, a key organism that has been shown to be implicated in intra-abdominal infection, particularly in regions with resistant strains (Di Carlo et al., 2011). Multidrug-resistant organisms make treatment regimens harder and necessitate a combination aggressive antibiotic therapy. The lab findings of the detection of some pathogens can influence not only antibiotic choice but also the requirement for surgical drainage, which is often a necessity for resolving an abscess. Detection of *Klebsiella pneumoniae*, for instance, could be employed to initiate more stringent infection prevention and other increased clinical vigilance because it can produce life-threatening infections. The findings on high-technology imaging modalities such as CT scans are complemented by laboratory information to make accurate diagnoses and plan therapy in pancreatic infectious disease. Correlation between the laboratory findings and imaging is used by the clinician to ascertain the extent of necrosis and any associated development of abscesses. Elevated inflammatory markers, in combination with imaging data, help to distinguish between the sole localized infections and those complicated or spreading systemically (Herrera et al., 2014). Additionally, percutaneous drainage guided by imaging can be employed as a consequence of these findings, which provides a minimally invasive technique of abscess treatment. Thus, combining lab results with imaging facilitates the ability for individualized treatment schedules to address both the anatomical and microbial presentation of pancreatic infections to achieve optimal therapeutic efficacy.

8.5. Drainage Techniques for Pancreatic Abscesses

Treatment for pancreatic abscess, especially for acute pancreatitis, is typically drainage procedures to prevent complications and promote healing. Open surgical procedures have been the default method all along; however, with current advancements, the trend is toward minimally invasive procedures, especially PCD. The procedure consists of using imaging guidance, i.e., ultrasound or CT scans, to insert a catheter into the abscess cavity. With this technique, clinicians can successfully drain infected necrotic material safely, leading to reduced bacterial load and symptom relief. Studies have proven PCD to be successful in more than half of patients, providing significant clinical improvement with no immediate need for surgery.

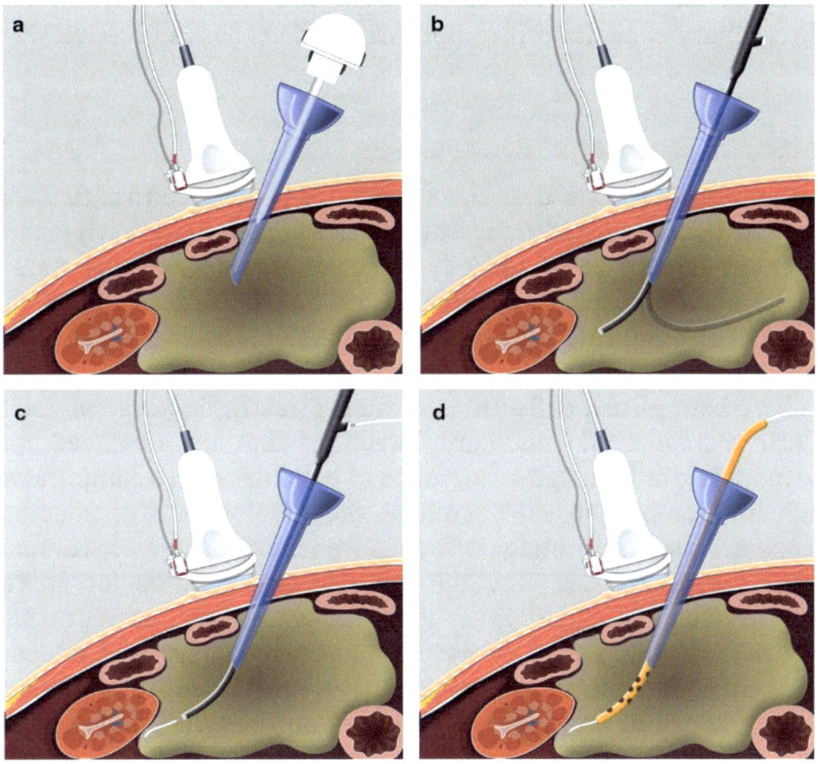

Figure 8.12. Drainage techniques for pancreatic abscesses.

Source: https://media.springernature.com/lw1200/springer-static/image/art%3A10.1186%2Fs13244-021-01087-2/MediaObjects/13244_2021_1087_Fig1_HTML.jpg.

Hence, PCD is a vital therapeutic measure in the treatment of severe pancreatitis, particularly in infected necrosis patients (Farooq et al., 2017). PCD is enhanced by strict monitoring and a focused approach to treatment. On insertion, the drainage catheter is stabilized and may be exposed to routine irrigation to maintain patency, especially if solid necrotic material is responsible for the blockage. After catheter placement, ongoing assessment by imaging modalities is essential to determine the resolution of the pancreatic abscess. The success criteria decrease the size of collection, infection control, and prevention of further surgery. PCD may not be entirely risk-free, and risks include infection, bleeding, and inadvertent injury to surrounding structures. Therefore, careful selection of candidates for PCD is critical; the practitioners should bear in mind not only the size and the character of the abscess but also the general clinical condition of the patients (Farooq et al., 2017). When PCD fails to yield satisfactory results or in the case of a deteriorating condition of the patient, surgical procedures such as necrosectomy may become necessary. Surgical intervention, however, is potentially more invasive and involves higher morbidity risks; therefore, it is generally reserved for those with refractory infection, organ failure, or PCD failure. The step-up treatment of severe acute pancreatitis emphasizes the use of PCD as the initial treatment option before more invasive interventions are applied. This strategy promotes a more conservative management philosophy that optimizes patient benefits by minimizing the risk of early surgical intervention. Last but not least, the drainage modality, PCD or surgical necrosectomy, should be chosen with due consideration of the clinical scenario, the presentation of pancreatic abscesses, and careful interdisciplinary consultation to optimize patient convalescence (Farooq et al., 2017) (Figure 8.12).

8.5.1. Indications for Drainage Procedures

In pancreatic abscesses and infections, drainage operations become central to effective management strategies in the case of them. Infected pancreatic necrosis patients greatly benefit from drainage interventions, particularly if they have clinically evident abscesses or large fluid collections. Early use of drainage techniques both alleviates symptoms and decreases the incidence of systemic infection due to localized disease. This approach is of utmost importance in cases where conservative therapy using medical interventions, including the administration of antibiotics, is not sufficient to treat the infection. By treating such collections of fluid directly, doctors can facilitate healing and reduce morbidity from complicated pancreatic infections that are advanced. Moreover, drainage procedures become more relevant in high-risk groups of patients, where complicated intra-abdominal infections can result in poor prognoses. Therefore, the development of infected necrosis should lead to a prompt consideration of drainage options, especially in case of worsening of the clinical condition or signs of sepsis. Abscess drainage can also be indicated for abscesses that extend into adjacent anatomical structures and cause systemic issues such as septic shock. Surgical and minimally invasive drainage procedures, therefore, are core resources in effectively handling the infections. Imparting these interventions judiciously is vital to improve patient outcomes given the fact that the epidemiology of these infections keeps on changing, most often being dominated by multidrug-resistant pathogens as per recent reports. In addition to mechanical decompression, drainage also provides improved accessibility of antibiotic therapy to the underlying microbial etiology. Polymicrobial flora is a frequent finding in infected pancreatic necrosis, for which an accommodative approach to antimicrobial stewardship is warranted. As described in the literature, conservative management strategies, though effective for the vast majority of conditions, might be insufficient to effectively treat the multifaceted nature of these deep infections. Intervention might involve percutaneous drainage or endoscopic approaches, both of which enable the specific delivery of therapies while also treating the site of infection. Overall, the problems associated with the conduct of drainage procedures not only indicate their clinical importance but also emphasize the need for ongoing research and refinement of therapeutic strategies for the treatment of pancreatic infections.

8.5.2. Methods of Drainage (Percutaneous, Surgical)

Treatment of pancreatic abscesses and infections generally involves successful drainage methods to alleviate the associated consequences of infected necrosis. Percutaneous drainage is now a preferred first-line treatment due to its minimally invasive method and satisfactory outcome in selected patients. The technique, made possible by imaging modalities such as ultrasound or CT, allows precise localization and evacuation of fluid collections. As Carrafiello et al. (2021) have observed,

CT-guided percutaneous drainage not only is less invasive than traditional surgery methods but also reduces morbidity and mortality rates. The effectiveness of the procedure is in the aspect that it addresses the abscess directly without the extensive exploration of the abdomen, thus allowing for a shorter healing time and reduced hospital stay for patients suffering from complications of pancreatic infections. When percutaneous drainage is unsuccessful or fails in certain situations, surgical drainage may be needed.

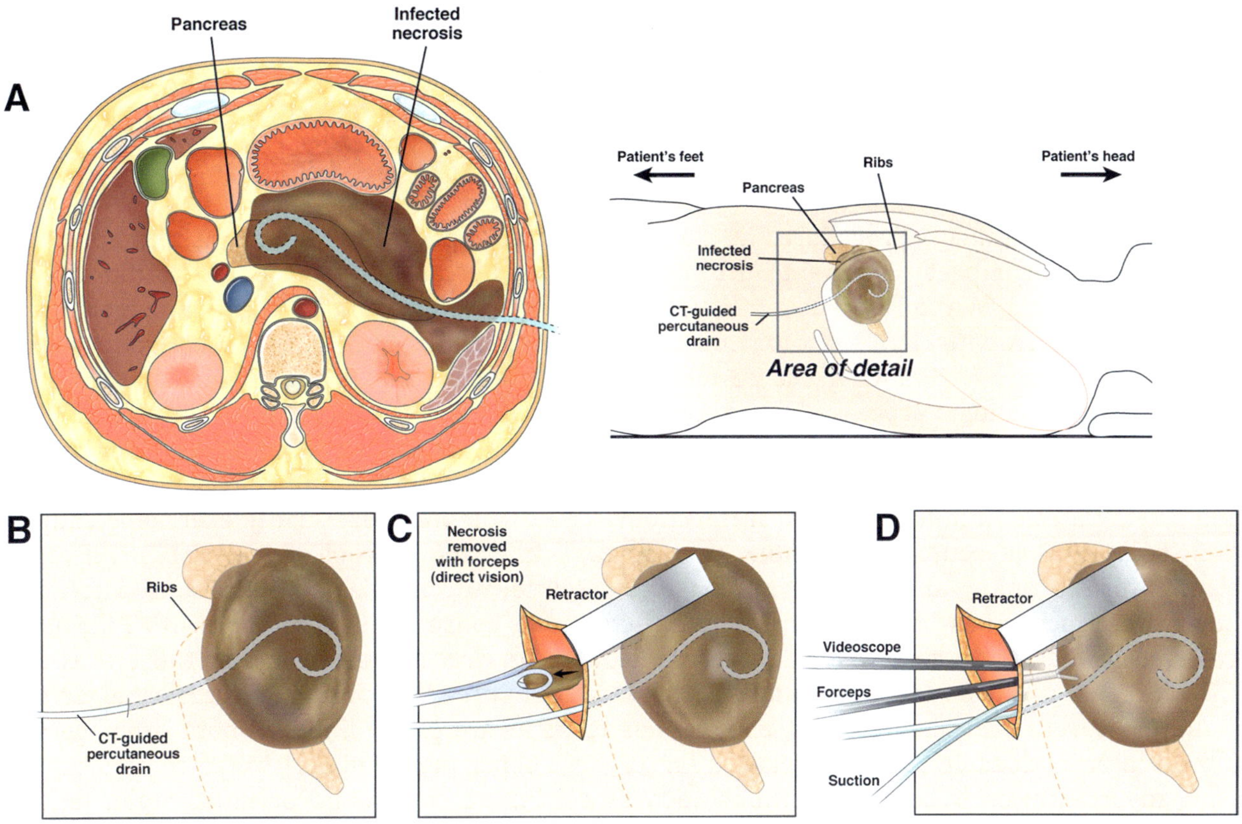

Figure 8.13. Surgical step-up approach consisting of percutaneous catheter drainage (PCD) and video-assisted retroperitoneal débridement (VARD).

Source: https://www.researchgate.net/profile/Alexander-Schaapherder/publication/258920606/figure/fig3/AS:267624466612233@1440818053337/Surgical-step-up-approach-Surgical-step-up-approach-consisting-of-percutaneous-catheter.png.

Surgical drainage would normally be reserved for those patients with large abscesses, organ failure, or clinical deterioration in spite of percutaneous efforts. Treatment by surgery involves open drainage or laparoscopy, which gives direct visualization of the abscess cavity and allows for thorough debridement of dead tissue. The preferred surgical method would depend on the general health of the patients and the severity of the condition. Surgery, while life-saving, is associated with more risks of complications compared to percutaneous techniques and therefore stringent patient selection for such an approach is required. This consideration is significant as complex intra-abdominal infections carry a poor prognosis, particularly in patients at high risk, as noted by

Sartelli (2010). Percutaneous and surgical drainage methods should be compared considering the evolving face of interventional radiology and its impact on the management of pancreatic infection. The technology developments in the field of imaging have significantly enhanced the safety and efficiency of percutaneous techniques to the extent that they are now available as the first-line treatment in the majority of cases. Second, the application of minimally invasive methodologies also aligns with the current healthcare trends which emphasize patient safety along with recovery outcomes. Clinicians should, however, exercise caution in observing the response of patients and be prepared to transition to surgical procedures as required. Lastly, using both methods based on the status of each patient and clinical history guarantees an effective treatment of pancreatic infection and abscess, hence enhancing the care of patients (Figure 8.13).

8.5.3. Complications Associated with Drainage

Complications of drainage procedures in the management of pancreatic infections and abscesses have a significant impact on patient outcomes and must be carefully considered at the time of treatment planning. While PCD has emerged as a significant intervention in the management of severe acute pancreatitis, its use is not free of risk. Complications of PCD, such as introduction of infection, bleeding, and hollow viscus perforation, can result from both the procedural technique as well as the pathologic process of the underlying disease. For instance, the risk of bleeding can be aggravated in instances of pre-existing coagulopathies, necessitating thorough monitoring and preventive measures. Further, catheter slipping complications may disrupt efficacy of drainage, thus playing a role in failure to control infections. These complications justify exercising caution when using PCD in acute management of pancreatic infection (Farooq et al., 2017). Informed selection of the timing and mode of drainage is essential to minimize complications. Literature shows that practice has been shifted in the direction of a conservative approach with PCD being preferred in the treatment of infected necrosis leaving surgical necrosectomy for those in whom PCD proves to be inadequate in stabilizing. This step-up approach provides a necessary algorithm to address severe acute pancreatitis, but one has to be aware of the limits of both drainage and surgical interventions. In addition, delay of surgery as a consequence of early reliance on drainage can inadvertently produce complications such as continued septicemia or multi-organ failure. Complications of drainage processes are in need of continuous evaluation in an attempt to optimize therapeutic methods and improve prognosis generally in patients with severe acute pancreatitis (Chen et al., 2025).

The introduction of MDROs places yet another layer on the clinical presentation of drainage procedures. With the rising rates of infection of resistant bacteria and other organisms in the case of severe acute pancreatitis, the efficacy of drainage processes is compromised, prolonging hospitalization and deteriorating patient outcomes. High rates of MDROs require that doctors conduct extensive microbial profiling and institute appropriate antimicrobial therapy, besides drainage procedures. Specifically, identification of causative organisms such as *Klebsiella pneumoniae* and *Pseudomonas aeruginosa* in infected pancreatic necrosis demands a personalized approach to antibiotic therapy, which in turn is associated with the success of PCD. In the management of pancreatic infections, the identification of the interface of drainage complications and microbial resistance is key in designing the right management modalities and ensuring patient safety (Chen et al., 2025).

8.6. Antibiotic Therapy for Pancreatic Infections

Treatment of pancreatic infection, particularly as infected necrosis, typically involves the use of targeted antibiotic therapy. This form of therapy is essential, remembering the increased risk of polymicrobial infections typical of acute pancreatitis complication. Prompt diagnosis and appropriate empirical antibiotic therapy can have a dramatic effect on patient prognosis. The use of broad-spectrum antibiotics such as imipenem or meropenem, administered prophylactically at admission, has been proven by research to be consistent with traditional treatment approaches for the prevention of infectious complications among severe pancreatitis patients (Farooq et al., 2017). Thus, early administration of the antibiotics is crucial in controlling the microbial load and ensuring the pattern of recovery among the patients. Repeated tracking of markers for infection, along with imaging studies, assists physicians in individualizing the choice of antibiotics to keep up with evolving microbial flora. Another significant shift in the treatment of pancreatic infection is an awareness of regional variation in causative pathogens. New evidence has emphasized the trend of rising MDROs, namely carbapenem-resistant *Klebsiella pneumoniae*, that have been demonstrated to present significant challenges in the treatment of pancreatic abscess and related infections (Di Carlo et al., 2011).

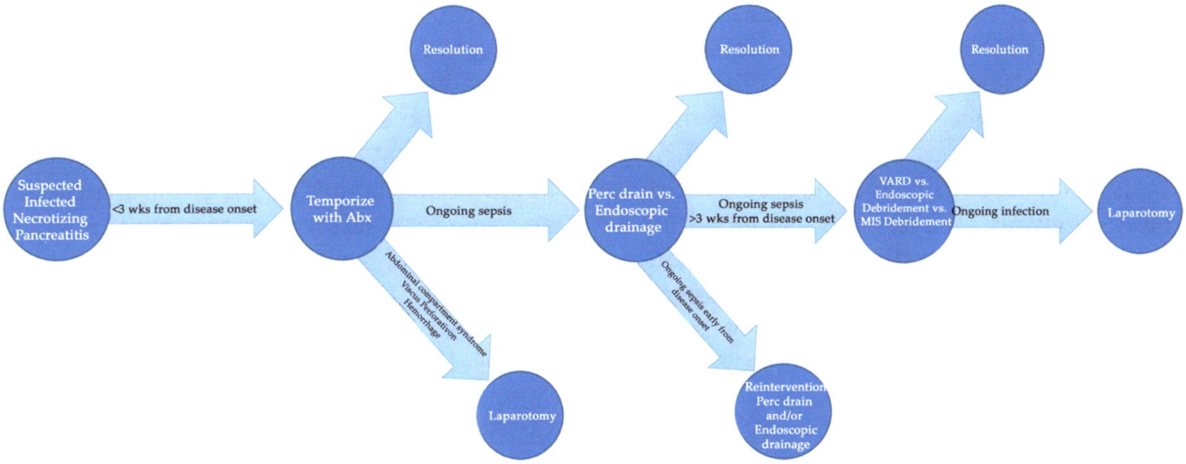

Figure 8.14. Step-up approach for the management of pancreatic necrosis.

Source: https://tsaco.bmj.com/content/tsaco/4/1/e000308/F6.large.jpg?width=800&height=600&carousel=1.

These infections, often established in the background of previous use or recent hospitalization with antibiotics, necessitate reevaluation of antibiotic treatment. The importance of individualized therapy based on microbiologic cultures and susceptibility testing cannot be overstated, since inexcusable use of antibiotics increases the trends toward resistance and undermines treatment attempts. In such a case, antibiotic treatment can be supplemented with newer agents such as colistin or tigecycline for resistant strains, highlighting the role of a combination approach in effectively treating such infections. Furthermore, image-guided intervention and antibiotic treatment are crucial in maximizing patient benefit. Percutaneous drainage of infected necrotic collections has a significant role to play in limiting infection as well as averted surgical intervention. This technique becomes particularly suited when it is combined with appropriate antibiotic therapy, which can enhance the effectiveness of drainage interventions and lower the risk of such complications as septicemia or persistent organ dysfunction (Farooq et al., 2017). Multidisciplinary treatment between infectious disease specialists and interventional radiology ensures a comprehensive approach that not only heals the causative infection but also enables successful fluid management within the abdominal cavity. Ultimately, a synergy strategy—integrating clinical decision-making, microbiological data, and intervention strategies—continues as the cornerstone in the management of pancreatic infection and its associated complications (Figure 8.14).

8.6.1. Overview of Antibiotic Options

Antibiotic therapy forms a critical component of treatment for pancreatic infections and abscesses from infected necrosis. Selection of antibiotics relies significantly on the microbial etiology of the infection, which is often polymicrobial in origin, i.e., organisms like *Escherichia coli*, *Klebsiella pneumoniae*, and multiple anaerobic bacteria. Emergence of multidrug-resistant (MDR) strains necessitates judicious antibiotic choice in a bid to realize successful outcome. Specifically, the combination of colistin and tigecycline has been encouraging in carbapenemase-producing bacteria infections like *Klebsiella pneumoniae*, as observed in recent studies (Di Carlo et al., 2011). Vancomycin may be included to protect resistant Staphylococcus aureus strains, since the more frequent development of MRSA has made the treatment more difficult. Along with monotherapy, the use of combination antibiotic regimens is typically prescribed for widening the spectrum of action and preventing resistance. This approach is most applicable in the case of severe infection of solid tumors or chronic neutropenic states, when patients' immune status is compromised (Rolston, 2017). In such cases, it is not unexpected for practitioners to implement empiric therapy based on local antibiograms to match the regime with prevailing resistance patterns. Moreover, the addition of recently introduced antibiotics or therapeutic drugs such as beta-lactam/beta-lactamase inhibitor combinations can offer alternatives in managing complex cases, increasing the chances of success. The effectiveness of antibiotic therapy is ultimately not only reliant on appropriate medication selection but also timely intervention and the adjuvant use of surgical drainage when necessary. Surgical procedures typically relieve purulent accumulations and allow antibiotics to penetrate more favorably into infected tissue. In addition, antimicrobial stewardship strategies newer to the literature emphasize limiting the duration of antibiotic treatment so as not to be causing further resistance in the hospital setting. Sustained observation for signs of infection resolution and potential complications is required, an expression of the moving equilibrium among clinical management, microbiologic results, and patient outcome in the treatment of pancreatic infections and abscesses.

8.6.2. Guidelines for Antibiotic Selection

In managing infected pancreatic necrosis and pancreatic abscesses, the selection of antibiotics plays a central role in determining the patient outcome. Microbial etiologic diversity necessitates individualized therapy. Gram-negative bacteria such as *Escherichia coli* and *Klebsiella pneumoniae*, and anaerobes with uncommon involvement of fungi, are among the common offending organisms in infected pancreatic necrosis. It is important that the initial antibiotic treatment provide broad-spectrum coverage against these bacteria, particularly in cases of suspected abdominal infection following acute pancreatitis episodes. Amoxicillin-clavulanate or piperacillin-tazobactam are often recommended first-line treatments because of their activity against a wide variety of likely pathogens.

The selection of antibiotics should be reevaluated forthwith on the basis of microbiological data obtained from cultures so that therapy is not rendered ineffective and nonspecific by too broad an antibiotic coverage, lest it risk the development of antibiotic resistance. Early intervention in the control of septic complications of pancreatic necrosis cannot be overstressed. When suspected or diagnosed with infected necrosis, clinicians should initiate the appropriate antibiotic treatment early since delay can lead to unnecessary morbidity and mortality. An important fact reveals that infection can increase acute pancreatitis mortality by as much as 80% (Ackerman et al., 2018). Treatment of infected pancreatic necrosis sometimes includes surgery and antibiotic therapy combined to achieve optimal outcome. Thus, an interdisciplinary team with involvement by infectious diseases specialists, gastroenterologists, and surgeons is required to design an integrated treatment plan. This exchange facilitates the successful identification of infection as well as optimization of antibiotic usage, which ultimately results in patient healing. Finally, antibiotic treatment adjustment should not just depend on culture and sensitivity results but also on patterns of resistance in the region. While antibiotic resistance increasingly becomes a pressing concern, professionals need to monitor locally prevalent microorganisms and resistance pattern in advance of initiating treatment (Ackerman et al., 2018). For instance, *Escherichia coli* and other Gram-negative bacilli tend to be resistant to usual drugs and thus need continuous monitoring and alteration of treatment protocols. Lastly, adhering to established guidelines for antibiotic choice, with room for clinician discretion based on patient-specific factors, will yield a better response to pancreatic infection. This multi-dimensional approach is intended to yield sustained infection remission, prevent complications, and guard against potential emergence of potentially more severe systemic presentation.

8.6.3. Challenges in Antibiotic Treatment

The challenge of applying antibiotic therapy in pancreatic infections and abscesses is further compounded by the emergence of antibiotic-resistant pathogens. With increasing microbial resistance, particularly among Gram-negative bacteria like *Pseudomonas aeruginosa* and ESBL-producing bacteria, clinicians are faced with formidable challenges to successful treatment. In the case of pancreatic infections where polymicrobial flora is typically present to further complicate the clinical picture, the application of standard empirical antibiotic therapies becomes all the more disappointing. This issue is particularly evident among patients presenting with clinical proof of infection subsequent to surgery or drainage operations. Adequate understanding of the resistance pattern of microbes is necessary, since inappropriate initial treatment lengthens the hospital stay and morbidity, making it crucial that real-time resistance data be utilized to guide clinical interventions. Furthermore, the geographical diversity in microbial patterns and resistance further complicates the management of pancreatic infections. For instance, bacteria found in a region of the country can have different resistance mechanisms than those that prevail in another region, as illustrated by the study of intra-abdominal infection in Tanzania that revealed differing patterns of susceptibility among isolates (Kitua et al., 2024). Thus, it is necessary that the clinicians keep in mind the local epidemiological trends in order to modify antibiotic therapy based on that. This subtle tactic plays a crucial role in the management of pancreatic abscesses, particularly where surgery is planned for drainage. A discrepancy between the directed antibiotic treatment and the microbial etiology not only prolongs disease duration but also has the potential to be a causative agent in postoperative complications with a potentially lethal outcome, making regional data imperative to guide treatment strategies. The appearance of resistant organisms complicates the situation surrounding antibiotic treatment further, with simultaneous ramifications for patient management strategies. Intra-abdominal infections from pancreatic necrosis and abscesses are bound to result in high morbidity and may entail complicated clinical scenarios where conventional antibiotic management may fail. As stated, the prevalence of resistant microorganism infections is on the rise, necessitating more invasive diagnostic measures, such as microbiological cultures and antibacterial susceptibility testing (Rolston, 2017). Moreover, management of infected necrosis may require interdisciplinary action that integrates advanced imaging with less invasive procedures to enhance drainage efficacy at the expense of reduced risks associated with surgery. Lastly, resolution of such challenges calls for strict compliance with infection control, antimicrobial stewardship, and continuing education among the clinical personnel to ensure optimal patient outcomes for pancreatic infection (Figure 8.15).

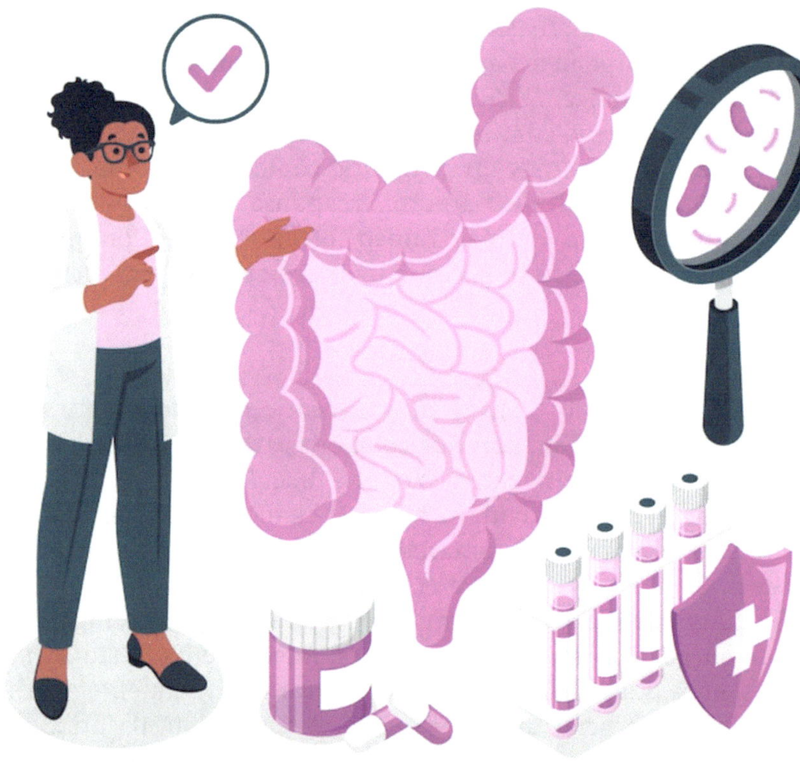

Figure 8.15. Challenges associated with antibiotic treatment in pancreatic infections and abscesses.

Source: https://cdn.medizzy.com/dsFAVWSzBw-EtL4AbMlb4ZZkGaQ=/680x491/img/posts/db50f71c-983d-4260-90f7-1c983d7260ef.

A CLOSER LOOK

PYOGENIC PANCREATIC ABSCESS MIMICKING PANCREATIC NEOPLASM

A pyogenic pancreatic abscess masquerading as a pancreatic neoplasm represents a daunting challenge to diagnosis due to similar clinical, radiologic, and even histologic features. These abscesses are most commonly late complications of acute necrotizing pancreatitis or, less frequently, may arise secondary to trauma, infection, or postoperative complications. Clinical presentation may be in the guise of abdominal pain, fever, weight loss, and malaise—presentation also characteristic of pancreatic malignancy, notably pancreatic adenocarcinoma (Figure 8.16).

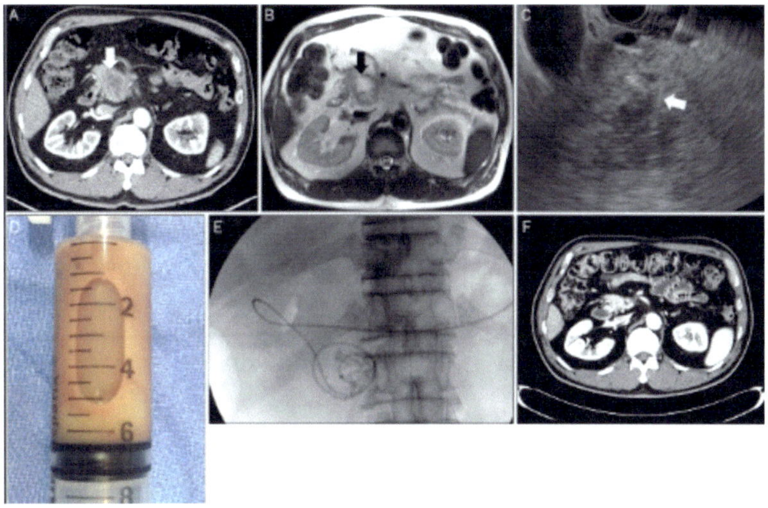

Source: https://external-content.duckduckgo.com/iu/?u=https%3A%2F%2Fai2-s2-public.s3.amazonaws.com%2Ffigures%2F2017-08-08%2Fbf7557b3c91dcfc1179a317bcb140268fcdd9096%2F2-Figure1-1.png&f=1&nofb=1&ipt=3348cc80b672213e12ada29e075faa7c6c9765fbc7874440bca40bbc1869dc2f.

Radiographically, pancreatic neoplasms and abscesses appear either as solid or mixed cystic-solid masses with ill-defined borders and heterogeneous contrast enhancement on radiology. Pancreatic neoplasms will have vascular encasement and ductal obstruction, but abscesses will have inflammation and fluid collection surrounding them. Certain abscesses, especially organized ones or chronic ones, may appear as well-walled complex masses, mimicking cystic neoplasias such as mucinous cystic neoplasm or solid pseudopapillary tumor.

EUS is important in their discrimination because it gives good visualization of internal architecture and allows fine-needle aspiration (FNA). In pyogenic abscess, FNA will most commonly yield purulent material with an abundance of neutrophils and bacterial growth on culture. Neoplastic lesions may contain atypical or malignant cells, mucin, and elevated tumor markers like CEA or CA 19-9. With these tools, however, there have been case reports of suspicion for cancer that led to unwarranted surgery, demonstrating the importance of proper evaluation before resection.

Treatment of a pyogenic pancreatic abscess is with appropriate antibiotic therapy according to culture and drainage of the abscess—either endoscopically or percutaneously, depending on location and complexity. Surgical drainage is necessary for unresolving or multiloculated infections. Treatment of pancreatic neoplasms, on the other hand, is varied depending upon histologic type and stage and encompasses surgical resection, chemotherapy, or both.

There is a requirement for clinicians to maintain a high level of suspicion for infectious etiologies, particularly in patients with pancreatitis or immunocompromise. Multidisciplinary assessment and prudent interpretation of clinical, radiologic, and cytopathologic data are required to avoid misdiagnosis and deliver proper management.

SUMMARY

Pancreatic infection and abscesses pose a significant clinical dilemma due to their multifactorial origins and the significant associated morbidity. Indications of infected necrosis tend to result in aggravation of the patient's clinical status, necessitating prompt and appropriate interventions aimed at reducing associated risks. Cautiousness is required when early recognition of the signs and symptoms of pancreatic infections is to be made, since early initiation of drainage and antibiotics is capable of greatly improving patient outcomes. The identification of microbial etiology with the isolation of causative pathogens becomes imperative in the provision of the best antibiotic treatment regimens, thereby leading to better management of these feared complications of acute pancreatitis. In addition, the controversy surrounding the method of drainage highlights the direction towards minimally invasive methods, which have been promising in reducing morbidity associated with traditional surgical interventions. The present management of infected pancreatic necrosis targets a staged approach where walled-off necrosis formation is established before the onset of invasive treatment. This paradigm shift is a landmark in patient management, an indication of research and developments in surgical techniques, as well as the value placed in individualized treatment options. These evolving methodologies identify the importance of an array of multidisciplinary care to deliver effective complication management following pancreatic disease. Finally, mortality rates in relation to severe acute pancreatitis and its complications are still of concern to medical practitioners. As indicated in the literature, risk factors influencing outcomes like age, having underlying pre-existing comorbidities, and infected necrosis need to be carefully evaluated in practice. Alteration of treatment strategies based on these risk factors can help clinicians predict the development of complications and improve survival rates. Ongoing research efforts that further clarify the pathology of pancreatic infections and maximize therapeutic methods are needed for the enhancement of treatment outcomes. Additional research in this field will ultimately allow for the development of more efficient interventions to suppress the heavy burden resulting from pancreatic infections, reaffirming the importance of scrupulous clinical research in advancing patient care (Husu, 2022).

The incidence of HIV-related acute pancreatitis has been considerably higher than among HIV-negative patients, as evidenced by a study in Durban, which showed that 38% of patients with acute pancreatitis were HIV-positive, compared to 16% HIV positivity among a trauma population. Such heightened incidence raises a serious set of questions on the mechanisms and microbial pathogenesis involved in pancreatic infections in HIV patients. It is also important to point out that the linkage of HIV infection with increased pancreatitis occurrence cannot be ruled out, particularly considering the unique aetiologies present in such infections, such as the large prevalence of drug-related aetiology for HIV-related types. Thus, the exploration of microbial communities and their clinical expression in HIV-infected patients and pancreatic infections is extremely promising for future studies, particularly regarding disease management and successful treatment strategies. In the prediction of results in cases of acute pancreatitis, application of traditional markers and scoring systems such as CRP and APACHE II score demonstrates varying performances in HIV-positive and HIV-negative patients. CRP was particularly found to be less reliable in the prediction of severe disease in patients with HIV, reaffirming the need for personalized prognostic approach for this specific group of patients. Parallel to this, the Glasgow score was relatively uniform in its predictive value in both groups, indicating a potential pathway of enhanced assessment methods for clinical use. This unravels the importance not only of evaluating conventional scoring systems in a generalized manner but also in customizing it to the particular needs of patients facing double odds to overcome both in pancreatitis and in concurrent HIV infection. In addition, management and treatment of pancreatic infection demand a well-established understanding of drainage and antibiotic therapy. Minimally invasive approaches have been successful, as indicated in literature on current techniques in management of acute and chronic pancreatitis. Surgical and radiologically guided drainage operations remain central to eliminating infected necrosis and preventing additional complications, which are common in severe pancreatitis. In contrast, the function of antibiotic therapy continues to be dynamic in accordance with changing microbial etiologies and antimicrobial resistance rates. Altogether, the foregoing observations underscore the need for an integrated therapeutic strategy that combines effective drainage with appropriate use of antibiotics for further augmenting the patient's prognosis in pancreatic infections and abscesses (Anderson et al., 2019; Husu, 2022).

KEY TERMS FROM THIS CHAPTER

- Acinar cells
- Amylase
- Antibiotic choice
- Antibiotic management
- Antibiotic therapy
- Antibiotic treatment
- Blood cell elevation
- Blood sugar balance
- Cholecystokinin (CCK)
- Combined strategy
- Elongated gland
- Endocrine tissues
- Escherichia coli
- Gastrointestinal pathology
- Glucagon
- Hollow viscus perforation
- Infection control
- Insulin

References

1. Herrera, D., Alonso, B., de Arriba, L., Santa Cruz, I., Serrano, C., & Sanz, M. (2014). Acute periodontal lesions. *Periodontology 2000*, *65*(1), 149–177. https://doi.org/10.1111/prd.12022Ackerman, D., Longo, S., Stawicki, S. P., et al. (2018). Septic embolism in endocarditis: Anatomic and pathophysiologic considerations. https://core.ac.uk/download/322436843.pdf (accessed on 26 May 2025).
2. Anderson, F. (2019). Acute pancreatitis in a high HIV prevalence environment: Analysis of prevalence, demographics, prognosticators and outcomes. https://core.ac.uk/download/322918164.pdf (accessed on 26 May 2025).
3. Antonelli, M., Arvaniti, K., Blot, K., Koen, et al. (2024). Epidemiology and risk factors for mortality in critically ill patients with pancreatic infection. https://core.ac.uk/download/604467599.pdf (accessed on 26 May 2025).
4. Wendt, S., Bačák, M., Petroff, D., Lippmann, N., Blank, V., Seehofer, D., Zimmermann, L., Lübbert, C., & Karlas, T. (2024). Clinical management, pathogen spectrum and outcomes in patients with pyogenic liver abscess in a German tertiary-care hospital. *Scientific reports*, *14*(1), 12972. https://doi.org/10.1038/s41598-024-63819-w (accessed on 26 May 2025).
5. Canadian Medical Association. (1990). *Volume 33, Issue 5*. https://core.ac.uk/download/215387822.pdf (accessed on 26 May 2025).
6. Chen, Y., Cui, Q., Cao, J., Wu, Q., Lu, P., Li, G., & Sun, N. (2025). Characterization of Pancreatic Infections in Patients with Severe Acute Pancreatitis: A Retrospective Study from 2019 to 2023. *Infection and drug resistance*, *18*, 199–207. https://doi.org/10.2147/IDR.S500916 (accessed on 26 May 2025).
7. Carrafiello, G., D'Amuri, F., De Filippo, M., Del Rio, P., Gentili, F., Maestroni, U., Pagnini, F., et al. (2021). CT-guided percutaneous drainage of abdominopelvic collections: A pictorial essay. https://core.ac.uk/download/534985866.pdf (accessed on 26 May 2025).
8. Dyrhovden, R. (2023). The use of 16S rRNA targeted next generation sequencing in diagnostics of polymicrobial invasive infections. https://core.ac.uk/download/580972375.pdf (accessed on 26 May 2025).
9. Farooq, J. M. (2017). A study of the role of percutaneous catheter drainage in the management of acute severe pancreatitis. https://core.ac.uk/download/288215927.pdf (accessed on 26 May 2025).
10. Gonik, B., & Pryde, P. G. (1994). Septic shock and sepsis syndrome in obstetric patients. https://core.ac.uk/download/pdf/8039226.pdf.
11. Husu, H. (2022). *Severe acute pancreatitis: mortality, complications, and surgical treatment*. [Doctoral Thesis, University of Helsinki]. Helsingin yliopisto. http://hdl.handle.net/10138/347732f (accessed on 26 May 2025).
12. Kitua, A. J. (2024). Microbial profile and antimicrobial resistance patterns of surgical intra-abdominal infections at a tertiary hospital in Tanzania: A retrospective cross-sectional study. https://core.ac.uk/download/653453349.pdf (accessed on 26 May 2025).
13. Luiten, E. J. T. (1998). Severe acute pancreatitis and selective decontamination (Results of a multicenter controlled clinical trial). https://core.ac.uk/download/18511253.pdf (accessed on 26 May 2025).

14. Madan, K. (2017). Assessment of outcome of percutaneous drainage in treatment of liver abscess. https://core.ac.uk/download/235661287.pdf (accessed on 26 May 2025).
15. Rolston K. V. (2017). Infections in Cancer Patients with Solid Tumors: A Review. *Infectious diseases and therapy*, *6*(1), 69–83. https://doi.org/10.1007/s40121-017-0146-1 accessed on 26 May 2025).
16. Saarinen, R. (2012). Juvenile parotitis. https://core.ac.uk/download/14925375.pdf (accessed on 26 May 2025).
17. Sáez, L. R. (2025). Pancreatitis: Treatment and complications. https://core.ac.uk/download/pdf/71823519.pdf (accessed on 26 May 2025).
18. Sartelli M. (2010). A focus on intra-abdominal infections. *World journal of emergency surgery : WJES*, *5*, 9. https://doi.org/10.1186/1749-7922-5-9. Di Carlo, P., Pantuso, G., Cusimano, A., D'Arpa, F., Giammanco, A., Gulotta, G., Latteri, A. M., Madonia, S., Salamone, G., & Mammina, C. (2011). Two cases of monomicrobial intraabdominal abscesses due to KPC--3 Klebsiella pneumoniae ST258 clone. *BMC gastroenterology*, *11*, 103. https://doi.org/10.1186/1471-230X-11-103

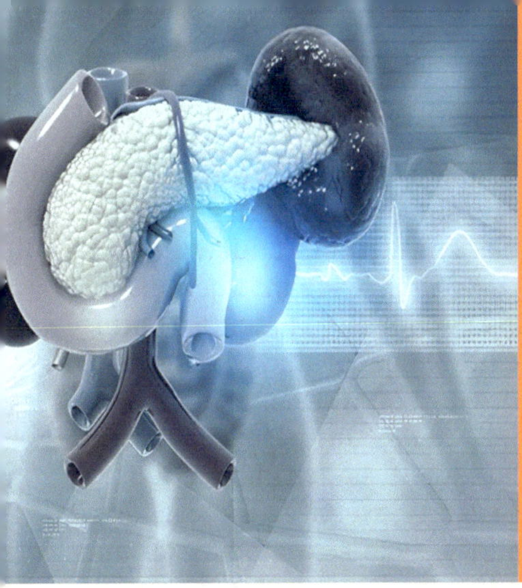

Chapter 9

PANCREATIC PSEUDOCYSTS

Contents

Introduction

The introduction to an essay is an essential groundwork, laying the foundation for arguments and ideas to come in the essay. It is where the reader is engaged and informed of the essay's central subject, the scope of the discussion, and the pertinence of the topic. Constructing a proper introduction takes not only the evident articulation of the main argument, but also explanation of context around the issue. Without context, it will be hard for readers to follow the logic behind the analysis. This complexity is additionally underscored by the necessity of getting one's structure in order in accordance with the scholarly norms of the particular issue at hand. In mathematics and philosophy, for instance, the truth can be philosophically nuanced, as witnessed through varying interpretations of logic systems that defy conventional understanding. Moreover, the introduction should brief readers on potential barriers they may face when engaging in an in-depth analysis of the topic. Many students, for instance, will find difficulty in transitioning from elementary descriptive writing to more complex forms of evaluative and synthetic discourse, says the debates within the pedagogical practice within the higher education arena. Major critical thinking skills such as synthesis and evaluation are normally deprived at the undergraduate level, wherefore essays are superficial and without understanding. This indicates the necessity not just to outline the basic thesis but also to provide instructions for more thorough engagement with the material. Including workshops supporting students' writing capabilities is an example of how certain teaching methods can facilitate deeper understanding of critical thinking, and that in turn stimulates more thorough academic work on written assignments, as indicated in student-control-oriented theme programs (Henri et al., 2015). On these grounds, an introduction should always finally be a bridge between the reader and the broader implications of the discussion in hand. The subjects under discussion are not necessarily exercises in academics but contribute to broader discourses across a wide range of disciplines, such as mathematics and quantum mechanics. The demonstration of Gödel's incompleteness theorems, for instance, reveals profound philosophical questions about the essence of truth and verifiability with implications of extensive nature in various fields of study (Anand et al., 2004). By situating the discussion within such influential intellectual contexts, the introduction not only attracts the reader but also establishes a basis for considering more intricate arguments that are to come. A strong, cohesive point of entry to the essay, its good beginning emphasizes the relevance and urgency of the issues with which it deals (Figure 9.1).

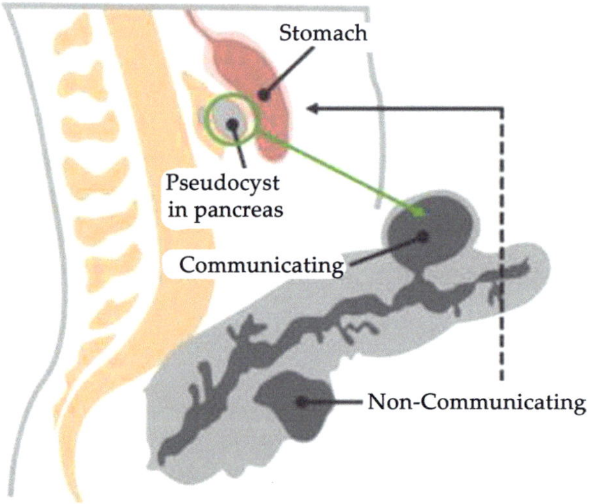

Figure 9.1. Pancreatic pseudocyst.

Source: https://d3uigcfkiiww0g.cloudfront.net/wordpress/blog/pics-en/uploads/Pancreativ-Pseudocyst-300x252.jpg.

Definition of Pancreatic Pseudocysts

Pancreatic pseudocysts are fluid-filled cystic cavities that typically occur as a complication of acute or chronic pancreatitis. Unlike true cysts, which are lined by epithelium, pseudocysts are not cell-lined but consist of necrotic tissue, inflammatory debris, and pancreatic secretions. These pseudocysts are often very large in size, ranging from a few millimeters to several centimeters, and can occur in variable positions such as within the pancreas or in surrounding structures. They are a biologic response to pancreatitis wherein enzymatic digestion of pancreatic tissue leads to entrapment of secretions within a fibrotic capsule formed by the responding tissue. Pancreatic pseudocyst knowledge is critical because they can be asymptomatic or cause complications based on their size and location. The treatment of pancreatic pseudocysts usually depends on their clinical presentation. Small asymptomatic pseudocysts usually do not need any intervention and can resolve spontaneously over time. Larger pseudocysts, especially symptomatic or complicated ones, usually require medical treatment. Endoscopic ultrasound (EUS)-guided therapy is an optimal technique of drainage for symptomatic pancreatic pseudocysts. A review of a study revealed satisfactory outcomes in treatment with a focus on the differentiation between debris-free pseudocysts and solid debris-filled pseudocysts. Technical success rates of drainage procedures are highly high, and technical success rate as high as nearly 97% has been identified in studies for fluid-filled pseudocysts, reflecting the efficacy of EUS-guided treatment in managing such conditions (Yang et al., 2017). In addition to initial therapy, implications of pancreatic pseudocysts also include recurrent potential recurrences and complications due to the development of pseudocysts, leading to frequent hospitalization and resource-greedy medical management. The risk in the clinical setting is elevated in the case of larger pseudocysts, which may require more intensive therapeutic management. Interestingly, treatment options for pancreatic pseudocysts are very heterogeneous on the basis of variable local practices and guidelines, an aspect that could be optimized with standardized guidelines. Awareness of the complexities involved in the treatment of pancreatic pseudocysts, including the risks of severe acute pancreatitis and the risk of multiple organ dysfunction, is crucial to improve patient outcome (Andersson et al., 2010) (Figure 9.2).

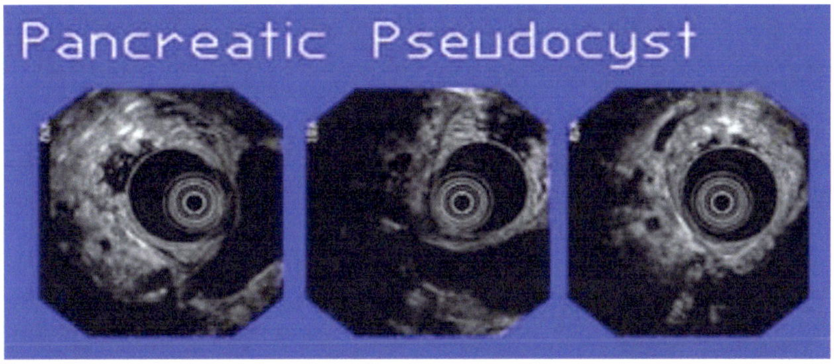

Figure 9.2. Pancreatic pseudocysts: Practice essentials, background, pathophysiology.

Source: https://external-content.duckduckgo.com/iu/?u=https%3A%2F%2Fimg.medscapestatic.com%2Fpi%2Fmeds%2Fckb%2F95%2F35795tn.jpg&f=1&nofb=1&ipt=04a9922c23c28c76a46c24321e3de08e7f023fb0175dcf187f0e9608f6c36a4c.

Importance of Understanding Causes and Natural History

Understand why environmental issues happen is key in formulating efficient measures against their impact. In regions such as Elfeta district in Ethiopia, the awareness of the cause of issues such as soil erosion like deforestation, intensification of cultivation, and population growth is critical in promoting sustainable agriculture. Farmers' perceptions of the causes greatly influence their engagement in conservation efforts. The study has shown that the variables of education, security of tenure, and training access enhance farmers' awareness of soil erosion processes. This improves people's participation in practicing conservation measures. People's participation in addressing the causes will enhance the effectiveness of soil and water conservation strategies and, in turn, sustain agricultural production and environmental integrity in the regions (Geleto et al., 2018). Its environmental history of ecological changes is as important for explaining contemporary environmental problems. The Quaternary period is an excellent example of the way climatic change has reshaped ecological assemblages and driven evolutionary processes. Awareness of these changes emphasizes ongoing conservation activities by highlighting the interconnectedness of species adaptation, population, and extinction occurrences. For instance, knowing the past impacts of climate change can allow scientists to extrapolate future ecological responses and inform biodiversity management plans. Having a view of history is important as it exposes trends that can provide valuable information about how ecosystems react to change. By knowing the natural history of previous climate change and how it impacted, scientists can enhance present conservation practices and ensure that ecosystems remain resilient within the framework of ongoing environmental change (Stewart et al., 2010). Really, a thorough understanding of what is causing and what is natural history of the environment is at the heart of successful stewardship and conservation. It not only enhances the understanding and sensitivity of local societies to immediate needs but also places the big environmental narrative behind policymaking and scientific measurement. Genealogies of evolutionary change and the drivers of ecosystems throughout history open our eyes to new broad ways of thinking, forcing us to consider long-term implications of immediate actions. This knowledge is key to constructing both ecological resilience and sustainable development. So, injecting a sense of causes and natural history into environmental policy and education has the ability to create responsible leaders and citizens who can respond to the needs of the environment of the day.

Overview of Treatment Options

The care of chronic wounds, particularly diabetic ulcers, is a significant challenge within the healthcare industry because traditional means do not effectively work. Diabetic ulcers and other chronic wounds require far-reaching management plans that include local as well as systemic factors that prevent healing. New therapies like nanotechnology applications have been suggested to possess great potential for betterment in the outcomes of wound care. Nanomaterials such as nanoparticles and nanofilms possess unique characteristics that can promote antimicrobial activity, prevent inflammation, and promote healing, becoming a deserving addition to ongoing treatment strategies. Although preliminary results from *in vitro* and *in vivo* studies are promising, more research is needed to assess the long-term impact of these new practices in clinical practice (Auerbach, 2023). In addition to nanotechnology, switchable polymeric particles are also new treatment systems that enhance drug delivery. By and large, polymethacrylate-based copolymers provide versatility in coping with various therapeutic complexities, particularly in diseases such as diabetes and inflammatory bowel disease. The polymers also exhibit pH-dependent solubility with capability to deliver drugs in a controlled fashion to accommodate specific locations within the body. This targeted approach not only increases the efficacy of therapies like oral insulin but also holds potential in optimizing therapies for numerous diseases via sustained drug delivery. With such advanced materials, healthcare practitioners are able to effectively manage long-term diseases and improve overall patient outcomes via customized treatment regimens (Dyess et al., 2020). Collectively, the treatment for chronic diseases is continually improving as newer materials and technologies become available. By utilizing the distinct qualities of nanotechnology and tunable polymer systems, medical practitioners can access new therapeutic avenues that were previously unavailable. Developmental breakthroughs in such treatments are a paradigm shift for treating chronic diseases, such as diabetic ulcers. As research evolves, the clinician needs to stay abreast of these advances in order to use the most effective approaches in treating patients. Such informed practice not only optimizes therapeutic impact but also the aim to maximize quality of life for patients with chronic conditions.

9.1. Causes of Pancreatic Pseudocysts

Development of pancreatic pseudocysts is most frequently linked with acute pancreatitis, which is inflammation of the pancreas. In acute pancreatitis, there are several etiologies that can lead to leakage of pancreatic enzymes into the local tissue, finally leading to local trauma. This damage may lead to the development of pseudocysts, which are walled-off fluid collections that may contain enzymes, necrotic debris, and other byproducts of inflammation. The precipitating insult to acute pancreatitis most commonly consists of gallstones, alcohol abuse, or other metabolic disturbances, such as hyperlipidemia. Additionally, given the increase in the occurrence of pancreatic injuries, there is a need to respond to the current lack of evidence for the treatment of these injuries, especially in evaluating the resultant pancreatic pseudocysts that may occur as a consequence of such injuries (Krige et al., 2017). Chronic pancreatitis is also a significant cause of pancreatic pseudocysts. Unlike the acute form, chronic pancreatitis is characterized by the ongoing destruction of pancreatic tissue, resulting in fibrosis and the formation of strictures in the ducts. These can lead to interference with the passage of pancreatic juices, resulting in increased pressure within the pancreatic ductal system and subsequently pseudocyst formation. This pathophysiologic mechanism illustrates the complexity of pancreatic disease, in which chronic inflammation not only results in loss of function but also potentially complications such as pseudocyst formation. Diagnosis and stratification of such cystic lesions are based on being able to distinguish benign from high-risk conditions, complicated by the increasing prevalence of pancreatic cystic lesions as encountered using imaging techniques (Antunes., 2020). Furthermore, symptoms such as trauma and surgery are also said to cause the formation of pancreatic pseudocysts.

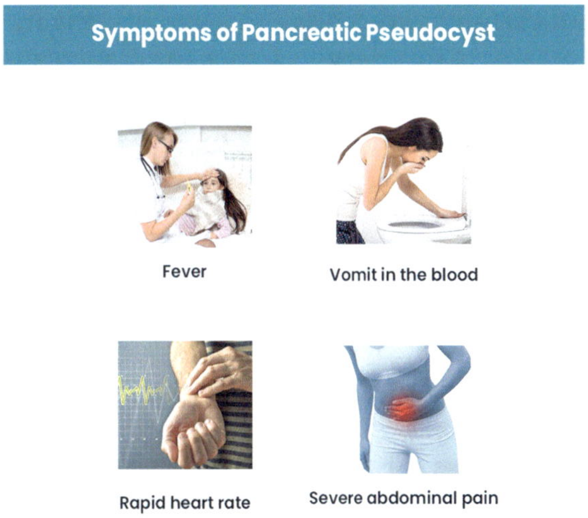

Figure 9.3. Symptoms of pancreatic pseudocyst.

Source: https://healthsoul.s3.amazonaws.com/uploads/660f9f90-af38-4b3a-b7b1-c73f7723bebf.jpg.

Pancreatic trauma, both blunt and penetrating, will inflict injury on the pancreatic parenchyma and pancreatic secretion leakage into adjacent spaces. Similarly, surgery involving the pancreas will indirectly compromise its function and anatomy and result in acute or delayed pseudocyst formation. All these causes, in collaboration, refer to the multifactorial pathogenesis of the formation of pancreatic pseudocyst, necessitating a general understanding of pathogenetic mechanisms. Physicians must employ advanced diagnostic methods, including imaging and biochemical analysis, to appropriately identify and manage patients at risk of pseudocyst complications, thus improving clinical results (Krige et al., 2017) (Figure 9.3).

9.1.1. Acute Pancreatitis

Acute pancreatitis is a severe clinical condition, wherein pancreatitis suddenly occurs with inflammation of the pancreas that may lead to serious complications. The illness has a tendency to be triggered by gallstones, alcoholism, and heavy intake of alcohol along with certain medications. Premature activation of the pancreatic enzymes leads to autodigestion and inflammation of the pancreatic tissue, which is the pathophysiology of acute pancreatitis. As the disease advances, patients may experience abdominal pain, nausea, and vomiting for which urgent medical care is needed. With the rising incidences of acute pancreatitis worldwide, knowledge regarding its etiology and presentation is now crucial to facilitate early intervention and improve patient outcomes (Constantin et al., 2014). The complexity of the condition further necessitates an elaborate approach to diagnosis as well as treatment strategies. Therapy of acute pancreatitis is individualized according to its severity ranging from mild to severe and potentially life-threatening forms. Most cases, approximately 25%, are severe and are characterized by irreversible damage in the nature of necrotizing pancreatitis. No absolute medical treatment for acute pancreatitis currently exists, and supportive therapy is therefore paramount. This is typically followed by pain management, fluid resuscitation, and nutrition, often changing over from parenteral to enteral feeding as the patient recovers. Recent studies underscore the need for early detection and timely intervention in improving morbidity and mortality rates associated with the disease (Constantin et al., 2014). Continuing research to maximize treatment regimens and develop new therapies targeting the root pathophysiology of acute pancreatitis is necessary. New insight into the molecular mechanisms of acute pancreatitis provides the prospect for the application of targeted therapies aimed at the suppression of the inflammatory processes involved. Latest advances in understanding the pathophysiology of the diseases have been spurred by the development of various animal models, which have enabled researchers to investigate the intricate acinar events that have been described in the initial stage of pancreatitis. Research with transgenic mice has enabled the study of specific genetic alterations, and additional information was gained regarding how certain genes induce the inflammatory cascade that characterizes the illness. This data is essential to the ultimate use in clinical interventions designed to enhance the severity of acute pancreatitis and reduce postoperative complications (Schäfer et al., 2005). With continued investigation of the condition by the medical community, there is hope that more potent therapy regimens shall be discovered, sooner or later, improving survival rates and enhancing the quality of life of these patients.

9.1.2. Chronic Pancreatitis

Chronic pancreatitis is recurrent inflammation of the pancreas that leads to possible irreversible damage and functional impairments. Unlike acute pancreatitis, whose symptoms recover completely after the initial inflammation, chronic pancreatitis is a progressive condition with various comorbid conditions that contribute to its severity. Its etiology most often involves prolonged alcoholism, genetic predispositions, and autoimmune disorders, all of which contribute to ongoing inflammation. These risk factors can also lead to chronic pain, malabsorption, and metabolic derangements, leading to a severe decrease in the quality of life of these patients. Since a chronic, degenerative illness, the implications are not only pancreas-specific but also systemic and need a comprehensive care and management plan. Treatment of chronic pancreatitis needs an integrated approach that addresses both the physiological and psychological aspects of the disease. Current modalities of treatment consist of a change in lifestyle, nutritional support, administration of analgesics for pain control, and, in some cases, surgery. Abstinence from alcohol and consumption of a low-fat diet are recommended for most patients to alleviate symptoms and slow disease processes. Interestingly, research has shown that patients with chronic pancreatitis are also at a greater risk of developing other chronic conditions such as diabetes and cardiac issues due to pancreatic dysregulation and malnutrition, making them more challenging to treat.

Treating these comorbidities requires coordinated interventions by the clinicians to provide patients with holistic care tailored to their personal needs, making interprofessional care crucial in achieving optimal health outcomes. Secondly, an understanding of the economic and sociocultural determinants of chronic pancreatitis is crucial in the organization of proper care. Patients under the financial belt may not be able to seek proper medical care or embrace desirable dietary changes, thus deteriorating their condition further. Stigma against alcohol use disorder also dissuades patients from seeking early medical interventions. Furthermore, social ecological systems and recovery capital models highlight the importance of a supportive community to deal with chronic conditions like pancreatitis. Research today supports the need for synchronizing physical healthcare with addiction treatment as it suggests that co-treated substance use and chronic illness management enhance recovery capacity and patient overall health, recognizing an important area to study further (Workman, 2011; Osborne et al., 2022) (Figure 9.4).

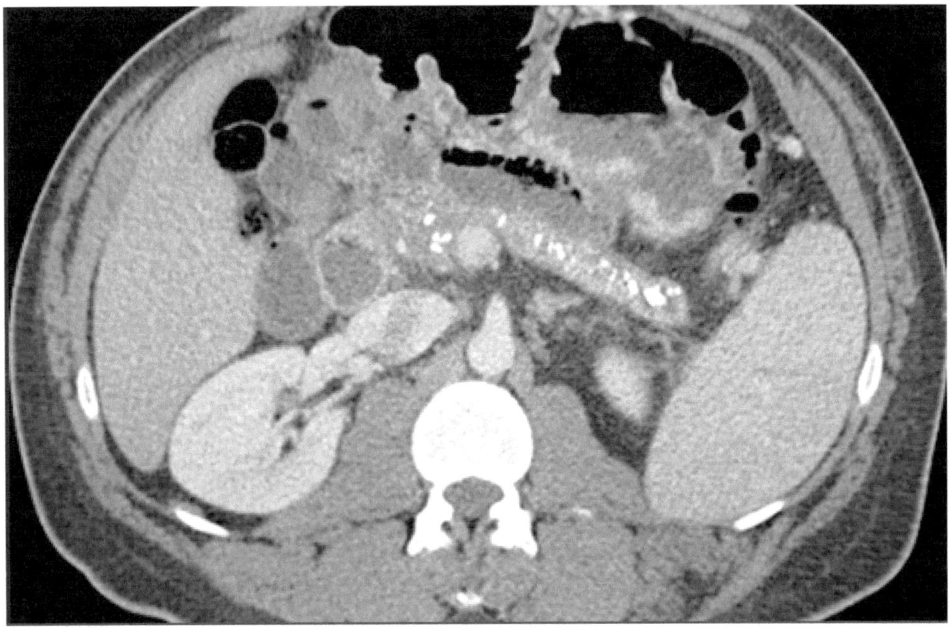

Figure 9.4. Management of chronic pancreatitis.

Source: https://external-content.duckduckgo.com/iu/?u=https%3A%2F%2Fwww.bmj.com%2Fsites%2Fdefault%2Ffiles%2Fsites%2Fdefautl%2Ffiles%2Fattachments%2Fbmj-article%2F2024%2F02%2Fchronic_pancreatitis_tomography_scan.jpg&f=1&nofb=1&ipt=1d644e9a7c4661472265229cb18c65f2ba448b1647ead229947257f65ea6c884.

9.1.3. Trauma to the Pancreas

Pancreatic injury, particularly following blunt abdominal trauma, is a significant clinical issue due to the difficulty in diagnosis and treatment. This vital organ with its roles in endocrine and exocrine function is susceptible to any kind of injury, ranging from contusion to duct transection. Clinical experience has drawn attention to isolated pancreatic duct injury as rare but hazardous if not diagnosed. The early diagnosis is reliant on the synergy of clinical observation and advanced imaging modalities, such as ultrasonography and CT scan, that are capable of detecting subtle pancreatic trauma. Delayed detection of pancreatic trauma leads to morbidity and has effects on the global prognosis and quality of the patient's life. Health care practitioners that handle abdominal trauma in trauma centers must be well versed with the complexities of pancreatic trauma (de Jonge et al., 2001). In managing the intricacies of pancreatic trauma diagnosis, a great leap has been made through vast research that reviews the outcomes of various treatment modalities. One of the primary fields of research is improving surgical procedures that optimize the preservation of pancreatic tissue during intervention. Evidence requires robust evidence to close gaps in knowledge regarding proper management strategies for complex pancreatic injuries. An analysis of a large cohort of patients treated at specialized trauma centers has revealed that strict adherence to conventional guidelines can yield good outcomes in pancreatic injury. The findings also underscore the imperative to address the development of consensus guidelines, which would condense clinical decision-making in the practice of trauma care, specifically pancreatic injuries (Krige et al., 2017). Lastly, the fate of treatment of pancreatic trauma depends upon constant research informing clinic practice and operative development. The conclusion of the current study highlights the need for early diagnosis facilitated by interprofessional collaboration between trauma surgeons, radiologists, and critical care physicians. Awareness of biochemical and physiological impacts of pancreatic injuries maintains clinical discussion and encourages the implementation of evidence-based guidelines. With advancements in the specialty, management protocols need to be optimized for maintaining pancreatic function with minimal surgical complications. Focusing on these aspects, healthcare practitioners will be able to enhance recovery rates in traumatic pancreatic injury patients, providing a foundation for advances in trauma surgery (de Jonge et al., 2001; Krige et al., 2017).

9.2. Natural History of Pancreatic Pseudocysts

Natural history of pancreatic pseudocysts is characterized by a heterogenous clinical course, based on etiology, size, and duration of symptoms. The most frequent underlying condition of acute pancreatitis often serves as the precipitating event of these fluid collections, and the most common etiologies are abdominal trauma and chronic pancreatitis. In the pediatric age range, studies show that 63.2% of patients with pancreatic pseudocysts have a background of trauma, reflecting the significant role played by injury in their etiology. This association is significant, with pseudocysts following trauma having a better prognosis, spontaneous resolution occurring in the majority of cases. Non-resolving pseudocysts are, however, likely to lead to further complications, such that treatment becomes essential. Knowledge of these factors enhances clinicians' ability to cure pancreatic pseudocysts and highlights the need for continued research into their natural history. Management of pancreatic pseudocysts varies depending on their presentation and on the risks of complications in each individual case. Despite some cysts healing spontaneously, surgical treatment remains a cornerstone of treatment in symptomatic or complicated cases. Evidence shows that procedures such as cystogastrostomy and cystojejunostomy are done, especially if pseudocysts are very painful or are felt to endanger adjacent structures. Surgical intervention has been effective and safe with good results for patients despite the morbidity. The experience from Zagazig University Hospital illustrates that while the majority of patients can be managed conservatively, surgery cannot be avoided when pseudocysts result in complications of infection or fistula development (Khalifa et al., 2018). A high-level understanding of the treatment options and outcomes is therefore required in managing this condition in its diverse patient populations and clinical settings. Recent advancements in endoscopic procedures offer hopeful alternatives for people with pancreatic pseudocysts, particularly those who are not candidates for surgery. Endoscopic drainage is an effective treatment, with high patient comfort and low morbidity and mortality risks associated with traditional surgery. Endoscopic intervention has been found to provide early symptom relief while offering improved recurrence rates compared to surgery (Ardengh et al., 2000). As the medical community strives to determine the efficacy of the various drainage approaches, the use of minimally invasive techniques in treatment algorithms is poised to characterize future treatment of pancreatic pseudocysts. Ongoing assessment of such approaches underscores the importance of maintaining a flexible approach to treatment algorithms so as to optimize patient advantage while minimizing against the underlying pathologic issues generated by such fluid collections (Figure 9.5).

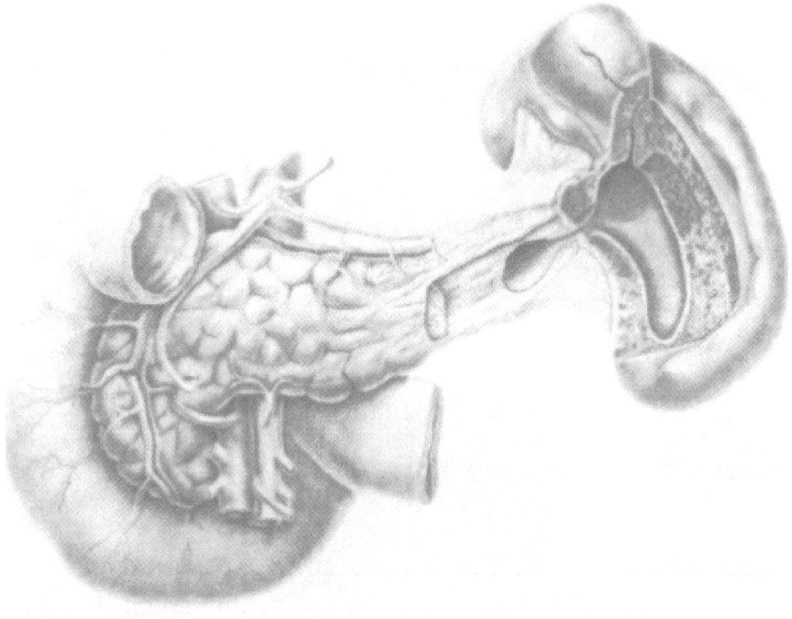

Figure 9.5. Intrasplenic dissection by pancreatic pseudocysts.

Source: https://external-content.duckduckgo.com/iu/?u=https%3A%2F%2Fwww.nejm.org%2Fna101%2Fhome%2Fliteratum%2Fpublisher%2Fmms%2Fjournals%2Fcontent%2Fnejm%2F1972%2Fnejm_1972.287.issue-2%2Fnejm197207132870204%2F20130816%2Fimages%2Fimg_medium%2Fnejm197207132870204_f1.jpeg&f=1&nofb=1&ipt=0fb749e79c63f409e9e28c6725920bd099ee2db452c6ced7da943e720ab85db7.

9.2.1. Development and Progression of Pseudocysts

Their development is most often a secondary expression of an underlying pathological process, typically associated with inflammatory or neoplastic processes within other organ systems. Cysts are most frequently characterizing fluid collections without true epithelial lining and, as such, are distinct from other cystic lesions. The course of pseudocysts can be especially noted in the setting of pancreatic disease, where the inflammatory process of acute pancreatitis can result in the development of these abnormalities.

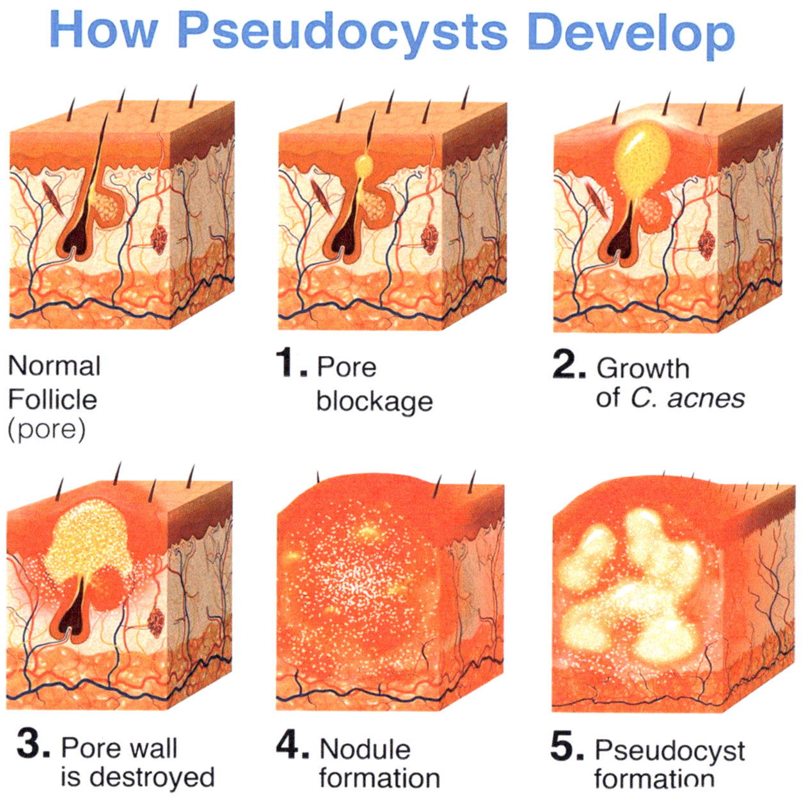

Figure 9.6. Development and progression of pseudocysts.

Source: https://www.acne.org/wp-content/uploads/2022/01/1750538743_06aHowPseudocystsDevelop.jpg.

As time passes and inflammation settles, a pseudocyst can increase in size and put pressure on adjacent tissues and organs, which can cause complications such as pain or obstruction. It is important for healthcare professionals to understand the developmental pathways of these structures in order to allow for early intervention that can avert additional morbidity from their development. The phase of pseudocyst progression is characterized by dynamic progression that is heavily influenced by the body's mechanism for healing. As the cyst develops, it is more likely to transform from inflammatory to a better-organized form, typically being a fibrous capsule encapsulating the fluid collection. This encapsulation may become complicated, particularly if the pseudocyst becomes large enough to encroach on nearby anatomical structures. For instance, mechanical obstruction or compression of abdominal organs by biliary tracts or production of gastrointestinal symptoms or jaundice can be seen in pseudocysts of the pancreas. Clinically, there should be follow-up of pseudocysts, as their pattern of growth can necessitate surgical intervention, particularly in cases with Persistent symptoms or complications as described in studies regarding delayed treatment effects and surgery outcomes for such lesions. Furthermore, management of pseudocysts depends on a fine line of intervention vs. observation, especially as concerns their associated risk factors responsible for their formation. Size of the pseudocyst, symptom status, and presence of comorbidities are specifically key factors that determine the decision-making process. Present guidelines favor an individual case-by-case approach with emphasis placed on the imaging and symptomatology role in directing the management trajectory. Such awareness of the intricate dynamics of pseudocyst development and maturation and potential complications can greatly improve clinical outcomes. As highlighted, priority for further exploration of pseudocyst-associated pathologies remains a priority, leading future priority to more intensive diagnostic and therapeutic intervention in the management of these complex entities (Manan et al., 2022; Núñez-Troconis, 2020) (Figure 9.6).

9.2.2. Potential Complications

In the healthcare sector, awareness of complications arising from medical interventions is a major aspect in patient safety and better results. Complications can arise from many different factors, including the complexity of treatment protocols, patient comorbidity, and drug interactions. In handling diagnostic challenges, it is essential to recognize that shared decision-making is a critical aspect of managing such potential complications. This collaborative, iterative exchange between patients and healthcare providers can reveal a patient's individualized needs and values, as highlighted by Berger et al. (2017). By engaging in this conversation, healthcare practitioners are then able to anticipate more accurately complications that could arise, whereby preemptive measures can prevent risks from developing. Overall, this proactive effort not only enhances patient trust but also results in better compliance with treatment protocols, affecting overall healthcare effectiveness positively. Another source of complexity in understanding potential complications is inherent uncertainty that comes with medical practices. Medical professionals usually work with cases of ongoing patient conditions that can lead to unforeseen events, and therefore, it is crucial for ongoing processes to be modeled correctly. Fox et al. (2004) assert that this modeling entails assessing how uncontrollable physical processes can influence the effectiveness and risk of treatment. For instance, a planned-out medical intervention could have different results based on immediate physiological responses that were not predictable upon initial screening. Therefore, healthcare professionals should always be on high alert and prepared to adjust, continuously observing the patient's condition and modifying treatment plans as a result. This type of flexibility not only helps in the control of short-term complications when they arise but also guards against long-term adverse impacts by ongoing communication with patients. Moreover, the consequences of potential complications extend beyond the immediate treatment of patients. They resound throughout the health care system, shaping clinical advice and practitioner education. As complications arise, the need to continuously update empirical knowledge is apparent, guiding better practices in diagnostic and interventional practices. The incorporation of patient-centered approaches is vital, as argued by Berger et al. (2017), to better equip protocols addressing these evolving complications. Education programs would emphasize not just the effectiveness of treatment but also risk factor recognition that leads to complications. By doing so, the healthcare community fosters a culture of continuous improvement and learning that ultimately works towards reducing complications and enhancing patient care. This emphasis on understanding and adapting to possible complications will be the framework for stronger healthcare practices in the future.

9.2.3. Spontaneous Resolution Rates

Spontaneous resolution rates are one of the central concepts in describing numerous conditions, especially in psychology and medicine. Spontaneous resolution rates is a term that describes the likelihood of a specific condition spontaneously remitting or improving without any type of intervention. In the case of certain medical diseases, it has been found that a significant percentage of patients experience spontaneous resolution.

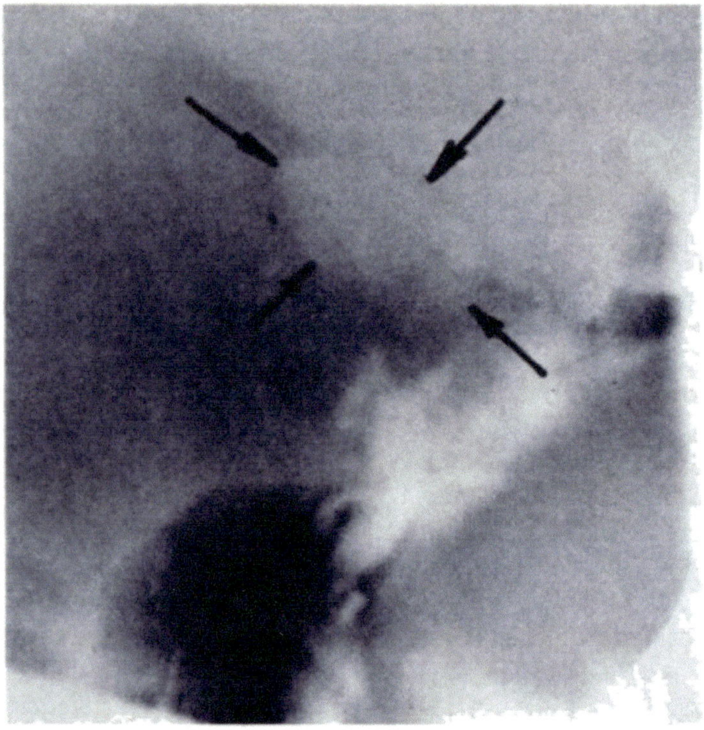

Figure 9.7. Spontaneous resolution of mediastinal pancreatic pseudocyst.

Source: https://external-content.duckduckgo.com/iu/?u=https%3A%2F%2Fjournal.chestnet.org%2Fcms%2Fattachment%2F4dd69ea8-461c-495c-9ef4-1c0c9db987b8%2Fgr2.jpg&f=1&nofb=1&ipt=76dbd8df3d47a56c8cdfc7dc5d5b1ec3ccb69e10a42f3e88db272d27a23e5052.

This process increases the stakes for monitoring patients because it has the ability to affect treatment avenues and health care budgets. Finding and analyzing these rates can lead to more effective decision-making in deciding to initiate or delay treatment, beckoning patient-centered approaches to clinical practice and optimizing overall outcomes. Furthermore, spontaneous resolution rates do not solely reside in physical illness but are equally relevant in the realm of mental illness. Research has shown that the majority of individuals with mild and moderate depression and anxiety will notice their symptoms spontaneously improve over time even without having received established treatment. This reality supports an attitude of caution regarding interventions because premature or aggressive intervention would threaten spontaneous recovery processes. By seeing these rates in mental health, clinicians can better determine patients who might benefit from supportive therapies, as a contrast to more intensive psychological or drug treatments, leading to a more nuanced treatment environment. In addition to their medical and psychological importance, spontaneous resolution rates may have potentially wider effects on social behaviors and market forces. For example, resolution of some social problems or conflicts may be possible without external intervention, indicating an internal potential for societies to autocorrect over time. This is also reflected in natural resources management, where emergence can be seen in the manner that communities develop their responses to changing conditions in water management practice and policy, as described by trends in irrigation management and conflict resolution in cases like India (Saleth, 2025). These dynamics require policies that facilitate these processes of spontaneous restoration, rather than undermining them, and strengthening the interlinkages between human behavior, resource management, and the natural environment (Figure 9.7).

9.3. Indications for Drainage

The term drainage is used by the medical field as a concept to encompass a wide array of clinical scenarios in which the drainage system is utilized to remove accumulated infection material or fluid that is needed for patient well-being. Indications for drainage could result from a myriad of etiologies that include but are not limited to the following: abscess, fluid collections, or certain trauma. Once abscesses have developed, they can be sites of localized infection that, left untreated, can become systemic. Surgical intervention with drainage aids in symptom alleviation, prevention of complications, and healing. The operation is particularly critical in the treatment of patients who carry a higher risk of sepsis, where prompt intervention can significantly enhance the outcome and restrict mortality from uncontrolled infection. The occurrence of fluid collections, i.e., those present in pleural effusions or post-operative seromas, is another primary indication for drainage. These conditions can disrupt normal physiology and lead to respiratory distress or discomfort. A big pleural effusion, for instance, can compress the lung and reduce the surface area available for gas exchange. Thoracentesis or chest tube insertion in such a case allows for the immediate drainage of excess fluid and thus normal pulmonary function and overall condition of the patients. Prompt diagnosis of such symptoms and follow-up drainage can be most crucial in avoiding longer-term complications such as pneumonia or pulmonary embolism, both of which can significantly hamper patient recovery. Furthermore, the importance of identifying and reacting to signs for drainage also extends to the field of surgical intervention. More specifically, treatment of disease involving vascular structures such as aortic aneurysms illustrates the advances in drainage techniques. With the evolution of surgical procedures have come possibilities to drain built-up fluids and in the process prevent calamitous results, such as aneurysm burst. Responsive drainage is not only successful but also proactive to reversing threats of expanding vascular diseases. As testified by the historical and ongoing developments in surgical practice, excellent drainage techniques establish a vital route towards enhancing patient outcomes and safety in a myriad of conditions, demonstrating the pivotal role of surgical innovation and leadership in this field (Bhogal et al., 2011). The necessity to regularly re-examine our tactics in the application of antibiotics and infection prevention, especially in innovative healthcare facilities, is an open issue within medical realms (Goss et al., 2000) (Figure 9.8).

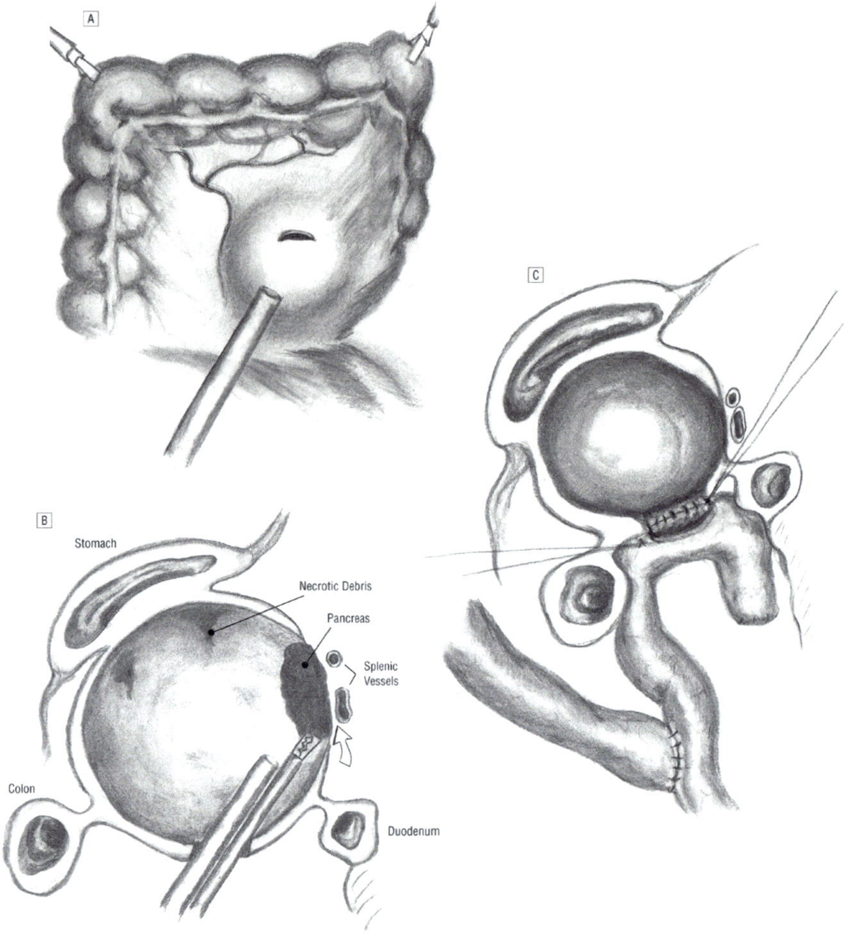

Figure 9.8. Internal drainage of giant acute pseudocysts.

Source: https://jamanetwork.com/data/journals/surg/9427/soa9040f1.png.

9.3.1. Size and Symptoms of the Pseudocyst

The size of a pseudocyst can have a profound influence on its clinical picture and management strategy. Presented most frequently as a complication of pancreatitis, pseudocysts may vary widely in size, ranging from a few centimeters to larger collections of greater than 10 centimeters. Small pseudocysts are asymptomatic and spontaneously resolve, while larger pseudocysts will cause dramatic symptoms due to their mass effect upon adjacent structures. Since the cyst will grow in size, it can compress nearby organs, which may produce abdominal pain, nausea, or vomiting. Of interest is that large cysts are more probable to develop complications of infection, perforation, or hemorrhage and therefore require close monitoring and, in most cases, treatment in order to prevent future health hazards. The symptoms of pseudocysts are nonspecific and therefore diagnosis is hindered. Patients may present with pain in the abdomen, which can mimic other diseases of the gastrointestinal tract and thus lead to diagnostic delays. The clinical picture can be further complicated by backache and early satiety. When infected or ruptured pseudocyst becomes a complication, symptoms can evolve to fever and leukocytosis. The symptomatic pseudocysts are treated clinically by observation with imaging, such as ultrasound or computed tomography, to assess the size and fluid properties and therefore lead to appropriate surgical or endoscopic treatment. Lastly, its recognition and correlation with cysts size is important in determining the correct therapy. Retrospective study findings emphasize the necessity of precise size and symptom evaluation for the management of pancreatic pseudocysts. For instance, research has shown that rates of symptomatic improvement are not significantly varied based on the presence or absence of solid debris in the fluid collection, and this seems to be consistent with an intricate relationship between features of the cyst and outcomes. In a series of patients receiving endoscopic treatment, technical success was high regardless of cyst size, although, for example, cyst contents might play a role in determining the likelihood of subsequent re-intervention (Yang et al., 2017). Further, the evidence indicates that larger pseudocysts might need more intensive treatment based on their related complications and reduced long-term resolution rates (Yang et al., 2016). Therefore, understanding the intricate interactions among size, symptoms, and outcome of treatment is of highest precedence to optimize the care of patients with pancreatic pseudocysts.

9.3.2. Presence of Infection or Complications

The development of infection or complications remains a cause of concern in the majority of medical conditions as they have a great influence on the outcomes of patients. In pancreatic illness, infection control can simply dictate the lines of recovery. Evidence has indicated that nutritional strategies, including those supplemented with fiber, play a crucial role in avoiding complications of acute pancreatitis. Notably, high prebiotic dietary intake has been linked to lower rates of pancreatic necrosis, systemic inflammatory response syndrome, and multiorgan failure. These are gains due to fibers ability to preserve intestinal homeostasis of the barrier, and thereby reduce risk for infection. A cautious focus, therefore, on dietary interventions can thus control the potential infections complicating pancreatic pathologies, demonstrating the intricate association between food and disease outcome, as noted by Ribichini et al. (2019). Complications of drug administration also are a cause of great concern, particularly in oncology drugs, as well as osteoporosis drugs. A great example is medication-related osteonecrosis of the jaw (MRONJ), which is a serious complication of antiresorptive and antiangiogenic agents that can seriously jeopardize the quality of life of patients. The multifactorial etiology of MRONJ is highlighted by the fact that there are several risk factors, including the drugs employed, types of patients, and timing of dental interventions, which must be cautiously considered. Effective prevention measures presuppose full understanding of risk factors. Coordination among dental and medical specialists will be necessary to identify preventive care that is proven to decrease the risk of developing MRONJ during treatment, in recognition of the need for a multidisciplinary approach in treating infection complication complications as described in Bedogni et al. (2018). Beyond nutritional and drug interactions, global management of complications will need to encompass a whole-patient comprehension of treatment. Underlying medical conditions, patient compliance with treatment, and the presence of available medical resources also contribute in influencing the risk for infection and complications. Patients with compromised immune systems, for instance, are at higher risk of infections, such that they need to be strictly monitored and have interventions instituted at once. Likewise, clear communication between medical practitioners, particularly for patient status changes and interventions, contributes significantly towards preventive care against future complications. Through fostering a culture of teamwork and openness, infection management and complications can be enhanced, with overall improved patient outcomes and quality of life. Such a holistic approach is imperative to the administration of the nuances that are present when infection and complications occur in the many healthcare environments (Figure 9.9).

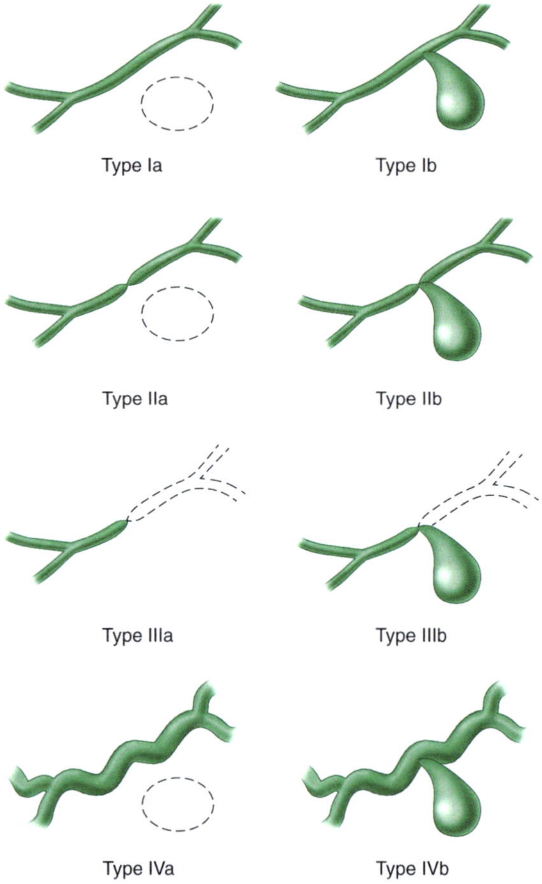

Figure 9.9. Pseudocysts and other complications of pancreatitis.

Source: https://storage.googleapis.com/dl.dentistrykey.com/clinical/PseudocystsandOtherComplicationsofPancreatitis/3_3s20B9780323402323000935.jpg.

9.3.3. Impact on Surrounding Organs

The impact on surrounding organs in the case of some diseases can be enormous and widespread, with a tendency to create cascades of effects on overall health and well-being. For instance, diseases that attack the genital areas in a specific way usually have consequences that transfer from local manifestations. The consequence can be realized not only in physical terms, through pain or disability, but also psychologically, altering an individual's attitude towards sex health and self-concept. This complexity underscores the inherent interconnectedness of body systems: an impairment in one area, such as the genitalia, may very well lead to complications relating to several other organs. The psychological impacts that ensue from these disorders have a tendency to cause a cycle of decline wherein physical and mental well-being are affected (Albu et al., 2015). Besides that, the impact on surrounding organs can equally be justified in terms of occupational health, that is, in facilities like crushing plants. The harmful condition that the workers in these industries expose themselves to most times results in occupational diseases that not only compromise respiratory function but equally weaken the working of other organs in the body. For instance, particulates and dust exposure lead to chronic respiratory diseases, which in turn reduce the oxygenation of principal organs, affecting cardiovascular and neurological functions. The environmental degradation resulting from these industries aggravates such health conditions, thereby rendering it a complex problem that not only impacts the labor force but also general community health. The necessity of safer techniques and the importance of regulatory processes cannot be overestimated in dealing with such connected health conditions (Bem et al., 2025). Treatment and prevention in response to the impact of localized diseases on nearby organs demand an integrative approach. The awareness of how localized conditions in one part of the body can lead to complications elsewhere underscores the importance of systemic health care. For example, treatment protocols must not only correct the presenting symptoms but also consider potential ramifications of such on kidneys, liver, or other organs, which can get stressed as a function of systemic response to localized pathology. Secondly, the psychological implications of such medical diseases have to be included in healthcare strategies, so that mental health would be considered a component of physical health. Overall, multidisciplinary treatment technologies incorporating medical, psychological, and environmental aspects play an important role in mitigating the extensive impacts on neighboring organs and in preserving general well-being (Albu et al., 2015).

9.4. Endoscopic Approaches to Drainage

The advancement of endoscopic procedures for drainage is an advancement of the minimally invasive surgical field. The procedures not only enhance the precision of drainage therapy but also reduce the extent of trauma compared to that of conventional surgical techniques. Clinicians can effect good treatment of abscesses, obstruction of the bile ducts, and pancreatic fluid collections through less invasive approaches and small incisions by utilizing endoscopic procedures.

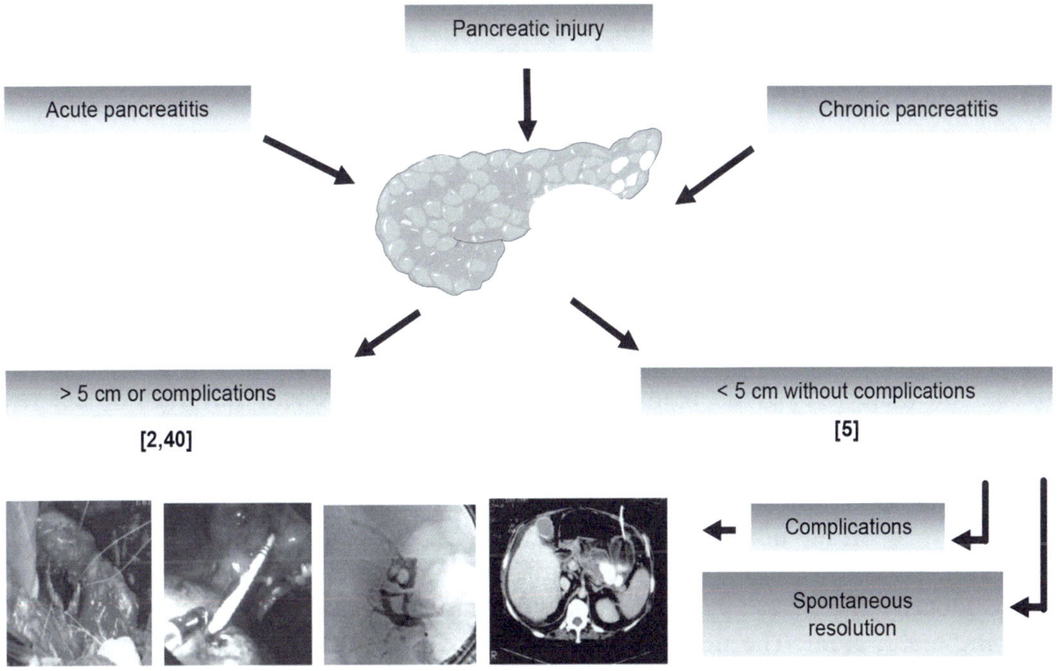

Figure 9.10. Comparison of surgical and percutaneous treatment modalities.

Source: https://pmc.ncbi.nlm.nih.gov/articles/PMC2020756/.

This move towards less invasive procedures is in line with the growing emphasis on patient safety and recovery time, allowing for faster rehabilitation and shorter inpatient stays. Additionally, as outlined in Advances in Minimally Invasive Surgery, these endoscopic procedures have a firm foundation in procedure guidelines and illustrations to back them and are therefore available to surgeons of any level of experience (Ayme et al., 2022). The success of endoscopic drainage techniques is also highly reliant on optimal patient selection and identification of suitable anatomical targets. Detailed understanding of the pathology of the underlying disease is equally crucial;

for instance, in the treatment of pancreatic pseudocysts, whether endoscopic drainage would be done or not would depend on such factors as size, location, and symptomatology. Further, precise imaging techniques, like ultrasound and computed tomography, are important for guiding the endoscopic process in terms of safety and effectiveness. Further development of such techniques with newer technologies and methodologies will enhance the effectiveness of endoscopic drainage further. It is important that surgical training keeps pace with such developments, prioritizing the place of Entrustable Professional Activities (EPAs) in maintaining residents as competent in such novel techniques (Amare, 2023). As numerous advantages are associated with endoscopic drainage procedures, complications and learning curve are yet concerns for practitioners. Complications like perforation or bleeding can occur, and this calls for a thorough knowledge of risks associated and management options. Additionally, the application of endoscopic drainage methods necessitates a technical skills base, which can be developed through formal residency training. By developing an outline of EPAs for endoscopy procedures, residency programs are able to prepare residents adequately to practice on their own, with both technical skill and the essential decision-making power required in complex surgical cases. Hence, an emphasis on continuous evaluation and enhancement of residency training programs is of utmost importance since it mirrors the quality of surgical care that patients receive (Amare, 2023) (Figure 9.10).

9.4.1. Techniques Used in Endoscopic Drainage

Endoscopic drainage techniques have transformed the management of gastrointestinal disease, allowing less invasive alternatives to standard surgery. EUS-guided cystogastrostomy is one such technique employed for drainage of pancreatic walled-off necrosis. The technique involves endoscopic ultrasound visualization of the collection of necrotic debris followed by puncture and stenting to establish drainage into the stomach. The minimally invasive nature of this procedure not only reduces patient morbidity but also lengthens recovery periods compared to open surgery. The effectiveness of such methods stems from a multidisciplinary approach, that harmonizes the skill of surgeons and endoscopists, the key qualification being to deliver treatment based on personalized patient requirements, as evidenced by the growing use of endoscopic drainage in practice (Bahdi et al., 2024). Yet another milestone in endoscopic drainage is the EUS-guided gastrojejunostomy, a solution to gastric outlet obstruction. The intervention allows for the creation of a bypass between the stomach and jejunum without requiring major surgery. It begins with an endoscopic ultrasound to identify the most appropriate site for anastomosis, followed by the placement of a lumen-apposing metal stent. The noninferiority of the technique compared to traditional surgical methods proves the worth of consistent innovation in minimally invasive procedures. It also underscores the importance of ongoing clinical follow-ups to interpret the long-term outcomes and effectiveness of these techniques across different patient populations (Bahdi et al., 2024). These results improve the dynamic field of endoscopic interventions, which is indicative of moving towards more patient-centered care. Expansion of endoscopic drainage techniques needs vigorous interdisciplinary collaboration in order to develop and refine therapy protocols. With the popularity of endoscopic sleeve gastroplasty as a procedure to treat obesity, it is evident that the field is rapidly changing with improvements in technology and procedures. These techniques are not only aimed at minimizing dislodge to the patient's physiology but also at facilitating quicker recovery and fewer complications with conventional surgeries. Secondly, the need for intensive studies aimed at ascertaining the effectiveness of these endoscopic surgeries is pivotal, as emphasized in expert discussion on minimally invasive procedures. With ongoing progress in endoscopic techniques, there is growing interest in patient choice as well as the associated risks, ultimately resulting in individualized treatment plans that optimize overall patient satisfaction and outcomes (Figure 9.11).

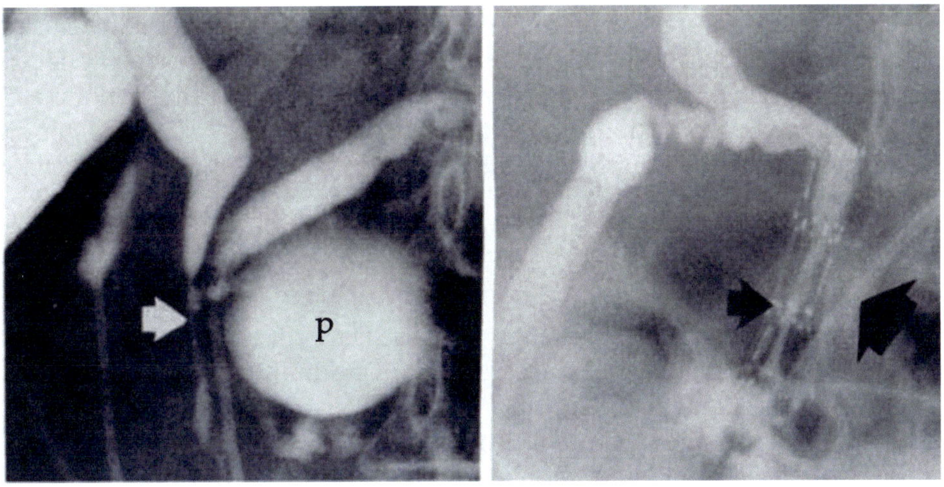

Figure 9.11. Endoscopic drainage of pseudocyst.

Source: https://external-content.duckduckgo.com/iu/?u=https%3A%2F%2Fwww.researchgate.net%2Fprofile%2FAbraham-Dachman%2Fpublication%2F21301782%2Ffigure%2Ffig10%2FAS%3A668277986562057%401536341296603%2FEndoscopic-drainage-of-pseudocyst-ERCP-of-47-year-old-woman-referred-for-treatment-of.jpg&f=1&nofb=1&ipt=928d66864818b0bc9f108ea7669dc0761207310e83973e55d181d39a7175fb38.

9.4.2. Advantages of Endoscopic Methods

Endoscopic procedures have changed the landscape of diagnostic and treatment interventions in medicine, offering several advantages compared to traditional surgical techniques. For instance, these minimally invasive procedures have reduced patient morbidity, shorten recovery time, and cause less postoperative pain. Compared to open techniques with large incisions, endoscopic procedures entail small incisions or natural openings, thus minimizing scarring and allowing rapid recovery. Besides, the precision in endoscopic procedures allows for accurate delivery of interventions, minimizing damage to neighboring tissues. As such, endoscopic procedures not only ensure greater patient comfort but also result in lower hospitalization costs and a shorter return to normal living, emphasizing their beneficial impact on healthcare efficacy. The technological advancements in endoscopic procedures have immensely contributed to diagnostic effectiveness, particularly with the diagnosis of gastrointestinal disease. Techniques such as Capsule Endoscopy (CE) are instances of such advancement, allowing visualization of the small intestine, which is least accessible with routine endoscopy. CE is confounded by challenges such as localization of pathologies, yet studies continue to further refine the process and provide more credible resultant information. Accordingly, important technologies targeting signal strength and localization precision are being developed in order to efficiently deal with these challenges, thereby promoting the overall efficacy of CE. As has been noted in available literature, the integration of sophisticated localization systems is core to transforming the diagnostic potential of wireless capsule endoscopy, which is dynamic at a very rapid rate (Ashour et al., 2017). Apart from diagnostics, endoscopic methods also offer new therapies, especially in the management of obesity. Methods like argon plasma coagulation have been promising in controlling complications following gastric bypass surgeries, such as dilation of anastomosis. Recent studies suggest that the procedure can effectively narrow the gastrojejunal anastomosis to allow further weight loss in obese patients who experienced relapse (Cantanhede et al., 2024). The results indicate that over 50% of regained excess body weight can be eliminated after treatment, which verifies the safety and effectiveness of this endoscopic treatment. These applications are indicative of the flexibility of endoscopic procedures, which are not only beneficial for diagnosis but also useful for treating various conditions, thus highlighting their key role in today's medical practice.

9.4.3. Limitations and Potential Complications

This exploration of limitations and potential complications is key in any empirical research, especially in maternal wellbeing and pregnancy risk assessments. One limitation comes from the utilization of historical and demographic data, which may not capture the full gamut of variables affecting pregnancy. For instance, even if ensemble learning techniques applied in childbearing potential prediction employ salient variables such as maternal age and history of previous pregnancy, other relevant variables like mental health and socio-economic status are often under-represented or altogether absent, resulting in biased predictions. Besides, the complex interaction between such variables is often out of exact modeling, thus hard to draw generalizable conclusions applicable across broad populations. These limitations not only impact the validity of the results but also diminish the potential of coming up with adequate interventions that could potentially significantly improve maternal and infant health outcomes since the demand for continuous improvement in the methodologies adopted in such analyses is very evident (Aziz et al., 2024). Furthermore, combining the application of ensemble learning methods, though very promising due to its potential of furthering predictive power, has its own set of obstacles. Every ensemble method poses challenges to interpretability and computational complexity. For example, while Ensemble Bagging Trees had a remarkable accuracy of 85.6%, the inability of ensemble methods to be inscrutable poses a challenge to healthcare workers to understand the underlying prediction mechanisms. This constraint can lead to decision-making mistrust, particularly where medical professionals require well-established reasoning for risk assessment to guide clinical decisions. Misinterpretation or miscommunication of results is also a risk that renders the clinical usefulness of such cutting-edge methods more difficult. Thus, developing such models into actionable use in actual practice requires balancing predictive precision with clear interpretative frameworks (Aziz et al., 2024). Last but not least, the multi-dimensionality of healthcare systems accentuates also the need for extensive outcomes assessments to capture the quality and cost-effectiveness of such new technologies. Limitations in data collection can undermine the ability to determine complete effects and overall impacts of multi-dimension treatment strategies. If certain health systems fail to incorporate or work effectively with fresh technology, this would potentially cause discrepancies that conceal the valuable insights based on ensemble learning models. This requirement emphasizes the importance of careful evaluations of healthcare technologies that are not just aimed at making valid predictions but also at the broader implications regarding the treatment of patients and resource allocation. The incorporation of thorough assessments could illuminate pathways for improving both efficacy and efficiency in healthcare delivery, reinforcing the message that comprehensive strategies address the limitations inherent in traditional approaches.

9.5. Surgical Approaches to Drainage

The advancement in surgical technique has played a core role in enhancing patient results with regard to drainage surgeries. Traditionally, open operation was conventional in cases of drainage need, such as abscesses or fluid collection. With the advent of minimally invasive techniques, surgical maneuvers have had to shift, and recovery time has been reduced along with complication rates. This is one component of a broader movement in surgery since patient-centered care brings about the least invasive methods for optimal results. With conditions like aortic aneurysms, in which the need for surgery is most critical, there is growing concern about risk in both minimally invasive and open surgery. As the literature has highlighted, both techniques are not only designed to correct but also to optimize the control of complications and thus reduce morbidity related to disorders such as thoracic and abdominal aortic aneurysms (Bhogal et al., 2011).

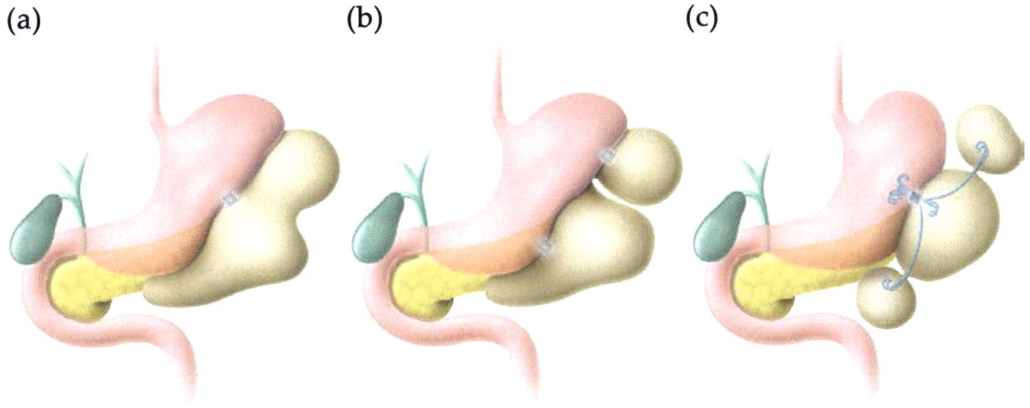

Figure 9.12. Pancreatic pseudocyst drainage.

Source: https://external-content.duckduckgo.com/iu/?u=https%3A%2F%2Fonlinelibrary.wiley.com%2Fcms%2Fasset%2F34654bd7-6eb1-49dd-b653-6e2a25ecfe2f%2Fjhbp146-fig-0005-m.jpg&f=1&nofb=1&ipt=009ed5b3e6ca946a50c61ea453e7812ba19d70c4917e0dc10cb3ded8c07ccca3.

The role of evidence-based practice in surgical management, particularly drainage methodologies, cannot be overestimated. Surgical practice guidelines such as those by the Italian Society of Colorectal Surgery aim to direct practitioners towards delivering the optimal care for their patients. Surgical practice guidelines condense a vast amount of clinical experience and research into decision-making guidelines for diverticular disease management, for example, such as the importance of urgent drainage procedure in complicated cases. By adhering to evidence-based practice guidelines, surgeons can easily modify treatment approaches to the specific circumstances of the patient, thus ensuring maximum overall treatment success. Such vigilance to standardized treatment also ensures that practitioners remain competent at identifying the necessity for surgical drainage and in choosing the best strategies for every case, again ensuring optimal positive patient outcomes (Annibale et al., 2015). Also, the role of technology and continuing education to reshape surgical practice in drainage is crucial. With advancement in techniques and technology, training in surgery must evolve to encompass such innovations so that the professionals are kept abreast with best practices. For instance, advances in imaging devices make precise localization of fluid collections possible, which is critical to planning drainage procedures. Additionally, the advent of robot-assisted technology in the context of minimally invasive surgery is representative of the direction towards enhanced surgeon capabilities and precision in drainage interventions. As the aspect of surgery continues to advance and adapt from experience, the necessity for the merging of technical proficiency and evidence-based medicine is apparent. Ultimately, this innovation represents a commitment towards enhancing patient safety and therapeutic outcomes in various domains of surgery, such as drainage interventions (Figure 9.12).

9.5.1. Types of Surgical Procedures Available

Surgical procedures may be generally categorized into various types based on their nature and purpose. A general categorization is into emergency and elective surgery. Elective surgery is planned ahead and typically involves non-life-threatening conditions, such as cosmetic procedures or joint replacements. Emergency surgery is not planned and is performed for the repair of life-threatening disorders, such as appendicitis or trauma. This differentiation is significant for both patients and healthcare workers, as it determines the urgency and logistical implications of surgical interventions. Understanding these categories enables patients to make informed decisions about their course of care and take into consideration the urgency and risk of surgery. Invasive vs. minimally invasive procedures is another classification of relevance. The traditional invasive procedures involved larger cuts and greater trauma to the body tissues, typically resulting in longer recovery times. In contrast, minimally invasive procedures use advanced techniques such as endoscopy or laparoscopic surgery, with minimal cuts and less interference with tissue. This second approach is likely to involve faster recovery, fewer pains, and shorter hospital stays, as an ideal solution for most patients. For instance, patients who receive procedures like laparoscopic cholecystectomy are likely to experience fewer complications and quicker rehabilitation than open surgery patients. As surgical technology improves, the trend clearly is shifting towards minimally invasive procedures, illustrating a broader trend in the surgical community towards better patient outcomes and satisfaction. Certain types of surgical procedures also illustrate the range of surgical practice. Orthognathic surgery, which corrects deformities of the jaw, is an excellent illustration of a specialty surgical process. Studies have shown that patients with craniofacial anomalies who receive orthognathic surgery experience individual challenges in treatment, such as prolonged hospital stays and higher complication rates, such as infections (Allareddy et al., 2018). These findings highlight the necessity for individualized surgical care to address individual patients' needs, especially in complex cases. Additionally, other surgeries such as orthopedic surgery, for example, knee arthroscopy, and cardiovascular procedures, i.e., angioplasty, emphasize how many different specialties demand bespoke techniques and recovery strategies. Overall, the range of surgeries available emphasizes the specialists and flexibility needed in modern medicine to accommodate the diverse needs of the client base (Allareddy et al., 2018).

9.5.2. Indications for Surgical Intervention

Surgical intervention typically enters the picture when conservative therapy fails to manage complicated medical diseases. One of the most important factors in surgical planning is determining the course and severity of the disease, particularly in diseases such as multidrug-resistant pulmonary tuberculosis. Results indicate that the addition of surgical procedures enhances the therapeutic response of patients who are not responsive to anti-tuberculosis chemotherapy. In studies, it was noticed that in patients who were being suggested for surgery, an early surgical phase would contribute immensely to overall effectiveness, with a potential curative rate of 60.6% in surgically treated patients, in comparison to traditional methods alone, which had high treatment failure rates (Ivashchenko et al., 2018). Consequently, the indications for surgery will thus need to consider both the clinical presentation of the disease and the patient's own treatment history. Acute appendicitis during pregnancy is a tragic demonstration of the overriding necessity of surgery in acute illness. While surgery in pregnancy is risky by nature, appendicitis is one of the most frequent non-obstetric surgical emergencies needing urgent treatment. Prompt surgical intervention is generally considered the gold standard, especially to prevent complications that may arise from a delayed treatment. Nevertheless, increasing evidence on managing uncomplicated appendicitis stresses the possibility of non-surgical methods, including antibiotic treatment, in lowering risks of surgical complications (Ajjarapu & Moreira, 2020). This specific example draws notice to the reality that, while surgery will be required in some cases, careful attention can bring other solutions into the picture which continue to achieve patient protection and clinical success. Beyond these examples, the bigger picture of surgical intervention looms large over much of medicine with many conditions needing surgical consideration. For instance, surgery is applied for malignancy, trauma, and other acute diagnoses, highlighting the importance of evidence-based surgical decision-making. With ongoing development in healthcare, there is still a requirement for precise analyses aimed at establishing which patients will benefit most from surgery. These are disease severity, stability of the patient, and potential operating risks and, as such, must be weighed carefully against results of surgery, affirming the importance of individualized care in the patient. As in both instances of pulmonary tuberculosis and appendicitis, properly considered indication for operating can have a significant impact on the overall prognosis and quality of life of the patient (Figure 9.13).

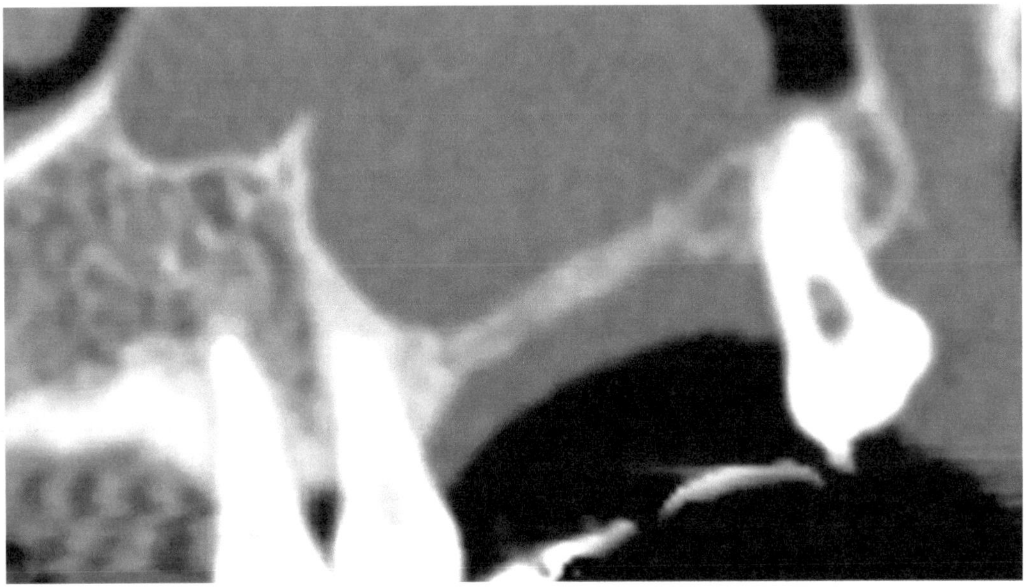

Figure 9.13. Surgical removal of pseudocysts in sinus floor augmentation.

Source: https://img.osteocom.me/img/5c2f854938b00c08b4c3c81b.

9.5.3. Risks and Benefits of Surgical Approaches

The trade-off between the risks and benefits within surgical procedures remains the main issue in modern medicine. Surgical operations, whether elective or emergent, have built-in risks such as infection, anesthesia-related complications, and prolonged recovery times. The threat of complications is an indicator of the necessity for healthcare practitioners to conduct thorough preoperative tests and consultations with patients. By examining individual health profiles, operating room teams will know how to identify patients who are most likely to have increased risks. This quantitative patient selection technique not only enhances safety but also benefits the decision-making process about surgical appropriateness since patients are ready to carefully consider their options. Therefore, even though surgical risks are extreme, they are an area of concentration for improvement in surgical training and patient care protocols. Surgical risks are generally outweighed by advantages when indicated properly. Successful surgeries can lead to improved quality of life, pain relief from debilitating symptoms, and healthier overall results. For instance, surgeries such as tumor excisions or joint replacements can greatly enhance patient mobility and comfort levels, allowing patients to resume normal activities. Furthermore, with advances in minimally invasive surgical techniques, recovery times and hospital stays have been reduced, eliminating some of the risks traditionally associated with surgical methods. However, claimed benefits must be grounded in robust statistical analysis to warrant assertions of efficacy. Economic research, such as that covered in healthcare rationing cases, can play a significant role in assessing the cost-effectiveness of procedures and distributing resources to procedures that create notable patient value (Frakes et al., 2017). For cesarean sections, benefits associated with direct skin-to-skin contact (SSC) with newborns after surgery illustrate the complexity in surgical risks and benefits. Research indicates that while cesarean sections are more likely to limit SSC access than are natural births, there are significant emotional and physiological benefits for early mother-child contact. Obstetric nurses are very supportive of SSC practices in accordance with the evidence that early contact facilitates bonding and increases successful breastfeeding rates. Yet, there are barriers to the routine use of SSC following cesarean procedures, which make care a necessary lacuna in practice and a need for obstetric care reforms. Surmounting such barriers optimizes surgical outcomes and strengthens the foundation of family-centered care within high-stakes medical environments (Balatero, 2018).

9.6. Comparison of Endoscopic and Surgical Approaches

The endoscopic versus surgical approach to medical interventions is a mature fulfillment of effectiveness, invasiveness, and patient outcomes. Endoscopic interventions are likely to offer minimally invasive interventions, which in turn are likely to result in shorter recovery periods and lower rates of complications. This can be exemplified by the use of chronic rhinosinusitis, where balloon catheter dilation (BCD) proves to be effective with minimal trauma to surrounding tissues. This is particularly useful to patients who may not tolerate the risks of more intensive surgical treatment. Furthermore, the use of stents, such as the Relieva Stratus™ MicroFlow spacer, illustrates advancements in the maintenance of sinus patency following endoscopic treatment. However, while BCD has beneficial effects, the use of the same adjunctively has so far failed to achieve significant improvements in the majority of cases, showing some limitations which require careful planning during intervention (Minni et al., 2018). On the other hand, conventional open surgical techniques, particularly for diseases like hiatal hernias, allow direct observation and manipulation of anatomical structures. Notably, laparoscopic methods permit proper repair of defects with proper assessment of the esophageal hiatus. Evidence shows that hiatal surface area measurement (HSA) with the aid of sophisticated imaging devices such as MDCT is capable of guiding surgical procedures appropriately. This is a quantitative method that offers a preoperative platform that may be absent in endoscopic methods because traditional imaging does not provide proper determination of the complexity of defects. Moreover, intraoperative outcomes obtained through laparoscopic methods can validate preoperative measurements and enhance outcomes through individually tailored surgical interventions (Boru et al., 2017). Finally, choosing between surgical and endoscopic methods relies on the interaction between the nature of the medical condition, patient characteristics, and the risks of each procedure. Endoscopic techniques typically constitute the first line of management for less invasive treatment with an emphasis on preserving tissue integrity. For more complex issues, however, surgery may become the only option in a bid to achieve optimal outcomes, particularly in refractory conditions. The evolving context of both approaches highlights the requirement for interdisciplinary practice, considering not only short-term patient outcomes but also longer-term effects such as symptom management and quality of life. Practitioners therefore must reconcile the advantages and disadvantages of each approach in order to formulate the optimal treatment plan tailored to individual patient needs and circumstances (Figure 9.14).

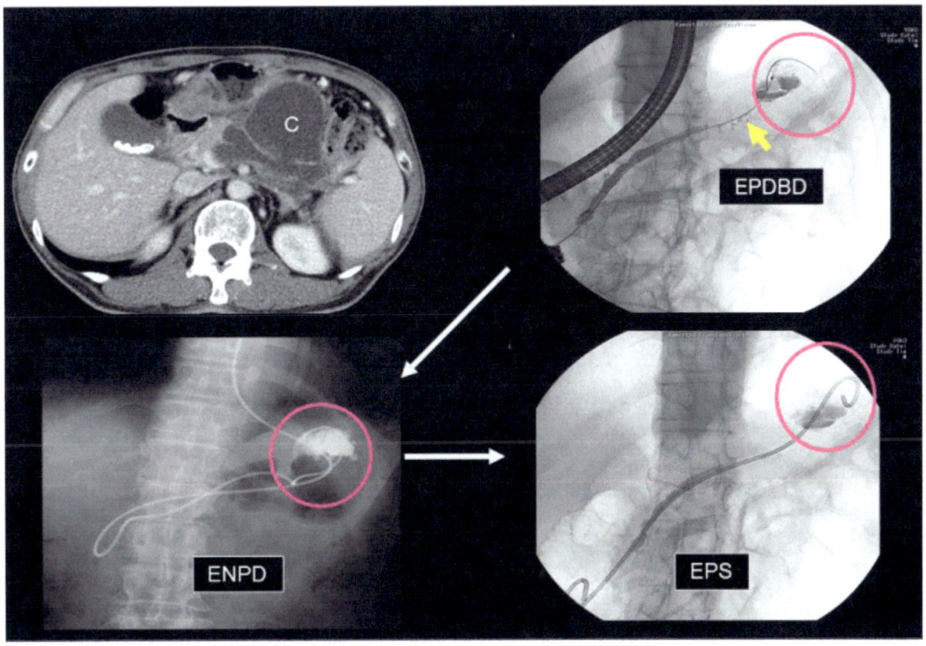

Figure 9.14. Usefulness and safety of endoscopic pancreatic duct balloon dilation.

Source: https://www.oatext.com/img/LPS-1-109-g007.gif.

9.6.1. Efficacy of Each Method

The power of different methods for pitch-class distribution analysis of music offers broad implications for tonal association and its role in perception. Recent work using the Discrete Fourier Transform (DFT) has emphasized the salience of certain components, 5, 3, and 2, that simplify the complexity of tonal analysis to an understandable two- or three-dimensional phase space. This relief is not only a technical convenience; it is also more enlightening about tonal perception, as it filters distributional data in a way that is consonant with auditory processing. In addition, DFT examination of probe-tone distributions reveals a subdominant bias shaped by temporal characteristics of behavioral paradigms, thereby validating that tonal hearing is context-specific.

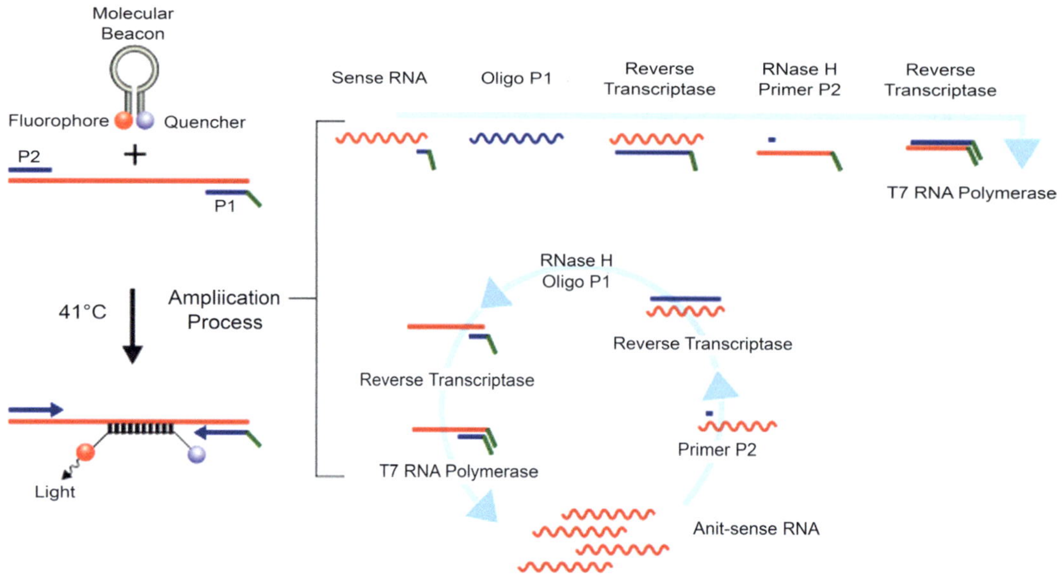

Figure 9.15. Quantitative nucleic acid sequence-based amplification (QT-NASBA).

Source: https://external-content.duckduckgo.com/iu/?u=http%3A%2F%2Fwww.premierbiosoft.com%2Fimages%2Ftech_images%2Fnasba_technology.jpg&f=1&nofb=1&ipt=437dc5c9226d3d1c213726e06f0426e4da0e8623707ec3d9b0d67d9e91a65b1b.

These findings reveal that the method's capacity to explain tonal relations is particularly powerful in natural listening contexts, resulting in a robust theoretical model of musical keys (Yust., 2017). Clinical epidemiology, quantitative molecular techniques (QMMs) achieve varying success in quantifying pathogen density, particularly in diagnosing diseases such as malaria caused by Plasmodium falciparum. Techniques such as quantitative real-time polymerase chain reaction (q-PCR) and quantitative nucleic acid sequence-based amplification (QT-NASBA) play a significant role in this direction. But traditional statistical calibration procedures are prone to provide inaccurate estimates of pathogen density as they do not reconcile between-assay variability. In contrast, a Bayesian mixed model solution represents a significant advancement since it allows for reconciliation of measurement variation across experiments and enhanced reliability of diagnostic sensitivity. This methodological advancement reveals the pressing need for robust statistical frameworks that can capture the complexities of QMMs and make valid epidemiological inferences (Gelman et al., 2015). This comparative analysis of these two methods—musical pitch-class analysis and pathogen density estimation—has broader implications for their respective fields. While the DFT is strong at elucidating tone structures and facilitating a rich image of music perception, Bayesian mixed models revolution clinical diagnostics by offering more precise data about pathogen distribution.

Each technique's potency stems not only from the used methodology but also from the particular applications in the given context and natural complexities of the data. Identifying the strength and weakness of every method, researchers can better transcend the complexity of both musical analysis and clinical diagnosis. Ultimately, this implicit knowledge regarding the efficacy of the method builds music theory and epidemiological studies as well, yielding a deeper understanding and improved practice in domains (Gelman et al., 2015; Yust., 2017) (Figure 9.15).

9.6.2. Recovery Times and Patient Outcomes

Recovery length and patient outcomes are principal signs in healthcare treatment evaluation, particularly in surgical treatment. The recovery length has the potential to have a significant influence on a patient's overall stay and future well-being. Emerging innovation in digital health interventions (DHIs) for remote postoperative monitoring has emerged as an impending catalyst for improving recovery outcomes. These technologies enable ongoing patient engagement and timely feedback, and they can shorten the recovery time by treating complications early and lowering readmission rates. While the potential exists, nonetheless, systematic review has shown that the majority of DHIs are still in nascent innovation phases and grapple with large-scale implementation and usually have little strong evidence for their effectiveness in lowering recovery times and improving patient outcomes (Bouamrane et al., 2023). Thus, while these digital innovations hold promising potential for enhancing patient care, further balanced evaluation in real-world settings is needed to inform best practice. Moreover, the intersection of recovery time and mental health serves to highlight the multidimensional nature of patient outcomes. Surgical patients are typically vulnerable to mental health issues such as depression and anxiety, which prolong recovery and hinder optimal outcomes. Evidence has shown that effective mental health treatment is able to improve overall recovery outcomes, so that treatment can result in improved mental health, reduced impairment in social and occupational functioning, and even increased employment rates among patients (Krekel et al., 2024). In so doing, integrating mental health care into postoperative care pathways could build an integrated model of recovery that facilitates both physical recovery and emotional resilience. Therefore, the understanding of recovery processes and mental health interactions is important for health care practitioners to optimize patient outcomes. With changing health care systems, the emphasis on maximizing recovery times alongside patient outcomes highlights the significance of coordinated models of care. These coordinated care models must involve not only medical and surgical aspects but also psychological management as well as rehabilitation services in an attempt to meet the holistic needs of the patients. The fusion of data-driven interventions and patient-centered care plans has the potential to increase recovery times by considerable margins. By tailoring interventions to individual patient profiles and needs, providers can facilitate accelerated recoveries and higher satisfaction with care received. Blending these innovative approaches is poised to lead to revolutionary improvements in postoperative care, opening the door to a paradigm shift towards ever-more patient-focused healthcare models driven by maximizing good outcomes. Thus, attention to recovery periods and patient results from an interdisciplinary approach has the potential to propel healthcare effectiveness and quality forward.

9.6.3. Cost-Effectiveness and Resource Utilization

The cost-effectiveness analysis in the medical context is paramount, particularly in the medical interventions where the usage of resources is of prime importance. The application of data mining models in the evaluation of alternative therapies for acute myocardial infarction is crucial in identifying the effect of the different treatment modalities on patient outcomes as well as concomitant healthcare spending. By leveraging insurance claim data for administrative purposes, researchers are able to build models that predict resource consumption for procedures such as thrombolytic therapy, percutaneous coronary intervention, and coronary artery bypass grafting. This new approach not only enhances the understanding of treatment efficacy but also alerts decision-makers about the economic viability of each procedure. These analyses demonstrate that by optimizing treatment strategies based on real-world data, healthcare systems can improve clinical performance and cost containment, necessitating continuous improvement in data mining methods in health economics (Ramos, 2011). In addition to controlling myocardial infarction, the shift of acute bacterial skin and skin structure infection (ABSSSI) treatment from the inpatient to the outpatient setting is another dimension of cost-effectiveness and utilization of resources. The introduction of oritavancin as a single-dose antibiotic marks the potential for huge cost savings and healthcare burden reduction. A matched cohort study in which oritavancin was given to patients compared with an evidence-based multi-dose regimen revealed that the former not only was able to keep up with clinical effectiveness but also was characterized by strong economic advantages. Specifically, patient per-capita costs were substantial at $2319, and days of therapy needed were markedly reduced. This disparity puts into sharp relief the fundamental necessity of comparing new interventions with existing benchmarks to optimize the use of health care resources, in terms of achieving maximum value at minimal cost (Galli et al., 2017). The experiences in both case studies emphasize the importance of incorporating cost-effectiveness analysis in health care practice and policy. Through considering resource usage and treatment outcomes across a variety of clinical situations, stakeholders are able to make sound decisions that balance both quality of care and cost. The consideration of the interaction between treatment methods and their cost implications enables healthcare workers to project resource requirements while maintaining standards of patient care. These analyses eventually lead to a more sustainable healthcare system, where planning resource usage can result in better health outcomes. With advancing medicine, the utilization of advanced analytical techniques and cost-effectiveness models will be paramount for coping with the complexities of modern medical practice (Ramos, 2011; Galli et al., 2017).

A CLOSER LOOK

DIAGNOSTIC DILEMMA WITH PANCREATIC PSEUDOCYSTS

Pancreatic pseudocysts can be a significant diagnostic dilemma, especially when they are cystic neoplasms or other pancreatic masses. Generally occurring as a complication of acute or chronic pancreatitis, pseudocysts are fluid accumulations wrapped in a fibrous and granulation tissue capsule but not epithelialized. The challenge is separating them from cystic neoplasms, such as mucinous cystic neoplasms (MCNs), intraductal papillary mucinous neoplasms (IPMNs), or even solid pseudopapillary tumors—since all can have a cystic appearance on imaging. Pseudocysts are usually homogeneous in nature and may have a background of pancreatitis, though this is not always evident or recorded, especially in subclinical disease or in patients with nonspecific symptoms. Imaging studies such as CT and MRI may be able to identify the presence of a cystic lesion but are unable to distinguish between pseudocysts and neoplastic cysts. Endoscopic ultrasonography (EUS) with fine-needle aspiration (FNA) may assist in establishing the diagnosis by analyzing cyst fluid for amylase, carcinoembryonic antigen (CEA), and cytology. High amylase and low CEA levels are suggestive of a pseudocyst, while high CEA levels may be suggestive of a mucinous neoplasm. However, overlap in biochemical profile is still possible, and false negatives or positives may be achieved. Misdiagnosis of a neoplasm as a pseudocyst can lead to unnecessary resection surgery, while missed diagnosis of a malignant cyst can delay treatment. Therefore, an absolute diagnostic process integrating clinical history, imaging, fluid analysis, and multidisciplinary assessment is required to accurately discriminate pseudocysts from other pancreatic cystic lesions and guide appropriate management (Bundock, 2015) (Figure 9.16).

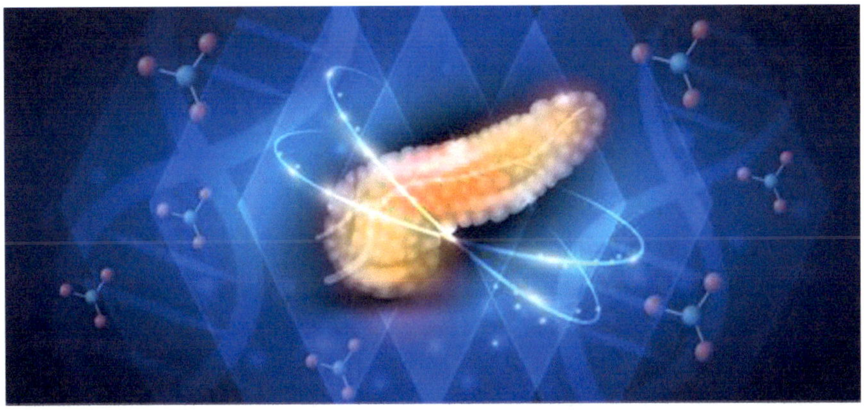

Source: https://external-content.duckduckgo.com/iu/?u=https%3A%2F%2Ftse1.mm.bing.net%2Fth%3Fid%3DOIP.vxD-4wfa1imtlFAOo8rYTQHaDZ%26cb%3Diwp2%26pid%3DApi&f=1&ipt=b150dc63d89c143246797d8d73a840ce1be4d5ddf905f8d3fe30f1f3e1a534b7.

SUMMARY

Every scholarly study is a point of decisive intersection where key points meet, projecting the themes addressed in the essay. To analyze this, the intricacies of internet privacy and information ownership have been represented in various theoretical foundations and case studies. The exploration of platforms like Facebook and the controversial Beacon ad feature are exemplary representation of the intricate issues that users encounter pertaining to their online information. This case not only recognizes concern by the user with commercial exploitation but also recognizes broader implications for privacy rights in the context of emerging technology. Thematic analysis of the response from the users sheds light on the interdependent dynamics that govern control and trust, affirming the argument that privacy remains a concern in a more globalized world, as argued by Cole et al. (2009). When examining the consequences of vagueness in legal theory, the outcomes can have a significant influence on future arguments concerning the philosophy of law. A close examination of how vagueness operates in legal contexts depicts a complex relationship between uncertainty and interpretation. Issues of legal indeterminacy and discretion become dominant themes that regulate judicial practice. These arguments illustrate a broader respect for the manner in which linguistic vagueness is embedded in the fabric of legal language, defying traditional understandings of the determinacy and clarity of law. Through such explicit connections, one can conclude that vagueness research not only illuminates legal interpretation but also addresses broader philosophical concerns, as cited by Silk (2019). Lastly, the convergence of insights gathered from these dialogues generates a deeper appreciation of online privacy and legal uncertainty. Where technology, personal data, and jurisprudence intersect, a cogent narrative is formed to illustrate that people will need protection in cyberspace and why there must be ongoing debate about it. Besides, knowledge of the implications of vagueness contributes meaningfully to legal discourse, enriching deeper understanding of how language affects law's meaning. Through these findings, researchers, policymakers, and technologists are forced into vigilance and anticipation of challenges inherent in the digital age and in law, thereby creating entry points for thoughtful discussion that propels both disciplines into the future.

The debate regarding the effectiveness of educational workshops is recognized to emphasize the important role guided instruction may have in improving student performance at the university level. That is, students tend to struggle with participating in higher-order thinking processes like evaluation and synthesis, which are essential for achieving success in advanced writing tasks. Studies indicated that the individuals who participated in a workshop for encouraging questioning and critical thinking not only gained a greater understanding of these ideas but also improved academically. It allowed students to select topics that were linked to their interests, and as this permitted them to create a personal interest in what they were doing, it can play a positive role in encouraging motivation and high levels of involvement in challenging activities (Henri et al., 2015). Therefore, the application of strategic workshops appears to be an effective intervention for the development of key academic abilities that are needed for achieving higher classification degrees. In theoretical physics, the discussion of philosophical foundations together with rigorous scientific investigation has created a very wide range of debates. The Mathematical Universe Hypothesis (MUH) and the External Reality Hypothesis (ERH) defy traditional assumptions by putting forward the concept that our physical reality exists independently of human perception and is, in effect, a mathematical abstract structure. It disrupts the paradigm to an extent that makes one rethink influential factors such as symmetry, randomness, and initial conditions, thereby making way for deeper comprehension of reality (Albrecht et al., 2007). Furthermore, language employed to explain these hypotheses generates avenues of thought concerning more abstract problems such as consciousness and alternate worlds, and thus bridges intellectual gaps between science and philosophy. Thus, these discussions not only advance us with respect to the understanding of physics but also overlap with broader questions of intellect. Finally, the presence of critical thinking skills instruction integrated throughout courses emphasizes the importance of an interdisciplinary education. By facilitating the engagement of students in a two-way process of acquiring content knowledge and skills, instructors are able to create more integrated learning experiences. This two-way emphasis can lead to a stronger academic environment in which students are encouraged to question and synthesize across disciplines, resulting in more responsive and reflective graduates. As noted in physics theoretical classes as well as learning workshops, it is imperative for mental growth to develop a curious mindset and ability to connect various ideas. Emphasis on these skills in curriculums reflects a shift towards more integrated learning habits that respond to contemporary academic requirements and prepare learners with skills for solving real-world issues (Albrecht et al., 2007; Henri et al., 2015).

KEY TERMS FROM THIS CHAPTER

- Acute pancreatitis
- Pancreatic duct
- Fibrous wall
- Hemorrhage
- Abdominal pain
- Ultrasound (USG)
- Chronic pancreatitis
- Encapsulated fluid collection
- Necrosis
- Infection
- Epigastric mass
- Computed tomography (CT)

References

1. Cantanhede, K. R. M., Cantanhede, R. M., Souza, P. F. D. de, Abbas, O. A. A., Medeiros, I. A. de O., Domingos, K. T. P. e S., Martins, D. S. L., Cordeiro, N. G., Gomes, M. L. S., & Borges, C. O. C. (2024). Effectiveness of argon plasma coagulation in the treatment of weight regain after roux-y gastric bypass: a cross-sectional prospective observational study. *International Journal of Nutrology*, *17*(1). https://doi.org/10.54448/ijn24111 (accessed on 26 May 2025).
2. Agcaoili, M. G. C. (2024). Best interests of the child in juvenile justice: Analysis of Malaysia, Philippines, and Thailand. https://core.ac.uk/download/618326451.pdf (accessed on 26 May 2025).
3. Agnihotri, A. K., Ailawadi, G., Barnhart, G. R., et al. (2016). Minimally invasive mitral valve surgery II: Surgical technique and postoperative management. https://core.ac.uk/download/323078625.pdf.
4. Ajjarapu, A. & Moreira, N. N., (2020) "Successful non-surgical management of acute, uncomplicated appendicitis in pregnancy: A case report", *Proceedings in Obstetrics and Gynecology* 9(3), 1–7. doi: https://doi.org/10.17077/2154-4751.1460 (accessed on 26 May 2025).
5. Albrecht, A., Church, A., Guth, A., Proca, A., Turing, A., Vilenkin, A., Vilenkin, A., et al. (2007). The mathematical universe. *arXiv preprint*. http://arxiv.org/abs/0704.0646 (accessed on 26 May 2025).
6. Albu, G., Georgescu, S. R., Sarbu, M. I., et al. (2015). Genital skin diseases and their expression in sexual functionality. https://core.ac.uk/download/144552324.pdf (accessed on 26 May 2025).
7. Allareddy, V., Fletcher, S., Metalwala, Z., et al. (2018). Orthognathic surgical outcomes in patients with and without craniofacial anomalies. https://core.ac.uk/download/213086834.pdf (accessed on 26 May 2025).
8. Amare, Equlinet (2023): Entrustable Professional Activities (EPAs) framework to inform surgical residency training programs in Ethiopia medical education. Dissertation, LMU München: Faculty of Medicine(accessed on 26 May 2025).
9. Yang, D., Amin, S., Gonzalez, S., Mullady, D., Hasak, S., Gaddam, S., Edmundowicz, S. A., Gromski, M. A., DeWitt, J. M., El Zein, M., Khashab, M. A., Wang, A. Y., Gaspar, J. P., Uppal, D. S., Nagula, S., Kapadia, S., Buscaglia, J. M., Bucobo, J. C., Schlachterman, A., Wagh, M. S., ... DiMaio, C. J. (2016). Transpapillary drainage has no added benefit on treatment outcomes in patients undergoing EUS-guided transmural drainage of pancreatic pseudocysts: a large multicenter study. *Gastrointestinal endoscopy*, *83*(4), 720–729. https://doi.org/10.1016/j.gie.2015.10.040 (accessed on 26 May 2025).
10. Yang, D., Amin, S., Gonzalez, S., Mullady, D., Edmundowicz, S. A., DeWitt, J. M., Khashab, M. A., Wang, A. Y., Nagula, S., Buscaglia, J. M., Bucobo, J. C., Wagh, M. S., Draganov, P. V., Stevens, T., Vargo, J. J., Khara, H. S., Diehl, D. L., Keswani, R. N., Komanduri, S., Yachimski, P. S., ... DiMaio, C. J. (2017). Clinical outcomes of EUS-guided drainage of debris-containing pancreatic pseudocysts: a large multicenter study. *Endoscopy international open*, *5*(2), E130–E136. https://doi.org/10.1055/s-0042-121666 (accessed on 26 May 2025).

11. Anand, B. S. (2004). Do Gödel's incompleteness theorems set absolute limits on the ability of the brain to express and communicate mental concepts verifiably? *arXiv preprint.* http://arxiv.org/abs/math/0407529 (accessed on 26 May 2025).

12. Andersson, B. (2010). Acute pancreatitis: Severity classification, complications and outcome. https://core.ac.uk/download/83707914.pdf (accessed on 26 May 2025).

13. Annevelink, E., Broeze, J., van Ree, R., et al. (2009). *Opportunities for Dutch biorefineries.* https://core.ac.uk/download/pdf/29248632.pdf (accessed on 26 May 2025).

14. Annibale, B., Bellini, D., Binda, G. A., Cuomo, R., et al. (2015). Practice parameters for the treatment of colonic diverticular disease: Italian Society of Colon and Rectal Surgery (SICCR) guidelines. https://core.ac.uk/download/54522076.pdf (accessed on 26 May 2025).

15. Antunes, S. de J. R. F. (2020). *Biomarkers for Classification and Risk Assessment of Pancreatic Cystic Neoplasms.* https://core.ac.uk/download/401085509.pdf (accessed on 26 May 2025).

16. Ardengh, J. C., Brant, C. Q., Ferrari, A. P., Libera, E. D., et al. (2000). Pancreatic pseudocysts transpapillary and transmural drainage. https://core.ac.uk/download/pdf/8088519.pdf.

17. Ashour, A. S., Dey, N., Sherratt, R. S., Shi, F., et al. (2017). Wireless capsule gastrointestinal endoscopy: Direction of arrival estimation-based localization survey. https://core.ac.uk/download/82920165.pdf (accessed on 26 May 2025).

18. Auerbach, E. (2023). Is nanotechnology an effective treatment for diabetic wounds? https://core.ac.uk/download/616444339.pdf (accessed on 26 May 2025).

19. Minni, A., Dragonetti, A., Sciuto, A., Rosati, D., Cavaliere, C., Ralli, M., Azimonti, D., Franzetti, A., & de Vincentiis, M. (2018). Use of balloon catheter dilation and steroid-eluting stent in light and severe rhinosinusitis of frontal sinus: a multicenter retrospective randomized study. *European review for medical and pharmacological sciences, 22*(21), 7482–7491. https://doi.org/10.26355/eurrev_201811_16289 (accessed on 26 May 2025).

20. Aziz, F., Buang, A., Mustamin, N. F., Nur, S., et al. (2024). Ensemble techniques-based risk classification for maternal health during pregnancy. https://core.ac.uk/download/622174248.pdf (accessed on 26 May 2025).

21. Ribichini, E., Stigliano, S., Rossi, S., Zaccari, P., Sacchi, M. C., Bruno, G., Badiali, D., & Severi, C. (2019). Role of Fibre in Nutritional Management of Pancreatic Diseases. *Nutrients, 11*(9), 2219. https://doi.org/10.3390/nu11092219 (accessed on 26 May 2025).

22. Bahdi, F., Donahue, T., Farooq, M., Issa, Y., et al. (2024). From scalpel to scope: How surgical techniques made way for state-of-the-art endoscopic procedures. https://core.ac.uk/download/635937301.pdf (accessed on 26 May 2025).

23. Balatero, J. S. (2018). *Obstetric Nurses' Perceived Barriers to Immediate Skin-to-Skin Contact After Cesarean Birth.* https://core.ac.uk/download/159401074.pdf (accessed on 26 May 2025).

24. Bedogni, A., Campisi, G., Di Fede, O., Fusco, V., et al. (2018). The dental management of patients at risk of medication-related osteonecrosis of the jaw: New paradigm of primary prevention. https://core.ac.uk/download/168406643.pdf (accessed on 26 May 2025).

25. Bem, J., & Bem, S. (2025). Impacts of activities in crushing plant on environment and occupational health of workers involved. https://core.ac.uk/download/pdf/6580102.pdf (accessed on 26 May 2025).

26. Berger, Z., Brito, J. P., Haskell, H., Hess, R., et al. (2017). Patient-centered diagnosis: Sharing

diagnostic decisions with patients in clinical practice. https://core.ac.uk/download/186331843.pdf (accessed on 26 May 2025).

27. Bhogal, R. H., & Downing, R. (2011). The evolution of aortic aneurysm repair: Past lessons and future directions. https://core.ac.uk/download/pdf/1631327.pdf.

28. Constantin VD, Carâp A, Socea B, Bobic S. Pancreatic Encephalopathy—A Rare Complication of Severe Acute Biliary Pancreatitis. *Journal of Mind and Medical Sciences*. 2014; 1(1):40-51. https://doi.org/10.22543/2392-7674.1005(accessed on 26 May 2025).

29. Boru, E. C., Guida, A., Iossa, A., Rengo, M., et al. (2017). 25th International Congress of the European Association for Endoscopic Surgery (EAES), Frankfurt, Germany, 14–17 June 2017: Oral presentations. https://core.ac.uk/download/141696623.pdf (accessed on 26 May 2025).

30. Bouamrane, M. M., Diehl, T. M., Harrison, E. M., Knight, S., et al. (2023). Readiness for implementation of novel digital health interventions for postoperative monitoring: A systematic review and clinical innovation network analysis. https://core.ac.uk/download/571260389.docx (accessed on 26 May 2025).

31. Bundock, K. A. (2015). *Doctor of Philosophy* [Doctoral dissertation]. https://core.ac.uk/download/276263678.pdf (accessed on 26 May 2025).

32. Carde, C., Diesmann, M., Hagen, E., Kuhlen, T. W., et al. (2018). VIOLA: A multi-purpose and web-based visualization tool for neuronal-network simulation output. https://arxiv.org/abs/1803.10205 (accessed on 26 May 2025).

33. Chandra, A., Fisher, E. S., & Skinner, J. S. (2008). Outcomes assessment and health care reform. https://core.ac.uk/download/71346829.pdf (accessed on 26 May 2025).

34. Cole, M., & Jamal, A. (2009). Rethinking privacy in social networks: A case study of Beacon. https://core.ac.uk/download/336548.pdf (accessed on 26 May 2025).

35. de Jonge, L., de Wit, L. T., Govaert, M. J., Obertop, H., et al. (2001). Fracture of the pancreas in two patients after a go-kart accident. https://core.ac.uk/download/pdf/82563672.pdf (accessed on 26 May 2025).

36. Dyess, J. (2020). *Research and Review of Polymethyl-Methacrylate Copolymers in The Development of Enhanced Pharmaceutical Delivery Systems*. https://core.ac.uk/download/322850900.pdf (accessed on 26 May 2025).

37. Fox, M., Howey, R., & Long, D. (2004). Validating plans with exogenous events. https://core.ac.uk/download/9015736.pdf (accessed on 26 May 2025).

38. Frakes, M. D., Frank, M. B., & Rozema, K. (2017). The economics of healthcare rationing. https://core.ac.uk/download/62571385.pdf (accessed on 26 May 2025).

39. Galli, A., Anastasio, P. J., Wolthoff, P., & Fan, W. (2017). Single-dose oritavancin compared to standard of care IV antibiotics for acute bacterial skin and skin structure infection in the outpatient setting: A retrospective real-world study. https://core.ac.uk/download/pdf/81881813.pdf (accessed on 26 May 2025).

40. Geleto, T. C. (2018). *Determinants for Farmers' Perception of Soil Erosion: The Case of Elreta District, West Shoa Zone, Oromia Regional State, Ethiopia*. https://core.ac.uk/download/234665260.pdf (accessed on 26 May 2025).

41. Gelman, A., Ouédraogo, A. L., Hoadley, B., Eisenhart, C., Fraser, C., Osborne, C., McCulloch, C. E., et al. (2015). Improving statistical inference on pathogen densities estimated by

quantitative molecular methods: Malaria gametocytaemia as a case study. https://core.ac.uk/download/159992778.pdf (accessed on 26 May 2025).

42. Khalifa, M. , Gobran, T. , Shreef, K. S. & Waly, A. (2015). Pancreatic pseudocyst in children. *Annals of Pediatric Surgery, 11* (2), 127-131. doi: 10.1097/01.XPS.0000462976.63254.c6. (accessed on 26 May 2025).

43. Goss, A., Jaunay, T., & Sambrook, P. (2000). Antibiotic prescribing practices by South Australian general dental practitioners. https://core.ac.uk/download/12748343.pdf (accessed on 26 May 2025).

44. Henri, D., Morrell, L., & Scott, G. (2015). Ask a clearer question, get a better answer. https://core.ac.uk/download/151157342.pdf (accessed on 26 May 2025).

45. Ivashchenko, V., Kalabukha, I., & Khmel, O. (2018). Estimation of reserves for improving the results of patients with multipresistant pulmonary tuberculosis in the application of surgical methods based on analysis of the efficiency of conservative treatment of a specified cohort. https://core.ac.uk/download/322516333.pdf (accessed on 26 May 2025).

46. Krekel, C., Oparina, E., & Srisuma, S. (2024). Talking therapy: Impacts of a nationwide mental health service in England. https://core.ac.uk/download/643235619.pdf (accessed on 26 May 2025).

47. Krige, J. 2017. A prospective evaluation to define optimal surgical strategies in the management of complex pancreatic injuries based on the analysis of patients treated at a major South African academic institution. University of Cape Town. (accessed on 26 May 2025).

48. Manan, M. R., Rahman, S., Komer, L., Manan, H., & Iftikhar, S. (2022). A multispecialty approach to the identification and diagnosis of nonaccidental trauma in children. *Cureus*. https://doi.org/10.7759/cureus.27276.

49. Ayme, Andrea & Suárez, Josseline & Ortega, Martin & Gualoto, Gualoto & Lima, Santillán & Campoverde, Adriana & Ticona, Alfredo & Vergara, Coello & Serrano, Gerzon. (2024). Advancements in Minimally Invasive Surgical Techniques: A Comprehensive Review. Salud, Ciencia y Tecnología. 3. 745. 10.56294/saludcyt2023745. (accessed on 26 May 2025).

50. Núñez-Troconis, J. (2020). Trichomonas vaginalis: Pathogenesis and its role in cervical cancer. *Investigación Clínica, 61*, 349–375. https://doi.org/10.22209/ic.v61n4a05.

51. Osborne, B. (2022). Examining the integration of physical health in the treatment of substance use disorders. https://core.ac.uk/download/597547496.pdf (accessed on 26 May 2025).

52. Ramos, Pedro, "Acute myocardial infarction patient data to assess healthcare utilization and treatments." (2011). *Electronic Theses and Dissertations*. Paper 1178. https://doi.org/10.18297/etd/1178(accessed on 26 May 2025).

53. Saleth, R. M. (2025). Strategic analysis of water institutions in India: Application of a new research paradigm. https://core.ac.uk/download/pdf/6481865.pdf (accessed on 26 May 2025).

54. Silk, Alex (2019). Theories of vagueness and theories of law. Legal Theory 25 (2):132-152. (accessed on 26 May 2025).

55. Stewart, E. R., & Thompson, G. R. (2016). Treatment of primary pulmonary aspergillosis: An assessment of the evidence. https://core.ac.uk/download/323070109.pdf (accessed on 26 May 2025).

56. Stewart, J. R. (2010). Understanding evolutionary processes during past Quaternary climatic cycles: Can it be applied to the future? https://core.ac.uk/download/4898204.pdf (accessed on 26 May 2025).
57. Schäfer, C., Tietz, A. B., & Göke, B. (2005). Pathophysiology of acute experimental pancreatitis: lessons from genetically engineered animal models and new molecular approaches. *Digestion*, *71*(3), 162–172. https://doi.org/10.1159/000086138 (accessed on 26 May 2025).
58. Workman, T. E. (2011). *Doctor of Philosophy* [Doctoral dissertation]. https://core.ac.uk/download/276264160.pdf (accessed on 26 May 2025).
59. Yust, J. (2017). Probing questions about keys: Tonal distributions through the DFT. https://open.bu.edu/bitstream/2144/39068/1/tonalDist_rev.pdf (accessed on 26 May 2025).

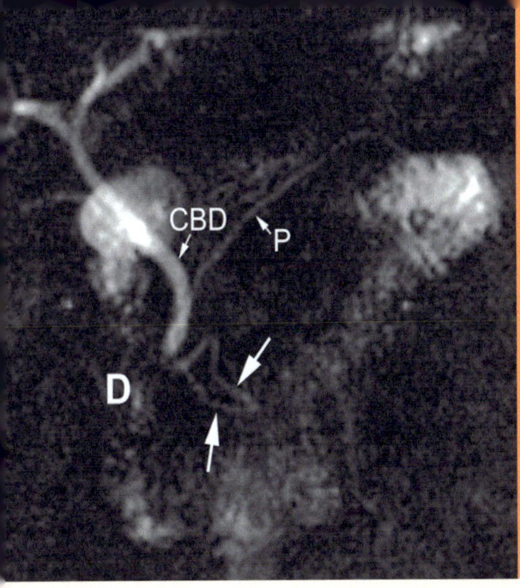

Chapter 10

CONGENITAL ANOMALIES OF THE PANCREAS

Contents

Introduction

Congenital pancreatic anomalies are a severe group of pediatric gastroenterologic illness with high health potential to affect. The pancreas, an essential abdominal organ for digestive and metabolic processes, may develop abnormally in embryogenesis to cause multiple structural malformations. Three of the most important diseases are pancreas divisum, annular pancreas, and choledochal cysts, both because they present single clinical challenges and because precise understanding of their pathophysiology is needed. These abnormalities usually do not become apparent until late childhood or adulthood, when signs of pancreatic dysfunction are detected. It is thus essential to look for the pathology of such conditions to ascertain important treatment interventions, as well as potential complications resulting from delayed diagnosis. Pancreatic congenital anomalies have clinical significance by their associations with severe complications, such as pancreatitis. A case in point is pancreas divisum, which is characterized by an inability of the fusion of the pancreatic duct, so that there may be ductal obstruction and subsequent inflammation. Understanding of the complex inter-relationship between congenital defects and impact on risk of pancreatitis bears importance, given that acute and chronic pancreatitis can be caused by more than one etiology, according to Rodrigo Sáez et al. (2025). These conditions not only deteriorate the health of patients but also impose great burdens on the health care system.

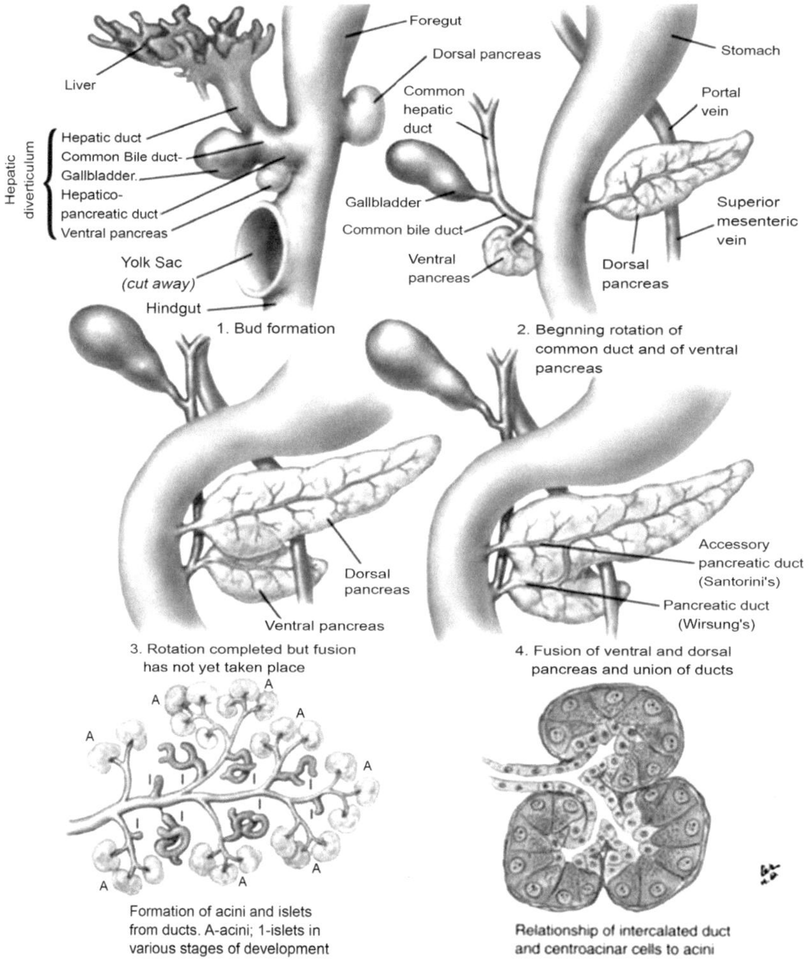

Figure 10.1. Congenital disorders of the pancreas.

Source: https://clinicalgate.com/wp-content/uploads/2015/04/B9781437714548000515_f051-001-9781437714548.jpg.

Therefore, an evaluation of these conditions should not only involve diagnostic strategies but also emphasize the need for early surgical interventions when required for improved patient outcomes. While treating congenital anomalies of the pancreas, it is important to consider the resective surgical modalities at hand and their resultant clinical implications. Surgical intervention may be a deciding point when it comes to the management of symptoms and prevention of long-term effects of conditions such as annular pancreas, where the duodenum is surrounded by the pancreas and blocked. Improved surgical techniques enhance the ability of healthcare providers to reverse the effect of such congenital anomalies effectively. Further, integrating sophisticated imaging technologies, facilitates improved assessment and diagnosis, and consequently timely intervention which can significantly alter prognoses. Under this multi-domain approach, knowledge of congenital anomalies and their management takes center stage among clinicians with the goal of providing the optimal care for afflicted patients, and consequently improving their quality of life (Figure 10.1).

Definition of Congenital Anomalies

Congenital anomalies, characterized by structural or functional abnormalities present at birth, significantly impact individual health and development. These anomalies arise from disruptions during critical periods of embryonic development, which can result from genetic mutations, environmental factors, or a combination of both influences. For the pancreas, congenital anomalies such as pancreas divisum, annular pancreas, and choledochal cysts demonstrate the manner in which these interruptions can lead to varying degrees of clinical significance. The pathophysiology of these abnormalities often determines careful diagnostic evaluation and a proper understanding of their embryological etiology. Diagnosis of congenital abnormalities not only helps in planning appropriate treatment but is also highly important in giving us information regarding the pathogenesis of these abnormalities. The clinical significance of pancreatic congenital anomalies cannot be overstressed, as they may lead to severe diseases impacting digestion and overall health. These include pancreas divisum, which may hinder the unobstructed flow of pancreatic secretions and then lead to repeated episodes of pancreatitis. An annular pancreas, in which pancreatic tissue encircles the duodenum, can lead to mechanical obstruction and resultant gastrointestinal disorders. Choledochal cysts, though sometimes asymptomatic, put patients at risk for cholangitis, pancreatitis, or even malignancy in adult life. Keeping these consequences in mind reinforces the need for early diagnosis and intervention. Above all, the association between such anomalies and long-term complications to health reiterates the necessity of continued research into their etiologies and impacts, as the high complication rates reported in related disorders (Rodrigo Sáez et al., 2025) attest. The therapeutic approach to pancreatic congenital abnormalities is inherently complex and varies with a range of surgical techniques and medical therapy appropriate to the particular anomaly. Illustrative examples include surgical intervention in the form of resection of ectopic pancreatic tissue for annular pancreas or transduodenal drainage for pancreas divisum to normalize drainage. Decision-making in treatment relies not only on the understanding of the anatomical variations but also on the potential complications ranging from infection to pancreatic necrosis. Ongoing advances in surgical techniques make the ability to handle these anomalies properly better, ultimately leading to improved patient outcomes. The challenges presented by these congenital malformations must be met to the end of fostering a better quality of life for the affected and highlights the continued worth of research and clinical ingenuity in the treatment of pancreatic congenital abnormalities.

Overview of the Pancreas and its Functions

The pancreas is an important organ that plays a vital role in the digestive and endocrine system of the human body. Behind the stomach, it releases digestive enzymes like amylase, lipase, and proteases, which break down carbohydrates, fats, and proteins in the small intestine. In addition to its digestive function, the pancreas has a crucial endocrine function by secreting hormones, mainly insulin and glucagon, that control blood glucose concentrations. The perfection of this coordination is crucial; their failure can lead to serious metabolic disorders, including diabetes mellitus, emphasizing the pancreas double function as exocrine and endocrine gland, controlling metabolic homeostasis and nutrient digestion. In addition to its role in digestion and endocrine secretion, the pancreas is susceptible to other congenital anomalies that can compromise its function. Pancreas divisum and annular pancreas are two well-known developmental anomalies, which tend to cause problems such as recurring pain in the abdomen, pancreatitis, or even obstructive jaundice. Their clinical significance is not just their potential to disrupt normal pancreatic function but also because they are associated with other gastrointestinal disease. Pancreas divisum, for instance, occurs when the pancreatic duct fails to fuse during fetal development and sets the person up for acute and chronic pancreatitis, complicating treatment. Recognition of these abnormalities enables more accurate understanding of their implications in pathophysiology and directs intraoperative decision-making in treatment guidelines. Selective operative procedures available to treat congenital pancreatic anomalies are diverse, based on the individual nature of each anomaly. Surgical interventions may involve procedural redo, such as the creation of a new drainage system for pancreas divisum or resection in more complex cases, such as annular pancreas. These interventions aim at symptom improvement and proper pancreatic function but are fraught with risk factors such as pancreatitis complications and post-operative infection and thus require proper patient selection and pre-operative workup. The successful management of these congenital anomalies hinges on a multidisciplinary plan that balances the intricacies of pancreatic function against the threat of complications, emphasizing the significance of clear understanding of the anatomy and pancreas physiology (Rodrigo Sáez et al., 2025).

Importance of Studying Pancreatic Anomalies

Identification of pancreatic anomalies is important for enhancing pediatric and adult healthcare. Pancreas divisum, annular pancreas, and choledochal cysts are congenital anomalies that have the potential to significantly affect an individual's health through varied clinical presentations. Early studies indicate that the anomalies have the potential to lead to pancreatitis and biliary obstruction among other complications, which calls for early diagnosis and intervention. Through systematic documentation and study of such conditions, as promoted by guidelines enumerated by the National Birth Defects Prevention Network, medical practitioners can improve the quality and validity of birth defects surveillance data, and thus contribute to more knowledge about the prevalence and etiology of pancreatic anomalies. This foundation paves the way for treatment approaches to counteract long-standing complications of these congenital defects, ultimately resulting in enhanced patient outcomes and quality of life. Furthermore, investigation into pancreatic anomalies enhances knowledge of their clinical significance, particularly with regards to surgery. Every anomaly presents with new challenges to be overcome, requiring modified surgical techniques such as pancreaticoduodenectomy or less complex methods of choledochal cyst treatment. The importance of selecting appropriate surgical methods is significant in terms of potential procedural complications and postoperative treatment. With growing education and awareness regarding such defects, the medical community is better positioned to prepare themselves for the nuances of surgical decision-making. Moreover, active research driven by efforts such as the Lancet Commission on Global Surgery highlights the importance of incorporating global health perspectives into the decision-making process for congenital anomalies as key public health issues warranting attention and investment. Finally, the analysis of pancreatic anomalies adds to the clinical setting as well as to avenues of future research. Understanding these conditions may lead to questions about their environmental and genetic risk factors, thus enabling early prevention and detection. This multidisciplinary collaboration is indicative of the overall movement towards personalized medicine, where knowledge gained from studying congenital anomalies can be transferable across a broad array of medical specialties, including genetics, gastroenterology, and surgery. By so doing, the practitioners may aim to instate more extensive surveillance programs designed to facilitate early detection of such anomalies since the rules by National Birth Defects Prevention Network (National Birth Defects Prevention Network Surveillance Guidelines and Standards Committee, 2025) prescribe. In doing so, a detailed exploration of pancreatic abnormalities adds to the overall aim of improving health outcomes in those born with congenital disorders, forming an integral link between research, clinical care, and patient advocacy (Figure 10.2).

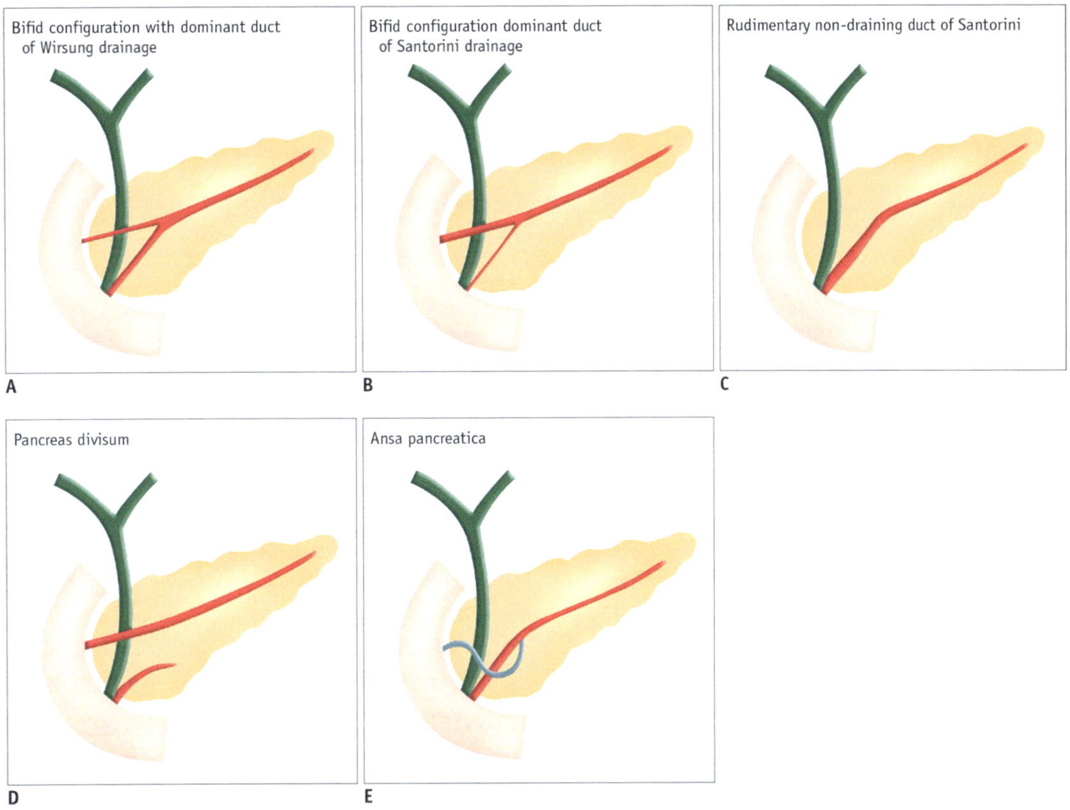

Figure 10.2. Congenital variants and anomalies of the pancreas and pancreatic duct.

Source: https://external-content.duckduckgo.com/iu/?u=https%3A%2F%2Ftse3.mm.bing.net%2Fth%3Fid%3DOIP.3gDF5Ga1B0-6qq9JEhbdOAHaFf%26pid%3DApi&f=1&ipt=35dcfa40d434deb8f3fd34c6d38f813c2bba9718a3289a33dcd9a9f3f2dd75f4.

10.1. Pancreas Divisum

The most frequent of all congenital pancreatic anomalies, pancreas divisum is due to failure of fusion of the dorsal and ventral pancreatic buds during embryonic development. The result is an anatomical separation of the ductal systems of the pancreas, each with its own drainage route into the duodenum through distinct papillae. Most patients with pancreas divisum are asymptomatic and become aware of their condition only when diagnosed incidentally on imaging studies obtained for reasons unrelated to pancreas.

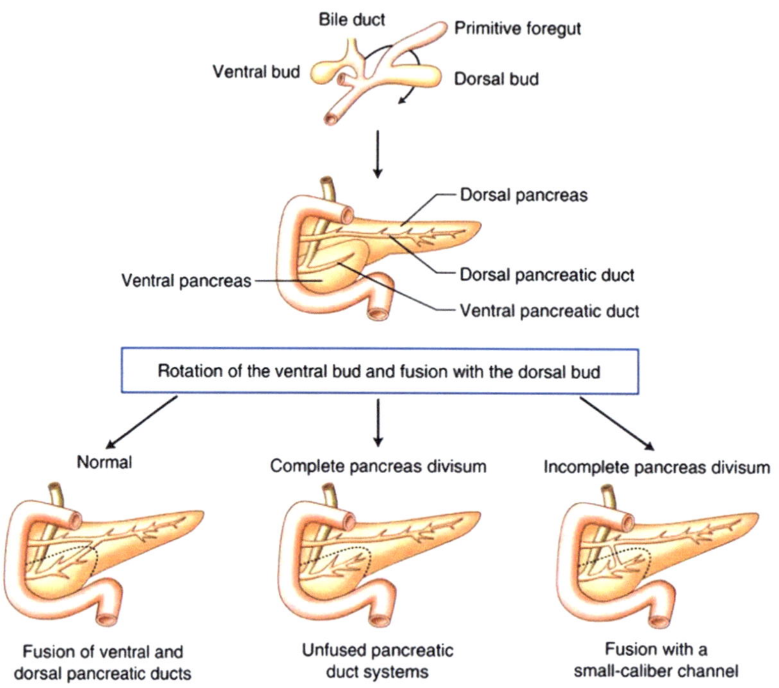

Figure 10.3. Pancreas divisum.

Source: https://arielmedicine.com/wp-content/uploads/2021/01/Anatomy-of-pancreas-divisum-1.png.

The anomaly, however, subjects the patient to some pancreatic diseases, such as acute recurrent pancreatitis, because the single drainage can cause obstruction at the minor papilla to result in increased intraductal pressure and inflammation. Understanding this pathophysiology is critical, as it has significant treatment and management implications for diseased patients (Fogel et al., 2019). Pancreas divisum is commonly thought of as a benign anatomical variant, but the potential that it is an etiologic factor in the downstream evolution of pancreatic disease is an intriguing point to explore and one that remains the subject of investigation. The pathogenesis of pancreas divisum and related diseases like chronic pancreatitis has been unclear; while some reports point toward a causative association, others are unable to show a definite correlation. The evidence suggests that certain patients with recurrent pancreatitis may be benefited by endoscopic management aimed towards the minor papilla, which may alleviate symptoms by facilitating more effective drainage of the dorsal pancreatic duct. Nevertheless, complete clinical reports are inadequate and consensus on the clinical significance and treatment of pancreas divisum patients is not present. The convergence of different research findings emphasizes the importance of case-to-case patient consultation on prognosis and treatment (Fogel et al., 2019). In the case of surgery, treatment strategies for managing consequences attributed to pancreas divisum have been evolving, with the interventions ranging from conservative treatment to surgical interventions. Endoscopic methods, such as sphincterotomy and minor papilla balloon dilation, are promising in alleviating symptoms for certain patients with recurrent pancreatitis. For failing cases of these interventions, surgical removal of the involved pancreatic segment is an option. But the absence of clear guidelines on the treatment of pancreas divisum calls for individualization, hence the need for multidisciplinary evaluation in determining the best course of action. Clinicians must weigh factors such as symptomatology, individual patient circumstances, and available treatment options in the development of a management plan so that patients are thoroughly informed about their condition and risks and benefits of potential interventions (Figure 10.3).

10.1.1. Description and Pathophysiology

Pancreas divisum pathophysiology is a relevant subject in the context of congenital pancreatic disease. It happens when the ventral and dorsal ducts of the pancreas do not fuse during embryogenesis, resulting in two separate drainage systems for the pancreas. While the majority of those with pancreas divisum are asymptomatic, there is debate regarding its potential role in worsening pancreatic illnesses, such as idiopathic recurrent acute pancreatitis and chronic pancreatitis. Current research into the connection between pancreas divisum and pancreatic pathology has yielded conflicting results. Scientists generally agree that while there is likely to be an association, the exact mechanisms by which pancreas divisum results in such pathologies are yet to be fully elucidated. This lack of certainty also emphasizes the importance of individualized therapeutic approaches in clinical management, particularly in planning surgery for such individuals (Fogel et al., 2019). On the other hand, annular pancreas refers to a congenital defect of the pancreas where pancreatic tissue encircles the duodenum, typically with resulting obstruction. This is due to impaired rotation of the ventral pancreatic bud during embryogenesis. Annular pancreas presents clinically in neonates and infants as vomiting, abdominal distension, and failure to thrive due to duodenal stenosis. If left untreated, it can lead to serious complications like intestinal obstruction and pancreatitis. Surgical decompression is generally indicated to decompress the obstruction, most commonly through excision of the surrounding tissue or duodenojejunostomy. Aside from immediate relief, the impact of this congenital anomaly extends beyond the perioperative course, with long-term follow-up necessary to manage any recurring gastrointestinal disturbances that follow surgical intervention (Park et al., 2021). Choledochal cysts are another notable congenital biliary tree and pancreatic interface anomaly. Choledochal cysts are dilatations of the common bile duct and potentially lead to complications such as cholangitis, pancreatitis, and even carcinoma risk of the biliary tree. The pathophysiology of choledochal cysts is generally related to embryologic maldevelopment defects of the biliary tract which can lead to dysfunctional drainage and bile stasis. Symptoms are unpredictable and can vary from asymptomatic childhood presentation to acute abdominal pain and jaundice. Patients require surgery, which most typically comprises total cyst excision and biliary tract reconstruction. Complete management is crucial not just for alleviation of acute symptoms but also for the avoidance of long-term sequelae of the congenital anomaly (Park et al., 2021).

10.1.2. Symptoms and Diagnosis

The clinical manifestation of pancreas congenital anomalies can be variable, even from asymptomatic to severe complications. In the case of pancreas divisum, which is the most frequent congenital pancreatic anomaly, most individuals remain asymptomatic throughout their lifespan. However, when symptoms do manifest, they can present as recurrent pain in the abdomen or pancreatitis that can mystify clinicians regarding their etiology. Uncertainty regarding the connection between pancreas divisum and pancreatic disease complicates diagnosis even further, necessitating thorough evaluation. The ultimate diagnosis is typically reliant on imaging techniques such as magnetic resonance cholangiopancreatography (MRCP) or endoscopic retrograde cholangiopancreatography (ERCP), which will illuminate the anatomical defects present in the patients pancreatic ductal system, thereby explaining the clinical presentation (Fogel et al., 2019).

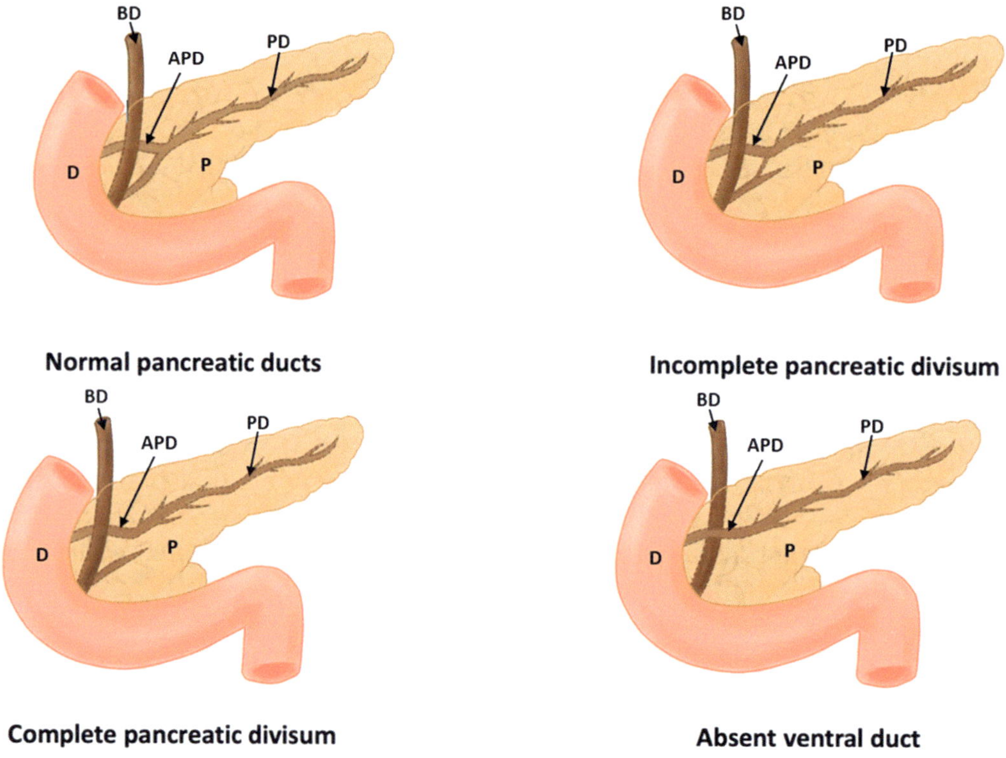

Figure 10.4. Incidence and clinical implications of anatomical variations in the pancreas and its ductal system.

Source: Orellana-Donoso M, Milos-Brandenberg D, Benavente-Urtubia A, Guerra-Loyola J, Bruna-Mejias A, Nova-Baeza P, Becerra-Farfán Á, Sepulveda-Loyola W, Luque-Bernal RM, Valenzuela-Fuenzalida JJ. Incidence and Clinical Implications of Anatomical Variations in the Pancreas and Its Ductal System: A Systematic Review and Meta-Analysis. *Life*. 2023; 13(8):1710. https://doi.org/10.3390/life13081710

In diseases such as annular pancreas, symptoms typically manifest in early infancy or early childhood and typically include gastrointestinal obstruction, vomiting, and poor weight gain. Diagnosis is typically made by imaging procedures, including abdominal X-rays and ultrasound, that may reveal the characteristic duodenal encirclement by pancreatic tissue. Recognition of these symptoms is critical for early treatment because untreated conditions can lead to significant complications, including bowel ischemia. Besides, choledochal cysts can also present with jaundice and abdominal pain, and therefore careful diagnosis using ultrasound or MRCP modalities can be warranted. The management of such congenital conditions is multifaceted and requires clinicians to reconcile clinical presentation with imaging and lab results to make accurate diagnoses and initiate early intervention (Park et al., 2021). The implications of diagnosing pancreatic anomalies such as these go beyond symptom management alone. A good understanding of the diagnostic criteria allows clinicians to create an optimal treatment plan appropriate to the individual patient's needs. For example, in patients with pancreas divisum who experience recurrent acute pancreatitis, therapeutic options may include endoscopic intervention at the minor papilla. Conversely, patients with annular pancreas may need surgery to treat duodenal obstruction. Thus, an accurate diagnosis not only illuminates the underlying pathological processes but also plays a huge role in treatment options and clinical outcomes. Early detection of symptoms and appropriate diagnostic approaches enable healthcare providers to avoid potential complications resulting from these congenital pancreatic anomalies (Fogel et al., 2019) (Figure 10.4).

10.1.3. Treatment Options and Management

The treatment of congenital anomalies of the pancreas may differ quite a lot according to the specific condition being treated. For example, pancreas divisum may be asymptomatic; however, when complications have developed, treatment options might include endoscopic or surgical measures. Evidence from recent literature suggests that endoscopic minor papilla intervention may be relieving in the context of recurrent acute pancreatitis due to pancreas divisum, though the absolute etiology of such pancreatic illness in this anomaly remains a bit controversial (Fogel et al., 2019). Decision-making for treatment must thus be patient-centered with an emphasis on a lengthy discussion of the potential risks and results of intervention versus observation, particularly in symptom-free patients. Physicians need to address such subtleties with care, considering both symptomatic presentation and patient background to guide their treatment strategy. Annular pancreas treatment, for example, frequently involves surgery due to the fact that the condition may cause duodenal obstruction. Surgery can involve duodenojejunostomy or pancreaticoduodenectomy, depending on the severity of the case and specific anatomical considerations.

Procedural choice often is determined by the patient's age, general health, and the presence of any other complicating conditions such as pancreatitis or duodenal perforation. Advances in minimally invasive techniques have been associated with improved outcomes postop and reduced recovery time, and this highlights the importance of individually tailored patient treatment protocols precisely fitted to each patient's unique circumstances. In some instances, endoscopic therapy may be an initial option, although surgical treatment remains the gold standard for the repair of the anatomical malformation and its sequelae. Choledochal cysts require more subtle and more aggressive management because they can cause serious complications like pancreatitis, cholangitis, and malignant potential of the bile duct. The most frequent treatment is surgical excision of the cyst, and in the majority of cases, it is followed by a biliary reconstruction procedure to enable the normal passage of bile. Early treatment is necessary, particularly in children, since the chances of complications from prolonged treatment are extremely high. The postoperative care can include observation for complications and follow-up after months or years for looking out for recurrence or new biliary pathology problems. Improved management of choledochal cysts has been brought about by the advancement of surgical techniques and the establishment of multidisciplinary groups of hepatopancreatobiliary surgeons, and a good understanding of both clinical and surgical modalities is of paramount importance (Park et al., 2021).

10.2. Annular Pancreas

Of all the various pancreas congenital anomalies, annular pancreas is significant for its particular anatomical complexities. Annular pancreas is an anomaly in which pancreatic tissue encircles the duodenum in a ring-like form and compresses the intestinal passage of material. Typically associated with other congenital anomalies, such as duodenal atresia or malrotation, annular pancreas may occur as a significant cause of neonatal intestinal obstruction. Symptoms typically present in infancy and include bilious vomiting, abdominal distension, and failure to pass meconium, which mandate early diagnosis and treatment.

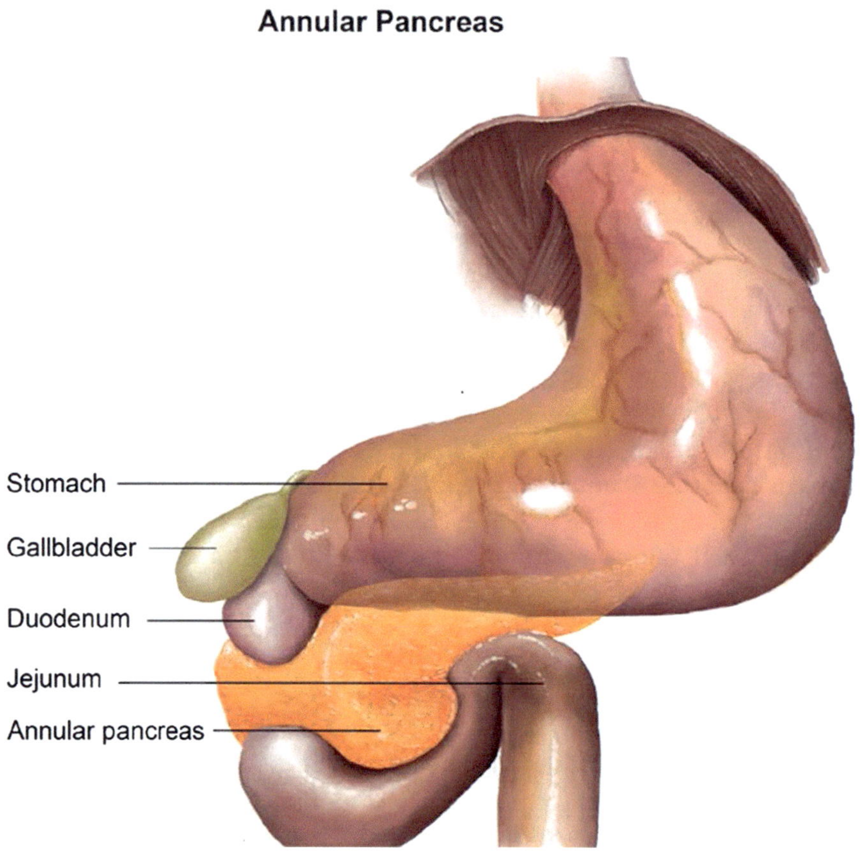

Figure 10.5. Annular pancreas.

Source: https://upload.medbullets.com/topic/109095/images/annular_pancreas.jpg.

According to literature published to date, the early recognition of annular pancreas is necessary because delayed treatment may cause severe morbidity and death in affected infants, especially when used in combination with other malformations at birth (Fogel et al., 2019). The relationship between annular pancreas and clinical outcomes is of utmost importance in deciding its impact on the care of the patient. Current evidence suggests that in the majority of instances, surgical intervention is required to mitigate the effect of duodenal obstruction, most often by duodenoduodenostomy or duodenojejunostomy procedures. Both procedures attempt to bypass the obstructed segment, restoring normal gastrointestinal function. The prognosis may still vary significantly based on the presence of other accompanying congenital anomalies. For instance, concomitant cardiac defects or low birth weight infants are bound to have poorer outcomes in surgery, aggravating conditions such as postoperative sepsis and prolonged hospital stays. Emphasis on early treatment and diagnosis is essential in the improved prognosis and quality of life for the affected infants since the rate of success in surgical intervention improves with early referrals (Fogel et al., 2019). Growth in neonatal surgical techniques has led to better global outcomes of children with annular pancreas. Development of advanced imaging technology made preoperative diagnosis possible, which allowed targeted surgical procedures in each patient. The establishment of special pediatric surgical units in tertiary centers also contributed significantly to better management. Studies have indicated that early surgical treatment, not just reduces the short-term risk of postoperative complications of intestinal obstruction, but also accommodates long-term growth and development of infants with the condition. Thus, multichannel practice approaches to address early diagnosis, surgical technique, and postoperative care from the basis of ideal annular pancreas management put a focus on continuous research into respective congenital anomalies to optimize therapy results (Karthik, 2010) (Figure 10.5).

10.2.1. Definition and Embryological Development

The pancreas, a vital digestive organ, is responsible for the production of enzymes and hormones required for digestion and metabolism. It is an exocrine and endocrine organ that has functions in gastrointestinal function through secretion of enzymes and glucose homeostasis regulation through control of hormones. The embryonic development of the pancreas is complex and starts in the fourth week of fetal life as an outcome of the foreguts endoderm. This organ forms from two distinct pancreatic buds: the dorsal bud, which forms the body and tail, and the ventral bud, which forms the head of the pancreas. Proper development and fusion of the two buds are critical; any disturbance during this process may lead to congenital anomalies, which have severe implications for the structure and function of the pancreas. It is during these developmental processes that insight into the anatomical variations and clinical significance of congenital anomalies is gained. During the development stages of embryologic development, a number of factors can have the ability to affect the development of the pancreas. Signal interaction between pathways such as the Notch and Hedgehog pathways plays an essential role in differentiation of pancreatic progenitor cells into endocrine and exocrine lineages. By eight weeks of gestation, the pancreas continues to undergo significant structural maturation, including establishing its vascular supply and ductal systems, which are essential to mature full grown function. Malformations such as pancreas divisum occur when the dorsal and ventral pancreatic ducts do not unite normally, resulting in distinct clinical presentations that may not be present until adulthood. Similarly, the annular pancreas results due to deranged rotation of the duodenum during fetal development, and a ring of pancreas forms which can be an obstructive entity (Beger et al., 2009). These conditions are reflective of a need for a properly ordered stage of embryological development to prevent congenital defects. Clinical correlates of pancreatic abnormalities based on embryological development are complex in nature. Congenital anomalies like choledochal cysts can compromise bile flow and induce cholangitis or pancreatitis. As imaging modalities improve, the anomaly is now diagnosed early in life so that intervention can proceed unhesitatingly. Treatment varies according to the anomalys nature and severity, ranging from least invasive maneuvers to more extensive resections. For example, pancreas divisum patients can benefit from endoscopic or surgical treatment if they experience recurring episodes of pancreatitis. It is important that the practitioners of health are aware of the embryological origin to ensure optimum patient care and develop appropriate surgical interventions. A complete comprehension of the causes of developmental pancreatic anomalies thus not only informs surgical practice but also enhances patient outcome via individualized therapeutic approaches (Beger et al., 2009) (Figure 10.6).

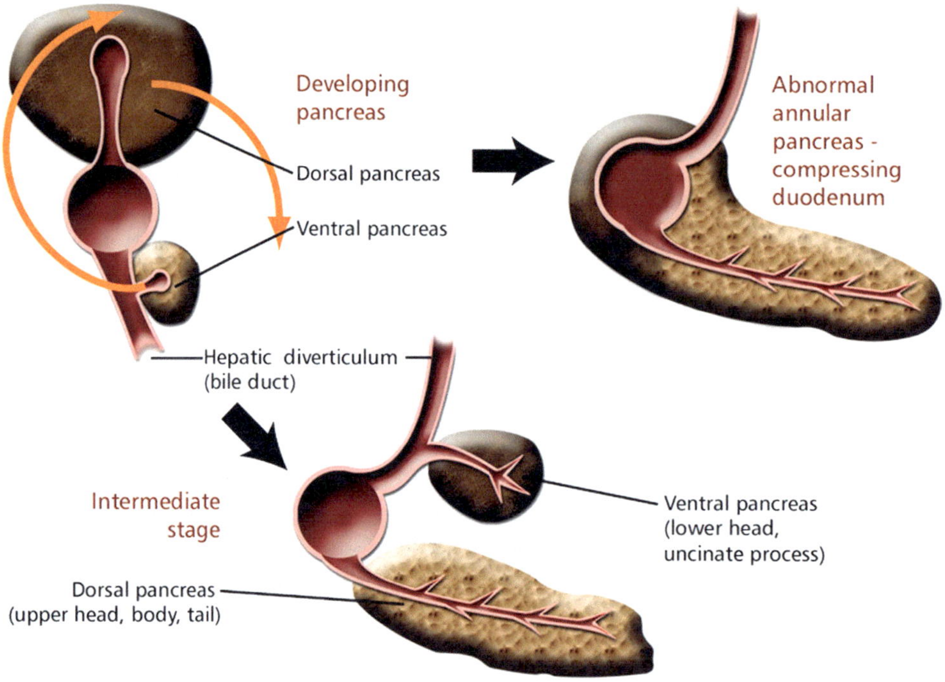

Figure 10.6. Embryonic development of pancreas.

Source: https://encrypted-tbn0.gstatic.com/images?q=tbn:ANd9GcS3C9ojcO0nOIitsMja-sM_RmR8vxoTFawxow&s.

10.2.2. Clinical Presentation and Complications

The clinical presentation of pancreatic congenital malformations can be highly diverse, depending on the type of malformation and the degree of anatomical derangement. Pancreas divisum, for instance, a relatively common congenital malformation, is frequently asymptomatic, and hence diagnosis is challenging, and it is of clinical importance. While pancreas divisum in some patients leads to idiopathic recurrent acute pancreatitis, pathophysiological mechanisms are essentially poorly understood. Existing literature shows a potential correlation with pancreas divisum and other pancreatic illness, but not consensus literature regarding its individual role in such illnesses. This lack of clarity speaks to the necessity for individualized clinical evaluation to allow clinicians to balance the patient's symptomology and treatment needs in an all-encompassing manner before any medical or interventional management (Fogel et al., 2019). Annular pancreas presents with a different clinical picture, especially in neonates, with duodenal obstruction. Annular pancreas occurs due to the rotation of the pancreatic tissue in an abnormal fashion during embryologic development. As such, a loop of pancreatic tissue encircles the duodenum. Infants affected by annular pancreas typically present with bilious vomiting, feeding intolerance, and abdominal distension. Surgical treatment, if diagnosed, can be required to remove the obstruction. Timing and approach to surgical intervention can have a profound impact on long-term results, and thus the imperative for early and accurate diagnosis in these cases is highlighted. Due to its unusual presentation and potential complications, maintaining watchfulness during clinical assessment is crucial in optimizing the management of patients with an annular pancreas. Choledochal cysts are another congenital anomaly that have severe clinical implications, primarily due to their risk of developing into complications like pancreatitis and cholangitis. The presentation is normally non-specific, and the typical triad of symptoms, jaundice, palpable mass, and pain, is seen in less than half of the cases (Torres et al., 2022). Thus, the employment of contemporary imaging studies for accurate diagnosis and classification is essential. Surgical intervention, which is most commonly excision of the cyst and hepaticoenterostomy, effectively excises the cyst and reduces the likelihood of subsequent complications. Due to the possibility of recurrent anomalies occurring, ongoing follow-up on these patients remains necessary in order to identify late sequelae and to ensure the optimal management for them during their lifetime. Such necessity underlines the appreciation of the clinical presentation and associated complications early during the management of choledochal cysts.

10.2.3. Surgical Interventions and Outcomes

The operative interventions to repair congenital anomalies of the pancreas, such as pancreas divisum, must take into account patient presentation and the unpredictability of the condition. Pancreas divisum is a congenital embryological abnormality that has been implicated in recurrent acute pancreatitis; the precise role of the condition in pancreatic pathology, however, is controversial. Although some studies reveal that therapeutic interventions like minimal papilla therapy can provide significant relief, the evidence does not show consensus as to whether surgical intervention is unavoidable for all patients with pancreas divisum. By the standards of the literature, it would be irresponsible to make a blanket recommendation without considering careful assessment of the patient's individual clinical status and potential outcomes of treatment, thus bringing to the fore the significance of lengthy patient discussion prior to treatment initiation (Fogel et al., 2019). On the other hand, choledochal cysts, including bile duct dilatations, typically mandate definitive surgical intervention due to their potential for severe complications such as cholangitis or malignancy. Excision of the cyst with subsequent hepaticoenterostomy is the typical therapy, which attempts to restore normal bile drainage and minimize recurrence. Although surgical outcomes are generally favorable, patients with choledochal cyst must be carefully observed for signs of postoperative complications and long-term recurrence. In a study, it has been found that lifelong follow-up is necessary as recurrence rates in such individuals are far greater than the general population, necessitating constant surveillance in postoperative management (Torres et al., 2022). From the point of view of assessing the effectiveness of surgical procedures, rigorous follow-up studies have to be conducted to identify the short-term and long-term effects of treatments of pancreatic anomalies. As a case point, the quality of patients' lives can be improved significantly when they are treated surgically for choledochal cysts, but these improvements need to be balanced in proportion to risks of potential complications. In pancreas divisum, where surgical management is more controversial, additional research is indicated to define the anomalous association with pancreatitis and, in turn, guide future therapeutic interventions. Patient heterogeneity and anatomical nuances call for a specialized type of surgical treatment to guarantee patient-specific requirements and clinical evidence-based treatment options to maximally optimize outcome within the spectrum of pancreatic congenital anomalies (Figure 10.7).

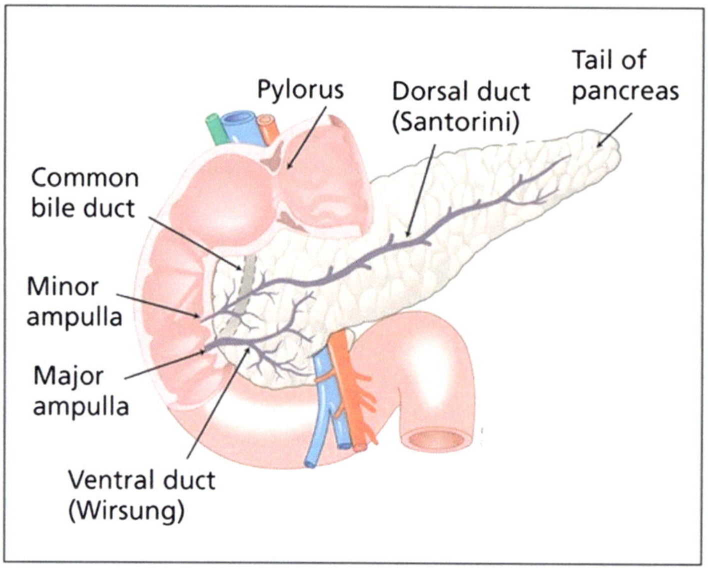

Figure 10.7. Pancreas divisum: a cause of idiopathic acute pancreatitis.

Source: https://encrypted-tbn0.gstatic.com/images?q=tbn:ANd9GcR5tAIB7rky7S6fbGANJRks4mZ9DPnj1-Dmjg&s.

10.3. Choledochal Cysts

Among the congenital malformations of the biliary and pancreatic system, choledochal cysts are noteworthy for their complex nature and clinical relevance. Choledochal cysts are biliary dilatations that can result in significant complications such as pancreatitis and biliary carcinogenesis. Pathogenesis of choledochal cysts is usually related to pancreaticobiliary maljunction (PBM), whereby the bile duct and pancreatic duct anomalously unite. This junction anomaly is the fundamental reason why choledochal cysts form and also appears to be an important risk factor for biliary cancer in affected individuals. Classification of choledochal cysts, as explained by Todani, categorizes them into various types based on their anatomical features, making diagnosis easier and guiding surgical interventions to prevent associated risks (Tüysüz, 2023). The clinical significance of choledochal cysts extends beyond their being an anatomical aberration; they have extremely significant implications for the management of the patient. Patients present with a variety of symptoms ranging from abdominal pain to jaundice and hence appropriate diagnostic evaluations are warranted. The imaging modalities of ultrasonography, MRI/MRCP, and CT scan have a pivotal role in making the diagnosis and grading of involvement of the biliary tract. Where routine imaging proves inadequate, nuclear hepatobiliary iminodiacetic acid (HIDA) scans are valuable for ascertaining the functional status of the biliary system. Accurate diagnosis is important since surgery is based on the Todani classification, thus requiring individually tailored treatment to yield optimal outcomes. Surgical excision, particularly to the lobar bifurcation level, is classically advised to prevent postoperative complications due to the residual cystic structures (Tüysüz, 2023). Importantly, surgical treatment of choledochal cysts must be performed with a clear vision of their anatomical and pathophysiologic implications. The localization of the cysts, often within the head of the pancreas, can render surgical access cumbersome and calls for careful dissection to avoid the injury of surrounding structures. Their use in the management of choledochal cysts has been promoted based on their advantages such as better visualization and minimal blood loss during surgery. Caution must be exercised against postoperative morbidity in terms of the formation of residual intra-pancreatic cysts, which may eventually increase the risk of malignant pancreatic neoplasms. Therefore, effective management of choledochal cysts needs a multidisciplinary strategy integrating surgical skills with careful follow-up management (Tüysüz, 2023) (Figure 10.8).

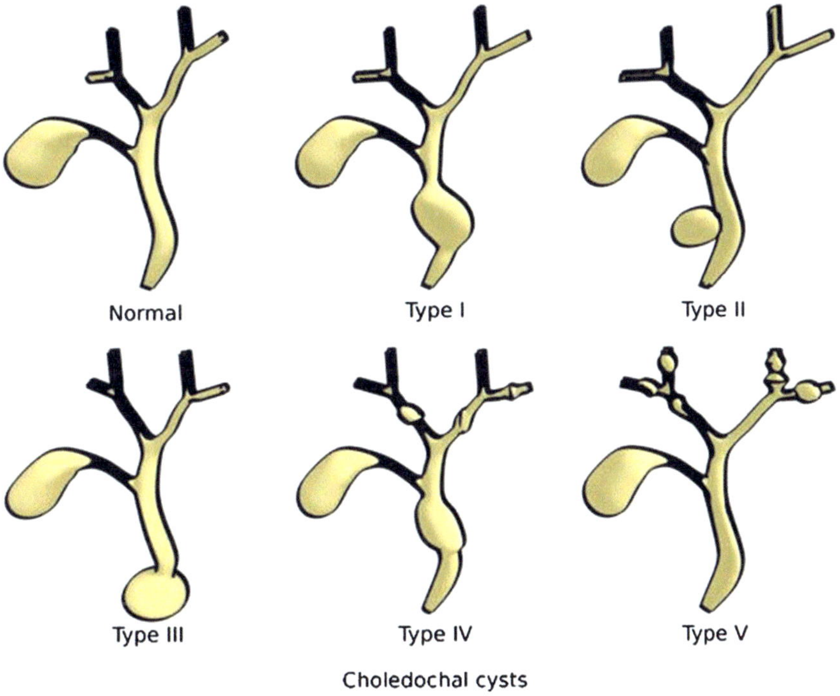

Figure 10.8. Choledochal cyst.

Source: https://www.amardeepchildrenhospital.com/wp-content/uploads/image-choledochal-cyst.jpg.

10.3.1. Types and Classification of Choledochal Cysts

Classification of choledochal cysts lies at the center of the implication of their clinical relevance and the choice of successful surgical interventions. The most widely embraced classification is that by Todani, categorizing them into five types based on anatomical features and morphological patterns. Type I cysts are characterized by cystic dilation of the common bile duct and are the most common type, while Type II are choledochal diverticula. Type III, or choledochoceles, are at the level of the duodenum and can influence pancreatic function due to their close relationship with the pancreatic duct. Type IV is seen as multiple cysts within the intrahepatic and extrahepatic bile ducts, while Type V, or Caroli disease, is seen as congenital dilatation of the intrahepatic ducts. Identifying these classifications enables treatment modalities to be tailor-made for each patient by health professionals, enhancing patient results and mitigating biliary-related morbidity from such disorders, as identified in discussion for these anomalies in literature (Tüysüz, 2023). The clinical significance of choledochal cysts is not limited to their classification; they have several severe complications, including cholangitis, pancreatitis, and biliary malignancies. One key characteristic of management is the recognition of the existence of PBM—a condition where the pancreatic duct and the biliary tree meet at an abnormal angle. The abnormal convergence is significant because it has been found to result in carcinogenesis of the biliary tree in patients with choledochal cysts, showing a clear connection between malformation and potential for malignancy. Their assessment is typically by imaging modalities such as ultrasonography, MRCP, and, based on the case, nuclear HIDA scanning. These testing modalities are instrumental in determining the extent of biliary involvement and PBM presence, which determines the appropriateness of surgical treatment (Tüysüz, 2023). Surgical treatment of choledochal cysts is mainly dictated by cyst type, PBM presence, and the patient's overall health status. The Todani classification determines surgery planning, with resection of the ill bile ducts and anastomosis to the intestine being the usual first choice in Type I and Type IV cysts. In the event that PBM happens, more aggressive techniques can be used for the purpose of possibly avoiding future complications like secondary malignancy. The operative setting is increasingly minimally invasive, with enhanced laparoscopic expertise providing promising results in terms of recovery and reduced morbidity. The drawbacks of left-behind intrapancreatic choledochal cysts also underscore the importance of complete surgical assessment, as remnants can create significant long-term health issues, revealing the sophistication involved in treating such congenital defects (Tüysüz, 2023).

10.3.2. Diagnostic Imaging Techniques

Diagnostic imaging procedures are at the forefront in treatment and diagnosis of congenital pancreatic abnormalities such as pancreas divisum, annular pancreas, and choledochal cysts. Non-invasive imaging tests such as ultrasound, computed tomography (CT), and magnetic resonance imaging (MRI) allow clinicians to obtain high-resolution images that reveal structural defects. Ultrasound is often the first imaging method due to its safety and effectiveness in early diagnosis, particularly with children. CT offers better visualization and can distinguish between different pancreatic conditions through detailed views of anatomy, thus making surgery easier to plan. MRI with MRCP is invaluable for examination of the pancreatic ductal system and associated biliary structures, and is performed accordingly for the diagnosis of choledochal cysts and pancreatic duct abnormalities, thus allowing subsequent therapeutic planning and interventions. In the decision regarding pancreas divisum, the role of diagnostic imaging is especially crucial. This condition, with the partial failure of fusion of the pancreatic ducts, is typically asymptomatic but may be a cause of recurrent pancreatitis in a small number of patients. Imaging techniques, particularly MRCP, can well outline the anatomy of the pancreatic ducts and identify variations suggestive of divisum. With the uncertain relationship between pancreas divisum and pancreatic disease, as mentioned in literature today, imaging not only assists in the diagnosis but also monitors potential complications like obstruction or pancreatitis (Fogel et al., 2019). Imaging findings need to be interpreted by clinicians alongside clinical symptoms in order to determine the necessity and urgency for intervention, thereby optimizing patient care and management. Their evaluation by imaging diagnosis further underscores their significance in practice. Choledochal cysts, for instance, may lead to obstruction of bile ducts or pancreatitis, for which precise imaging is required to delineate their anatomy and to assess associated risk. Ultrasound establishes the initial overall impression, which is then supplemented by detailed information from CT and MRI on the site and size of the cysts. Similarly, diagnosis of annular pancreas , a condition of infrequent malformation wherein pancreatic tissue envelops the duodenum , can be properly established with imaging modalities able to demonstrate the association between duodenum and the adjacent structures. Because surgical intervention may be necessary in symptomatic cases, the use of extensive imaging is important for diagnosis as well as for planning the surgery, thus improving patient outcomes (Park et al., 2021) (Figure 10.9).

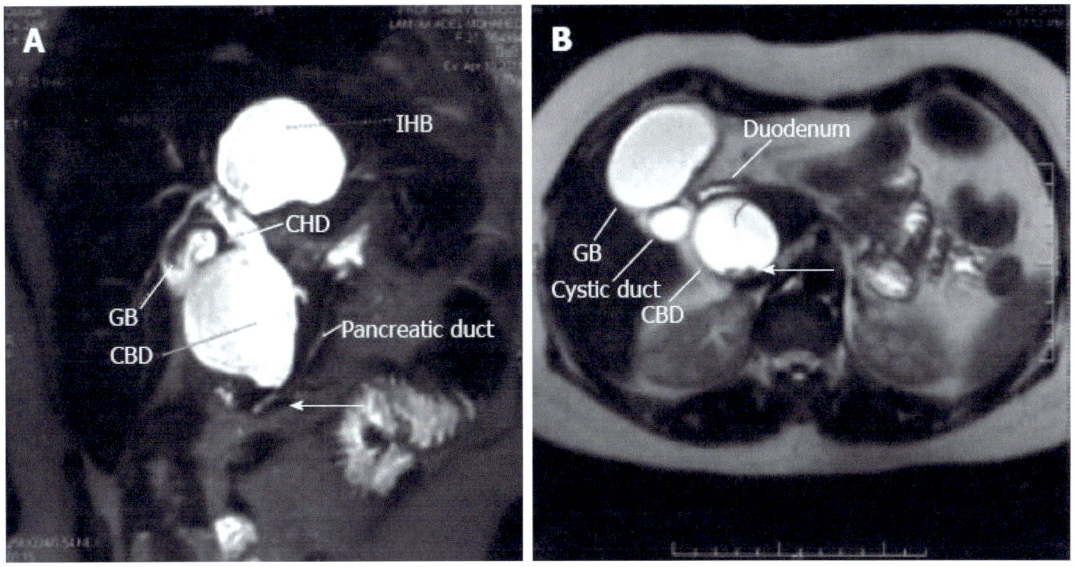

Figure 10.9. Diagnosis and management of choledochal cyst.

Source: https://external-content.duckduckgo.com/iu/?u=https%3A%2F%2Ff6publishing.blob.core.windows.net%2F3d3a966a-67be-4408-a340-3aa92a1b9142%2FWJG-20-7061-g002.jpg&f=1&nofb=1&ipt=84cacd29e27998eb94aa62f38636a261d5635abc523e57e2fac91365aa21b802.

10.3.3. Treatment Strategies and Prognosis

The management options for pancreatic congenital anomalies, specifically pancreas divisum, annular pancreas, and choledochal cysts, are greatly influenced by the degree of symptoms and the characteristics of each anomaly. For example, pancreas divisum, usually asymptomatic, can sometimes never be treated surgically. In symptomatic cases, though, which include recurrent pancreatitis or obstructive symptomatology, endoscopic or surgical intervention can be necessary to allow drainage. An annular pancreas can also lead to duodenal obstruction, necessitating surgical resection or bypass therapy for the relief of gastrointestinal discomfort and prevention of malnutrition. Treatment should be tailored individually, with attention not only to the anatomical defects but also to the overall condition of the patients, which can influence operative success and postoperative recovery. The outcome following surgical treatment of these pancreatic anomalies is likewise generally good but very variable in patients and between individual diseases. For instance, individuals with annular pancreas on operation typically experience excellent relief of symptoms and can regain normal function postoperation. For choledochal cysts, early surgical intervention reduces the risk of subsequent complications such as pancreatitis, cholangitis, or cancer of the biliary tract to provide better long-term outcomes. However, repeated symptoms do occur in some patients, especially with concomitant pancreatic or biliary disease. Therefore, an accurate understanding of potential complications and long-term care is extremely necessary to give optimal patient care, which only makes treatment individualization necessary. New therapeutic strategies and advances in surgical methodology continue to enhance the treatment of pancreatic congenital abnormalities. Current research indicates that minimally invasive surgical methods, like laparoscopic procedures, provide shorter recovery times and reduced rates of complications but without compromising the high level of efficacy. These developments are poised to revolutionize the treatment model, especially for those conditions that previously had to be treated with open surgeries, thereby enhancing the overall patient experience and outcome. Future research and concurrence among operating surgeons will be essential to harmonize these treatment strategies in various institutions, eventually leading to improved prognosis and quality of life for patients with congenital pancreatic anomaly (Park et al., 2021).

10.4. Clinical Significance of Congenital Anomalies

Congenital pancreatic abnormalities, such as pancreas divisum, annular pancreas, and choledochal cysts, are of significant clinical relevance as they can have a potential effect on the function of the pancreas as well as the overall health of the patient. The presence of such abnormalities ruptures the anatomy and physiology of the gastrointestinal tract and can lead to a variety of complications, such as pancreatitis, obstructive jaundice, or even malignancy. For instance, pancreas divisum, which is characterized by failure of pancreatic ducts to unite, is recognized as the most prevalent congenital pancreas anomaly but whose clinical relevance remains questioned. While generally asymptomatic in the majority of cases, recent studies have considered an apparent role in the pathogenesis of recurrent acute pancreatitis, thus warranting attention in meticulous assessment in the clinical presentation of patients with unclear pancreatic symptoms (Fogel et al., 2019). In the setting of clinical diagnosis and care, the nuances of each pancreatic anomaly must be appreciated. Annular pancreas, for example, is secondary to the abnormal rotation of the ventral and dorsal pancreatic buds during embryogenesis and can lead to duodenal obstruction in infancy. Its presentation will most likely necessitate surgical correction to reverse and restore normal gastrointestinal function. Similarly, choledochal cysts or bile duct cystic dilations will cause such complications as cholangitis and biliary cirrhosis unless they are treated. Both of these diseases illustrate the importance of early diagnosis and treatment, since early surgical treatment has a greatly improved outcome. The advancement in imaging modalities and surgical techniques remains key to the management of these congenital anomalies, thereby optimizing patient outcomes and prognoses (Park et al., 2021). Additionally, ongoing debate regarding the clinical relevance of these congenital anomalies spurs ongoing research and interprofessional interaction. The nature of congenital pancreatic anomalies necessitates profound understanding that transcends several medical disciplines, e.g., surgery, gastroenterology, and radiology. Current literature, e.g., for pancreas divisum, suggests growing interest in its description in relation to pancreatic disease and evaluation of potential management, although agreement has yet to be achieved (Fogel et al., 2019). As more information is released, particularly through collaborative efforts from the medical community, the expectation is to have clear guidelines and treatment protocols established. These developments will lead to improved quality care being provided to patients and form the foundation for subsequent educational models in fellowship programs, where up-and-coming surgeons and clinicians will be properly equipped to handle such complex cases (Park et al., 2021) (Figure 10.10).

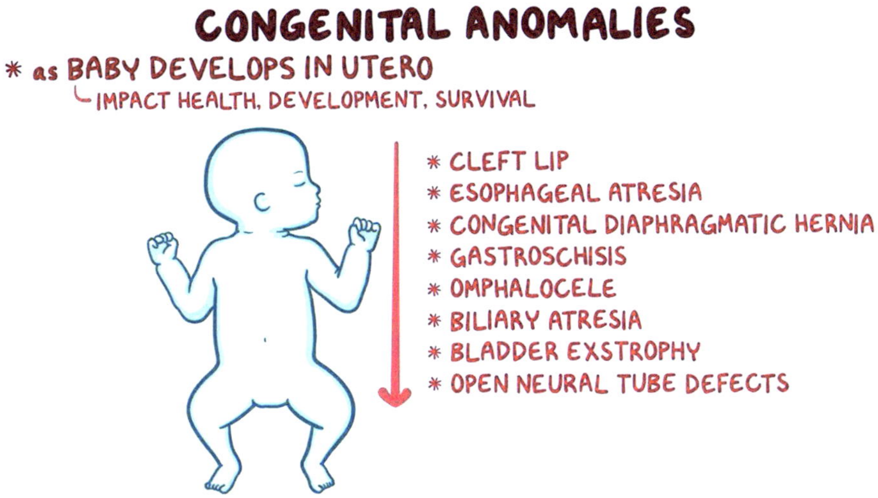

Figure 10.10. Clinical significance of congenital anomalies.

Source: https://external-content.duckduckgo.com/iu/?u=https%3A%2F%2Fosmose-it.s3.amazonaws.com%2FbcSAJX3gTrSDjk-Yg4SkvCGyQ_u-CZ2y%2F_.jpg&f=1&nofb=1&ipt=d1233bcd094cd218659762841b7b8c7f17560658a99c7a6482d19e21700b9e54.

10.4.1. Impact on Digestive Health

The digestive function of patients with congenital anomalies of the pancreas is frequently compromised, and this may lead to a broad range of gastrointestinal abnormalities. Pancreas divisum, annular pancreas, and choledochal cysts may block the normal course of digestive enzymes and bile, leading to malabsorption, recurring abdominal pain, and pancreatitis. For example, in pancreas divisum, the inability of pancreatic secretions to be well-drained by the major duct can cause raised pressure and inflammation and lead to chronic pain and gastrointestinal disorders. The significance of these gastrointestinal problems is further increased within pediatric populations, where early intervention and management are crucial for ensuring growth and development. Without appropriate surgical options, as well as individualized management plans, patients are at risk for long-term consequences on their GI function and quality of life (Krishnan et al., 2016). More fundamentally beyond the necessity for surgery of GI complications of these pancreatic abnormalities is a comprehensive strategy involving the observation and management of related GI conditions such as gastroesophageal reflux and intolerance to feeds. Such patients have been found to complain of reduced quality of life according to repeated symptoms and restrictions in diet. Literature has emphasized the importance of a well-designed strategy for gastrointestinal treatment in children with congenital defects with special attention to continuity of care in transitioning into adolescence and adulthood. Proper dietetic advice, methods of feeding, and symptom management are required in order to safeguard such patients against the adverse effect on their nutrition level and overall health, further justifying the need for a multidisciplinary care pattern in the treatment of such cases. Moreover, ensuring psychological welfare through regular medical checkup and adequate counseling is still the paramount in combating the multidimensional effect of congenital pancreatic anomalies on digestive health. It is only logical that patients would be apprehensive about food limitation, the uncertainty of gastrointestinal symptoms, and the risk involved in potential surgical interventions. With the provision of a health care setting that encourages openness and empowers patients, clinical practitioners can play a significant role in mitigating the psychological burden of chronic gastrointestinal disorders. The ongoing development of evidence-based guidelines, as documented in the study by specialists in the management of gastrointestinal complications, is an important step towards creating structured care pathways to enhance digestive health outcomes in patients with congenital pancreatic anomalies (Krishnan et al., 2016).

10.4.2. Association with Other Congenital Conditions

The association of congenital anomalies of the pancreas, such as pancreas divisum, annular pancreas, and choledochal cysts, with other congenital anomalies can yield important data on the etiology and clinical implications of these anomalies. Pancreas divisum, the most frequent among them, is proven to be one of the potential factors in the development of pancreatic disease, whereas recent studies present contradictory results on the presence of this association. Interestingly, while most of the people are without symptoms, there is some evidence in a few studies to indicate an association between pancreas divisum and conditions like recurrent acute pancreatitis, i.e., there would be a need for additional research to establish the underlying pathophysiology that would link such anomalies with broader clinical presentations (Fogel et al., 2019). Clarification of such associations could lead to more effective therapeutic interventions and delineate shared embryologic pathways responsible for both pancreatic malformations and such concomitant associated congenital defects. Similarly, annular pancreas, where pancreatic tissue encircles the duodenum, has been linked with other gastrointestinal defects like duodenal atresia and other midgut defects. Annular pancreas is usually found in association with other congenital syndromes, and it is also conceivable that this is part of a spectrum of developmental defects and not an isolated phenomenon. A careful observation of annular pancreas patients typically identifies associated disorders like Down syndrome and congenital heart disease, emphasizing the influence of genetic and environmental factors during embryogenesis.

The association between annular pancreas and these congenital defects complicates clinical management in these patients by necessitating a multidisciplinary strategy to treat the pancreatic anomaly along with its potential systemic implications. Choledochal cysts, a significant congenital pancreatic anomaly, are associated with a number of syndromic disorders, including Caroli disease and cystic fibrosis. Complications of pancreatitis and cholangitis may occur secondary to the cysts, further complicating the clinical picture. Coexistence of choledochal cysts with other congenital lesions requires screening and evaluation of affected patients on a large scale since the association can affect prognosis and management. For instance, the finding of a choledochal cyst in childhood may lead to looking for syndromic associations when presenting symptoms or supporting clinical findings suggest extension beyond the regional lesion. Recognition of these associations is valuable to the practitioner because early diagnosis and treatment could significantly alter disease course in patients with congenital lesions of the pancreas, as well as improve overall health outcomes (Figure 10.11).

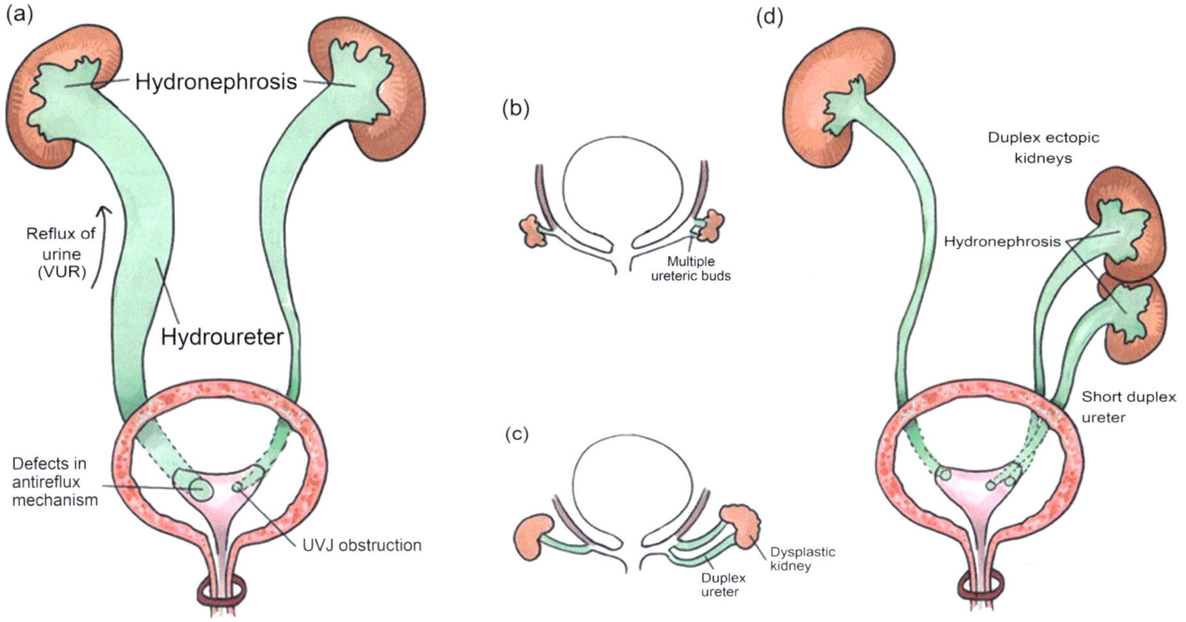

Figure 10.11. Common congenital anomalies of the ureter.

Source: https://www.researchgate.net/profile/Hila-Milo-Rasouly/publication/235621569/figure/fig4/AS:267892004487188@1440881839623/Common-congenital-anomalies-of-the-ureter-a-Two-main-causes-of-hydronephrosis-and.png.

10.4.3. Long-Term Health Implications

The long-term health effects concerning congenital anomalies of the pancreas, such as pancreas divisum and annular pancreas, are immense and multifaceted. They can disrupt normal pancreatic function and lead to other gastrointestinal issues. For example, pancreas divisum can impair ductal drainage and recur with episodes of abdominal pain and pancreatitis. Over time, such attacks can lead to the development of chronic pancreatitis, which means recurrent inflammation, that gradually impairs pancreatic function and thereby induces diabetes mellitus. The long-term health of such patients may, therefore, be compromised, as they are at risk of both metabolic illness as well as pancreatic malignancy in adulthood. It is therefore crucial to have knowledge of these implications during the management and follow-up of the patient. In assessing the long-term outcome in choledochal cyst patients, not only should one consider the primary surgical interventions but also the possibility of post-surgical complications developing. Though surgical resection can arrest symptoms and prevent ensuing bile duct obstruction, with advancing age, the risk of cholangiocarcinoma emerges significantly. Series have demonstrated that early intervention plays a critical role in preventing such an occurrence, but long-term follow-up is nonetheless required. Recurrent imaging and monitoring may be necessary to detect malignancy at an earlier, more manageable stage. Patients may also suffer from complications related to recurrent pancreatitis—

most commonly obstructive at the pancreatic duct—resulting from prolonged biliary obstruction or postoperative complications. Effective overall care planning is thus necessary in managing short-term as well as long-term health effects in such patients. In addition to the immediate complications of congenital pancreatic abnormalities, patients are also saddled with broader psychosocial impacts from chronic illness. The frequent medical interventions, hospitalizations, and dietary modifications necessitated by disease like chronic pancreatitis may strain mental well-being and quality of life. Furthermore, an increased rate of depression and anxiety has been observed in long-standing gastrointestinal illness patients. These psychological factors can exacerbate physical disease, leading to a vicious cycle of deteriorating wellbeing. Effective management strategies must incorporate mental attention alongside treatment of the physical, acknowledging that long-term consequences for health of pancreatic congenital malformations encompass more than clinical presentation but also emotional and psychological strength in an individual. Addressing these various dimensions of health is essential in providing holistic care to patients with such long-term diseases.

10.5. Surgical Options for Management

Surgical interventions are of utmost importance in congenital anomalies of the pancreas, particularly in disorders such as pancreas divisum, annular pancreas, and choledochal cysts. Pancreas divisum, although generally asymptomatic, can lead to significant clinical implications, like recurrent pancreatitis. Therapies for this typically include treatment of the minor papilla, i.e., decompression of the obstructed minor papilla where pancreas divisum is anatomically divided. In the absence of ultimate evidence of effectiveness relative to other treatment modalities, consideration needs to be given to the individual patient's expectation and clinical context. Recent literature has emphasized the mysterious role of pancreas divisum in pancreatic disease and suggests that more research is required to balance surgical management with individualized requirements, with diligent preoperative discussion and assessment emphasized (Fogel et al., 2019). Annular pancreas is a congenital defect in which pancreatic tissue encircles the duodenum and shows certain challenges during surgery. The defect will lead to obstruction of the duodenum, with initial symptoms of bilious vomiting and failure to thrive, especially among infants. Surgical procedures for it typically involve either pyloroplasty or duodenoduodenostomy aimed at relieving the obstruction and ensuring normal gastrointestinal function. In cases of high risk for pancreatic damage or for malnutrition, more extensive operations may be necessary. As annular pancreas pathophysiology continues to be better understood, other variables such as the presence of concomitant anomalies will also play a role in surgical decision-making. Ultimately, however, the procedure must then be considered individualized, making use of both the anatomic rules and the patient's physiological needs in order to provide optimal outcomes. Choledochal cysts with cystic dilatation of the bile duct represent a surgical challenge. The definitive procedure is cyst removal with hepaticoenterostomy, or liver transplantation in carefully selected cases, if there is a severe impairment of the liver or cirrhosis of the biliary tree. Surgery not only prevents symptom alleviation but also prevents later complications such as recurrent pancreatitis and cholangiocarcinoma. Although the typical triad of presentation—pain, mass, and jaundice, is not typically present, imaging does have to take an important role in guiding treatment and diagnosis. Because there is a risk for recurrence and also associated complications with choledochal cysts, patients require life-long follow-up, and this actually emphasizes the importance of having a good surgical plan that includes follow-up and management of any potential postoperative complications (Torres et al., 2022) (Figure 10.12).

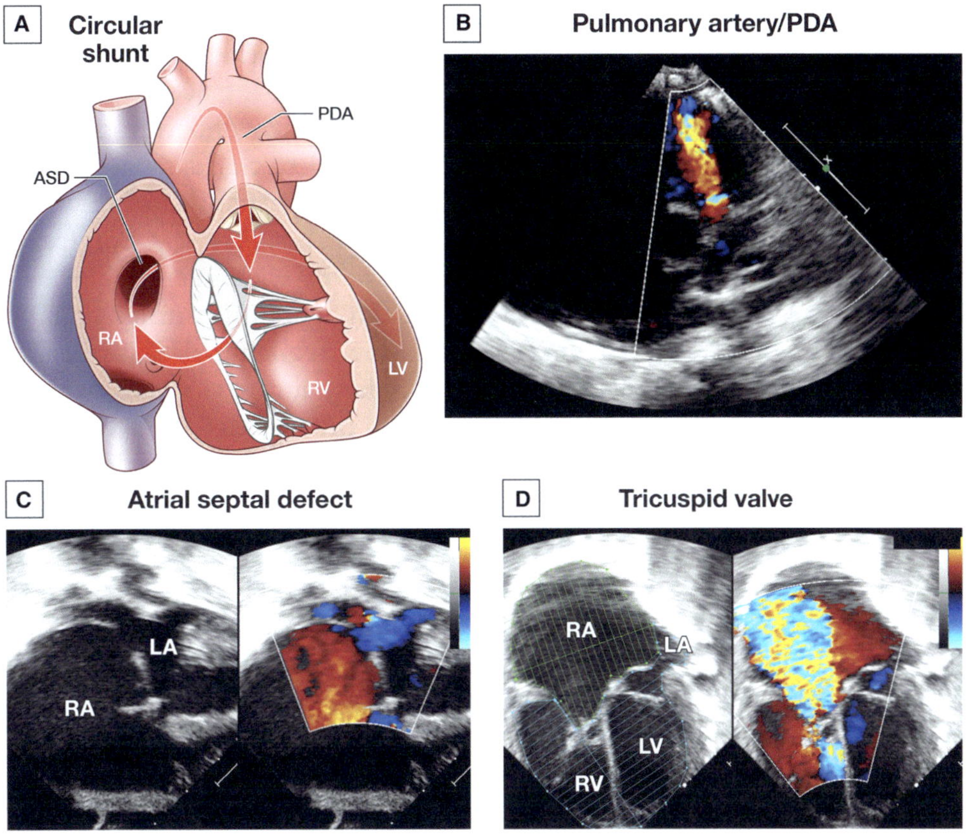

Figure 10.12. Surgical management of neonatal Ebstein anomaly with a circular shunt.

Source: https://www.jtcvs.org/cms/attachment/eca279e4-20b7-4bd1-b387-03d69748c8dc/gr1_lrg.jpg.

10.5.1. Indications for Surgical Intervention

Where congenital anomalies of the pancreas are concerned, the decision to proceed to surgery is frequently made on the basis of symptom severity and overall impact on the function of the pancreas.

In diseases such as pancreas divisum, the most common congenital anomaly, the majority of patients are asymptomatic. Yet, patients with recurrent acute pancreatitis or chronic pancreatitis can be benefited by surgery to reduce pain or prevent ongoing pancreatic injury. Doubts about the etiologic role of pancreas divisum require careful consideration of the individual's clinical setting since operative indications rely heavily on the presence of symptomatic disease rather than the anomaly. Current literature indicates that treatment, including minor papilla therapy, may be helpful but does not have a clear course of management (Fogel et al., 2019). Annular pancreas is typically treated surgically due to the risk for duodenal obstruction. Patients who present with bilious vomiting, abdominal distension, or failure to gain weight typically require surgery. Surgical intervention is usually duodenoduodenostomy or bypass to reestablish gastrointestinal tract continuity. Early diagnosis and treatment are critical to avoid severe complications like perforation and pancreatitis if the annular pancreas is not treated. The complexity of the anomaly emphasizes how careful consideration of the surgical approaches most appropriate for each patient's specific anatomical presentation needs to be taken. By removing the obstruction early, surgeons can prevent potential long-term sequelae of this congenital anomaly, validating the role of surgical intervention in optimized patient results (Park et al., 2021). Choledochal cysts are a condition where surgery is absolutely indicated. These congenital dilatation abnormalities of the biliary tract are complicated by such things as cholangitis, pancreatitis, and malignancy risk. Surgical management is typically aimed at cyst removal and reconstructive surgery, which re-establishes normal bile drainage and limits the frequency of complications. The timing of intervention is important; early surgical correction has improved results and decreases the frequency of severe complications in the long term. Therefore, clinicians must also be very vigilant during the diagnosis and treatment of choledochal cysts so that they can initiate early surgical intervention, thus enhancing the long-term welfare and health of those afflicted by this anomaly. This necessity underscores the central role of surgical procedures in medical care for congenital pancreatic anomalies (Park et al., 2021).

10.5.2. Common Surgical Procedures

Surgery remains an integral component of the management of congenital pancreatic anomalies, particularly in pancreas divisum, annular pancreas, and choledochal cysts. Every one of these anomalies presents with specific surgical challenges as well as personalized techniques for avoiding adverse effects and optimal outcomes. For instance, in pancreas divisum, where the ductal system does not normally unite but results in impaired drainage, surgical intervention typically includes pancreatic ductal stenting or accessory papilla sphincterotomy. Both of these interventions are intended to improve pancreatic drainage and prevent recurrent pancreatitis, a condition that is common in individuals with this congenital anomaly (Sajith et al., 2008). By correcting the primary anatomical defect, surgeons can significantly alleviate the long-term consequences of this congenital abnormality. In the case of annular pancreas, where the pancreas encircles the duodenum, surgical approaches are more extensive due to the risk of obstructive signs like biliary colic and duodenal obstruction. The most appropriate procedure generally includes corrective operations like duodenoduodenostomy or duodenojejunostomy with the focus to resolve such symptoms and restore gastrointestinal continuity. Cautiousness is essential because poorly performed surgical procedures lead to complications like pancreatitis, bowel obstruction, or even nutritional deficiency. Decision-making in such cases must weigh the need for symptom relief against the potential for subsequent complications due to surgical intervention (Sajith et al., 2008). To this end, a properly planned surgical intervention is crucial to enhancing the quality of life of annular pancreas patients. Furthermore, choledochal cysts, being a cystic dilatation of the bile duct, necessitate surgical treatment to prevent issues such as cholangitis, pancreatitis, or malignancy. The standard surgical treatment for choledochal cysts is complete resection of the cyst and bile duct reconstruction for drainage into the duodenum. There are numerous surgical techniques, including Roux-en-Y hepaticojejunostomy, that have gained more prominence due to their efficacy in preventing recurrence and complications. Surgical management not only addresses the immediate danger of the anomaly but also prevents future pancreatitis and other biliary disease from retained biliary sludge and stagnant bile (Singh et al., 2023). Therefore, proper surgical management is essential for the treatment of choledochal cysts and its complication (Figure 10.13).

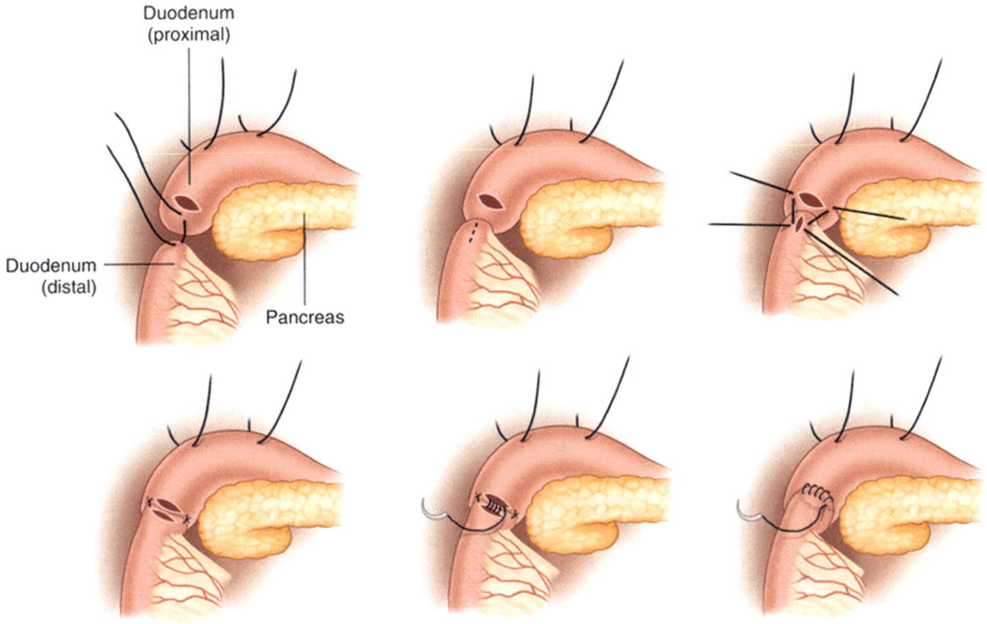

Figure 10.13. Duodenal Atresia Repair.

Source: https://i0.wp.com/thoracickey.com/wp-content/uploads/2017/06/A272754_1_En_20_Fig16_HTML.gif?fit=823%2C517&ssl=1.

10.5.3. Postoperative Care and Follow-Up

Appropriate postoperative care and follow-up are essential aspects of managing pancreas congenital anomalies such as pancreas divisum, annular pancreas, and choledochal cysts. Postoperative observation is essential in the detection of early signs of potential complications like infection, surgical site complications, or pancreas insufficiency. Follow-up visits allow healthcare providers to assess recovery to ensure patients are able to regain normal pancreatic function. For instance, in pancreas divisum, which may lead to recurring abdominal pain or pancreatitis, postoperative evaluations must include imaging scans to evaluate the patency of the ductal systems and determine whether there is residual issue. Prevention of complications is of paramount importance in improving long-term results because these anomalies predispose patients to severe health consequences if not managed correctly during the postoperative period. Apart from routine evaluation, imaging plays an important role in postoperative follow-up of children who have had pancreatic surgery. Through methods such as ultrasound, CT, and MRI, clinicians can monitor the structural integrity of the pancreas and detect complications early before they become life-threatening. Owing to the high sensitivity and specificity of these imaging techniques, particularly in children, they pave the way for early intervention and adjustment of postoperative care regimens, as necessary. Most notable is the utilization of MRI and ultrasound due to them being non-ionizing, thus reducing radiation dosage to the young patient. This emphasis on careful imaging and follow-up comes with the study of the significance of ensuring appropriate postoperative assessment, again pointing to the success that comes with proper follow-up and ensuing quality of life and clinical results in patients with congenital pancreatic abnormalities (Nievelstein et al., 2010). Further, patient and family education and communication form critical elements of postoperative care. Family education about the nature of the congenital anomaly, the surgical procedure performed, and possible postoperative complications prepares them to recognize warning signs that require immediate medical intervention. Nutritional counseling is also critical following pancreatic surgery, particularly for conditions like choledochal cysts where biliary function can be compromised. Proper dietary management may diminish postoperative symptoms and hasten recovery. Open communication can enable professionals to support the families in the recovery process more efficiently. This combined method emphasizes the complexity of the management of pancreatic congenital anomalies and the necessity of comprehensive follow-up measures to maximize optimal patient outcomes, particularly within the advanced postoperative setting (Johansson, 2023).

10.6. Case Studies and Clinical Outcomes

Clinical outcome assessment of congenital pancreas anomalies is the top priority for the improvement of patient care and operation. An illustrative case of pancreas divisum demonstrates the complexity in clinical decision-making. Although pancreas divisum is the most common congenital malformation of the pancreas, most patients are asymptomatic, which makes it hard to realize its clinical significance. Evidence suggests a potential pathogenic role in recurrent acute and chronic pancreatitis, but this view is not shared (Fogel et al., 2019). There is a need for therapeutic intervention, thus, minor papilla therapy and surgery, to be individualized based on individual patients based on their individual clinical presentation. Moreover, extensive deliberations on the advantage and disadvantage of intervention are required as there is no evidence from literature of a single treatment plan for pancreas divisum-related pancreatic disorders. Case studies are useful in gaining insights into the clinical importance and treatment methods in the instance of annular pancreas and choledochal cysts. For instance, annular pancreas can cause duodenal obstruction and require surgical drainage to remove symptoms and prevent complications. The nature of the anomaly demands comprehensive preoperative assessment, typically cross-sectional imaging to better delineate anatomy. Choledochal cysts and management are deserving of study due to the possibility of malignant transformation over time. Literature indicates a clear correlation between cyst type, size, and onset of subsequent cholangiocarcinoma (Johansson, 2023). The surgical procedure, either by excision and reconstruction or alternative techniques, is determined based on cysts' characteristics, with a focus on the importance of an equitable response to every case based on both existing clinical evidence as well as future potential. To enhance knowledge of congenital anomalies of the pancreas, ongoing research of case studies and clinical outcomes is necessary. Observation of intraductal papillary mucinous neoplasm (IPMN) shows significant clinical observations that may be related to other anomalies. Current data indicate that IPMN patients with anatomical ductal abnormalities, such as meandering main pancreatic duct, are at increased risk of having associated complications, suggesting recognisable patterns that may alter clinical management (Johansson, 2023). Long-term follow-up of these patients accentuates the imperative to establish robust surveillance protocols to monitor the evolution of pancreatic disease. Such observations reconfirm the multifaceted character of congenital malformations and the imperative to follow up with tailored management plans based on accretive clinical information and case study evidence. By enhancing communication between multidisciplinary teams, congenital pancreatic abnormalities can be made much better, guiding those who have possibly harmful conditions into effective and timely treatments (Figure 10.14).

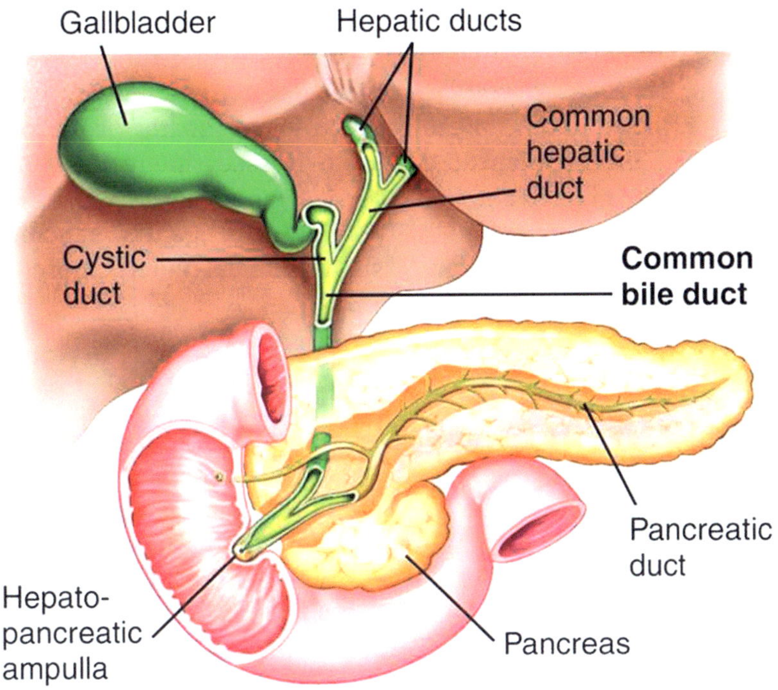

Figure 10.14. Cholangiocarcinoma development of the pancreas.

Source: https://www.creative-biolabs.com/vaccine/images/Cholangiocarcinoma-Vaccines.jpg.

10.6.1. Review of Notable Case Studies

The study of congenital pancreatic anomalies through representative case studies provides valuable information towards the understanding of the clinical significance and surgical treatment of disorders such as pancreas divisum, annular pancreas, and choledochal cysts. One such interesting case study of pancreas divisum had a patient with recurrent acute pancreatitis despite the fact that the disorder is the most common congenital anomaly of the pancreas. This case brought to the limelight the debate about the relationship between pancreas divisum and pancreatic disease, as delineated by existing literature that has struggled to arrive at a cause-and-effect determination (Fogel et al., 2019). The question of the treatment for this patient underscored the importance of personalized medical consultation, pointing out that procedures may vary based on the specific patient parameters and expectations. Equally, landmark case histories of annular pancreas have similarly consolidated the potentiality of ancillary complications like intestinal obstruction and pancreatitis. In a particular case, an infant with this condition was operated upon, which would reveal the intricate nature of this pancreatic anomaly within a clinical context. These cases indicate the importance of early diagnosis coupled with expeditious treatment in order to forestall drastic consequences like malnutrition and failure to thrive. Moreover, the surgical options frequently hinge on the patients age and general condition, thus making it more complex for healthcare practitioners to make an informed decision. The implications drawn from these case studies make it imperative that there be a multidisciplinary approach so as to effectively treat not just the congenital anomalies but also the resultant conditions that follow. Further, choledochal cysts are another exceedingly common congenital anomaly that deserves close scrutiny through such landmark case studies. The treatment of choledochal cysts has evolved extensively over time, from conservative to aggressive surgical intervention. A striking case brought into focus the successful laparoscopic removal of the cyst, a technique that came into widespread practice due to its noninvasive nature and superior recovery pattern. Besides, investigation of the case provided further proof to the use of imaging modalities such as PET/CT and sophisticated radiologic assessments in accurate diagnosis and formulating surgical strategies for such anomalies. Moving ahead into further discussions regarding individualized case study analysis of notable cases in other congenital pancreatic anomalies, it is obvious that treatment strategies developed based on full clinical understanding are most important for the aim of enhancing patient outcomes and care.

10.6.2. Analysis of Treatment Effectiveness

The evaluation of the effectiveness of treatment of pancreas abnormalities during the congenital period, such as pancreas divisum, is not facilitated by variability of the conditions' clinical presentation. Pancreas divisum, the most common congenital pancreatic malformation, is typically asymptomatic and therefore presents challenges in proving its clinical significance and necessity for treatment. Current literature indicates there is no general agreement concerning pancreas divisum and other pancreatic illnesses, particularly recurrent pancreatitis. Therapeutic management in the form of minor papilla treatment has been considered helpful in some patients with recurrent acute pancreatitis, but the evidence is not in total agreement since treatment effectiveness is questionable (Fogel et al., 2019). This dilemma underscores the need for individual patient assessment, where cure may be largely dependent upon unique clinical circumstances. In annular pancreas, treatment through surgery is normally called for due to duodenal obstruction and resultant complications. Surgical interventions most frequently employed are duodenojejunostomy or bypass operations, which decompress the obstructing encircling pancreatic tissue. Effectiveness of these interventions is often well-established; however, long-term outcomes may vary based on the surgical technique used, and overall health of the patient. Rehabilitation following surgery is imperative, with direct implications for rates of recovery and functional status. As suggested by recent reports, while the short-term outcome of surgery in annular pancreas is usually excellent, follow-up and management of complications such as malabsorption and pancreatic insufficiency must remain a priority. Multidisciplinary effort is required to ascertain the overall success of the treatment regime in patients with these anomalies. Choledochal cysts too are a congenital anomaly for which separate analysis regarding the success of treatment is warranted. Surgical removal of the cyst, usually in the form of a Roux-en-Y hepaticojejunostomy, is the preferred treatment method and has yielded encouraging success rates. Complications do occasionally occur, though, including cholangitis or secondary biliary cirrhosis, even following successful surgical treatment. The efficacy of treatment in the alleviation of choledochal cysts also relies on early diagnosis and timely treatment, which will notably decrease the risk of long-term complications. Current studies highlight a significant correlation between timing of operative intervention and overall health outcome in affected patients, with the suggestion that delayed treatment might adversely affect efficacy and prognostic outcomes. Continued evaluation through follow-up therapy is crucial for understanding long-term effectiveness of procedures employed in choledochal cyst treatment and for directing future therapeutic protocols (Fogel et al., 2019) (Figure 10.15).

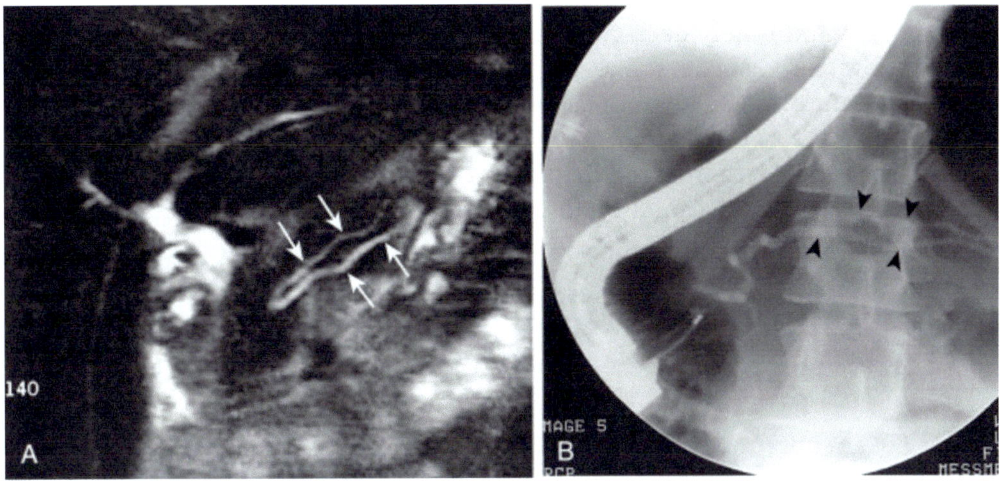

Figure 10.15. Anomalies and anatomic variants of the pancreas.

Source: https://external-content.duckduckgo.com/iu/?u=https%3A%2F%2Fi0.wp.com%2Fradiologykey.com%2Fwp-content%2Fuploads%2F2019%2F06%2Ff096-010ab-9781455751174.jpg%3Fw%3D960&f=1&nofb=1&ipt=cfc23b7683e65e6ca3ea86b7719fab0e7fce8dceed943250c1576e7adaaec11d.

10.6.3. Lessons Learned from Clinical Experiences

Clinical practice provides valuable lessons that enable understanding and control of congenital anomalies of the pancreas, such as pancreas divisum, annular pancreas, and choledochal cysts. These are usually conditions that need a multidisciplinary intervention, an aspect emphasizing cooperation between pediatricians, surgeons, and radiologists. For instance, in pancreas divisum, evidence shows that its association with spells of pancreatitis emphasizes the importance of careful follow-up and early interventions. It is crucial to be able to recognize such complications; clinical evidence indicates that recurrent abdominal pain patients can be benefited by early imaging investigations to avoid severe consequences from untreated illness. As noted, necrosis and infection complications of acute pancreatitis have high mortality and morbidity, thus acute recognition and strategic management are necessary (Rodrigo Sáez et al., 2025). The surgical corrective options that can be used for congenital pancreatic anomalies must similarly be done with a solid understanding of the clinical implications imposed by these abnormalities. In particular, treatment of choledochal cysts is more focused on individualized interventions aimed at each patient's unique presentation. Clinical experience reveals that numerous choledochal cysts will become malignant unless intervened upon, thus necessitating immediate intervention. Surgeons not only learn from the operation technique but also from the outcome of what they have determined, and their methods become better with time. Constant monitoring of the outcome of surgery enhances the best practice in the management of such anomalies and enhances the overall patient outcome and success of the surgery (National Birth Defects Prevention Network Surveillance Guidelines and Standards Committee, 2025). Also, practice lessons of clinical experience extend beyond direct patient care to the significance of comprehensive birth defects surveillance systems. The surveillance guidelines organizations such as the National Birth Defects Prevention Network have adopted are evidence of prioritization of high-quality data in order to acquire better knowledge of congenital anomalies.

By promoting accurate and timely data collection, such systems allow exploration of the etiologic and preventive factors for disorders like the annular pancreas. Experience in clinical practice informs the development of these guidelines, underscoring the need for consistent definitions and methods in birth defects surveillance. In applying these lessons to medical practice, the medical community advocates for growth in early diagnosis, treatment practice, and patient management of congenital pancreatic disease (National Birth Defects Prevention Network Surveillance Guidelines and Standards Committee, 2025).

A CLOSER LOOK

A RARE CONGENITAL ANOMALY OF THE PANCREAS

It is a rare congenital anomaly of pancrease that comprises annular pancreas, a developmental condition where pancreatic tissue encircles the second part of duodenum and may result in varied grades of duodenal obstruction. It results from premature incomplete rotation or misplacement of the ventral pancreatic bud during embryogenesis. Though it may be diagnosed in the neonate with duodenal obstruction symptoms—bilious vomiting, feed intolerance, or failure to thrive—most only come to be diagnosed as adults, when they have abdominal pain, nausea, vomiting, pancreatitis, or even duodenal ulcers. Some people may be asymptomatic, and the anomaly is discovered by chance on imaging or surgery for other reasons. Radiologic studies like upper gastrointestinal series can show a characteristic "double bubble" in neonates or duodenal stenosis in adults. CT and MRI can detect pancreatic tissue encircling the duodenum, but more detailed imaging may be required by endoscopic ultrasound (EUS) or MRCP. Annular pancreas can also be associated with other congenital anomalies, e.g., Down syndrome, tracheoesophageal fistula, or congenital heart disease. Treatment is determined by symptom severity. Symptomatic cases rarely require treatment, while symptomatic duodenal obstruction generally requires treatment in the form of surgical bypassing maneuvers such as duodenojejunostomy or gastrojejunostomy, rather than resection of the overlying pancreatic tissue to avoid pancreatic injury. In adults, if annular pancreas causes chronic pancreatitis or obstructive symptoms, treatment can be more complex and tailored based on the patient's clinical condition. Although rare, knowledge of annular pancreas is critical to surgeons, gastroenterologists, and radiologists since its presentation variability can imitate other gastrointestinal disease, and it is essential to make accurate diagnosis to avoid unnecessary procedures or inappropriate treatment. This anomaly depicts the richness of embryologic development and how it impacts gastrointestinal anatomy and physiology (Figure 10.16).

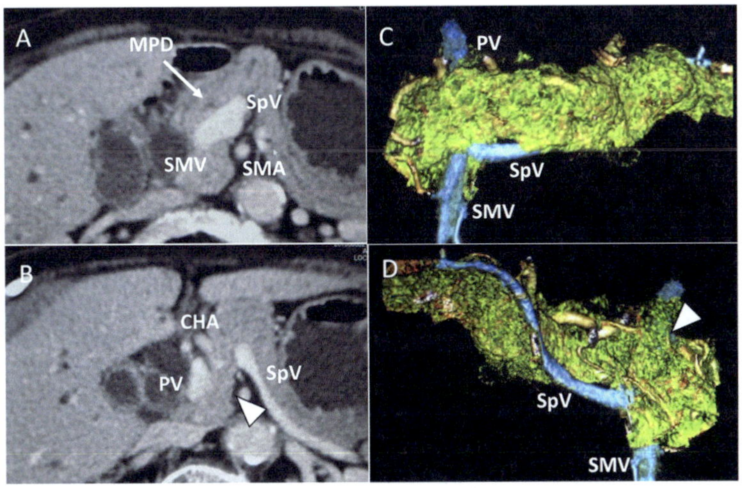

Source: https://www.americanjournalofsurgery.com/cms/10.1016/j.amjsurg.2016.11.018/asset/26a66529-096e-4336-86e3-8f0ce748db2b/main.assets/gr2_lrg.jpg.

SUMMARY

The study of congenital anomalies of the pancreas, including pancreas divisum, annular pancreas, and choledochal cysts, discloses that each condition presents unique challenges in diagnosis and treatment. The pancreatic anomalies have significant clinical effects, and timely and accurate identification is essential to prevent complications. Conditions such as pancreas divisum, whose abdominal pain and pancreatitis recurrence can be prevented if treated, indicate the importance of knowing the anatomy and physiology of the pancreas in clinical practice. The outcome for the afflicted can be radically altered by measures of early intervention, including surgical intervention, and thus doctors must be vigilant in detecting symptoms and likelihood of such abnormalities. In addition, clinical significance of such congenital anomalies cannot be overstated as they are associated with a plethora of complications that will complicate the care of the patients. For example, choledochal cysts are likely to result in biliary obstruction and acute or chronic pancreatitis, conditions with high-risk potential for ensuing pancreatic damage and worsening health status. The differences in the natural histories for the anomalies highlight the value of individualized management in therapy. Particularly, surgical interventions in cases of diseases like annular pancreas may be decisive for preventing severe complications and providing the patient with an improved prognosis. Having knowledge about individual pathways of each disease allows for more individualized treatment programs and improved symptom management. The ramifications of pancreatic congenital anomalies extend far beyond single cases and influence general healthcare dynamics. As diagnostic imaging technology improves, which higher imaging as utilized, increasingly becomes the norm, the identification and characterization of these conditions will be enhanced, and clinical decision-making will be enhanced. Besides, with increasing research uncovering the complexities associated with disease complications such as acute pancreatitis, characterized by varying levels of severity and high mortality rates as described in Rodrigo Sáez et al. (2025), the need for comprehensive management methods becomes apparent. A multi-disciplinary intervention through surgical management, medical treatment, and ongoing research, thus, becomes imperative in addressing complications from such congenital abnormalities. The ultimate goal is to improve patient outcomes and foster healthier pathways among individuals with these diseases.

The research on congenital pancreas abnormalities such as pancreas divisum, annular pancreas, and choledochal cysts brings into focus significant insights into their clinical significance and workings. Pancreas divisum with its dysfunctional ductal system can make the patient prone to chronic pancreatitis due to ineffective drainage of pancreatic enzymes. On the other hand, the annular pancreas, where pancreatic tissue encircles the duodenum, can be linked with gastrointestinal tract obstruction and requires careful surgical process. Choledochal cysts, biliary duct malformations, tend to present in childhood and risk bile duct obstruction and cholangitis. These diseases require knowledge of their embryonic origin to enhance diagnosis and treatment protocols. The clinical environment requires a multidisciplinary approach, incorporating surgical oncology, gastroenterology, and radiology to ensure proper management protocols and improved patient outcomes, highlighting the need for extensive knowledge in congenital pancreatic anomalies (Park et al., 2021). Surgical management is case-dependent depending on the nature of the anomaly and its clinical presentation. In pancreas divisum, endoscopic management in the form of sphincterotomy can be symptom-alleviating in some cases, while more severe cases can consist of surgical bypass or resection. Annular pancreas typically needs duodenoduodenostomy or duodenojejunostomy as corrective surgeries for decompression. On the other hand, choledochal cysts are usually treated by excision of the cyst and biliary tree reconstruction to prevent issues such as malignancy. These surgical interventions, while successful, are fraught with risks of the procedure and are likely to result in postoperative complications that should be watched closely. A full understanding of these surgical options, translated to individual patient needs, is necessary for doctors to effectively handle the issues posed by such congenital defects. The significance of such congenital defects transcends their immediate clinical relevance; they also hold promise for enhancement in surgical education and establishing standards in gastroenterological surgery. The integration of a strong curriculum that addresses these anomalies in hepatopancreatobiliary fellowship training, as recommended by consensus among various professional societies, has the capability to standardize educational output and maximize clinical competency (Park et al., 2021). It not only equips new surgeons with the proficiency to manage such cases effectively but also allows for optimum interdisciplinary collaboration between experts. Through an emphasis on best practices and evidence-based therapeutic approaches, we are empowered to produce more beneficial long-term outcomes for the individuals suffering from such congenital pancreatic abnormalities, solidifying the role of continual education in surgical technique advancement.

KEY TERMS FROM THIS CHAPTER

- Embryology
- Dorsal pancreas
- Annular pancreas
- Ectopic pancreas
- Hypoplasia
- Abnormal rotation
- Biliary obstruction
- Abdominal pain
- Pancreatic buds
- Ventral pancreas
- Pancreas divisum
- Agenesis of pancreas
- Accessory pancreatic duct
- Duodenal obstruction
- Pancreatitis
- Jaundice

References

1. Park, K. M., Rashidian, N., Mohamedaly, S., Brasel, K. J., Conroy, P., Glencer, A. C., He, J., Passeri, M. J., Katariya, N. N., Alseidi, A., & TrainHPB research group (2021). Unifying the Hepatopancreatobiliary Surgery Fellowship Curriculum via Delphi Consensus. *Journal of the American College of Surgeons, 233*(3), 395–414. https://doi.org/10.1016/j.jamcollsurg.2021.06.004 (accessed on 26 May 2025).
2. Torres, M., Becerra, M., Calderón, B., Salinas, I., Ruiz, M., & Ventura, J. (2023). Choledochal Cyst: Clinical Features, Diagnosis and Treatment Perspectives. IntechOpen. doi: 10.5772/intechopen.106451(accessed on 26 May 2025).
3. Beger, H. G., Buchler, M. W., Kozarek, R., Lerch, M. M., Neoptolemos, J. P., Warshaw, A. L., & Whitcomb, D. C., et al. (2009). *The Pancreas*. John Wiley & Sons. https://play.google.com/store/books/details?id=CGhTz-I3S1gC&source=gbs_api (accessed on 26 May 2025).
4. Krishnan, U., Mousa, H., Dall'Oglio, L., Homaira, N., Rosen, R., Faure, C., & Gottrand, F. (2016). ESPGHAN-NASPGHAN Guidelines for the Evaluation and Treatment of Gastrointestinal and Nutritional Complications in Children With Esophageal Atresia-Tracheoesophageal Fistula. *Journal of pediatric gastroenterology and nutrition, 63*(5), 550–570. https://doi.org/10.1097/MPG.0000000000001401
5. Fogel, E., Gutta, A., & Sherman, S. (2019). Identification and management of pancreas divisum. https://core.ac.uk/download/286317809.pdf (accessed on 26 May 2025).
6. Johansson, K. (2023). *Intraductal papillary mucinous neoplasm of the pancreas : a study with magnetic resonance imaging*. Helsingin yliopisto. https://helda.helsinki.fi/bitstream/handle/10138/356294/Johansson_Katarina_dissertation_2023.pdf?sequence=1&isAllowed=y(accessed on 26 May 2025).
7. Karthik, S. B. (2010). *Evaluation of Prognostic Factors in Neonatal Intestinal Obstruction*. https://core.ac.uk/download/235656705.pdf (accessed on 26 May 2025).
8. National Birth Defects Prevention Network Surveillance Guidelines and Standards Committee. (2025). *Guidelines for Conducting Birth Defects Surveillance*. https://core.ac.uk/download/144164626.pdf (accessed on 26 May 2025).
9. Nievelstein, R. A., Robben, S. G., & Blickman, J. G. (2011). Hepatobiliary and pancreatic imaging in children-techniques and an overview of non-neoplastic disease entities. *Pediatric radiology, 41*(1), 55–75. https://doi.org/10.1007/s00247-010-1858-5
10. Sáez, L. R. (2025). *Pancreatitis: Treatment and Complications*. https://core.ac.uk/download/pdf/71823519.pdf (accessed on 26 May 2025).
11. Sajith, K. G. (2008). *Clinical Profile and Genetic Studies in Recurrent Acute Pancreatitis: A Five-Year Study*. https://core.ac.uk/download/235655137.pdf (accessed on 26 May 2025).
12. Singh A, Prakash S, Rustagi SM. Anatomical Description of the Duct System of the Pancreas: A Cadaveric and Magnetic Resonance Cholangiopancreatography Study. Journal of Medical Academics 2022; 5 (1-2):6-11.**DOI:** 10.5005/jp-journals-11003-0119
13. Tüysüz, U. (2023). Characteristics, Diagnosis and Treatment of Choledochal Cysts. IntechOpen. doi: 10.5772/intechopen.109023 (accessed on 26 May 2025).

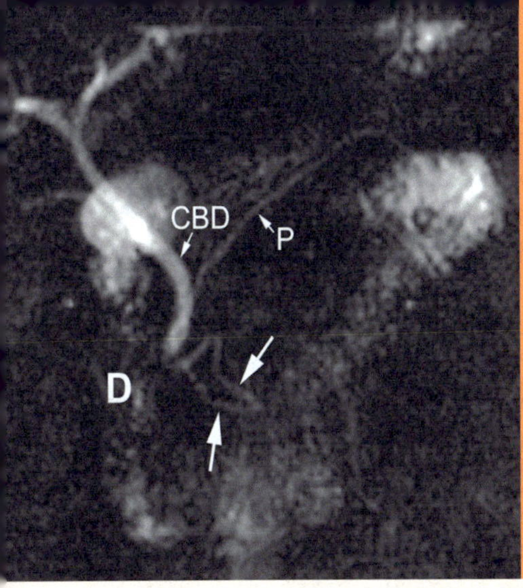

Chapter 11

PANCREATIC DUCTAL ADENOCARCINOMA

Contents

Introduction

Pancreatic ductal adenocarcinoma (PDAC) is a highly aggressive type of metastatic malignancy with a poor prognosis and rising incidence globally. Due to its peculiar pathology, it is challenging to diagnose at the early stage, and patients tend to be at the late stage at presentation, significantly reducing treatment possibilities and survival rates. As a multifactorial disease, PDAC is brought about by various risk factors, from lifestyle choices such as obesity and smoking to genetic dispositions that must be examined in depth. Syndromes with genes, such as Lynch syndrome and hereditary pancreatitis, particularly emphasize the family history in the development of PDAC. With its mortality rate usually outweighing its prevalence, it is essential to map the total scenario of PDAC in order to make clinical practices more optimal and early diagnosis and treatment patterns more efficient. The complexity involved in the diagnosis of pancreatic ductal adenocarcinoma necessitates an interdisciplinary approach to diagnosis that usually incorporates both imaging modalities and histopathological examination. Application of the TNM staging system is crucial in determining the extent of the disease, impacting treatment options from curative surgical interventions to palliative modalities. The system provides a standardized framework to determine the presence of primary tumors (T), lymph node involvement (N), and metastasis (M), which are predictors of overall prognosis for affected patients. Furthermore, technological advances in imaging modalities, such as MRI and endoscopic ultrasound, have enhanced diagnostic accuracy and facilitated greater delineation of tumor characteristics, with new potential for customized treatment regimens. Through this consolidation of staging foundations, health care professionals are aiming to implement timely and effective treatments against this tenacious enemy. With the evolving treatment paradigm for pancreatic ductal adenocarcinoma, it is important that one keeps in mind the dyad between surgery and palliation. Surgical resection is the optimal curative strategy for locally confined PDAC; however, the majority of patients are diagnosed at a stage where surgery cannot be attempted anymore. Palliative care then emerges as an essential second choice, prioritizing symptom control and quality of life over curing. Both treatments present their own difficulties and necessitate a refined understanding of the wishes and clinical context of the patient. The ongoing development of multidisciplinary therapy, fueled by continuing research and clinical trials, holds promise for the identification of new therapies that can optimize overall outcomes for patients grappling with this pernicious disease. In this multi-faceted setting, integration of evidence-based approaches will be instrumental in maximizing PDAC treatment and patient care (Figure 11.1).

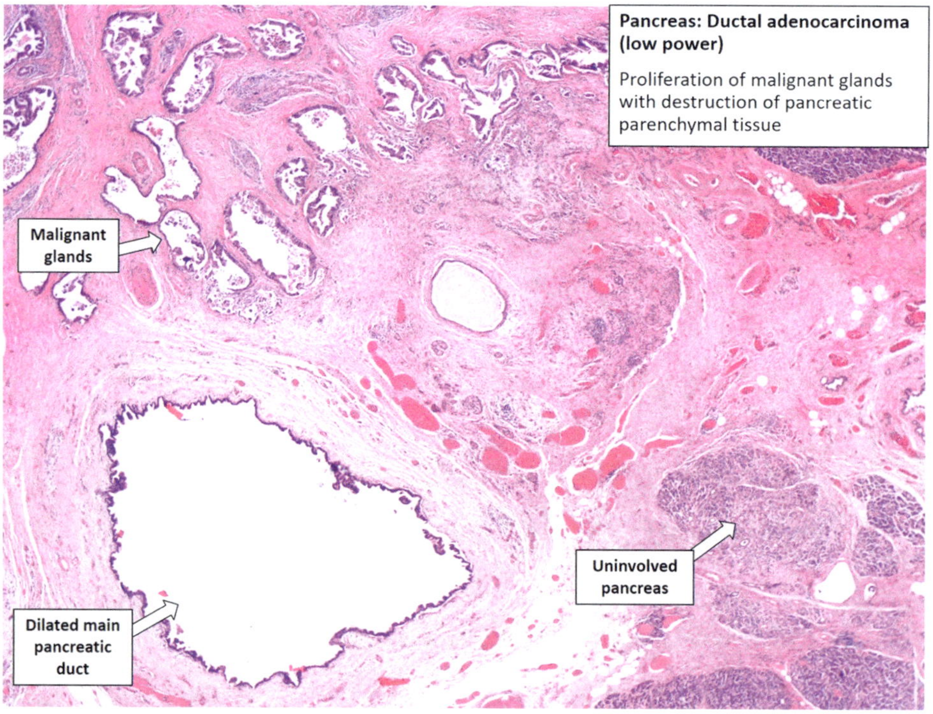

Figure 11.1. Pancreas – Adenocarcinoma.

Source: https://external-content.duckduckgo.com/iu/?u=https%3A%2F%2Fmedicine.nus.edu.sg%2Fpathweb%2Fwp-content%2Fuploads%2F2018%2F04%2FPancreas-Ductal-adenocarcinoma-lp.jpg&f=1&nofb=1&ipt=9cb24c696f12798a302d56a4e32e762cddd62d35b9059f3222f0eaa8aff8cde7.

Definition of Pancreatic Ductal Adenocarcinoma (PDAC)

PDAC is the most frequent form of pancreatic cancer and accounts for approximately 90% of all pancreatic tumors. PDAC originates from pancreas ductal epithelial cells and is defined by its malignancy and poor prognosis. PDAC prefers to occur in an advanced stage, thereby making diagnosis and treatment much more challenging. The disease is typically insidious, and symptoms like weight loss, pain in the abdomen, and jaundice typically occur late when the cancer is well-established. Further, the histological characteristics of PDAC typically come with a desmoplastic reaction that leads to dense stromal tissue that inhibits the therapeutic effect. A clear understanding of PDAC's definition and characteristics can help with effective risk assessment and early intervention plans that are crucial to improving patient outcomes. The etiology of PDAC is polygenic with several genes, environment, and lifestyle factors playing a combined role in its pathogenesis. Recognized risk factors are chronic pancreatitis, diabetes mellitus, and extensive tobacco use, which collectively account for the vast majority of instances. Additionally, familial genetic syndromes such as familial pancreatic cancer and Lynch syndrome also result in PDAC formation, indicating the involvement of genetic predisposition in its pathogenesis. The global burden of the disease demonstrates the importance of specific education regarding risk factors and the benefit of early diagnosis. Addressing these aspects is particularly important in view of the low survival rate, as less than 10% of patients survive five years after diagnosis. Thus, a thorough understanding of the risk factors for PDAC is a premise for prevention as well as development of screening programs. As PDAC is also a significant issue in diagnosis and treatment, staging of the disease is a key element in treating pancreatic cancer. The Tumor, Node, Metastasis (TNM) system of Tumor, Node, Metastasis is the most widely employed tool for staging and provides a standard framework to assess the scope of the disease. Accurate staging is paramount in establishing appropriate surgical options against palliation, defining treatment, and ultimately patient prognosis. The multifaceted nature of PDAC demands a multidisciplinary approach, with a role being played by surgical oncologists, medical oncologists, and radiologists in individualizing therapy. Emerging evidence highlights the role of chemotherapy in the adjuvant and palliative settings, which maintains the need for comprehensive treatment strategies that incorporate novel advancements on both surgical techniques and systemic therapies (Verslype et al., 2007). The need to understand how PDAC is staged and classified is therefore essential for clinicians to enhance survival rates and optimize care pathways.

Importance of Studying Pancreatic Cancer

Understanding the complexity of pancreatic cancer, here PDAC, is imperative due to its terrible impact on patients and the health care system. One of the deadliest cancers, PDAC presents with nonspecific symptoms, which lead to late diagnosis when the chances of treatment are slim. The importance of research on this cancer does not lie just in basic studies; it encompasses the development of effective screening methods, diagnostic reagents, and treatment regimens targeting earlier intervention. With a bleak 5-year survival rate of around 10%, the need for raising awareness and research dollars for studies that can discover the underlying mechanisms of the disease and lead to better outcomes in treatment is imminent. With scientists discovering the biology of PDAC tumors, they can unlock the potential for targeted therapeutic approaches that target specific genetic mutations and risk factors of the disease. Research into the risk factors and genetic syndromes of pancreatic ductal adenocarcinoma is a significant component of present research. Familial syndromes such as hereditary pancreatitis and Lynch syndrome carry an increased risk of developing PDAC, and hence genetic counseling and testing are essential in such populations. A thorough understanding of such associations enables healthcare providers to implement early surveillance practices and preventive strategies in high-risk patients. Also, since information regarding environmental causes, such as smoking and obesity, is growing and will keep growing, public campaigns may be aimed at reducing instances of pancreatic cancer. The intersection of genetic data and lifestyle illustrates the intricate character of the disease and justifies research on pancreatic cancer as a method for preventing future diagnoses and improving patient treatment. In addition, advancement in diagnostic techniques and staging procedures, such as the TNM system of staging, is very important for optimizing patient outcomes in pancreatic ductal adenocarcinoma. Proper and early diagnosis through imaging procedures and biomarkers allows adequate staging, which is an integral part in the establishment of optimal treatment modalities, surgical or palliative. Establishment of a robust core curriculum in surgical oncology, as has been demonstrated by much of the European medical societies' work, demonstrates a requirement for healthcare providers to be educated in the novel knowledge and skills required to successfully manage this aggressive cancer. Continuing medical education and evidence-based therapy not only improves survival but also improves quality of life in PDAC patients. As ongoing clinical research brings forward new evidence, the integration of these findings into practice will be essential to combating the relentless nature of this aggressive disease (Van der Hage et al., 2021) (Figure 11.2).

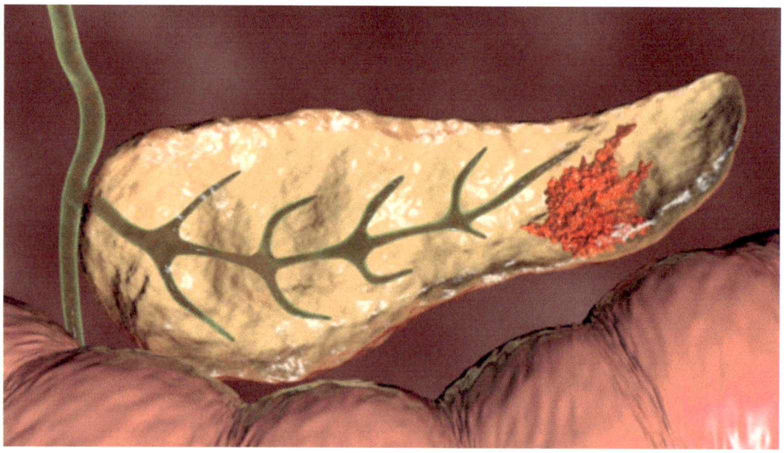

Figure 11.2. Pancreatic cancer reveals potential therapeutic targets.

Source: https://external-content.duckduckgo.com/iu/?u=https%3A%2F%2Fwww.genengnews.com%2Fwp-content%2Fuploads%2F2020%2F09%2FSep15_2020_Getty_1215121166_Pancreas-scaled-e1600198791887.jpg&f=1&nofb=1&ipt=49927d80b3c6d20dce3b4818254fbcc8d244290e617d7a7397ee23dd1aa47c31.

11.1. Risk Factors

The aetiology of pancreatic ductal adenocarcinoma (PDAC) is multi-factorial with intrinsic and extrinsic factors contributing to its aetiology. Among all the modifiable risk factors, smoking has proven to be the most powerful, with evidence indicating that smokers have a two to three-fold increased risk of PDAC when compared to non-smokers. In addition, obesity and physical inactivity have been linked with an increased risk of cancer and suggest that metabolic syndrome plays a significant role in pancreatic carcinogenesis. Chronic pancreatitis, commonly due to heavy alcohol consumption, also raises the risk. Clarifying these lifestyle variables is significant in prevention because interventions aimed at decreasing smoking, healthy weight, and moderate alcohol consumption can significantly reduce PDAC incidence among populations at risk. Apart from lifestyle factors, genetic syndromes also increase risk to pancreatic ductal adenocarcinoma, proving the complex relationship between genes and environment. Syndromes such as hereditary pancreatitis, Peutz-Jeghers syndrome, and Lynch syndrome have already been strongly associated with heightened risk of PDAC development. Genetic mutation in the BRCA2 gene also plays a significant role, proving that family history can dictate screening guidelines and prevention. The identification of these genetic associations underscores the necessity for genetic testing and counseling in individuals with a family history of pancreatic cancer. Early detection and surveillance procedures can be crucial in high-risk patients, enabling timely interventions that can improve prognosis and reduce mortality from this highly fatal cancer. Finally, understanding the risk factors of pancreatic ductal adenocarcinoma not only directs prevention but also drives practice in diagnosis and management. Multidisciplinary care has to be incorporated, particularly in optimizing surgical and palliative treatment for patients with this disease. A multidisciplinary strategy involving surgical oncology, medical oncology, and supportive care specialties is central to managing PDAC effectively, as deliberations by specialists suggested in recent years. The complexities of PDAC necessitate continued research and clinical trials to better stage, manage, and test because such efforts can enhance patient outcomes and survival (Verslype et al., 2007; Van der Hage et al., 2021) (Figure 11.3). The challenge is to bring this information into practice and achieve simultaneous improvements in patient-centered care for patients suffering from this deadly cancer.

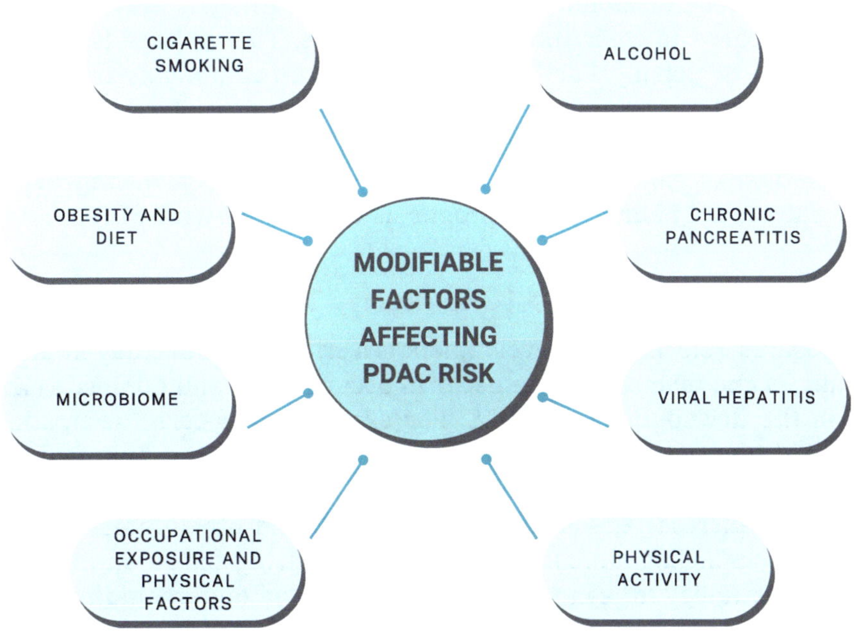

Figure 11.3. Rick factor for pancreatic ductal adenocarcinoma (PDAC).

Source: Michalak N, Małecka-Wojciesko E. Modifiable Pancreatic Ductal Adenocarcinoma (PDAC) Risk Factors. *Journal of Clinical Medicine*. 2023; 12(13):4318. https://doi.org/10.3390/jcm12134318

11.1.1. Lifestyle Factors (Smoking, Diet, Obesity)

Lifestyle risk factors including obesity, diet, and smoking play a large role in causing PDAC. Smoking as an established risk factor is responsible for about 20% of the incidence of pancreatic cancer worldwide. The tobacco smoke harbors carcinogens that induce genetic mutations, promote tumor cell proliferation in the pancreas, and facilitate pancreatic cancer development. The synergistic effect of smoking with other determinants like obesity also raises the risk. Of special interest, studies have found that obese smokers have a higher risk of developing this aggressive cancer than those who do not smoke or who are healthy weight. Because lifestyle changes have the ability to decrease such risks, public health interventions designed to prevent smoking and improve diet are essential to incorporate into cancer prevention activities. Diet is a critical element of pancreatic cancer risk profile, and certain dietary habits have been related to increased and decreased risk. Higher intakes of red and processed meat have been related to higher risk because of the application of nitrates and preservatives that have carcinogenic effects. In contrast, high levels of fruit, vegetables, and whole grains might have protective effects against cancer development. This is because of antioxidant and phytochemical composition that decreases oxidative stress and promotes cell wellness. Furthermore, a balanced diet assists in maintaining weight, which is an important factor because obesity has been associated with enhanced pancreatic cancer risk. As such, a nutrition education focus may be able to provide individuals with the power necessary to make improved dietary choices, which could decrease overall risk for PDAC. Obesity is increasingly coming to be recognized as a crucial lifestyle determinant of the development of pancreatic ductal adenocarcinoma. Being overweight is associated with many changes in metabolism, including insulin resistance and long-term inflammation, that may elevate cancer risk. Studies show that individuals with higher body mass indexes (BMIs) possess a hugely elevated risk for developing pancreatic cancer compared to their thinner counterparts. This linkage is noteworthy given the rising incidence of obesity globally. Furthermore, obesity can complicate treatment and outcomes since it often coexists with other associated conditions such as diabetes, also linked to elevated risk of pancreatic cancer. Obesity must be tackled with tailored interventions in physical activity and diet in the fight against pancreatic cancer because, aside from reducing risk, these measures can also improve outcomes of surgery and prognosis of patients with PDAC.

11.1.2. Environmental Exposures (Chemicals, Toxins)

Environmental exposures' role in PDAC development is a critical area of study in the field of oncology. A number of chemicals and toxins that also occur in occupational and domestic environments have been implicated in the development of PDAC. For example, long-term occupational exposure to certain pesticides and industrial chemicals such as benzene has been linked to pancreatic cancer development. In addition, tobacco smoke contains numerous carcinogens, and apart from inducing lung cancers, they also increase the risk of getting PDAC and other intestinal cancers. All these environmental risk factors highlight the importance of recognizing and reversing exposure to noxious agents as a preventive strategy for cancer. Lastly, an integrated understanding of these risk factors can assist in establishing guidelines to reduce the overall risk of pancreatic cancer in order to achieve improved public health. In exploring the complex interplay between environmental exposures and PDAC, the role played by infections in the causation of cancer cannot be overlooked. Studies have indicated that viral and bacterial infections may have a significant effect on cancer risk and contribute to approximately 16% of total cancers worldwide as observed in the year 2008. While not related to PDAC directly, pathogens such as Helicobacter pylori have also been implicated in other gastrointestinal cancers, which point towards a complex relationship involving environmental influences. Besides that, long-standing infections can give rise to oncogenic mechanisms that ultimately predispose one to pancreatic cancer through the mechanisms of immune suppression and inflammation. This requires inclusive infection prevention strategies such as vaccination and public health policy to block pathogenic exposures that indirectly increase the risk to cancers like PDAC. The integration of environmental exposure information into PDAC risk assessment propels the science towards a comprehensive understanding of cancer etiology. The acknowledgment that lifestyle, occupation, and geography all contribute to exposure to carcinogens can lead to targeted prevention. For instance, populations with higher industrial pollution can have regulations implemented to limit emission and sanitize air quality, thereby reducing cancer risk. Additionally, the detection and monitoring of specific environmental toxins associated with PDAC occurrence would be beneficial to initiate early prevention and education. As continued advances in cancer research are made, the inclusion of data on environmental exposure will become essential to further individualize diagnostic criteria and staging methods, directly affecting treatment plans—spanning surgical interventions to end-of-life palliative measures—encouraging more individualized care management of pancreatic ductal adenocarcinoma (Figure 11.4).

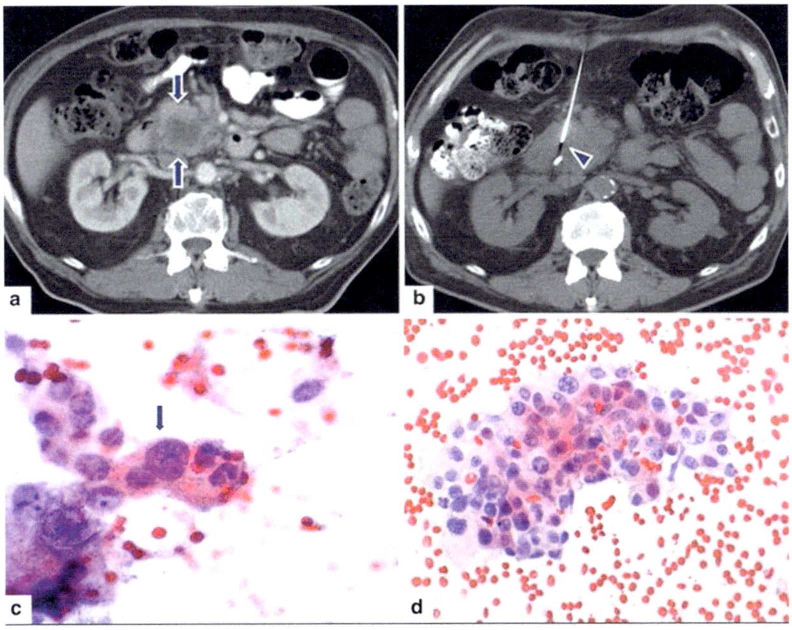

Figure 11.4. Pancreatic ductal adenocarcinoma (PDAC) radiology.

Source: https://i1.wp.com/radiologykey.com/wp-content/uploads/2017/04/A313896_1_En_11_Fig85_HTML.gif?fit=638%2C495&ssl=1.

11.1.3. Age and Gender Predispositions

Age and sex predispositions are key epidemiological factors in PDAC that influence incidence rates as well as prognostic outcomes. Epidemiological studies demonstrate a steep increase in the incidence of PDAC among older people, particularly among individuals aged 65 years and above, indicating the association between rising age and development of the malignant cancer. Age-related mechanisms, such as the acquisition of genetic mutations and loss of immune function with age, also contribute to augmented cancer risk. Additionally, there is a gender disparity in PDAC incidence, which is 1.5 times higher among men than women. This may be due to variations in lifestyle factors, hormonal influences, and environmental exposure to carcinogens. It is essential to grasp these sex and age dynamics to individualize prevention approaches and optimize treatment across different populations (Hoyer, 2021). Moreover, sex and age propensities extend beyond the rates of incidence because they closely relate with survival as well as response to treatment modalities. Research has indicated that younger patients have better prognoses, perhaps because of better physiological reserve and the capacity to recuperate better from surgery. Older people present with comorbidities that make treatment decisions more complicated and worsen outcomes. Biological gender differences, including hormonal and gene expression influences, also affect the efficacy of treatments. Studies have shown that women can potentially have a relatively improved survival overall compared to men, indicating the complex interplay between sociocultural and biological determinants. These findings emphasize the importance of an introspective approach to PDAC treatment, particularly since the development in personalized medicine persists (Lewis et al., 2018). At a wider view, the understanding of the significance of gender and age vulnerabilities could further facilitate the implementation of public health programs for education and early intervention. Specially tailored programs with a focus on gender- and age-related risk factors can facilitate persons and healthcare workers taking preventive action more aggressively. In addition, screening protocols may be improved through stratification according to these demographics in order to enable targeted interventions that will maximize early detection rates and treatment outcomes. Policymakers and health organizations may utilize this data to effectively inform resource allocation and engage in community outreach activities that address the needs of various age and gender groups. By addressing these predispositions in depth, the medical fraternity can work together towards alleviating the PDAC burden through early diagnosis and individualized treatment avenues (Hoyer, 2021).

11.2. Genetic Syndromes

The role of genetic syndromes in PDAC is an area of greatest relevance to understand the pathology and potential prevention of this cancer. Certain inherited syndromes, such as familial pancreatitis and Lynch syndrome, have been found to significantly increase the risk of pancreatic cancer. For instance, inherited pancreatitis patients have a lifetime cumulative risk of up to 40% for PDAC, and this shows how genetic susceptibilities play a crucial role in cancer etiology. This characteristic demonstrates the need to heighten surveillance in these vulnerable patients, since early diagnosis is vital for improving prognosis. This is emphatic evidence that genetic syndromes are not merely control variables but pivotal factors in the etiology and treatment of pancreatic cancer. Additionally, the diagnostic environment of pancreatic cancer has a direct proportion with advances towards understanding genetic syndromes. Although there are no direct screening tests for PDAC currently, existing recommendations advocate intensive monitoring of individuals with hereditary risk factors. This is motivated by the realization that genetic susceptibility may lead to late-stage and ill-prognosed cancers. Advanced imaging technologies like MRI and endoscopic ultrasound are now essential in the identification of early-stage cancers in individuals who are genetically predisposed. However, there remains a challenge regarding specificity and reliability with such technologies, with ongoing research focused on biomarkers and novel technologies for the early detection of cancers. The intersection of genetic syndromes and diagnostic technology is a significant area that could lead to better early detection and response to treatment. Efforts at research in genetic syndromes applicable to pancreatic cancer go as far as therapeutic use, where the understanding of genetic backgrounds can influence treatment planning. For instance, individuals carrying BRCA1 and BRCA2 gene mutations can be given targeted therapy, e.g., PARP inhibitors, that offer renewed promise to patients who previously had poor prospects. Development of personalized medicine on the basis of genotypic information is increasingly being part of PDAC management. With more progress being made, the incorporation of genetic testing into therapeutic strategies will further maximize surgical and palliative treatment and contribute to improved patient outcomes. This paradigm shift places more emphasis on the necessity to approach genetic syndromes as not only risk factors but also as integral elements in the overall treatment regime for pancreatic ductal adenocarcinoma, moving towards an integrated approach to the management of cancer (Figure 11.5).

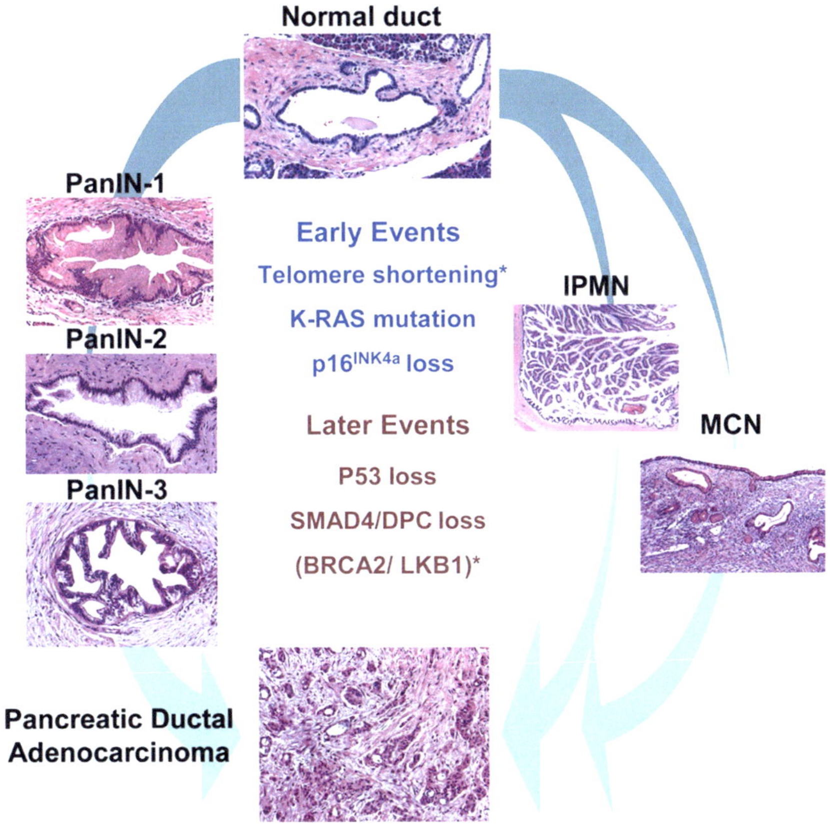

Figure 11.5. Genetics and biology of pancreatic ductal adenocarcinoma.

Source: https://genesdev.cshlp.org/content/20/10/1218/F2.large.jpg.

11.2.1. Hereditary Pancreatitis

Among the pathophysiologies of pancreatic illnesses, hereditary pancreatitis is unique in having a high association with an increased risk for PDAC. The underlying genetic illness is primarily due to PRSS1 gene mutations encoding for the protein trypsinogen. Mutations lead to abnormal activation of trypsin that induces recurring episodes of acute pancreatitis, chronic inflammation, and eventually ductal pancreatic changes that can potentially lead to malignant transformation of the patient. Research has pointed out that those with hereditary pancreatitis are at a lifetime risk of developing PDAC between 40%–50%, which is considerably higher compared to the rest of the population. Subsequently, recognition of hereditary pancreatitis not only aids in the early identification of high-risk patients but also emphasizes the importance of careful surveillance measures to allow earlier diagnosis of any malignant lesions, as in keeping with the overall goal of improving patient outcomes in the management of pancreatic cancer (Zerón et al., 2009). Moreover, the importance of hereditary pancreatitis extends beyond its direct medical consequences as it impacts both genetic counseling and management strategies. Individuals who have such a history in the family are generally recommended to participate in genetic testing and family screening. These steps are paramount because a high proportion of hereditary cases result from an autosomal dominant pattern of inheritance. Early identification with the assistance of effective screening may enable clinicians to manage chronic pancreatitis adequately and diligently monitor the development of pancreatic cancer. Endoscopic ultrasonography and other imaging techniques play a significant role in the identification of precursor lesions, such as pancreatic intraepithelial neoplasia, that may develop in high-risk individuals, thereby ensuring the maximum chance of timely surgical resections. The inclusion of such steps can lead to preemptive treatment that may critically alter the course of disease evolution in patients who are genetically predisposed (Zerón et al., 2009). The association of hereditary pancreatitis and subsequent risk for PDAC necessitates long-term multidisciplinary management in patients. Treatment strategies must walk the fine line of maintaining pancreatic function and minimizing cancer risks. While signs for surgical treatments, such as prophylactic pancreatectomy, are warranted in selected high-risk patients, palliative treatment also has important roles for patients with distant disease. Complex integration of symptom management, active follow-up, and patient education will be required to optimize outcomes in the at-risk group. Additionally, ongoing studies of the molecular and genetic etiology of hereditary pancreatitis will continue to lead to new treatments that may further enhance prevention measures or therapeutic strategies for these patients. The presentation of hereditary pancreatitis thus transcends current clinical management and deals with broader endeavors in maximizing cancer screening and improving long-term outcomes in treating pancreatic ductal adenocarcinoma (Biagini et al., 2014).

11.2.2. Familial Atypical Multiple Mole Melanoma (FAMMM) Syndrome

FAMMM syndrome is an inherited disorder that highly increases the risk of melanoma, a life-threatening skin malignancy. FAMMM syndrome patients typically develop many atypical moles and a family history of melanoma, which may indicate a genetic tendency. Mutations in genes related to this syndrome are primarily in tumor suppressor genes such as CDKN2A. Evidence has indicated that those with a family history have a greatly elevated risk not only for melanoma but also for other types of cancer, including PDAC and breast cancer. This correlation is of relevance in the context of screening practices in high-risk patients for pancreatic cancer. In fact, initial surveillance in individuals with FAMMM syndrome can permit prompt action against melanoma and provide insight into risks of pancreatic cancer as well, highlighting the interdependence of genetic syndromes and cancer (Biagini et al., 2014). The implication of FAMMM syndrome is not only for melanoma but also for greater awareness of pancreatic ductal adenocarcinoma. Cancer registries and family studies demonstrate that patients with this syndrome are more likely to develop pancreatic cancer, and this fact provokes controversy about multi-cancer screening policies. Hence, medical professionals should embark on an aggressive role in managing FAMMM syndrome patients, employing rigorous screening techniques to detect potential malignancies at the earliest level. EUS presents as a valuable resource for the early detection of pancreatic cancer, having high sensitivity for most lesions, including those in genetically predisposed patients. With our increasing knowledge of the genetic basis of cancer, including the identification of cancer-predisposing alleles, their application to clinical practice can improve the prognosis of high-risk patients by allowing earlier cancer detection and hence improved survival (Butler, 2025). Furthermore, the overlap between FAMMM syndrome and pancreatic ductal adenocarcinoma puts focus on the need for focused education and counseling regarding genetic risk. Those families and patients who are afflicted with this syndrome should be educated not only about their heightened risk for melanoma but also about its impact on other cancers, including PDAC. Genetic counseling can be helpful to de-mystify the nature of risks as well as surveillance recommendations that are recommended. In addition, being aware of their own personal cancer susceptibilities can make families more active participants in screening programs, thereby enhancing early diagnosis and control. As continuing studies further illuminate the genealogical undertones of FAMMM syndrome and its association with other cancers, ongoing debate among the medical community about the benefits of surveillance combining them will be necessary (Biagini et al., 2014) (Figure 11.6).

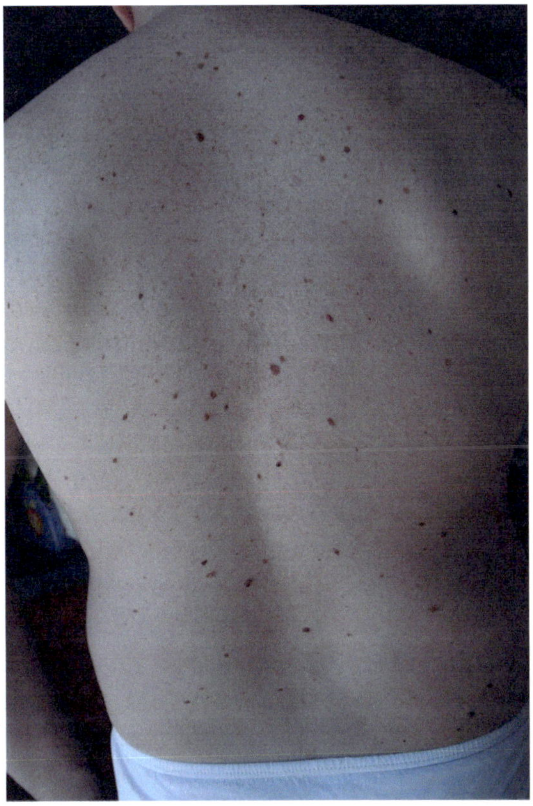

Figure 11.6. Familial atypical multiple mole melanoma (FAMMM) syndrome.

Source: By 0x6adb015 - Own work, CC BY-SA 3.0, https://commons.wikimedia.org/w/index.php?curid=16325455

11.2.3. Lynch Syndrome and its Association with Pancreatic Cancer

Lynch syndrome, or hereditary non-polyposis colorectal cancer (HNPCC), is an autosomal dominant genetic disorder with mutations in the DNA mismatch repair genes. Lynch syndrome has a significantly elevated risk of several cancers, including colorectal, endometrial, and ovarian cancer. Interestingly, emerging evidence now suggests that carriers of Lynch syndrome also have a risk for PDAC. Despite PDAC having been generally accepted as a disease in its own right with independent risk factors, the inherent genetic mutations of Lynch syndrome are likely to predispose the affected individuals to the pathophysiology of pancreatic cancer.

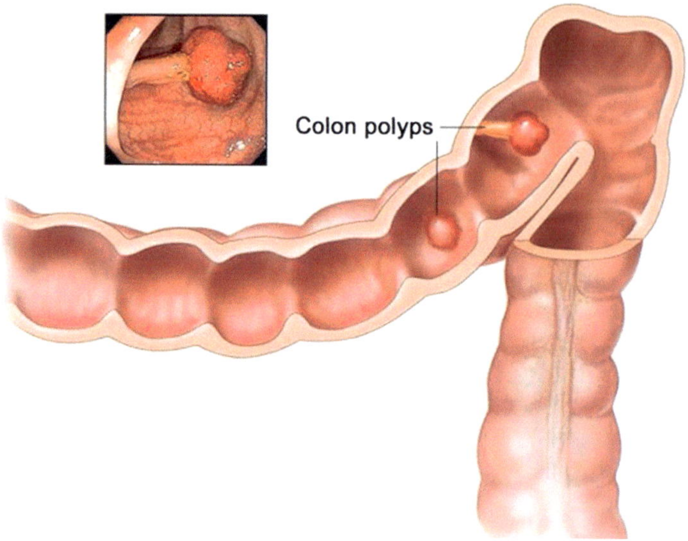

Figure 11.7. Lynch syndrome.

Source: https://external-content.duckduckgo.com/iu/?u=https%3A%2F%2Fmedlineplus.gov%2Fimages%2FPX0001QS_PRESENTATION.jpeg&f=1&nofb=1&ipt=8d9029e4449cf632a42089dd77e99f2addd174786e6c1830a3ac5fc13faf60c1.

The pathogenetic mechanisms are usually through the accumulation of genetic lesions due to the defective repair process of DNA that is typical of Lynch syndrome and this raises the risk of developing malignancies in organs other than the pancreas as well. Recent studies have elucidated the provocative association of pancreatic cancer with Lynch syndrome, highlighting the importance of genetic testing for vulnerable groups. Although the lifetime risk for pancreatic cancer in individuals with Lynch syndrome is not as precisely determined as that for colorectal cancer, projections have been presented that the risk does indeed escalate considerably. For instance, the lifetime risk for pancreatic cancer in Lynch syndrome patients may range from 2%–10%, considering many variables such as the type of gene mutation and family background. This points towards active surveillance and management practices in Lynch syndrome patients, just like for colorectal cancer. Greater understanding and recognition of this association can pave the way for improved diagnostic approaches and targeted therapeutic interventions, ultimately determining patient outcomes. The mention of Lynch syndrome in the grand discussion of PDAC risk factors indicates the interplay of complex genetic predisposition with environmental influences. This identification also paves the way for more personalized screening algorithms as well as aligns with current advances in personalized medicine in an effort to make treatment more specific depending on individualized genetic profiles. With continued advances in science, the development of gene expression signatures potentially has even more to offer regarding prognosis and response to therapy in people with Lynch syndrome and pancreatic cancer. With the current guidance and understanding of the genetic and molecular characteristics of cancers like pancreatic adenocarcinoma, continued research into Lynch syndromes would be an essential component in the optimization of therapeutic protocols and reduction of morbidity associated with this very malignant cancer (Eurola,Iacobelli et al., 2012; Eurola,, 2022) (Figure 11.7).

11.3. Diagnosis

Diagnosis of PDAC is extremely difficult for the most part due to the diseases inherent asymptomatic nature during its early stages. Most patients are not visible with symptoms until the cancer has developed a progressed form, resulting in poor prognosis and limited intervention options. Delayed presentation of clinical signs in the majority is prognostic of metastasis, complicating interventions. Furthermore, there is currently no absolute screening or diagnostic test for PDAC, which renders it very challenging to detect at an early stage. Present research focuses on identifying individuals at risk, like those who have inherited genetic syndromes, for whom intensive surveillance measures may help lead to earlier diagnosis. Relying on clinical presentation alone for diagnosis serves to only augment the requirement for improved detection tools in clinics, and therefore there is a necessity for new avenues in diagnosing pancreatic cancer (Søreide et al., 2023). New technologies bring about some optimism for enhancing the diagnosis of pancreatic cancer. Tumor biomarkers and "omics" technology like genomics and metabolomics are being pursued with promise to enhance early detection. However, all this progress comes with its set of challenges, particularly concerning the reliability and cross-validation of the potential diagnostic markers. The majority of proposed biomarkers are still in rudimentary stages, facing issues of restricted external validation and significantly lower accuracy when cross-validated outside initial data sets. This limitation raises questions concerning the efficacy of ongoing research and points to a need for continuous enhancement of diagnostic processes. Also, the use of biopsies at diagnosis complicates things further since they may not precisely represent the disease at an earlier, more treatable stage (Søreide et al., 2023). Hence, the evolution of diagnostic advancement is not only beneficial but also inevitable to improve patient outcomes. Moreover, integrative diagnostic approaches are being developed that capitalize on imaging and analytics advancements. Techniques such as radiomics, where many features are being extracted from the images, and machine learning algorithms are promising to detect pancreatic cancer earlier than the current methods do. Such advancements in technology can enable physicians to detect disease features that might not be detected by the human observer, thus improving the accuracy of diagnosis. Furthermore, "liquid biopsies" – procedures that analyze the body's liquids like blood or urine for cancer marks – are under exploration as new non-invasive methods of early diagnosis. If they were taken up into practice, these methods might bypass some of the false positives associated with current screening methods, and therefore outweigh the harms and contribute to overall good from screening. This shift towards new diagnostic devices is likely to significantly influence the treatment approaches utilized in treating PDAC in the future (Søreide et al., 2023) (Figure 11.8).

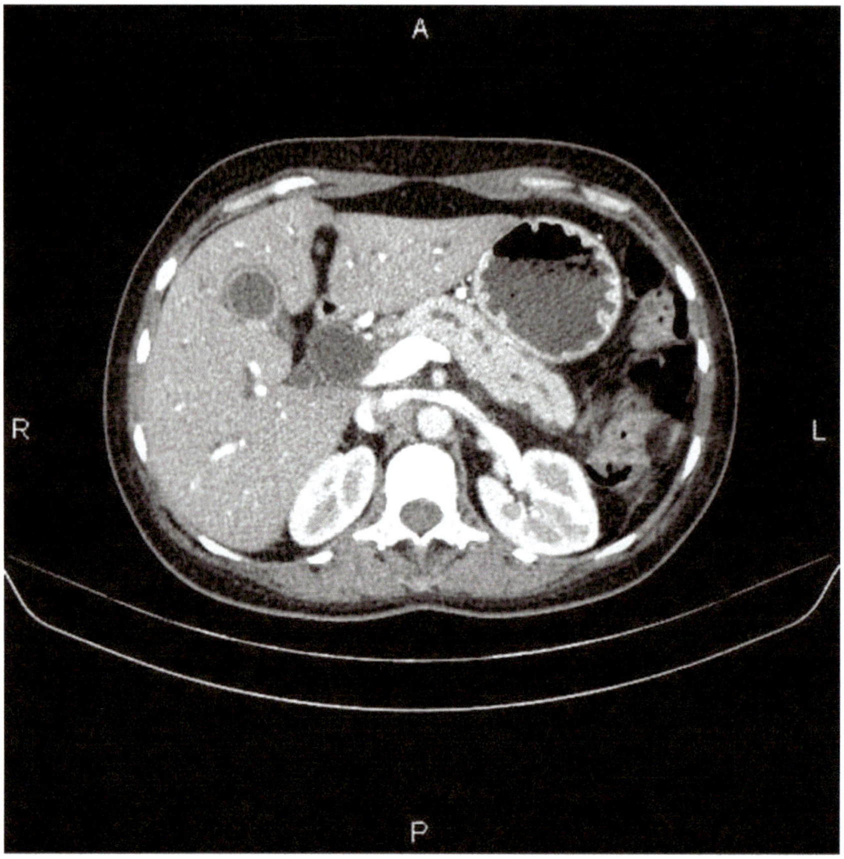

Figure 11.8. Diagnosis of pancreatic ductal adenocarcinoma (PDAC).

Source: https://prod-images-static.radiopaedia.org/images/56804193/63._big_gallery.jpeg.

11.3.1. Symptoms and Clinical Presentation

The symptomatology of PDAC is often indolent, with vague or nonspecific symptoms referable to more common gastrointestinal illnesses. The earliest symptoms can be nonspecific, including weight loss, anorexia, and fatigue. Over time, more classic symptoms become evident, among them jaundice, a yellowing of the eyes and skin due to bile duct obstruction. Other presentations include symptomatic abdominal pain that is typically back-radiating and accompanied by changes in stool, such as steatorrhea, which indicates fat malabsorption. Such complexity typically leads to delayed diagnosis, which makes early therapeutic efforts difficult, which are essential in an effort to improve patient outcomes. Therefore, the clinical presentation should raise a heightened suspicion of pancreatic cancer, especially in high-risk populations, driving the need for greater understanding amongst healthcare workers (Agarwal et al., 2017). In advanced stages of PDAC, on consideration of the clinical presentation, the symptoms progress to become more severe and intense. Patients experience worsening epigastric pain and can present with ascites if the tumor begins to invade the nearby structures or metastasize to distant organs. Anorexia and nausea are common causes of substantial weight loss, affecting quality of life and general state of health. Notably, the occurrence of obstruction of the biliary tract due to tumor involvement results in severe pruritus and can progress to cholangitis, an acute infection that demands prompt medical treatment. The heterogeneity of symptoms highlights the importance of a sharp diagnostic approach, often complemented by high technology imaging to establish the extent of disease progression, especially in light of any impending surgical intervention (Cannavale et al., 2016). The treatment team must be well-equipped to handle such shifting clinical contexts effectively. As a whole, the clinical course and symptoms of pancreatic ductal adenocarcinoma are primary indicators of disease progression, and medical practitioners need to react with knowledgeable haste. Because early presentation is often nonspecific complaint, education of the typical symptoms will be essential in order to optimize early diagnosis. Because symptomatic worsening generally reflects advanced disease, an understanding of this spectrum not only makes optimal therapeutic intervention selection easier but also directs palliative intervention. Incorporation of knowledge into practice is essential not just to improve survival but also to enhance patients' quality of life throughout the disease (Cannavale et al., 2016; Agarwal et al., 2017). Health care professionals must improve symptom perception and management in order to overcome the challenges of this aggressive malignancy effectively.

11.3.2. Imaging Techniques (Computed Tomography (CT), Magnetic Resonance Imaging (MRI), and Endoscopic Ultrasound (EUS))

Imaging modalities have a central place in the staging and diagnosis of PDAC. Cross-sectional images based on CT scans allow accurate visualization of the pancreas as well as other structures. CT is particularly helpful in assessing the extent of the disease, including local invasiveness and metastasis, which are major determinants in planning treatment modality. CT scans can also give clues about vascular involvement, an important determinant in surgical candidacy. Advanced technologies such as multi-phase CT and contrast material use enhance sensitivity in the detection of pancreatic masses and associated lesions. This characteristic is paramount given PDAC's covert course, where tumors do not present symptoms until late stages (Podină et al., 2025). CT is, therefore, an oncologist's equally valuable tool, not only being beneficial in initial diagnosis but also in tracking disease progression. Another essential imaging modality employed in managing pancreatic cancer is MRI. It provides superior soft tissue contrast, which is particularly advantageous in distinguishing pancreatic tumors from adjacent organs and tissues. MRI is especially useful in circumstances where CT cannot be so sure or in patients requiring additional evaluation following an abnormal CT outcome. It is noteworthy that MRI can also help identify potential liver metastases and assess peritoneal spread, offering a comprehensive view of the diseases extent. Due to its non-ionizing nature, MRI is particularly beneficial for young patients or those requiring multiple imaging studies throughout their treatment journey. Furthermore, innovations like diffusion-weighted imaging contribute to sensitivity for fine tissue changes detection, further cementing its role in the diagnostic algorithm (Podină et al., 2025). Together, MRI contributes significantly to creating a comprehensive picture of PDAC that informs treatment planning. EUS stands out for its particular ability to visualize the pancreas and surrounding structures in fine detail. Being as minimally invasive as it is, EUS allows for real-time visualization, which boasts the benefit of picking up small lesions that are not yet evident on CT or MRI scans. With fine-needle aspiration (FNA), EUS can also be used to allow for the retrieval of tissue samples, enabling histological diagnosis of PDAC. This technical advantage is actually beneficial in pancreatic cancer diagnosis due to the challenge posed by its typically insidious presentation. EUS is also pivotal in delivering therapeutic interventions, such as biliary stent placement for obstructions. Integrating interventional and diagnostic capabilities, EUS becomes an essential element in PDAC therapy (Mauro et al., 2025). As imaging technology continues to evolve, integration of EUS images with images taken on CT and MRI can allow for more comprehensive treatment methods, ultimately helping the patient (Figure 11.9).

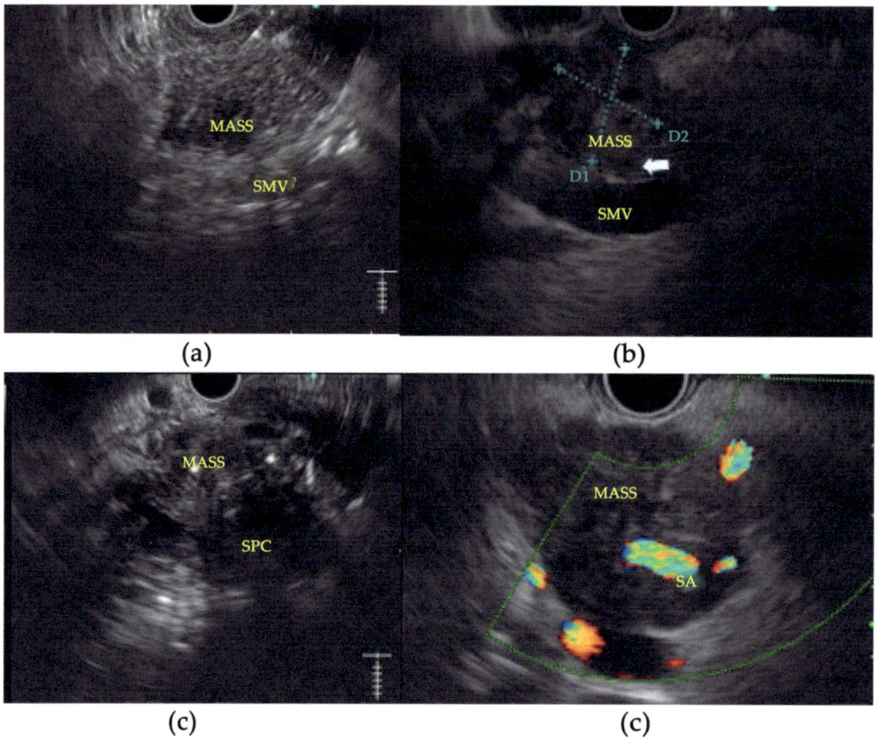

Figure 11.9. Role of endoscopic ultrasound (EUS) in the diagnosis of pancreatic ductal adenocarcinoma (PDAC).

Source: https://pub.mdpi-res.com/diagnostics/diagnostics-14-00078/article_deploy/html/images/diagnostics-14-00078-g001.png?1703822957.

11.3.3. Biomarkers and Laboratory Tests

Biomarkers play a critical role in early diagnosis and treatment of PDAC, particularly in a condition with delayed presentation and adverse outcome. Among the several biomarkers detected, carbohydrate antigen 19-9 (Ca19-9) has been most widely used in the clinical setting for detection and monitoring of PDAC. However, its usefulness as a standalone diagnostic reagent is minimal, especially since high levels can occur in other diseases and lead to false positives. More current studies have examined more recent candidate markers such as Thrombospondin-2 (THBS2) and Human Chitinase 3-like 1 (YKL-40), alongside Ca19-9. A noteworthy finding has been that a panel of several analytes containing these markers has found higher diagnostic performance than standard measurements, highlighting the promise of more successful early detection tools in PDAC patients (Mortimer, 2024). Not only is diagnostic testing essential for PDAC diagnosis but also for staging and determination of appropriate treatment. Staging by TNM classification system calls for accurate measurement of tumor size, nodal involvement, and metastases. Imaging studies supplement biomarker analysis by providing visible evidence of disease progression, allowing clinicians to risk-stratify patients according to disease burden. Recent advances have included the addition of new imaging techniques and machine learning diagnostics such as Fourier Transform Infrared (FTIR) spectroscopy, which have been shown to have extremely high diagnostic sensitivity in the ability to differentiate malignant from non-malignant tissues. Advanced diagnostic methods can ultimately lead to early surgery or simplified palliative care interventions, thus aligning treatment with the phase of the patient's disease (Verslype et al., 2007). The integration of biomarkers and laboratory tests into clinical approaches can also facilitate the creation of customized treatment regimens for PDAC patients. With the evolving trend of therapeutic interventions like chemotherapy and chemoradiotherapy, accurate diagnostic evaluations have become the pillar of selecting the treatment. Biomarker-directed therapy holds the potential to tailor treatments based on the individual characteristics of each tumor, possibly with enhanced outcomes and quality of life. Clinical trial enrollment also remains a vital component of learning and practice formation in the PDAC management. Whereas ongoing research aims to validate the clinical usefulness of emerging biomarkers alongside streamlined laboratory tests, the importance of an interdisciplinary initiative, translating these advances into practice, cannot be overstated (Mortimer, 2024).

11.4. Staging Tumor, Node, Metastasis (TNM)

The staging of PDAC by the TNM classification is of great significance in determining therapy and prognosis of the patient. The TNM classification segregates tumors into three parameters of significance: tumor size (T), regional lymph node involvement (N), and metastasis at a distant site (M). All these parameters provide information regarding the spread of the disease and influence therapy indirectly. Accurate staging is not only valuable to determine resectability—where surgery may be an option—but also to guide palliative care interventions in the patient with advanced disease. The elegance of the TNM system facilitates more precise evaluation of the extent of disease, so that health professionals can tailor management options that best suit each patient's individual circumstances. Inclusion of radiological evaluations like MRI and MRCP in the TNM staging system adds further to diagnostic specificity and treatment planning. Reports suggest that these imaging techniques are able to successfully define the tumor's nature and evaluate its resectability over surgical results, with high sensitivity and specificity rates (Turowska et al., 2009). Such accuracy helps clinicians in the selection of candidates for surgery, which is the most effective cure for resectable PDAC. In addition, imaging can stage patients based on their staging and greatly assist in creating an awareness of their general prognosis. Incorporation of new imaging techniques into the traditional TNM system therefore, mirrors the evolving character of treatment for pancreatic cancer. In addition to the traditional staging groups, more recent studies indicate the incorporation of tumor grade into the TNM system to improve prognostic accuracy. Data reveal that high-grade tumors, regardless of the AJCC stage, correlate with poorer survival outcomes, suggesting that grade could serve as an independent predictor of prognosis in PDAC (Wasif et al., 2010). By refining the staging process with this additional parameter, clinicians can achieve a more accurate stratification of patients, potentially influencing treatment decisions and enrollment in clinical trials. Adding tumor grade to TNM staging not only discusses the biological behavior of pancreatic neoplasms but also enhances the capacity for individualized treatment plans, thereby enhancing the intricacies and heterogeneities related to this challenging malignancy (Figure 11.10).

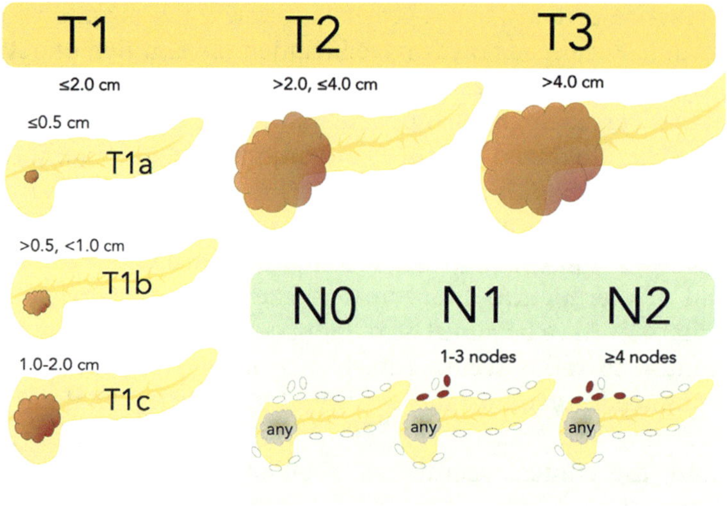

Figure 11.10. Staging tumor, node, metastasis (TNM) in pancreatic ductal adenocarcinoma (PDAC).

Source: https://ars.els-cdn.com/content/image/1-s2.0-S0748798320301165-gr1.jpg.

11.4.1. Explanation of the Tumor, Node, Metastasis (TNM) Classification System

TNM staging system is an orderly system that the oncologists utilize to stage cancer, here they are staging PDAC. The TNM stands for Tumor size (T), Node status (N), and Metastasis (M). One should assess the main tumor; it is to establish the extent of the adjacent tissues and organs invaded. In PDAC, this assessment can specifically be problematic because tumors are largely infiltrative in their growth patterns, complicating both surgical planning and patient prognosis. Similarly, accurate staging is essential because treatment will be directed by it and survival will be prognosticated. Tumor size measurement—to encompass the various T classifications, is the foundation of this strict assessment process, establishing the general extent of the disease at diagnosis. Node involvement, labeled as "N" in the TNM classification, assesses the presence and extent of cancer dissemination to lymph nodes. In patients with PDAC, assessment of regional lymph node involvement is essential in determining resectability as well as overall prognosis. Lymph node status has been recognized as one of the best predictors in cancer treatments, including PDAC. The staging ranges from N0, or lack of lymph node involvement, to N1, when regional nodes are affected. Clinically, the identification of lymphatic spread greatly affects treatment, frequently dictating if a patient can receive curative surgery or which adjuvant treatments are given. Current studies have highlighted the value of accurate staging of lymph node involvement in PDAC because it is correlated with outcomes depending on the intervention type and timing (Brosens et al., 2018). The final component of the TNM system, "M" for Metastasis, refers to whether the cancer has or has not metastasized to other body parts. This is critical to the staging of PDAC, where an increased likelihood of metastatic spread significantly influences therapies and prognoses. For instance, M0 indicates the absence of distant metastasis but M1 indicates the presence of metastasis. This is significant because patients with metastatic PDAC have a significantly poorer prognosis compared to those with localized disease. The detection of all sites of metastasis is essential in treatment planning since patients can be directed towards palliative care instead of curative intent in the event of distant metastasis. Proper understanding of TNM classification facilitates clinicians to formulate specific treatment strategies that are appropriate for the stage and complexity of the diseases, ultimately leading patients towards appropriate therapeutic interventions (Turowska et al., 2009).

11.4.2. Importance of Staging in Treatment Planning

Staging is also relevant to treatment planning for PDAC because it provides critical information on the extent of disease spread. By employing the TNM staging system, in which T indicates the tumor size, N lymph node involvement, and M the presence of metastasis, physicians can determine the optimal treatment modalities for the patient. Small tumors, for instance, may be resected, and surgery remains the only cure for PDAC. Conversely, individuals with more advanced disease may require palliative interventions aimed at symptom control rather than curative intent. Through accurate determination of the stage of disease, medical providers may tailor treatment modalities to maximize the potential for favorable patient outcomes while preventing unnecessary intervention. In addition, awareness of the pancreatic cancer stage increases the likelihood of predicting and advising patients. The difference between local and metastatic disease, for example, can have significant impacts on treatment possibilities and survival.

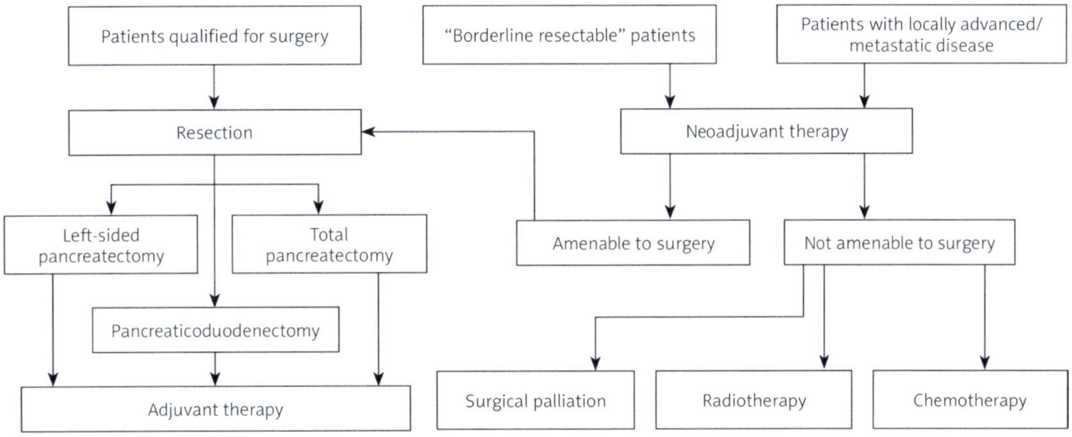

Figure 11.11. Treatment plan for pancreatic ductal adenocarcinoma in different stages.

Source: https://www.researchgate.net/profile/Julita-Kulbacka/publication/305507485/figure/fig1/AS:386757863460864@1469221668861/Treatment-plan-for-pancreatic-ductal-adenocarcinoma-in-different-stages-of-disease.png.

Those with earlier diagnoses, in which the tumor is confined to the pancreas, generally have more favorable outcomes, particularly if resected with promptness. More advanced stages, by contrast, may lead to consideration of palliative therapy and the maximization of quality of life. Therefore, accurate staging not only directs clinical practice but also determines the risk and expectation disclosure to patients and families in a way that informed and effective involvement in their care process is enabled. In addition, the improvement of staging and treatment plans highlights the need for periodic updated standards in surgical oncology. International curricula development in surgical oncology is a move towards the standardization of training and education, thus equipping healthcare providers with the awareness to adapt to the limitations of staging and treatment planning. Harmonization is essential as the cancer burden increases worldwide, calling for an appropriately qualified surgical oncology professional. As practice standards evolve with the implementation of evidence-based care, the need for accurate staging in treatment planning will remain a cornerstone in optimizing patient outcomes in addition to harmonizing therapy with the prevailing knowledge base in pancreatic ductal adenocarcinoma treatment (Are et al., 2016; Van der Hage et al., 2021) (Figure 11.11).

11.4.3. Prognostic Implications of Different Stages

In the setting of PDAC, an understanding of disease staging plays a critical role in the determination of the prognostic value to the patient. Staging, characteristically reported as being in terms of the TNM system, designates the size of the tumor, the extent of involvement by lymph nodes, and metastatic disease. Each stage is linked to specific clinical presentation and survival, with earlier stages (I and II) having much better prognoses compared with late-stage (III and IV) disease. Current literature affirms that proper identification of such disparate stages can direct therapy approaches, permitting differential treatment considerations between potential surgical resections for tumor extirpation and palliative treatments for control of advanced disease symptoms. Thus, early-stage diagnosis and treatment remain paramount in optimizing patient survival and overall quality of life (Van der Hage et al., 2021). Further, prognostic relevance of PDAC stages is also complicated by the coexistence of risk factors and genetic syndromes. Literature indicates that patients with certain genetic predispositions, such as BRCA mutation or Peutz-Jeghers syndrome, may have peculiar challenges regarding prognosis vis-à-vis their disease stage. For instance, individuals with inherited syndromes present with more extensive disease at diagnosis, which can seriously jeopardize their chances of survival even within the same TNM stage groupings. This nuance guides oncologists to more personalize surveillance and treatment regimens, considering tumor stage as well as inherent genetic predisposition. This complex approach underscores the importance of comprehensive assessment in an effort to optimize treatment outcomes in diverse patient populations (Van der Hage et al., 2021). Finally, the dramatic contrast in survival between various phases of PDAC underscores the importance of continued research and optimization of diagnostic techniques. Development in imaging and discovery of biomarkers becomes increasingly crucial in achieving earlier diagnosis of PDAC, thus allowing timely surgical intervention. Statistical evidence from research indicates that stage I patients have a five-year survival rate of almost 39%, while stage IV patients have rates as low as 3%. This is not only an indication of the profound impact staging has on prognostic result, but it also indicates a broader imperative to encourage medical practitioners to voice concern over higher awareness and screening, particularly in at-risk groups. Resolution of these imbalances ultimately has the potential to change the existing treatment paradigm, maximizing patient outcomes through early-stage intervention (Van der Hage et al., 2021).

11.5. Surgical Treatment

Surgical treatment remains an integral part of PDAC treatment, particularly for resectable disease. The gold standard in surgical treatment for PDAC is the Whipple procedure, also known as pancreaticoduodenectomy, which entails the removal of the head of the pancreas, accompanied by segments of the small intestine, bile duct, and commonly, the gallbladder. Surgical removal can potentially transform survival in carefully selected patients. However, surgery success is based on proper staging and a multidisciplinary assessment of each case, ensuring that the advantages of the procedure outweigh the risks taken. Furthermore, training in surgical oncology aims at standardizing skills among surgeons to enhance surgery outcomes, corroborating the need for a well-rounded education in cancer treatment, as reiterated by recent publications supporting reconstructing curricula in surgery (Van der Hage et al., 2021).

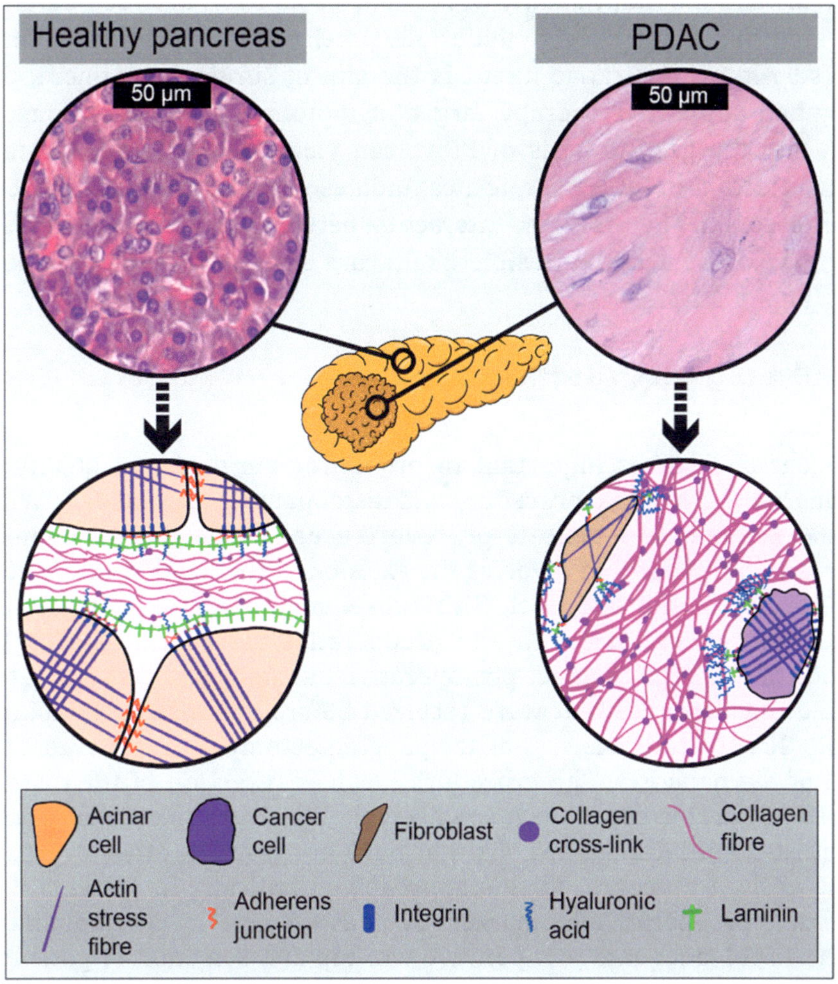

Figure 11.12. Pancreatic ductal adenocarcinoma (PDAC): Relating biomechanics and prognosis.

Source: MacCurtain BM, Quirke NP, Thorpe SD, Gallagher TK. Pancreatic Ductal Adenocarcinoma: Relating Biomechanics and Prognosis. *Journal of Clinical Medicine*. 2021; 10(12):2711. https://doi.org/10.3390/jcm10122711

With pancreatic cancer, timing and location of surgical therapy are paramount. In patients with localized disease, surgical resection can be the only chance for long-term remission. Yet, high locoregional failure rate of PDAC requires a strict approach to adjuvant therapy following surgery. Chemotherapy and chemoradiotherapy have been shown to improve outcomes if administered post-surgical resection. This multidisciplinary orientation highlights the strength of an integrated team, which can provide best treatment pathways including postoperative care and other therapies appropriate to a patient's disease profile. This is also supported by participating in clinical trials, which contributes to the evolving evidence base for treatments, reaffirming the role of surgery in the overall therapeutic framework (Verslype et al., 2007). Not all PDAC patients are, however, suitable for surgery because of several factors, such as the advanced stage of the tumor or the presence of severe comorbidities. In their case, the focus shifts to palliative treatment as a required necessity to manage symptoms and maintain quality of life. The separation between surgical and palliative treatment draws attention to the need to undertake precise staging and an intimate knowledge of the diseases course. Although curative intent is the aim of surgical treatment, palliative therapy via chemotherapy and supportive therapy targets symptom relief and prolongation of survival. Ongoing research into the genetic basis of PDAC can yield novel therapeutic targets as well as perhaps direct the selection of future surgical candidates and maximize palliative interventions in noncandidates for resection. Therefore, the interaction between surgery and palliative interventions requires ongoing development and a flexible healthcare system to address patients' needs in an effective manner (Figure 11.12).

11.5.1. Types of Surgical Procedures (Whipple Procedure, Distal Pancreatectomy)

Surgical management of PDAC is important in promoting survival and quality of life, and two common operations are the Whipple procedure and distal pancreatectomy. The Whipple procedure, or pancreaticoduodenectomy, is a delicate procedure usually indicated for tumors arising in the head of the pancreas. This procedure involves the excision of the head of the pancreas, duodenum, gallbladder, and portion of the bile duct with subsequent repair of the gastrointestinal tract. Research indicates that patient selection and preoperative assessment during Whipple surgery are important since they directly impact postoperative outcome and survival rate, particularly in the case of neoadjuvant therapies that were received before enhance resectability and prognosis (Wetterauer et al., 2023). Nevertheless, distal pancreatectomy is applied to tumors located in the body and tail of the pancreas. The procedure involves resection of the distal segment of the pancreas and, in some specific cases, even splenectomy. The distal pancreatectomy is particularly effective in the situation of localized lesions that have not invaded other organs. Several studies have reported the desired outcomes in this approach, specifically in patients with lower tumor burdens and favorable preoperative biomarkers such as CA 19-9 levels (Mortimer, 2024). Similar to any operation in PDAC, adequate preoperative workup and selection of patients are important, with the benefit of surgery outweighing possible hazards. While both the Whipple procedure and distal pancreatectomy bear indications and implications of their own, they both underscore the role of surgery in the management of PDAC. Choice between procedures typically is based on the site of the tumor, extent of disease, and factors related to the patient, including overall health and goals of treatment. The evolution in surgical techniques and preoperative care modalities, including the use of neoadjuvant treatment, reflects increased understanding of the disease and offers the hope of improved patient outcome following surgery (Wetterauer et al., 2023). Because of this, these resections are central to the cure in localized disease as well as to the assessment of the efficacy of adjunctive treatments within the overall therapeutic regimen of pancreatic ductal adenocarcinoma.

11.5.2. Criteria for Surgical Candidacy

Surgical candidacy is established in PDAC patients based on a meticulous assessment of various clinical, anatomical, and molecular factors. The initial step is the staging of the cancer based on TNM classification, which reflects the extent of spread of the tumor and potential for resectability. Patients are candidates for surgery only if they present with resectable tumors, and these typically have localized disease without vascular invasion or distant metastasis.

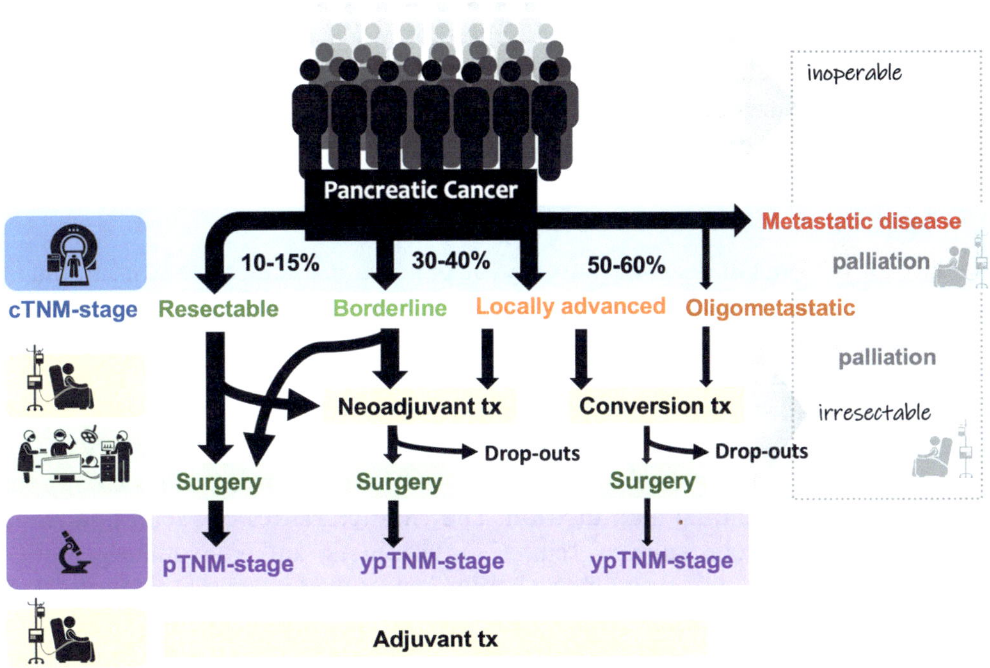

Figure 11.13. TNM-staging for pancreatic adenocarcinoma.

Source: https://ars.els-cdn.com/content/image/1-s2.0-S0748798320301165-gr2.jpg.

Furthermore, diagnostic modalities such as imaging studies—CT scan and MRI, are of critical importance in determining the behavior of the tumor and the involvement of surrounding organs. The determination is underlined by the necessity of obtaining adequate surgical margins because studies have shown that a margin clearance greater than 1.5 mm is crucial in long-term survival, contributing to the blend of surgical proficiency and comprehensive preoperative evaluation. Beyond conventional imaging and clinical staging, the inclusion of molecular biomarkers in candidacy determination for surgery is a new frontier in PDAC treatment. S100A4 and S100A2 have been identified as independent markers of prognosis, offering more advanced information about tumor behavior and possible responsiveness to treatment. Stratification of patients by these biomarkers significantly enhances preoperative decision-making, being able to predict who is most likely to be benefited by surgical resection as opposed to palliative therapy. Preoperative molecular prognostic nomograms integrating tumor size with expression of biomarkers, for instance, can more accurately predict survival outcomes compared to models derived using clinical factors only. Such advances are in line with the trend toward personalized medicine, which increasingly informs therapeutic strategies in oncology, such as in the case of such refractory cancers as pancreatic cancer. Furthermore, the patient's general condition and functional status are unavoidable variables in determining fitness for surgery. Deliberate preoperative assessment, such as comorbidity, nutritional status, and psychosocial preparedness, are unavoidable in order to guarantee that patients can undergo the stress of surgical therapy. Poor performance status or severe comorbidities can preclude patients from curatively planned surgery, and thus modify the treatment priority toward managed care or palliative therapy. Furthermore, surgical expertise plays a crucial role in successful resection of PDAC, where complex surgical maneuvers, such as minimally invasive surgery and prolonged pancreatectomy, are seen to influence patient outcome. The recent literature emphasizes the importance of a strategy that includes multidisciplinary care consisting of oncologists, surgeons, and supportive care teams to ensure best treatment pathways according to patient-specific criteria (Figure 11.13).

11.5.3. Postoperative Care and Complications

Postoperative care for patients undergoing surgery for pancreatic ductal adenocarcinoma is important due to the high potential for complications associated with this disease. After Whipple surgery, patients usually face serious issues regarding pain management, nutrition, and assessment for postoperative complications like pancreatic fistula, delayed gastric emptying, and infections. Pain management is very crucial, and ineffective pain control results in longer hospital stays and prolonged recovery. Moreover, nutritional impairments are caused by the process of surgery and the disease itself and demand strict planning of the diet and potential supplementation to support patients in recovering strength and avoiding malnutrition. The characteristics of such impairments require a multidisciplinary care between surgical teams, nutritionists, and pain management experts to improve recovery after surgery and support the healing process of patients (Andersson et al., 2022). Apart from postoperative complications during the operation, long-term complications also have a significant effect on the quality of life in postoperative pancreatic ductal adenocarcinoma patients. The majority of patients will have recurring symptoms of pancreatic insufficiency, which manifest as malabsorption, weight loss, and diabetes secondary to disturbed endocrine function. Follow-up is mandated from time to time to assess the nutrition of the patients and treat any metabolic complications that arise. The emotional impact of a cancer diagnosis and major surgery also should not be underestimated. Patients may require the use of mental health resources to address anxiety, depression, and emotional distress as they heal from their experience. The synergistic effects of these physical and emotional consequences amplify the need for a comprehensive postoperative care plan that addresses all aspects of patient health and recovery (Are et al., 2016). In addition, evolving standards for surgical oncology training and postoperative care identify the necessity for the effective management of complications. An inadequate area of training for surgical oncologists is a cause for inconsistency in postoperative care, which can translate into variation in outcomes across institutions and geographically. Developing a global curriculum in surgical oncology, as commenced by the Society of Surgical Oncology, aims to standardize significant competencies in the management of postoperative care and complications. Such guidelines are critical to improving the postoperative quality of patients with pancreatic ductal adenocarcinoma. By educating surgical teams on better practices and including multidisciplinary care, overall rates of surgical complications can be avoided, resulting in maximizing survival rates and quality of life in this high-risk patient group (Are et al., 2016; Andersson et al., 2022).

11.6. Palliative Treatment

In pancreatic ductal adenocarcinoma (PDA) treatment, palliative care also plays an important role, especially because this cancer is usually diagnosed in advanced stages where curative surgery is no longer possible. The primary aim of palliative care is symptom diminishment, enhancement of the quality of life, and provision of psychological support to patients and their families. In view of the unique symptomatic burden of PDA, including severe pain, weight loss, and gastrointestinal disturbances, palliative treatment is generally a broad-based strategy that incorporates pharmacotherapy, enteral feeding, and psychosocial care.

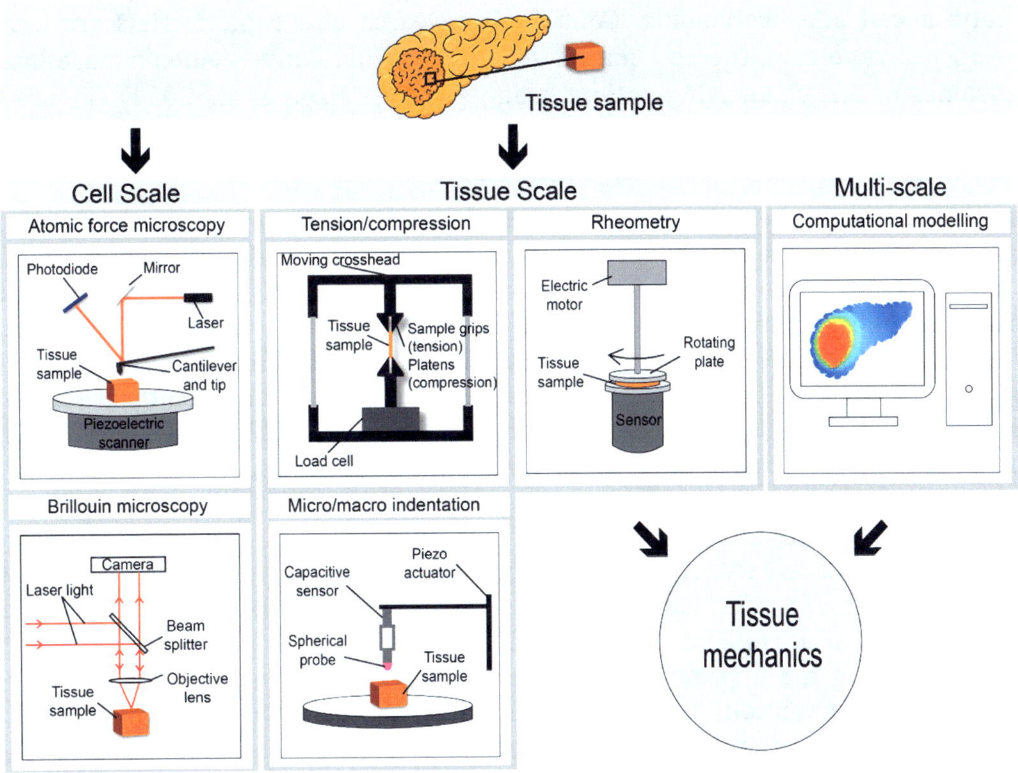

Figure 11.14. Targeted therapy for pancreatic ductal adenocarcinoma.

Source: MacCurtain BM, Quirke NP, Thorpe SD, Gallagher TK. Pancreatic Ductal Adenocarcinoma: Relating Biomechanics and Prognosis. *Journal of Clinical Medicine*. 2021; 10(12):2711. https://doi.org/10.3390/jcm10122711

These comprehensive regimens enable symptom alleviation and overall enhancement of the quality of life in the patients such that quality of life rather than mere prolongation becomes the objective. Current evidence confirms the effectiveness of various palliative therapy modalities in PDA patients. Chemotherapy has also been shown to enhance survival and symptoms within both adjuvant and palliative situations, with agents like gemcitabine yielding positive outcomes when administered together with other drugs like erlotinib or platinum-containing compounds (Verslype et al., 2007). Combination therapy not only optimizes pharmacologic effect but also helps in the control of complications of advanced disease. Moreover, palliative radiotherapy has some other benefits, particularly for locally advanced disease when surgery is out of the question. Best practice is a coalition of health workers who can customize treatment strategies to address the requirements of every patient while giving effective humane care. Providing palliative care to PDA patients requires an integral system including constant assessment and adjustment of the treatment plan. Continuous monitoring of symptomatic progression allows healthcare providers to modify palliative therapies effectively, focusing on patient comfort. Additionally, establishing open communication between the patient and care team is essential in addressing emotional and psychological concerns, which often accompany a cancer diagnosis. Through establishing a supportive culture of compassion, palliative care can significantly enhance the quality of life for those living with pancreatic ductal adenocarcinoma. Continuing research and clinical trials are essential to further develop palliative care, thereby contributing to the cumulative evidence base intended to optimize outcomes in this challenging patient group (Van der Hage et al., 2021) (Figure 11.14).

11.6.1. Goals of Palliative Care in Pancreatic Cancer

The aims of palliative treatment for pancreatic cancer are varied, primarily aiming to enhance patient quality of life in cases of poor prognosis. Among these are the alleviation of symptoms accompanying the illness and its treatment, such as pain, nausea, fatigue, and emotional distress. Unlike curative treatment, where survival prolongation is the focus without consideration of the discomfort and emotional state, palliative treatment prioritizes them. This patient-focused approach encourages open communication between patients, their loved ones, and healthcare professionals in order to adequately address both physical and psychosocial problems. Research has proven that the introduction of palliative care early can lead to higher patient satisfaction, reduced hospitalization, and even increased survival in some cases, testifying to its indispensable role within the overall treatment of pancreatic ductal adenocarcinoma (Huang et al., 2020). Apart from symptom management, the palliative care teams are responsible for designing multidisciplinary care according to the patient's requirements. The teams consist of oncologists, palliative care specialists, social workers, and dietitians who collaborate to provide holistic care. For pancreatic cancer patients, it may include designing the appropriate nutrition intervention to manage cachexia as well as designing pain relief interventions that include pharmacological as well as non-pharmacological measures. Moreover, palliative care facilitates advanced care planning to ensure that the treatment decisions are in line with the patient's values, preferences, and goals throughout their experience with cancer. Such an interdisciplinary arrangement ensures that the patient receives personalized care that honors their dignity and preferences (Agarwal et al., 2017). In addition, the role of palliative care encompasses bereavement support to the families following death. The psychological burden of pancreatic cancer is not limited to the patient, and it is therefore essential that palliative care services incorporate family support and grief counseling resources. This comprehensive model serves to address not only the patient's affliction but also the family's effects from acute illness. By integrating a holistic model of palliative care that treats the entire cancer journey from diagnosis to survival issues to end-of-life decisions, medical care professionals can significantly enhance overall patient experience for pancreatic cancer. Thus, this supportive infrastructure must be recognized as an invaluable component of oncology therapy, complementing the requirement for early implementation of palliative approaches even in situations with aggressive treatments (Agarwal et al., 2017; Huang et al., 2020) (Figure 11.15).

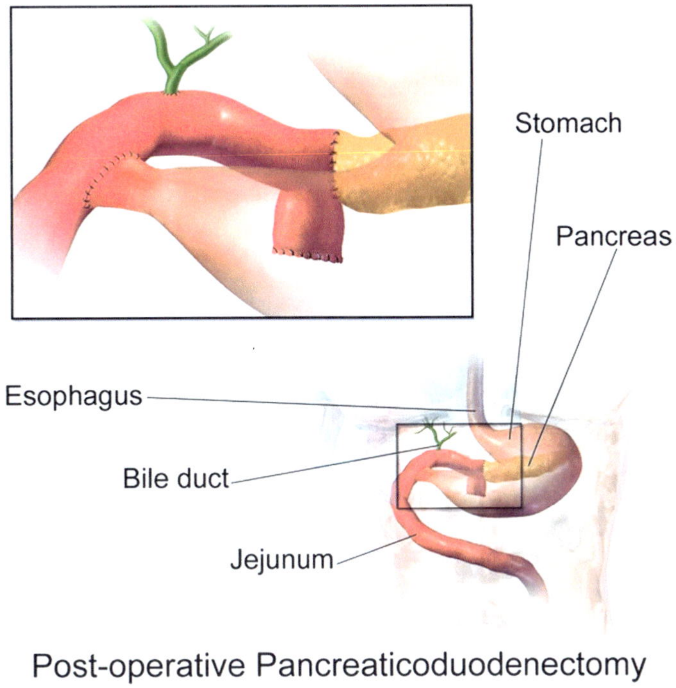

Figure 11.15. Palliative therapy.

Source: https://cdn.storymd.com/optimized/koXkaNFEA8/thumbnail.webp.

11.6.2. Pain Management Strategies

Effective pain management is essential in those with PDAC since the condition is associated with extreme pain and distress. Pain complexity typically necessitates the use of a multidisciplinary team composed of oncologists, pain specialists, and palliative care teams. The practitioners collaborate to create tailor-made management plans addressing the multiple reasons for pain that patients experience, and these include a combination of cancer and treatment side effects. Pharmacological management, such as the use of opioids and adjunctive interventions, is significant for pain reduction, but equally significant is maintaining constant assessment and adjustment of these interventions to meet the patient's evolving needs. An active, evidence-based strategy, as suggested by current guidelines, is necessary to maximize the quality of life of patients during treatment (Martin-Perez et al., 2021). For PDAC, as well, non-drug approaches to pain control are equally significant. The approaches, for example, of psychosocial support, physiotherapy, and complementary treatments like acupuncture or mindfulness, can optimize the effectiveness of traditional means of pain alleviation. Such interventions can ease not only the physical aspects of pain but also the psychological and emotional weight that accompany a cancer diagnosis. Evidence points to the importance of addressing these holistic needs, and the potential to increase the experience of agency and overall care satisfaction. The inclusion of such non-pharmacological interventions into pain management programs is best practice and consistent with the imperative of multi-dimensional patient support, as posited by Verslype et al. (2007). The context and timing of interventions during pain management may also significantly affect patient outcomes. For the cases of PDAC treated with surgery, early treatment can prevent chronic pain, which is still a significant issue after the procedure. Palliative treatments become particularly critical when curative interventions are no longer possible and attention shifts to enhancing quality of life through symptom control. The evolving pain profile in PDAC necessitates regular re-evaluation and flexibility from healthcare providers, in such a way that the plans for managing pain are informed about patient preferences and treatment responses. Especially, as clinical controversies have shown, this adaptability is a component for improved outcomes and can involve participation in clinical trials for the exploration of new means of managing pain for future use (Verslype et al., 2007).

11.6.3. Supportive Therapies and Quality of Life Considerations

Supportive therapies in PDAC are crucial in all ways of enhancing patients' quality of life, especially advanced disease where curative treatment is no longer available. Supportive therapies are a great number of interventions designed to palliate disease and disease treatment symptoms and complications. Pain relief is a good example since most of these patients exhibit considerable distress caused by tumor growth and metastasis. Integrating palliative care teams can provide a multidisciplinary intervention that places top value on pain and symptom management in addition to conventional medical treatment.

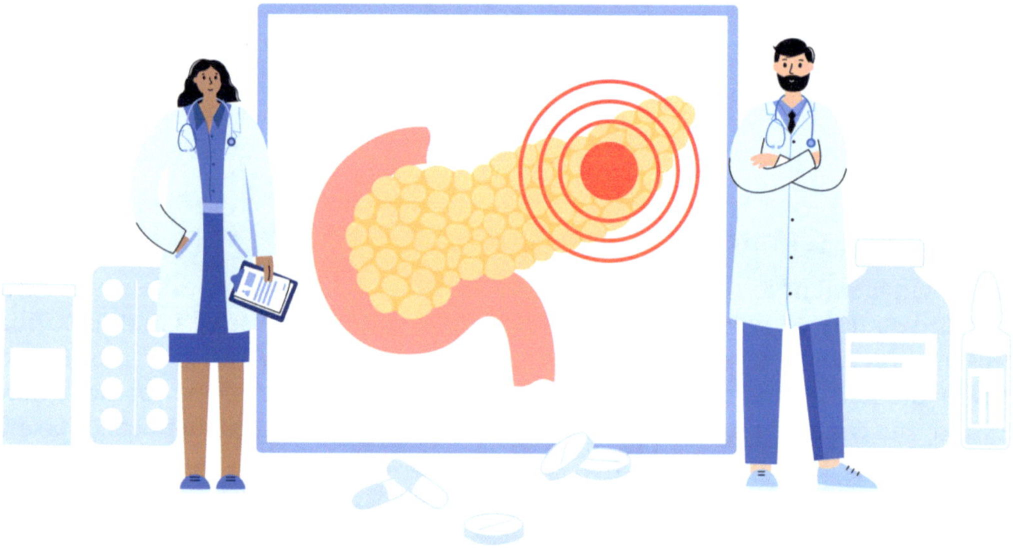

Figure 11.16. Supportive therapies and quality of life considerations in pancreatic cancer.

Source: https://cancercoach.co/wp-content/uploads/2020/11/pancreatic-cancer.jpg.

In addition, correction of nutritional deficiencies by way of dietary guidance has the potential to reverse weight loss and cachexia, which occur commonly among PDAC patients due to the disease and resultant metabolic disturbances. These supportive measures not only improve the physical health but also psychological and emotional care, resulting in an overall quality of life. Moreover, the psychological distress of PDAC diagnosis and subsequent treatment process has immense impacts on patients and families as well. Psychosocial support services within the treatment framework are required in order to manage anxiety and depression, which are prevalent among such patients.

Services that involve counseling, support groups, or mental health care give patients vital coping skills, a feeling of community, and emotional strength. Interestingly, these services are also given to caregivers, who have their own stressors attending to the patient. As underscored by relevant literature, the use of long-term supportive therapies has been associated with improvement in subjective well-being among patients and thus confirming the belief that PDAC treatment extends beyond physical symptoms. Mental health management is thus a crucial component of integrative cancer treatment. Finally, as much as survival rates in PDAC remain low, focus on the quality of life, particularly in patients receiving palliative treatment, can lead to dramatic implications. The exploration of supportive therapies, including pharmacological and non-pharmacological interventions, is notable for their focus on the management of advanced disease. Evidence shows that the patients who get multimodal care, which may include chemotherapy in combination with symptom care, report greater overall satisfaction with their treatment. Besides, as shown in treatment strategies for oligometastatic disease studies, tailored surgical treatments also enhance survival in particular patients, opening doors to improved quality of life. Thus, it is imperative that clinicians put emphasis on supportive therapy, integrating it into treatment regimens, in order to eventually enhance the quality of life for patients with PDAC management challenges (Ghidini et al., 2019; Holmberg, 2022) (Figure 11.16).

A CLOSER LOOK

STAGES OF PANCREATIC CANCER

Pancreatic cancer is usually staged based on the TNM system (Tumor, Node, Metastasis) that gives a measure of the magnitude of spread of the disease and guides treatment planning. The stages range from Stage 0 (carcinoma in situ) to Stage IV (metastatic disease). In Stage 0, there is cancer only in the surface layers of the pancreatic duct cells and not in deeper tissues or in lymph nodes or distant organs. It is an early or premalignant phase that is seldom clinically detected but can be found incidentally in individuals who are at high risk and are under surveillance. Stage I is divided into IA and IB based on tumor size. Stage IA is employed if tumors are smaller than 2 cm and confined to the pancreas, and Stage IB is employed if tumors are greater than 2 cm but confined to the pancreas. No lymph node involvement and metastasis yet, and surgical excision offers the best promise of cure (Figure 11.17).

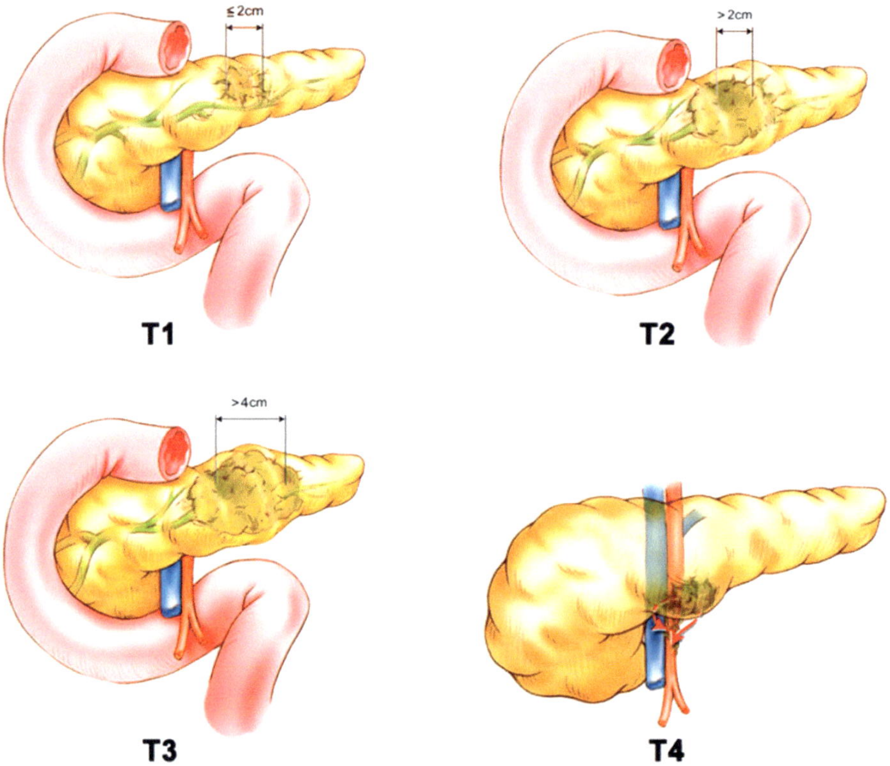

Source: https://pathology.jhu.edu/build/assets/pancreas/_lgImg/pancreas-tumor-illustrations.jpg.

Stage II pancreatic cancer is local tumor growth outside the pancreas or microscopic regional lymph node spread. Stage IIA includes tumors that grow outside the pancreas without vascular invasion of large arteries or veins and no nodal involvement. Stage IIB means cancer in regional lymph nodes but without vascular invasion. These patients are typically still considered resectable, although lymph node metastasis will reduce long-term survival. Stage III pancreatic cancer is typically considered locally advanced and unresectable since the tumor has infiltrated large vasculature, such as the superior mesenteric artery or celiac axis. While no distant spread to the body has occurred, involvement of critical vasculature makes surgical resection difficult. Treatment in this stage usually includes chemotherapy and/or radiation to attempt downstaging the tumor (Mortoglou, 2024).

Stage IV is the highest stage and indicates that cancer has metastasized to distant organs, usually the peritoneum, liver, or lungs. Metastatic pancreatic cancer patients cannot be surgically treated and are treated with systemic therapies such as chemotherapy, targeted therapy, or immunotherapy in exceptional cases. Prognosis deteriorates markedly with advancing stage, and overall 5-year survival for pancreatic cancer remains low, most notably in Stage IV, where it is less than 5%. Early detection and staging are crucial to optimizing the outcome of treatment, and studies into biomarkers, imaging, and molecular profiling are continually improving early diagnosis and therapeutic strategies (Idachaba et al., 2019).

SUMMARY

Overview of PDAC, it is interesting to discuss the rationale for its unfavorable prognosis despite advances in the understanding of its biological basis. The lack of early diagnosis advances renders most patients, approximately 90%, diagnosed with late-stage disease, thus limiting the potential of available treatment. The main thrust of ongoing research is to find new biomarkers for early detection, which has the potential to drastically change patient outcomes. These developments may bring with them windows into personalized therapeutic regimens, foretelling precision oncology to be a key means to navigate the complexities of PDAC. If we do not accord priority to these novel strategies, the socioeconomic burden induced by pancreatic cancer will continue to increase, further substantiating the requirement for more advanced diagnostic and therapeutic regimens (Andersson et al., 2022). Furthermore, understanding of surgical and palliative treatment clinical results provides insight into patient survival and quality of life. Though the only curative treatment present, surgical resection is applicable only to a limited number of patients. Trends indicate performance status and disease stage are among factors determining outcomes after surgery. In contrast, in palliative patients—usually with end-stage disease—treatment objectives focus on symptom relief and quality of life conservation. The literature at hand is evocative of variability in survival rates and recurrence patterns between neoplastic PDAC conditions and other cancers, as evidenced by the intraductal papillary mucinous neoplasm (inv-IPMN) study with favorable rates presented (Holmberg, 2022). These differences emphasize the need to adapt treatment protocols considering patient profiles, reaffirming the importance of informed decision-making that considers patient values. Overall, pancreatic ductal adenocarcinoma is a very complicated disease process that necessitates risk assessment, genetic predisposition, appropriate staging, and an elegant appreciation of treatment options. Future research must not only focus on high-risk patients and potential genetic syndromes but also prioritize developing protocol-based interventions that address the complexity of PDAC. Advances in early detection, coupled with investigation into improved molecular characterization of tumors, could lead to more aggressive efforts in managing this potent disease. Lastly, a dynamic between rigorous scientific inquiry and clinical practice holds center stage in revolutionizing PDAC management and improving prognostic outcomes for patients who suffer from this devious cancer (Andersson et al., 2022).

The finding of PDA reveals a complex interaction of predisposing risk factors and genetic factors that account for the onset and progression of the disease. Notably, modifiable risk factors related to lifestyle such as smoking, obesity, and diabetes emerge as significant factors that increase the risk for PDA. In addition, genetic syndromes like Peutz-Jeghers syndrome and hereditary pancreatitis identify the hereditary nature of the condition, meaning that a patient's family history is a highly significant factor for susceptibility. This multifactorial perspective of PDA emphasizes the need for comprehensive preventive strategies through both genetic screening and lifestyle adaptation, as well as an understanding of the heterogeneous character of the disease that can vary hugely from patient to patient (Sundaresan et al., 2022). Pancreatic ductal adenocarcinoma diagnosis and staging are the most crucial steps in the decision of appropriate therapeutic approaches. The TNM system, quantifying tumor size, nodal status, and metastasis, is at the core of staging and guides treatment planning. Early detection remains challenging because the disease often is asymptomatic in the early stages. Technical breakthroughs in imaging and biomarkers are key advances toward improved diagnostic accuracy. Biomarkers produced through tumor biology research can increase detection levels, and in clinical applications, they have the potential to transform patterns of disease management to a great extent. Lastly, standardizing diagnostic procedures with precise staging procedures can improve prognosis outcomes and enable timely interventions for patients (Yee et al., 2019). Treatment for pancreatic ductal adenocarcinoma highlights the difference between surgical intervention and palliative care. Surgical extirpation, when feasible, has the best hope for long-term survival; yet, the majority of patients are seen at stages beyond surgical cure. In these instances, palliative therapy strives to palliate, rather than cure, symptoms and improve quality of life, with a particular focus on sensitive care. Choice of therapy must be based on a full understanding of the patient's illness, desires, and biological behavior of the tumor. With the ongoing advancements in research, the application of precision medicine approaches to therapy regimens becomes increasingly important. This shift may involve personalized therapies and innovative combinations of drugs targeting individual tumor biomarkers, but also additional enhancement of the therapeutic strategies' effectiveness and the psychosocial aspects of patient treatment (Yee et al., 2019; Sundaresan et al., 2022).

KEY TERMS FROM THIS CHAPTER

- Age-related mechanisms
- Biological gender differences
- Biomarkers
- Body mass indexes (BMIs)
- Cancer risk
- Endoscopic ultrasound
- Evidence-based therapy
- Fat malabsorption
- Fine-needle aspiration (FNA)
- Gene mutation
- Genetic counseling
- Genetic illness

References

1. Idachaba, S., Dada, O., Abimbola, O., Olayinka, O., Uma, A., Olunu, E., & Fakoya, A. O. J. (2019). A Review of Pancreatic Cancer: Epidemiology, Genetics, Screening, and Management. *Open access Macedonian journal of medical sciences*, *7*(4), 663–671. https://doi.org/10.3889/oamjms.2019.104 (accessed on 26 May 2025).
2. Agarwal, D. M., DeWitt, J., Eagleson, M., Easler, J., et al. (2017). A multidisciplinary approach to pancreas cancer in 2016: A review. https://core.ac.uk/download/129149165.pdf (accessed on 26 May 2025).
3. van der Hage, J., Sandrucci, S., Audisio, R., Wyld, L., Søreide, K., ESSO core curriculum contributors, Amaral, T., Audisio, R., Bahadoer, V., Beets, G., Benstead, K., Berge Nilsen, E., Bol, K., Brandl, A., Braun, J., Cufer, T., Dopazo, C., Edhemovic, I., Eriksen, J. G., Fiore, M., ... Zahl Eriksson, A. G. (2021). The ESSO core curriculum committee update on surgical oncology. *European journal of surgical oncology : the journal of the European Society of Surgical Oncology and the British Association of Surgical Oncology*, *47*(11), e1–e30. https://doi.org/10.1016/j.ejso.2021.10.003 (accessed on 26 May 2025).
4. Andersson, R., Ansari, D., Haglund, C., Seppänen, H., et al. (2022). Pancreatic cancer—The past, the present, and the future. https://core.ac.uk/download/551684805.pdf (accessed on 26 May 2025).
5. Are, C., Berman, R. S., Wyld, L., Cummings, C., Lecoq, C., & Audisio, R. A. (2016). Global Curriculum in Surgical Oncology. *Annals of surgical oncology*, *23*(6), 1782–1795. https://doi.org/10.1245/s10434-016-5239-7 (accessed on 26 May 2025).
6. Biagini, M. R., Galli, A., & Lami, G. (2014). Endoscopic ultrasonography for surveillance of individuals at high risk for pancreatic cancer. https://core.ac.uk/download/301569814.pdf (accessed on 26 May 2025).
7. Biankin, A. V., Casolino, R., Golan, T., Hall, M. J., et al. (2023). Germline BRCA testing in pancreatic cancer: Improving awareness, timing, turnaround, and uptake. https://core.ac.uk/download/593670877.pdf (accessed on 26 May 2025).
8. Martin-Perez, E., Domínguez-Muñoz, J. E., Botella-Romero, F., Cerezo, L., Matute Teresa, F., Serrano, T., & Vera, R. (2020). Multidisciplinary consensus statement on the clinical management of patients with pancreatic cancer. *Clinical & translational oncology : official publication of the Federation of Spanish Oncology Societies and of the National Cancer Institute of Mexico*, *22*(11), 1963–1975. https://doi.org/10.1007/s12094-020-02350-6 (accessed on 26 May 2025).
9. Brosens, L., Dijk, F., Fariña-Sarasqueta, A., Koens, L., et al. (2018). Dilemmas for the pathologist in the oncologic assessment of pancreatoduodenectomy specimens. https://core.ac.uk/download/154410315.pdf (accessed on 26 May 2025).
10. Butler, J. V. (2025). Factors which influence penetrance in familial pancreatic cancer. https://core.ac.uk/download/80775755.pdf (accessed on 26 May 2025).
11. Cannavale, A., Santoni, M., Gazzetti, M., Maher, B., Fanelli, F., Fiocca, F., & Catalano, C. (2016). Updated Management of Malignant Biliary Tract Tumors: An Illustrative Review. *Journal of vascular and interventional radiology : JVIR*, *27*(7), 1056–1069. https://doi.org/10.1016/j.jvir.2016.01.149(accessed on 26 May 2025).

12. Verslype, C., Van Cutsem, E., Dicato, M., Cascinu, S., Cunningham, D., Diaz-Rubio, E., Glimelius, B., Haller, D., Haustermans, K., Heinemann, V., Hoff, P., Johnston, P. G., Kerr, D., Labianca, R., Louvet, C., Minsky, B., Moore, M., Nordlinger, B., Pedrazzoli, S., Roth, A., ... Zalcberg, J. (2007). The management of pancreatic cancer. Current expert opinion and recommendations derived from the 8th World Congress on Gastrointestinal Cancer, Barcelona, 2006. *Annals of oncology : official journal of the European Society for Medical Oncology, 18 Suppl 7,* vii1–vii10. https://doi.org/10.1093/annonc/mdm210 (accessed on 26 May 2025).

13. Chang, D. (2011). *Biomarkers of Phenotype, Prognosis and Response to Therapy in Pancreatic Cancer* [Doctoral dissertation, University of New South Wales]. UNSWorks. https://unsworks.unsw.edu.au/bitstreams/e46d22ad-63c0-45ee-832e-82950d0198c1/download (accessed on 26 May 2025).

14. Eurola, A. (2022). *Treatment Response and Thromboembolic Complications in Neoadjuvant-Treated Pancreatic Cancer* [Doctoral dissertation]. https://core.ac.uk/download/541342377.pdf (accessed on 26 May 2025).

15. Franceschi, Silvia and Herrero, Rolando (2014) Infections. In: Hall, Andrew J., Newton, Robert, Qiao, You-Lin, Stewart, B. V. and Wild, C. P., (eds.) World Cancer Report 2014. World Cancer Report . International Agency for Research on Cancer , Lyons , pp. 105-114. (accessed on 26 May 2025).

16. Mendieta Zerón, H., García Flores, J. R., & Romero Prieto, M. L. (2009). Limitations in improving detection of pancreatic adenocarcinoma. *Future oncology (London, England)*, *5*(5), 657–668. https://doi.org/10.2217/fon.09.32

17. Ghidini, M., Petrillo, A., Salati, M., Khakoo, S., Varricchio, A., Tomasello, G., Grossi, F., & Petrelli, F. (2019). Surgery or Locoregional Approaches for Hepatic Oligometastatic Pancreatic Cancer: Myth, Hope, or Reality?. *Cancers*, *11*(8), 1095. https://doi.org/10.3390/cancers11081095(accessed on 26 May 2025).

18. Søreide, K., Ismail, W., Roalsø, M., Ghotbi, J., & Zaharia, C. (2023). Early Diagnosis of Pancreatic Cancer: Clinical Premonitions, Timely Precursor Detection and Increased Curative-Intent Surgery. *Cancer control : journal of the Moffitt Cancer Center*, *30*, 10732748231154711. https://doi.org/10.1177/10732748231154711 (accessed on 26 May 2025).

19. Holmberg, M. (2022). *Invasive Intraductal Papillary Mucinous Neoplasm and Pancreatic Ductal Adenocarcinoma: A Comparison in Clinicopathology and Long-Term Outcome* [Doctoral dissertation]. https://core.ac.uk/download/541039934.pdf (accessed on 26 May 2025).

20. Hoyer, K. (2021). *Molecular Biological Characterization of Resectable Pancreatic Ductal Adenocarcinoma* [Doctoral dissertation]. https://core.ac.uk/download/479349145.pdf (accessed on 26 May 2025).

21. Huang, L. (2020). *Investigation of Treatment Modalities and Outcomes Concerning Pancreatic and Gastric Cancer Patients in Europe and the US* [Doctoral dissertation]. https://core.ac.uk/download/287790221.pdf (accessed on 26 May 2025).

22. Iacobelli, S., Iovanna, J., et al. (2012). *Diagnostic, Prognostic and Therapeutic Value of Gene Signatures.* https://core.ac.uk/download/53299347.pdf (accessed on 26 May 2025).

23. Lee, N., & Yee, N. (2019). *Cancer Biomarkers and Targets in Digestive Organs.* https://core.ac.uk/download/478119209.pdf (accessed on 26 May 2025).

24. Lewis, S. (2018). *Sociodemographic and Pancreatic Cancer Survival Rate* [Doctoral dissertation]. https://core.ac.uk/download/217231241.pdf (accessed on 26 May 2025).

25. Wasif, N., Ko, C. Y., Farrell, J., Wainberg, Z., Hines, O. J., Reber, H., & Tomlinson, J. S. (2010). Impact of tumor grade on prognosis in pancreatic cancer: should we include grade in AJCC staging?. *Annals of surgical oncology, 17*(9), 2312–2320. https://doi.org/10.1245/s10434-010-1071-7

26. Mauro, A., Faverio, C., Brizzi, L., Mazza, S., Scalvini, D., Alfieri, D., Cappellini, A., et al. (2025). Multidisciplinary therapeutic approaches to pancreatic cancer according to the resect ability status. *Journal of Clinical Medicine, 14*. https://www.semanticscholar.org/paper/a2406ee46bcff8ad59e409904593b897dca87b3b (accessed on 26 May 2025).

27. Mortimer, M. (2024). *Contemporary Approaches to The Diagnosis and Management of Pancreatic Ductal Adenocarcinoma: Examining the Role of Biomarkers in Aiding Early Diagnosis* [Doctoral dissertation]. DOI (Published version): 10.23889/SUthesis.66243(accessed on 26 May 2025).

28. Mortoglou, M. (2024). *MicroRNAs in Pancreatic Ductal Adenocarcinoma: New Approaches for Better Diagnosis and Therapy* [Doctoral dissertation]. https://core.ac.uk/download/596424369.pdf (accessed on 26 May 2025).

29. Nichols, L. (2021). *The Utility of a Novel Blood-Based Biomarker in The Diagnosis of Pancreatic Cancer* [Doctoral dissertation]. https://core.ac.uk/download/479457592.pdf (accessed on 26 May 2025).

30. Podină, N., Gheorghe, E. C., Constantin, A., Cazacu, I., Croitoru, V., Gheorghe, C., Balaban, D., et al. (2025). Artificial intelligence in pancreatic imaging: A systematic review. *United European Gastroenterology Journal, 13*, 55–77. https://www.semanticscholar.org/paper/ba90db863b28e1bb6b1b9576c8eaba98bbe0cf51 (accessed on 26 May 2025).

31. Sundaresan, S., Çetin, F., Birge, Ö., Sharan, M., Mathur, R., Kumar, M., Rana, K., et al. (2022). Clinical diagnosis and management of squamous cell carcinoma. In *IntechOpen eBooks*. https://doi.org/10.5772/intechopen.94812.

32. Turowska, A., Lebkowska, U., & Walecki, J. (2009). Evaluation and treatment decision of pancreatic tumors by use of MRI with MRCP imaging. Polish Journal of Radiology, 74(1), p. 7–15.(accessed on 26 May 2025).

33. Wetterauer, N. (2023). *Der Nutzen Von Prädiktiven Faktoren Zur Identifikation Von Patienten Mit Primär Nicht Resektablem Adenokarzinom Des Pankreas, Welche Von Einer Sekundären Resektion Profitieren* [Doctoral dissertation]. https://core.ac.uk/download/555540498.pdf (accessed on 26 May 2025).

34. Yee, N. S., Lee, N. P., Zhang, Y., Zarrabi, K., Hou, W., Madajewicz, S., Choi, M., et al. (2019). *Cancer Biomarkers and Targets in Digestive Organs*. MDPI. https://doi.org/10.3390/books978-3-03921-464-8.

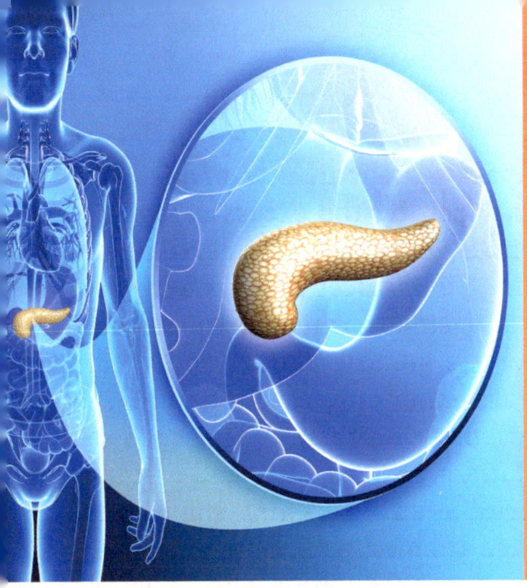

Chapter 12

PANCREATIC NEUROENDOCRINE TUMORS (PNETS)

Contents

Introduction

The view of pancreatic neuroendocrine tumors (PNETs) is a fascinating but problematic situation in oncology, with clinically and biologically heterogeneous behaviors. Compared with the more common exocrine pancreas cancers, PNETs are of neuroendocrine cell origin and classified into functioning and non-functioning categories, largely based on their endocrine activity. Functional tumors, that is, insulinomas and gastrinomas, secrete hormones leading to unusual clinical syndromes, whereas non-functioning tumors typically remain silent until late disease, thus ensuring the diagnosis and treatment in a timely fashion difficult. This distinction emphasizes the need for an intimate familiarity with the specific biological pathways of these tumors, their presentation, and the consequent specific therapeutic approaches required for successful control. The multidisciplinary care of PNETs requires advice from greater than one specialty and is therefore the rationale underlying the provision of support for a more collaborative healthcare model. The most commonly presenting functional PNETs are insulinomas and gastrinomas, both of which significantly impact patient quality of life due to their state of being hormonally active. Insulinomas are characterized by the excess secretion of insulin, resulting in hypoglycemic attacks, whereas gastrinomas generate Zollinger-Ellison syndrome, which requires gastric acid hypersecretion and debilitating peptic ulcer disease. Surgical management of the tumors is not only required but also medical management principles to correct the symptomatic excess hormone. As research continues and there is greater understanding of the pathophysiology of the tumors, new guidelines for therapy are emerging. Evidence proves the importance of biochemical diagnostics in such a condition, presenting a systemic approach to PNET treatment and negation of clinical results through individual interventions (Kos-Kudła et al., 2017). Non-functioning tumors, however, remain clinically undetectable until reaching significant size or metastasis, hence posing a challenge in their treatment. Such tumors' patient might come with nonspecific signs or abdominal pain, and therefore warrant close observation and imaging evaluation. Surgical resection is the cornerstone treatment in PNETs for either functional activity; the advanced disease, however, is treated with new therapies such as peptide receptor radionuclide therapy and targeted molecular therapy. The therapeutic progress has ameliorated prognosis in patients presenting with the tumors (Cardona et al., 2019). This comprehensive review will steer through the different categories of PNETs, present their medical and surgical management, and finally make a valuable contribution toward ensuring better care for the patients involved in the fast-progressing area of neuroendocrine oncology (Figure 12.1).

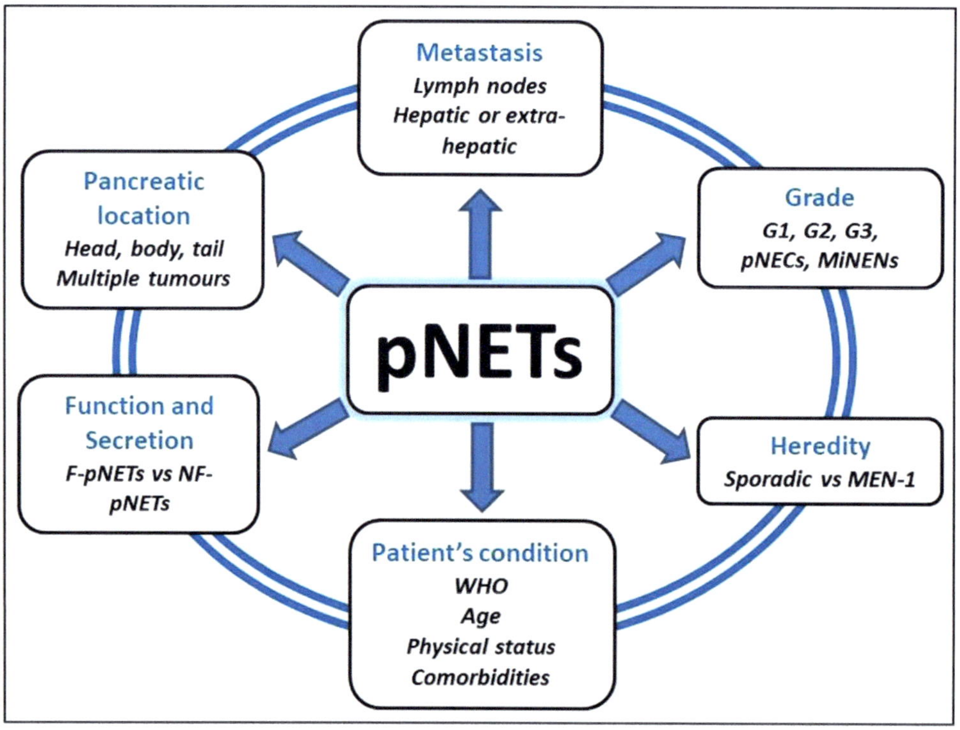

Figure 12.1. Pancreatic neuroendocrine tumors (PNETs).

Source: de Ponthaud C, Menegaux F, Gaujoux S. Updated Principles of Surgical Management of Pancreatic Neuroendocrine Tumours (pNETs): What Every Surgeon Needs to Know. *Cancers*. 2021; 13(23):5969. https://doi.org/10.3390/cancers13235969

Definition of Pancreatic Neuroendocrine Tumors (PNETs)

PNETs are a distinct group of neoplasms arising from the endocrine cells of the pancreas. In contrast to the more common pancreatic adenocarcinomas, the PNETs are classified based on their origin in neuroendocrine cells that are responsible for the production of hormones. This classification renders the PNETs to be different in their behavior, presentation, and treatment. The World Health Organizations (WHO) 2017 classification emphasizes the importance of accurate diagnosis of these tumors since their grading and staging have a direct bearing on the prognosis and management. Thus, PNETs are separated into functioning and non-functioning tumors, primarily based on their ability to secrete hormones resulting in particular clinical syndromes. It is important to understand this difference in order to design focus-specific intervention strategies that take into account the specific physiological impacts these tumors may exert on the health and well-being of patients (Cuccurullo et al., 2021). Functioning PNETs produce hormones that can lead to particular clinical characteristics, while non-functioning tumors are not producing excess hormones, often presenting late for diagnosis. Among the various functioning tumors, insulinomas, gastrinomas, and VIPomas are some of them. Insulinomas secrete insulin, with presentation being attacks of hypoglycemia, whereas gastrinomas cause hypersecretion of gastric acid, with presentation in the form of Zollinger-Ellison syndrome. VIPomas secrete vasoactive intestinal peptide, causing profuse watery diarrhea and electrolyte imbalance. Non-functioning PNETs, however, might be silent until there is huge tumor burden, since early detection cannot be done. Proper management of both types is required because the choice between surgical resection, locoregional therapies, and systemic therapy largely hinges upon the tumor's functional status and disease stage, underlining the clinical relevance of properly dividing PNETs (Gill et al., 2017). That, in recent decades, the incidence of PNETs increased highlights the necessity of greater knowledge and more precise diagnostic tools. Studies have emphasized the role of biomarkers, such as microRNAs, in the forecasting of clinical behavior and clinical outcomes of such tumors. For instance, it has been noted that some microRNAs have been identified to be linked with metastatic potential as well as patient prognosis generally, and more importantly, between those with locoregional disease and those with distant metastasis. Identification of microRNA-3653, with differential expression in metastases, is a promising biomarker for monitoring disease development. Continued research into molecular markers and their correlation with tumor behavior is important since it may lead to the development of more targeted therapies as well as improved prognostic models in the treatment of PNETs, hence improving patient outcomes (Gill et al., 2017).

Importance of Distinguishing Between Functioning and Non-Functioning Tumors

Non-functioning and functioning PNETs differ in a manner that is essential to the clinical strategy for diagnosis and treatment. Functioning tumors, for example, insulinomas or gastrinomas, secrete excessive hormones, which lead to typical symptoms like hypoglycemia or Zollinger-Ellison syndrome, respectively. Detection of such symptoms allows early medical intervention and the control of hormone-related complications effectively. On the other hand, non-functioning tumors do not produce significant amounts of hormones and often have nonspecific symptoms or remain asymptomatic until very advanced. Early detection and treatment are therefore critical because non-functioning PNETs can remain hidden and become more challenging to treat, highlighting the need for accurate classification in treatment planning and strategies for patient management (Cuccurullo et al., 2021). The functional implications of their separation follow them into management and prognostic outcome. Functioning PNETs typically need a disparate treatment plan, with medical treatments to control hormone secretion, but surgical resection is still considered in both if feasible. Surgical management of non-functioning tumors is aimed at reducing tumor burden and maximizing symptomatic control, but it can differ significantly depending on tumor grade and stage. While functioning tumors usually respond with good prognostic outcomes in the case of early diagnosis, non-functioning tumors can be more indolent in nature which eventually can mean metastasis, making management difficult (Brighi, 2022). This distinction addresses the importance of not just accurate diagnosis but the structured, multi-disciplinary management strategy for optimal patient outcomes (Brighi, 2022). Furthermore, advancements in diagnostic methods, such as imaging studies and biomarkers, have significantly improved discrimination of working vs. non-working tumors, thus enhancing clinical decision-making. More understanding of the molecular and genetic characteristics of PNETs provides valuable information about potential target therapies as well as planning individualized treatment plans. For instance, the discovery of single biomarkers may be able to help predict the behavior of these tumors and hence a more tailored treatment approach. Research also continues to determine the prognostic value of a number of genetic mutations and their correlation with response to therapy, such as that evaluating MGMT-promoter methylation status in relation to temozolomide regimens (Brighi, 2022). Finally, the distinction is not strictly theoretical; it lies at the heart of offering the best, individualized patient care in the complex landscape of PNET treatment (Figure 12.2).

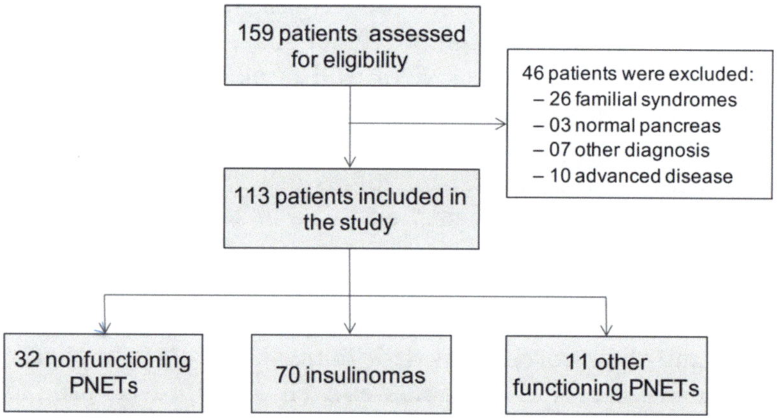

Figure 12.2. Non-functioning pancreatic neuroendocrine tumors (PNETs).

Source: https://external-content.duckduckgo.com/iu/?u=https%3A%2F%2Fminio.scielo.br%2Fdocumentstore%2F2317-6326%2F6stgSGfXQQcBXjztkCPMgbK%2F94b6319eb8573051d5468fc8ab35caca18ee2008.jpg&f=1&nofb=1&ipt=82cc52445f296f6a8582b0cc520dcc8ee0992638f1b63a9a9e294b34cfd330c6.

12.1. Classification of Pancreatic Neuroendocrine Tumors (PNETs)

The subclassification of the PNETs has practical significance for the creation of effective diagnostic and therapeutic modalities. According to the World Health Organization (WHO) classification, the

PNETs are divided based on their functional status and histopathological features. The functioning tumors, such as insulinomas, gastrinomas, and VIPomas, are characterized by the secretions of the hormones leading to some clinical features, such as hypoglycemia and Zollinger-Ellison syndrome, respectively. Conversely, non-functioning tumors are not typically hypersecretory of hormones and are asymptomatic unless they are extremely large or metastasized. This difference is important in the treatment and prognosis of disease since the behavior and course of functioning tumors can be significantly different from tumors that do not secrete hormones, and thus correct classification is very important in clinical practice (Kos-Kudła et al., 2017). Additional PNET classification analysis, nonetheless, needs an assessment of their grade and stage, as these play a central role in prognosis and proper planning for management. The neuroendocrine tumor grade can then be determined based on mitotic rate and necrosis, with this having an influence on the interpretation of the global disease. Low-grade tumors are more likely to yield favorable outcomes, whereas high-grade forms may lead to unfavorable disease behavior and poor prognoses. Histopathologic classification not only enables better understanding of tumor biology but also influences the treatment paradigm that may include surgery resection or the administration of targeted therapies (Kos-Kudła et al., 2017). The integration of biochemical markers, imaging, and histology is pivotal in the generation of individualized treatment strategies that are in line with the multidisciplinary management of PNET. Dissimilarities in the classification system also reflect upon a multidisciplinary treatment modality. Even as surgical treatment remains the anchor for local disease, the treatment paradigm of PNETs shifts with advances in medical technology and surgical techniques. Having strict diagnostic criteria consisting of biochemical assays, imaging studies, and the emergent need for immunohistochemical verification of diagnoses is the foundation of effective patient management. The growing body of clinical evidence allows the integration of biotherapy, molecular targeted agents, and peptide receptor radionuclide therapy into therapeutic paradigms, particularly in patients with advanced or metastatic disease. In doing so, understanding the intricate classification of PNETs forms teamwork among clinicians dedicated to optimal patient outcomes (Cuccurullo et al., 2021) (Figure 12.3).

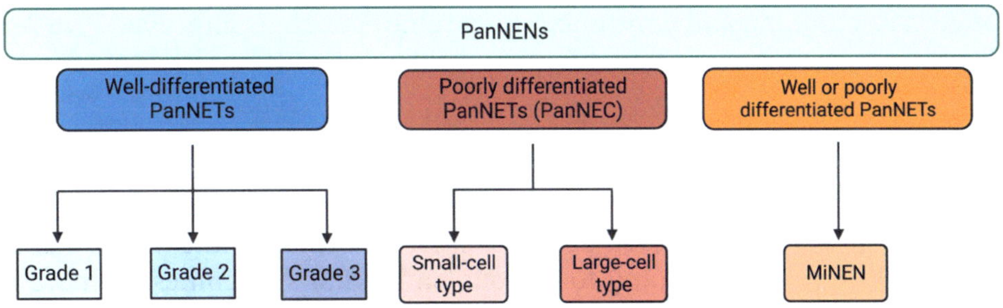

Figure 12.3. An Insight on Functioning pancreatic neuroendocrine neoplasms (PNETs).

Source: Bevere M, Gkountakos A, Martelli FM, Scarpa A, Luchini C, Simbolo M. An Insight on Functioning Pancreatic Neuroendocrine Neoplasms. *Biomedicines*. 2023; 11(2):303. https://doi.org/10.3390/biomedicines11020303

12.1.1. Functioning Versus Non-Functioning Tumors

The distinction between functioning and non-functioning PNETs is key to understanding their clinical presentation and management. Functioning tumors secrete hormones actively, leading to characteristic clinical syndromes based on the hormone secreted. Insulinomas, for instance, secrete excess insulin with resulting hypoglycemia, whereas gastrinomas lead to Zollinger-Ellison syndrome with hypersecretion of gastric acid on a large scale. The signs and symptoms that these functioning tumors present can be significantly influencing patients quality of life and need to be addressed with a differentiated approach to medical management. Non-functioning tumors, however, never secrete any active hormones and most commonly leave patients asymptomatic unless the tumor is significantly large or metastatic. The absence of endocrine activity makes it more challenging to diagnose because these tumors are diagnosed only incidentally when patients undergo imaging for unrelated purposes. Diagnosis of a functioning PNET is an integration of clinical evaluation, biochemical testing, and imaging tests to confirm overproduction of specific hormones. Diagnosis of a NET-associated functioning syndrome is both clinical in nature and biochemical evidence for increased levels of hormone, as outlined in ENETS recommendations. The different hormonal syndromes can result from various types of tumors, including insulinoma, gastrinoma, and VIPoma, each requiring individual diagnostic protocols and treatment strategies. For instance, in diagnosing insulinoma, fasting insulin and glucose tolerance tests are used, while gastrin elevation in gastrinoma can be determined by serum gastrin assays. Effective management of such functioning tumors must necessarily be an interdisciplinary effort, where the services of endocrinologists, surgeons, and oncologists must be consulted and individualized therapeutic regimens must be formulated combining both tumor control and hormone-related symptoms. Conversely, treatment for non-functioning tumors generally revolves around surgery, owing to their tendency towards delayed diagnosis. Surgical resection is still the mainstay of management since it is capable of curing localized tumors and stopping disease progression. This is because non-functioning PNETs are usually detected late, leading to metastasis at presentation in most patients, which makes it challenging to decide on treatment. For these patients, therapies include medical treatments for tumor growth, such as somatostatin analogs, peptide receptor radionuclide therapy, and chemotherapy, as noted in PNET treatment modalities (Andrysiak-Mamos et al., 2014). Surgery use in non-functioning PNETs must be evaluated individually, with significant consideration for disease spread and overall clinical status of the patients. Finally, a thorough understanding of the differences between functioning and non-functioning tumors enables improved PNET management, enabling medical professionals to tailor interventions that optimize patient outcomes (Bartsch et al., 2023).

12.1.2. Types of Functioning Tumors

Functional PNETs are characterized by their ability to secrete hormones into the bloodstream, forming a characteristic clinical profile pertaining to various endocrine syndromes. Tumors are generally classified based on the exact hormones secreted, e.g., insulin, gastrin, vasoactive intestinal peptide (VIP), etc. Insulinomas, for example, are the most common functional neuroendocrine tumors and cause hypoglycemia due to the hypersecretion of insulin. Contrarily, gastrinomas produce Zollinger-Ellison syndrome, which presents with extremely potent peptic ulcers and hypersecretion of gastric acid. The clinical relevance of these endocrine-functioning tumors demonstrates the importance of accurate diagnosis and individually managed therapy because their hormonal secretion not only determines the tumor histology but also impacts therapy management, such as surgery and medical therapy targeting hormone release control (Andrysiak-Mamos et al., 2014). Gastrinomas, among the numerous varieties of functioning PNETs, are a particular challenge in both diagnosis and treatment. Tend to be found in either the pancreas or the duodenum, these tumors release large quantities of gastrin, a hormone that stimulates acid secretion from the stomach. Patients can range from having symptoms of abdominal pain and diarrhea to frank ulcers. Diagnosis is typically established by biochemical examination to determine the presence of hypergastrinemia, supplemented by imaging techniques such as endoscopic ultrasound (EUS) or computed tomography (CT) to localize tumors. Therapy for gastrinomas is commonly multifactorial, in that a balance between surgical resection of the localized tumor and treatment with proton pump inhibitors or somatostatin analogs to suppress symptoms and reduce acid secretion is attempted. Because gastrinomas are complex, the treatment for these tumors involves a multidisciplinary team to ensure that patient outcomes are optimized and complete care is delivered (Andrysiak-Mamos et al., 2014). VIPomas, being rarer than insulinomas and gastrinomas, are another critical type of functioning PNETs. Upon secretion of vasoactive intestinal peptide, these tumors can lead to a syndrome known as WDHA (Watery Diarrhea, Hypokalemia, and Achlorhydria). The typical presentation is copious watery diarrhea secondary to the secretory action of VIP on the intestine and secondary electrolyte imbalance. Assay of elevated serum levels of VIP and imaging techniques for tumor localization are the diagnostic procedures. Treatment is most effective if the lesion is removed surgically, particularly if the lesion is discrete. In metastases, symptomatic control with somatostatin analogs can be achieved by medical treatment to improve quality of life. In general, familiarization with the varied forms of functioning tumors in the spectrum of PNET is important for the proper design of effective individualized treatment protocols and improving patient care (Bartsch et al., 2023) (Figure 12.4).

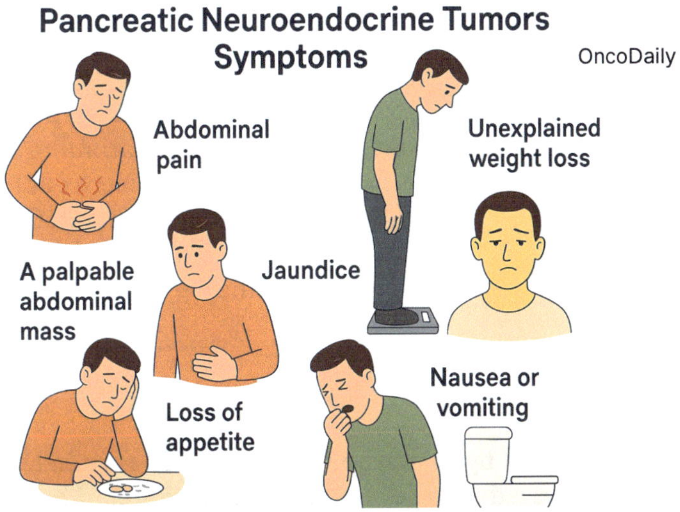

Figure 12.4. Symptoms of pancreatic neuroendocrine tumors (PNETs).

Source: https://oncodaily.com/oncolibrary/cancer-types/pancreatic-neuroendocrine-tumors.

12.1.3. Role of Histological Classification

Histological classification is especially important in the case of PNETs, and it classifies the types of tumors based on morphology, differentiation, and functional status. Classification aids doctors in making accurate diagnoses, which is essential to determine the best treatment regimens. The World Health Organization classification of 2017 especially separates neuroendocrine tumors into well-differentiated, moderately differentiated, and poorly differentiated ones with certain prognostic value. Functional tumors such as insulinomas and gastrinomas exhibit hormonal activity that has a very significant impact on clinical presentation and management streams. Non-functioning tumors, by contrast, are often asymptomatic until late in the disease, and underscore the very important role of histological detection to allow appropriate clinical responses. By validating the tumor subtype with biochemistry and imaging coupled with histopathological analysis, clinicians are able to develop tailored patient management plans essential to therapeutic success (Kos-Kudła et al., 2017). Besides aiding diagnosis, histological classification is used in making prognostic predictions and influencing therapeutic decisions. Grade and stage of PNETs, established by histological examination, are crucial in predicting patient outcomes and survival rates. Higher-grade tumors will tend to need aggressive treatment regimens, including surgery and adjuvant treatment, whereas lower-grade tumors will respond well to less aggressive therapies. This PNET gradient is the basis for the multidisciplinary approach to treatment, which must incorporate specialists who are trained in medical and surgical management. Endocrinologists, oncologists, and operating teams must collaborate to overcome the difficulties created by functioning compared with non-functioning tumors. The improved understanding derived from histological classification then finally enhances the quality of care given to patients, as it is tailored to the specific nature and behavior of each patient's tumors (Kos-Kudła et al., 2017). Moreover, the evolution of imaging technologies and molecular targeted therapies enhanced the significance of histological classification in managing PNETs. Sophisticated imaging technologies allow more accurate depiction of tumor characteristics and receptor profiles, which have a significant impact on available treatments. As an illustration, the presence of somatostatin receptors delineates patients' inclusion criteria for peptide receptor radionuclide therapy such that histological classification becomes categorically mandatory for determining a patient's therapeutic regimen. In addition, integration of immunohistochemical markers has enhanced diagnostic precision, such that differentiation between tumor types based on levels of receptor expression has become possible. This continuing evolution in histological assessment not only enhances the therapeutic environment of the treatment of PNET but is also an important component in clinical research, guiding the development of new therapies as dictated by the individual tumor biology. Enhanced patient care outcomes can thus be directly attributed to diligent integration of histological classification into the therapy framework (Cuccurullo et al., 2021).

12.2. Insulinoma

Insulinoma, a PNET, is characterized by inappropriately secreted insulin leading to hypoglycemia. It is most often characterized by a triad of observations: presentation of hypoglycemia, a documented low level of glucose, and relief with ingestion of glucose. Patients may be confused, irritable, or even become comatose with hypoglycemia. The prevalence of insulinoma is relatively low, at 1–4 per million per year, typically in the age range 40–60 years. Given the tendency for insulinomas to be small and asymptomatic until extensive disease development, early and accurate diagnosis is critically important to allow appropriate management, facilitating discrimination from other causes of hypoglycemia that may have a similar clinical presentation (Andrysiak-Mamos et al., 2014). Diagnostic testing for insulinoma involves biochemical evaluation with fasting insulin and glucose levels, and imaging tests such as CT or magnetic resonance imaging (MRI) to identify the tumor. Advanced imaging techniques such as EUS can also prove useful in identifying small tumors that would otherwise be missed. In addition, immunohistochemical assays are instrumental in making a definitive diagnosis. Of specific mention, histopathologic diagnosis via immunohistochemistry not only establishes the direction of treatment but also facilitates the grading of tumor, which is crucial to predict patient outcome (Andrysiak-Mamos et al., 2014). A multidisciplinary approach is therefore usually recommended involving endocrinologists, surgeons, and radiologists to coordinate the care of the patient. Surgical resection of insulinoma remains the treatment of choice, particularly in patients with a localized mass. The nature of the surgery may range from enucleation of the tumor to distal pancreatectomy depending on the size and location of the tumor. In unresectable insulinomas or in those who are nonsurgical candidates, treatment with diazoxide or octreotide can control symptoms by inhibiting insulin secretion. In more complex cases, peptide receptor radionuclide therapy (PRRT) may be utilized as an experimental treatment. Effective management not only alleviates symptoms but also enhances quality of life, validating the necessity of individualized therapeutic regimens based on tumor characteristics and patient-specific factors (Bartsch et al., 2023) (Figure 12.5).

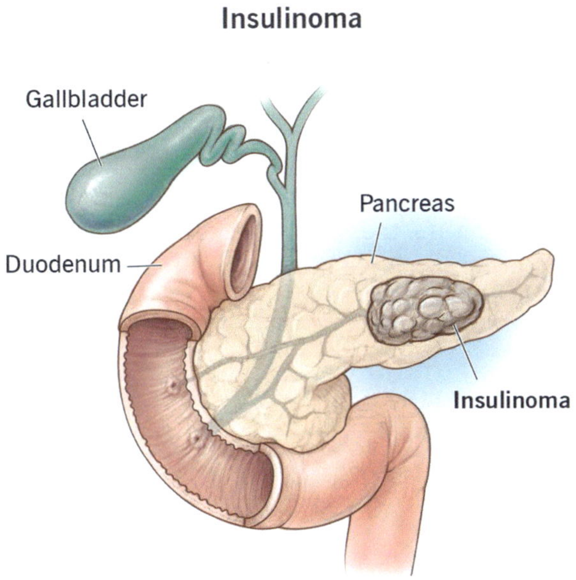

Figure 12.5. Insulinoma.

Source: https://my.clevelandclinic.org/-/scassets/images/org/health/articles/22217-insulinoma.

12.2.1. Pathophysiology and Symptoms

The pathophysiology of the PNETs is complex and reflects multiple genetic alterations and endocrine secretions that lead to various clinical presentations. The two types of tumors are functioning and non-functioning, with the former secreting hormones such as insulin, gastrin, and VIP. Excessive secretion of these hormones leads to characteristic syndromes with varying manifestations. For instance, insulinomas are responsible for causing hypoglycemia, with symptoms of weakness, confusion, and sweating during attacks, while gastrinomas can result in Zollinger-Ellison syndrome, which is characterized by peptic ulcers due to hypersecretion of gastric acid. Alternatively, non-functioning PNETs are not hormone secretors and remain asymptomatic until late in their course, then produce nonspecific symptoms such as abdominal pain or weight loss, which render early diagnosis and management planning challenging (Kos-Kudła et al., 2017). For functioning PNETs, in their symptomatology, the endocrine environment created by the secretions of the tumor becomes the area of focus in order to understand patient presentation. Insulinomas, for instance, are the most common functioning PNET and cause episodic hypoglycemia, leading to dizziness, seizures, and, in some instances, loss of consciousness. The symptoms improve after intravenous glucose administration, thus providing a clue towards diagnosis. Similarly, gastrinomas are associated with recurrent peptic ulcer disease and can lead to abdominal pain and gastrointestinal hemorrhage secondary to inappropriate acid secretion. VIPomas, although less common, produce enormous watery diarrhea, hypokalemia, and achlorhydria, and lead to a significant amount of morbidity if not diagnosed and treated early. The diverse clinical presentation of the tumor underlines the need for an elaborate knowledge of its pathophysiological mechanisms (Andersen et al., 2024). In addition to the immediate effects of hormone secretion, the pathophysiology of PNETs is also attributable to intrinsic properties of the tumor and also due to the interaction of genetic factors. Sporadic PNETs are most prevalent, but multiple endocrine neoplasia type 1 (MEN1) and other familial syndromes also predispose individuals to developing these tumors. Recurrent somatic mutations have been identified by genetic sequencing in important genes, including MEN1, and in cell proliferation and survival pathways. Discernible differences are observed between functioning and non-functioning tumors in terms of the presence of genetic changes, with more common recurrent alterations in pathways such as phosphoinositide 3-kinase and receptor tyrosine kinase signaling being found in non-functioning tumors. Information on these changes becomes significant to establish probable therapeutic targets and untangle the intricate biology of PNETs to ultimately impact both medical and surgical practice (Kos-Kudła et al., 2017) (Figure 12.6).

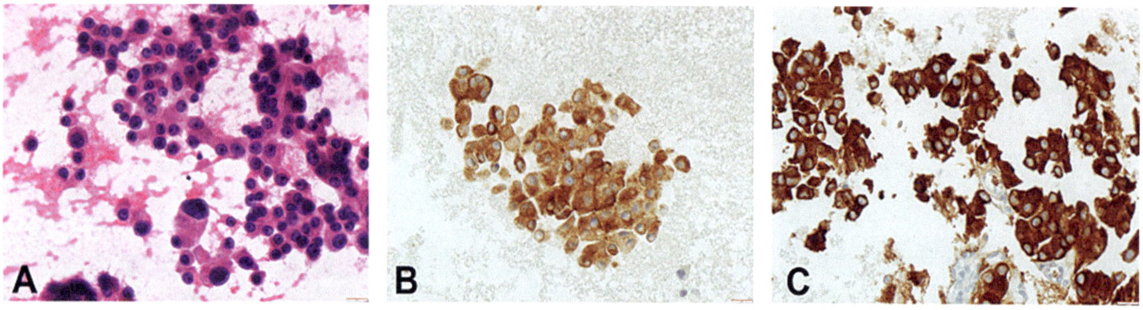

Figure 12.6. Vasoactive intestinal peptide tumor as the cause of persistent diarrhea.

Source: Lopes S, Alves M, Rodrigues P (September 13, 2022) Vasoactive Intestinal Peptide Tumor as the Cause of Persistent Diarrhea: A Diagnostic Challenge. Cureus 14(9): e29130. doi:10.7759/cureus.29130

12.2.2. Diagnosis and Imaging Techniques

Diagnosis of PNETs calls for a coordinated approach that combines biochemical studies with advanced imaging techniques. Biochemical markers, made up of serum concentrations of some neuroendocrine hormones, form the pillars of diagnostic studies. The markers may convey the clinician information regarding the functional status of the tumor, particularly in the case of insulinoma or gastrinoma, where hormonal secretion leads to specific clinical syndromes. However, biochemical studies by themselves are unable to make the diagnosis or stage accurately, and that is where imaging finds application. EUS, CT, and MRI are critical in imaging the tumor anatomy, its relationship with surrounding structures, and in screening for metastases. A combination of these modalities is required for an educated and accurate diagnosis that will allow for appropriate therapeutic planning and management (Andrysiak-Mamos et al., 2014). In imaging, EUS has proven to be an extremely valuable modality due to its high sensitivity in detecting small tumors, often less than 2 cm in size, that are missed on other imaging studies. In addition to cross-sectional imaging of the pancreas, EUS provides fine-needle aspiration biopsy, taking tissue for histopathological examination and immunohistochemical investigation. This histological diagnosis is important in that it can distinguish among various subtypes of PNETs and their biologic behavior and dictate management strategies. CT scanning, commonly used for staging and preoperative evaluation, offers a broader view, with information regarding vascular involvement and distant spread, while MRI may be reserved for selected cases or in patients requiring repeated imaging without ionizing radiation exposure (Kos-Kudła et al., 2017). Thus, prudent selection of imaging modalities is imperative in the management of PNETs. The evolving picture of diagnostic imaging in PNETs also encompasses newer functional imaging techniques such as positron emission tomography (PET) scans and somatostatin receptor scintigraphy that assist in tumor localization with improved specificity. These functional imaging studies are particularly useful for assessing the tumors that may be less evident on routine CT or MRI, thereby enhancing detection rates and providing information regarding tumor biology. Somatostatin receptor imaging, for example, has direct therapeutic implications, particularly PRRT in patients with somatostatin receptor-positive neoplasms. This multi-disciplinary approach emphasizes the necessity for a multi-disciplinary team skilled in the interpretation of biochemical and imaging data to optimize patient management and outcomes in patients with PNETs (Andrysiak-Mamos et al., 2014). With ongoing technological advancements, ongoing revision of the diagnostic approach will be necessary to improve patient care and effectiveness of treatment.

12.2.3. Treatment Options: Medical and Surgical

Treatment of PNETs is also varied, with both surgery and drug intervention. Surgery comes first, especially where the tumor is resectable and localized. Surgical resection is ideal to facilitate cure, especially for functioning tumors such as insulinomas that are normally safe to remove due to their generally small size and slow growth. However, surgical management is complicated further by the late presentation of the diseases, which often leads to late diagnosis. Therefore, while patients with insulinoma present early, others with other functional tumors like gastrinoma or VIPoma will have a more significant issue of metastasis at presentation, further limiting the range of the available surgical interventions. Hence, early intervention and diagnosis surgery are decisive in improving outcomes for PNET patients (Adamiec et al., 2024). Management of PNETs is tailored to the unique functioning syndrome of each tumor type, employing pharmacologic interventions against targeted hormone secretions. For instance, symptomatic control is crucial in conditions like gastrinoma, where acid reduction with proton pump inhibitors must be used to control gastric hypersecretion and symptom relief. Somatostatin analogs octreotide and lanreotide have also been effective in the inhibition of hormone release and symptom control in patients with a range of functioning PNETs. The drugs also inhibit the growth of the tumor and are employed in the case of non-resectable tumors. More novel targeted therapies, including mTOR inhibitors and tyrosine kinase inhibitors, are also being found beneficial in advanced PNET management, allowing for a more personalized management approach (Bartsch et al., 2023). The combination of both therapeutic and surgical approaches is essential to the overall management of pancreatic neuroendocrine tumors. When inoperability occurs secondary to tumor size or metastasis, medical therapies have a major role to play. Therapies such as PRRT are rising as viable alternatives, particularly in non-functional tumors or in the event of failure of traditional therapy. They attempt to improve the quality of life with tumor control. Scientific research continues to advance and perfect novel therapeutic agents and techniques, proving that PNET treatment options are dynamic. As with all cancer treatments, a multidisciplinary team of surgical oncologists, endocrinologists, and medical oncologists is crucial in the management of this rare and complex group of tumors (Adamiec et al., 2024) (Figure 12.7).

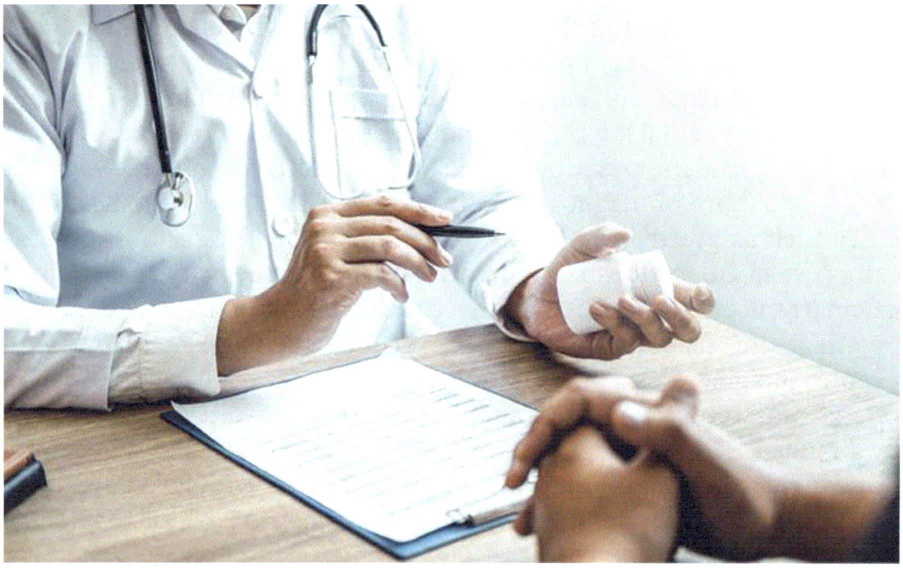

Figure 12.7. Treatment options for pancreatic neuroendocrine tumors (PNETs).

Source: https://pancan.org/wp-content/uploads/2025/03/blog-image-1.jpg.

12.3. Gastrinoma

Gastrinomas, being one of the functioning PNETs, are characterized by pathologically elevated secretion of gastric acid due to hypergastrinemia. They typically present along with Zollinger-Ellison syndrome, which is a severe peptic ulcer disease caused by overproduction of acid. Gastrinomas typically lie within the gastrinoma triangle, an area demarcated by the duodenum, pancreas, and biliary tree. Unlike the other PNETs, gastrinomas can be quite diagnostic challenges with varying difficulty of detection at times until advanced disease stages due to the nonspecific nature of abdominal pain and diarrhea. Application of newer imaging techniques such as EUS and CT can raise diagnostic precision to enable early treatment and management, since the revised guidelines for diagnosis developed by the Polish Network of Neuroendocrine Tumors highlight the importance of effective imaging in the diagnosis of gastrinoma (Andrysiak-Mamos et al., 2014). Both medical and surgical therapies are used in the treatment of gastrinoma and therefore require a multimodal approach by qualified specialists. Surgical resection remains the preferred treatment whenever feasible, especially for gastrinomas that are confined to the pancreas or duodenum. These procedures are intended to achieve a total tumor resection to remove the symptoms of gastric acid hypersecretion. For patients with unresectable gastrinomas or with metastatic disease, treatment with medical therapy is necessary. Proton pump inhibitors (PPIs) to control acid secretion and somatostatin analogs to inhibit gastrin release are therapeutic choices. These therapies require continuous readjustments based on response from the patient, highlighting the importance of treatment individualization in the effective treatment of gastrinomas (Bartsch et al., 2023). Furthermore, follow-up therapy and long-term care of gastrinoma patients require careful monitoring of hormonal levels and clinical symptoms to assess treatment efficacy. Regular biochemical evaluations will show any re-occurrence of tumor activity or treatment side effects so that patient condition changes can be addressed promptly. The virulence of gastrinomas, with their ability to become malignant and metastasize, illustrates the need for ongoing research into new treatment options and diagnostic markers. As new advancements continue in targeted molecular treatments and peptide receptor radionuclide therapy, the latter has the potential for maximum results in the treatment of gastrinoma and, ultimately, the quality of life of affected patients (Andrysiak-Mamos et al., 2014) (Figure 12.8).

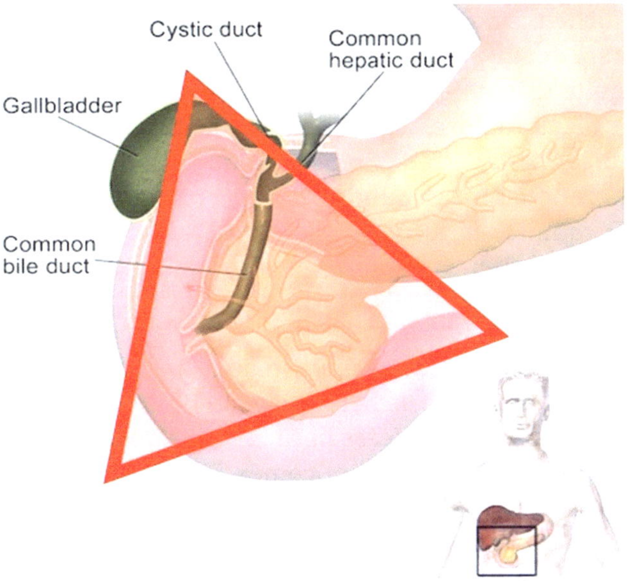

Figure 12.8. Gastrinoma.

Source: https://oncodaily.com/pub/uploads/2024/05/Gastrinoma-Triangle.jpg.

12.3.1. Characteristics and Clinical Presentation

The clinical presentation and characteristics of PNETs vary considerably based on their functional status and hormone secretion. Functioning tumors such as insulinoma, gastrinoma, and VIPoma secrete excess hormones that lead to characteristic clinical syndromes. Insulinomas, for instance, secrete hyperinsulinemia, leading to episodes of hypoglycemia with related features of sweating, palpitations, and confusion. On the other hand, gastrinomas cause Zollinger-Ellison syndrome, where the hypersecretion of gastrin causes recurrent peptic ulcers and gastrointestinal discomfort. Clinical manifestations for such tumors are often nonspecific and need cautious evaluation to avoid misdiagnosis and effective management interventions being applied. Recognition of these specific symptoms is crucial for intervention on time, as the sequelae of untreated hormonal derangements can lead to severe morbidity and overall quality of life (Bartsch et al., 2023). Presentation of non-functioning PNETs is also classically different. These tumors are not hormone-secreting and thus have a silent behavior commonly until advanced. The patients may present with nonspecific signs such as abdominal pain, weight loss, or obstructive jaundice, and it is hard to diagnose them because these are also presentations of other gastrointestinal disorders. Imaging is key in the diagnosis of non-functioning PNETs and techniques such as endoscopic ultrasound, computed tomography, and magnetic resonance imaging assist in the detection and characterization of the tumor (Andrysiak-Mamos et al., 2014). The indolent nature of some non-functioning PNETs can lead to late diagnosis, and therefore, it is extremely important that clinicians have a very strong suspicion, particularly in the presence of risk factors or familial syndromes of neuroendocrine neoplasms. Lastly, the importance of histopathological examination cannot be overemphasized to differentiate between functioning and non-functioning PNETs. Immunohistochemical examination is also central to the diagnosis confirmation and determination of the tumor's differentiation and grade, which affects management decisions. Clinical presentation also guides further diagnostic work-up in the form of biochemical examination to evaluate tumor markers for specific hormone syndromes. Multidisciplinary team practice is also central to optimal management, as treatment of functioning tumors is quite different from that of non-functioning tumors. Surgery remains the treatment of choice for localized tumors, while medical therapy, like peptide receptor radionuclide therapy, would be the choice in advanced disease (Andrysiak-Mamos et al., 2014; Bartsch et al., 2023). Treatment is contingent on a correct understanding of the tumor's behavior and presentation, and this demonstrates the complex nature of PNETs.

12.3.2. Diagnostic Challenges and Biomarkers

Diagnosis of PNETs is difficult and needs a multi-modal approach involving clinical evaluation, imaging, and biochemical investigations. The heterogeneity of presentation between functioning and non-functioning tumors also renders the process harder. Functioning PNETs, such as insulinomas and gastrinomas, present with typical hormonal syndromes, resulting in earlier diagnosis. In contrast, non-functioning tumors are typically asymptomatic until presentation at a late stage, resulting in delayed diagnosis and poorer prognosis. The absence of typical presenting symptoms additionally slows down diagnostic workups, traditionally making physicians reliant on high-technology imaging modalities and biomarkers for proper diagnosis. As highlighted by ENETS guidelines, biochemical investigation, such as measurement of hormone levels, is vital for differentiation of these types of tumors and also treatment strategy formulation, with respect to the unique therapeutic aspects of each (Bartsch et al., 2023). The ongoing advancements in understanding the molecular foundations of PNETs have brought the potential value of biomarkers to the forefront of the diagnostic and prognostic arenas. MicroRNA (miRNA) dysregulation has also emerged as the key player in the pathogenesis of PNET, with miRNAs being implicated in correlation with disease advancement and metastatic activity. For instance, miR-3653 has been reported to be markedly elevated in metastatic disease compared with localized disease patients, possibly as a prognostic marker (Gill et al., 2017). These molecular markers, in addition to facilitating improved stratification of patients, also provide insights into the biological behavior of tumors. With such biomarkers, healthcare practitioners can provide enhanced diagnostic accuracy and modulate treatment modalities based on the aggressiveness of the tumor type, achieving improved personalization of patient care. Even with the promise that biomarkers like miRNAs hold, challenges remain in using them in clinical practice. The heterogeneity of PNETs is the basis for variation in the expression of biomarkers, making it challenging to standardize diagnosis criteria. Moreover, there must be continued efforts towards establishing the clinical relevance of candidate biomarkers in various patient groups and tumor types. Despite being encouraging, information on biological markers in PNETs remains poor, and thus, hardwork must be put in place towards developing solid protocols that integrate these biomarkers into clinical practice. Besides, further research is imperative to explore the relationship between some biomarkers and treatment outcomes, ultimately optimizing prognostication and treatment decision-making Gill et al., 2017; (Bartsch et al., 2023). As technology advances, the resolution of these imaging challenges will optimize early diagnosis and treatment efficacy in patients with PNET (Figure 12.9).

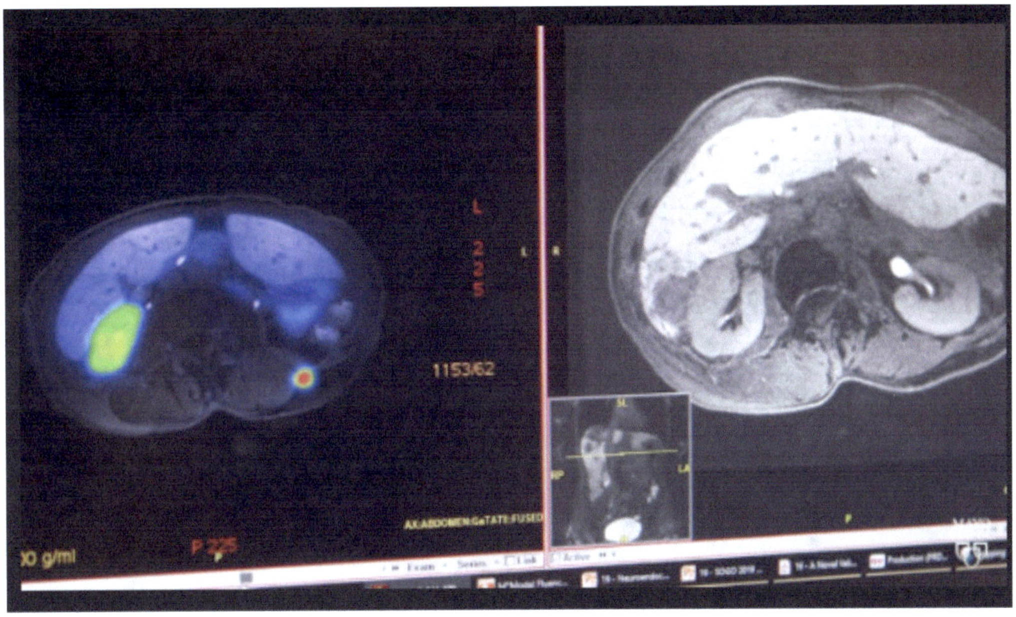

Figure 12.9. Diagnosis of pancreatic neuroendocrine tumors (PNETs).

Source: https://external-content.duckduckgo.com/iu/?u=http%3A%2F%2Fres.cloudinary.com%2Fbroadcastmed%2Fimage%2Ffetch%2Fq_auto%2Cc_fill%2Cw_1300%2Ch_731%2Cg_faces%3Acenter%2Cf_auto%2Fhttp%3A%2F%2F55933-bcmed.s3.amazonaws.com%2Fbcp%2Fimages%2ForlVideoAssets%2FimgSource%2Fmac_pnets.png&f=1&nofb=1&ipt=d7ebf7b7ab7341e612accb184188ff64dc6b1b5ee9e4478dce4000b392c26078.

12.3.3. Management Strategies: Pharmacological and Surgical

Treatment of PNETs is a multidirectional process combining pharmacologic and surgical treatment, specifically targeting tumor function. The functional tumors, such as insulinomas, gastrinomas, and VIPomas, usually present with certain problems due to their capacity to secrete hormones, leading to consequent clinical symptoms. For instance, insulinomas secrete excess insulin that leads to repeated hypoglycemia. Pharmacologic treatment therefore, typically begins with diazoxide or octreotide to control symptoms. Surgical excision remains the gold standard of these tumors whenever feasible, as cure is also an option with total resection. Integration of all the above measures is necessary because the type of tumor, that is, functioning or not, is mainly responsible for determining the line of management (Kos-Kudła et al., 2017). Non-functioning pancreatic neuroendocrine tumors (NFPETs) may be asymptomatic at onset, for which there may be a delay in diagnosis. The management of NFPETs is primarily aimed at the size, location, and potential spread of the tumor. Surgery is the first line of treatment in the event of local disease as it provides the chance of curative resection, thereby improving patient prognosis. For those patients with unresectable or metastatic disease, treatment is done with pharmacotherapy in the form of targeted therapy and chemotherapy. The use of somatostatin analogues is also beneficial, controlling tumor growth and alleviating some symptoms of tumor burden. Thus, differentiation between functioning and non-functioning tumors requires personalized management strategies that utilize both surgical and drug interventions in a judicious manner (Cuccurullo et al., 2021). The evolving pattern of therapeutic intervention also highlights the position of individualized medicine in PNET management. The evolution of molecular target therapies and PRRT has revolutionized the treatment method, particularly in advanced disease. These treatments are aimed at capitalizing on some of the specific molecular characteristics of neuroendocrine tumors to optimize therapeutic impact and minimize side effects. The role of the multidisciplinary team cannot be overstressed under such a scenario; oncologists, surgeons, radiologists, and endocrinologists must collaborate to optimize therapeutic care. Such cooperation ensures patients receive comprehensive care that is attuned to the nuances of their afflictions. Thus, the union of surgical and pharmacological management approaches is still significant in addressing the multifactorial etiology of PNETs and improving patient outcomes (Kos-Kudła et al., 2017) (Figure 12.10).

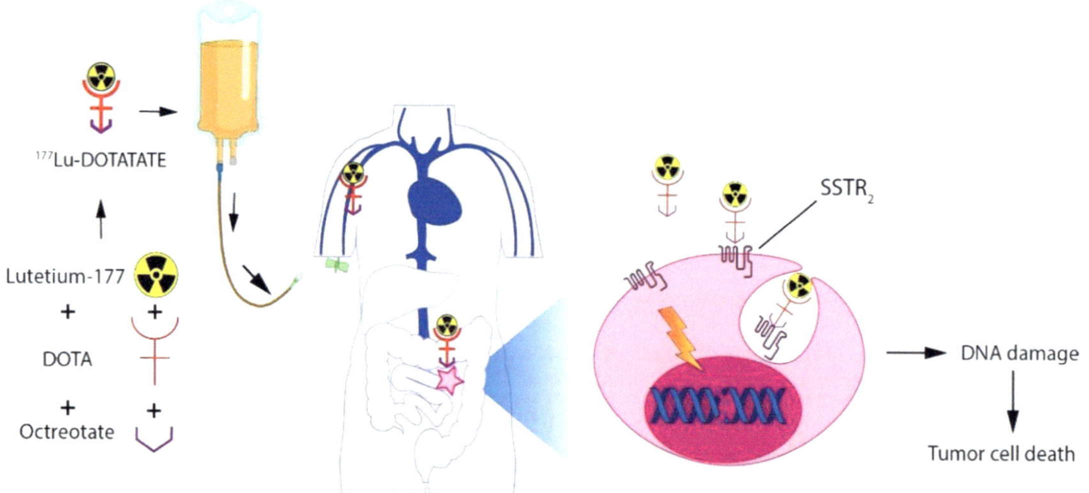

Figure 12.10. Peptide receptor radionuclide therapy (PRRT) of pancreatic neuroendocrine tumors (PNETs).

Source: Becx MN, Minczeles NS, Brabander T, de Herder WW, Nonnekens J, Hofland J. A Clinical Guide to Peptide Receptor Radionuclide Therapy with ^{177}Lu-DOTATATE in Neuroendocrine Tumor Patients. *Cancers.* 2022; 14(23):5792. https://doi.org/10.3390/cancers14235792

12.4. VIPoma

PNETs' pathophysiology and clinical presentation are diverse, with VIPoma standing as one of the unique ones due to its special presentation and pathophysiology. VIPoma originates from the pancreatic islet cells that secrete VIP, and it plays a critical role in maintaining intestinal fluid and electrolyte secretion. The classic presentation of patients with VIPoma is with a syndrome of WDHA secondary to an increase in levels of VIP. This hypersecretion leads to severe disturbances of fluid homeostasis, ultimately leading to dehydration and electrolyte imbalance, which is of prime clinical significance in the treatment of this rare tumor. Since the initial presentation is often subtle and the magnitude of complications is enormous, prompt diagnosis of VIPoma remains a great challenge in the clinical practice, highlighting the importance of vigilance on the part of clinicians (Adamiec et al., 2024). Diagnosis of VIPoma is a multidisciplinary exercise that fuses clinical examination with high-tech imaging. Laboratory tests confirm elevated serum VIP, typically along with assessment of electrolytes, the most frequent being potassium, which is generally low due to the secretory demands of the disease. Imaging tests such as CT and MRI are important in establishing the tumor size and detecting metastases, particularly to the liver, a common site of spread. As approximately 40%–80% of PNET patients have metastatic disease at presentation, including individuals with VIPoma, detecting metastatic lesions is important for staging and planning treatment (Aurello et al., 2018).

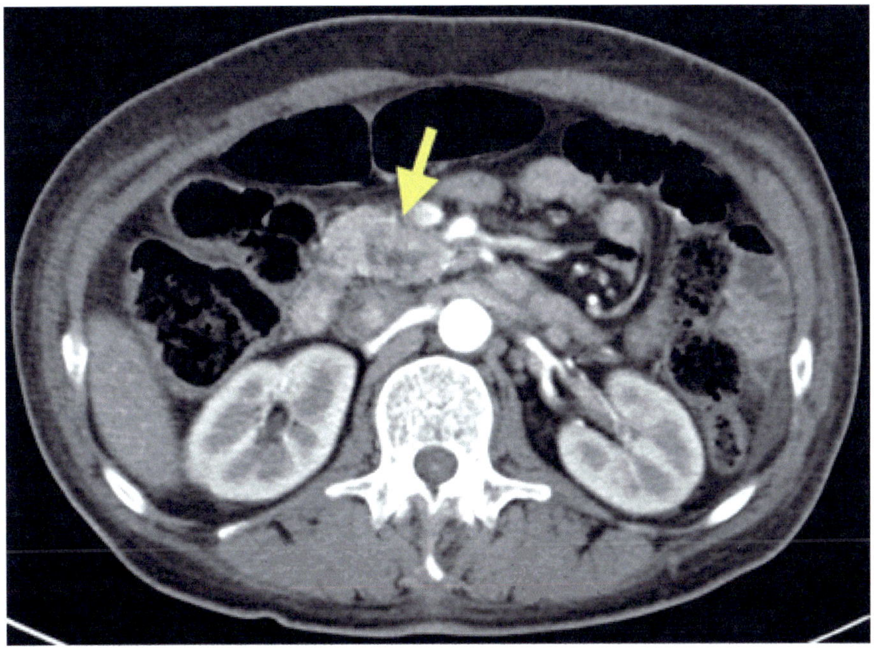

Figure 12.11. VIPoma with multiple endocrine neoplasia type 1.

Source: https://external-content.duckduckgo.com/iu/?u=https%3A%2F%2Fcasereports.bmj.com%2Fcontent%2Fcasereports%2F2015%2Fbcr-2015-213016%2FF1.medium.gif&f=1&nofb=1&ipt=791df8091c2197f38a9158267a8a35a2321be24d0525bb55681f37af6b29cf35.

Following diagnosis, the therapeutic maneuvers are symptomatic treatment along with the surgical removal of the tumors, provided the disease is localized. VIPoma treatment is peculiar due to its virulent nature and late presentation. Surgical removal remains the treatment of choice in the case of the localized tumor with chances of a curative outcome. However, most of the patients present with advanced disease along with liver metastases, which severely complicates treatment strategies. In such cases, a combination of therapies can be used, for example, somatostatin analogs to help reduce symptoms of VIP hypersecretion. Furthermore, therapies of a targeted nature, like everolimus or sunitinib, have proven useful in the management of progressive metastatic disease, significantly prolonging patient survival and improving quality of life. However, the development of patient-individualized treatment regimens that are appropriately balanced between aggressive disease treatment and supportive care remains significant to enhance the outcomes of patients (Adamiec et al., 2024) (Figure 12.11).

12.4.1. Overview of Vasoactive Intestinal Peptide (VIP)

VIP is a neuropeptide that has a critical role to play in several of the body's physiological functions, most significantly gastrointestinal function and neuroendocrine regulation. It is mainly produced in the intestines and has significant actions to relax smooth muscle, dilate blood vessels, and control secretory activity. In PNETs, VIP is best noted when referring to VIPoma, a rare and dedicated functioning tumor. VIPoma leads to a clinical syndrome characterized by fecund diarrhea, electrolyte imbalance, and flushing due to hypersecretion of VIP.

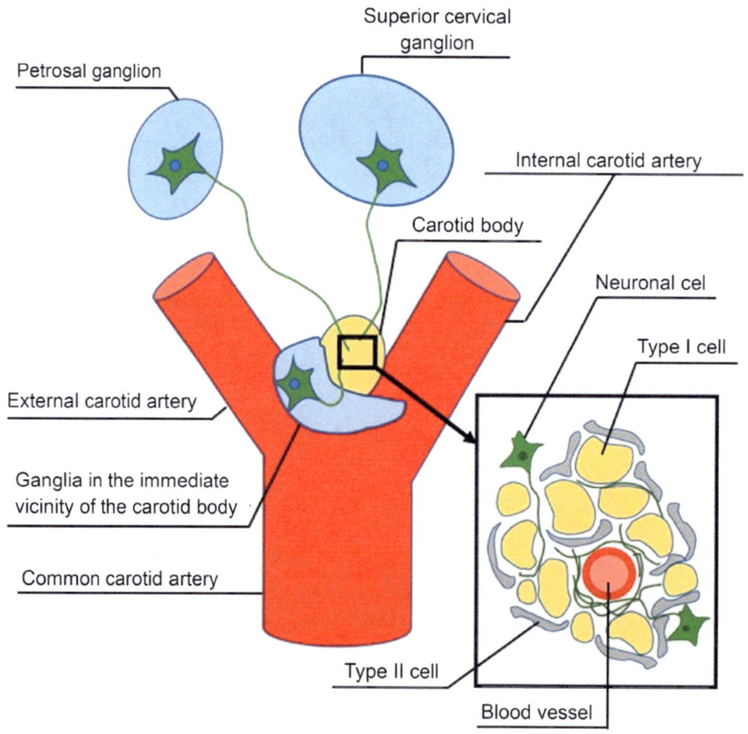

Figure 12.12. Vasoactive intestinal polypeptide (VIP).

Source: Gonkowski, Slawomir. 2020. "Vasoactive Intestinal Polypeptide in the Carotid Body—A History of Forty Years of Research. A Mini Review" *International Journal of Molecular Sciences* 21, no. 13: 4692. https://doi.org/10.3390/ijms21134692

An understanding of the biological activity of VIP not only accounts for its activity in normal physiology but also illuminates symptomatic presentation and the underlying challenge of diagnosis and treatment of VIP-secreting tumors. Interestingly, VIP is recognized for its multiplicative effects beyond gastrointestinal smooth muscle effects. It plays a role in glucose metabolism, digestion, and even hormonal homeostasis and thus is an endocrine multifaceted player. Multipotentiality is especially significant when evaluating patients with PNETs, particularly those presenting with signs of overproduction of hormones. In VIPoma, for example, VIP secretion leads to inappropriate activation of intestinal secretions, causing massive diarrhea that complicates the clinical presentation and hides the underlying diagnosis. Moreover, the role of VIP in systemic vasodilation may cause hypotensive episodes in patients and demands an integrated treatment strategy for symptom management and planning, along with timely consideration as set out in current guidelines (Andrysiak-Mamos et al., 2014; Adamiec et al., 2024). Besides, the management of VIPoma is also difficult due to the need for a multidimensional therapeutic regimen capable of treating the tumor itself as well as the resulting metabolic dysfunction. Surgery remains the cornerstone of therapy wherever feasible; nevertheless, they usually present in very advanced stages, and thus, the options are limited. Where surgery is not possible, medical management measures—like somatostatin analogues and targeted therapies, are of great significance in curtailing the effects of VIP overproduction. Coordination among multidisciplinary teams is also crucial to ensure optimal patient outcomes in view of the participation of PNET management challenges, the intricacy of VIP function, and the diverse presentation of these tumors' related symptoms. The intricate interaction between VIP and its pathological connotations emphasizes the importance of continued investigation of newer therapeutic alternatives (Andrysiak-Mamos et al., 2014; Adamiec et al., 2024) (Figure 12.12).

12.4.2. Clinical Features and Diagnosis

The clinical presentation of PNETs is diverse and will be dependent on whether the tumors are functional or non-functional. Functioning tumors will be presenting with their hormone secretion, which produces typical clinical syndromes such as hyperinsulinemia with insulinomas or elevated gastrin in gastrinomas. Patients with insulinomas are likely to present with episodes of hypoglycemia, which may result in sweating, confusion, or even loss of consciousness. On the other hand, gastrinomas have been known to evoke Zollinger-Ellison syndrome, with refractory peptic ulcers and secondary chronic diarrhea owing to hypersecretion of gastric acid. Non-functional tumors, on the other hand, usually secrete no hormone, and their clinical features often arise due to mass effect or metastasis, presenting with abdominal pain, weight loss, and jaundice as tumors increase or invade neighboring structures, illustrating the diverse presentations of these neoplasms. Diagnosis of PNETs is primarily based on biochemical, imaging, and histopathological analyses. Biochemical analysis is significant, particularly for the identification of hypersecretion of hormones. For instance, measurement of serum insulin is used for the diagnosis of insulinoma, while elevated gastrin levels are used to confirm gastrinoma. Advanced imaging techniques such as CT, MRI, and somatostatin receptor scintigraphy (SRS) play a crucial role in the localization of the tumors and in defining their extent, which enables differential diagnosis between functioning and non-functioning tumors. Histopathological diagnosis through biopsy is also of paramount importance, as it provides absolute proof of PNET type and grade for ideal tailoring of clinician management. Multi-disciplinary management cannot be over-pursued, providing maximum benefit through the convergence of experts belonging to various disciplines for global patient care. Existing guidelines emphasize using updated diagnostic and treatment guidelines for the management of PNETs, including national and international guidelines. According to Bartsch et al. (2023), the guidelines highlight the significance of biochemical workup, imaging investigations, and histopathological confirmation to navigate the complex landscape of PNET diagnosis and management. Furthermore, they emphasize the significance of multidisciplinary input by healthcare professionals with expertise in neuroendocrine tumors, which is pivotal while developing individualized treatment strategies for patients. Surgical therapy remains a corner stone of treatment for the majority of cases, particularly resectable disease. Other treatment options such as biotherapy, peptide receptor radionuclide therapy, and molecular targeted therapies expand the clinical treatment for PNETs, as outlined in Kos-Kudła et al. (2017). This multi-systemic treatment is essential to address the unique issues presented by functioning as well as non-functioning PNETs correctly.

12.4.3. Treatment Approaches: Medical Management and Surgery

The treatment of PNETs needs an individualized approach which takes into account the tumor's peculiar nature, for example, its functionality. For functioning tumors like insulinomas, gastrinomas, and VIPomas, relief of the clinical manifestations caused by hypersecretion of the hormone is usually tackled with medical therapy. This may include the use of drugs such as octreotide or lanreotide, which are somatostatin analogues that cause suppression of hormone secretion and relief of clinical symptoms. Furthermore, such agents also stabilize the tumor in some patients to enable a bridge to more definitive procedures.

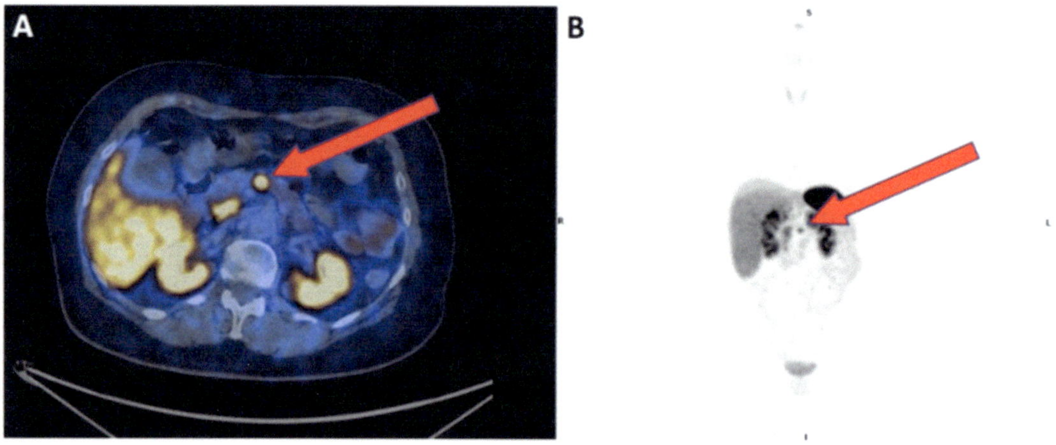

Figure 12.13. Role of PET/CT and therapy management of pancreatic neuroendocrine tumors (PNETs).

Source: Calabrò D, Argalia G, Ambrosini V. Role of PET/CT and Therapy Management of Pancreatic Neuroendocrine Tumors. *Diagnostics*. 2020; 10(12):1059. https://doi.org/10.3390/diagnostics10121059

ENETS guidelines emphasize the provision of individualized treatment timetables for PNETs, particularly well-differentiated and grade 1–3 PNETs, emphasizing the sophisticated interplay between medical treatment and surgery in the course of treatment of such tumors (Bartsch et al., 2023). Surgical resection remains the cornerstone of potentially curative therapy in locally confined PNETs. If the tumors are detected at an early stage and not metastasized, surgical resection can lead to remarkable improvements in patient outcomes as it effectively removes both the original mass and also localized metastases. The operation is typically done via Whipple procedure or distal pancreatectomy, respectively, depending on the size and location of the tumors. However, the late-diagnosis difficulty renders this therapeutic option out of reach to the majority of patients. As studies highlight, even in those patients diagnosed with insulinoma, the timing of surgery is critical, and the earlier it is undertaken, the better the outcome rate (Adamiec et al., 2024). Hence, enhancing awareness and diagnostic methods for PNETs is crucial to enhance the potential for surgical success and patient prognosis. In cases of unresectable tumors due to distant metastasis or local progression, the focus is on medical treatment to manage the disease and symptoms. Targeted agents, such as mTOR inhibitors (e.g., everolimus) and tyrosine kinase inhibitors (e.g., sunitinib), have shown to manage the tumor growth and symptoms in advanced disease. PRRT has also proven to be effective for some patients, those with somatostatin receptor-positive cancers. The method not only targets the tumor but also minimizes damage to the surrounding healthy tissue, and thus is a huge advancement in the toolkit of treatment. Lastly, the integration of surgical and medical therapies, as is ordered by each tumors behavior and the patients health, is the best way in curing PNETs, enhancing overall survival rate and quality of life in patients (Bartsch et al., 2023) (Figure 12.13).

12.5. Non-Functioning Pancreatic Neuroendocrine Tumors (NF-PNETs)

NF-PNETs represent a special category of the broader category of pancreatic neuroendocrine tumors. NF-PNETs do not secrete sufficient amounts of hormones to produce clinically significant symptoms or syndromes, as opposed to their functioning counterparts. Patients are often not symptomatic until the tumor becomes sizable or metastatic, which makes it hard to diagnose them in an early stage. This more malignant behavior of NF-PNETs emphasizes the need for vigilance and regular screening in high-risk populations, particularly in light of their capacity to grow rapidly compared to functioning tumors. Management of NF-PNETs requires extensive familiarity with both their biology and the diagnostic challenges that arise from the absence of obvious hormone-related signs and symptoms. An integral aspect of NF-PNET management is the techniques employed in diagnosis to assess tumor behavior. Biochemical diagnostic workup, though not as prominent as in working cases, consists of imaging tests such as CT scans, MRI, and EUS, which are important in the assessment of the tumors size, site, and metastasis. Furthermore, histopathological confirmation by immunohistochemical tests is important to assess the tumors nature and grade, which will decide on the ensuing management plans. The Polish Network of Neuroendocrine Tumors emphasizes the use of a multidisciplinary team of professionals with expertise in the treatment of these neoplasms to achieve comprehensive care using the resources of oncologists, surgeons, radiologists, and pathologists (Andrysiak-Mamos et al., 2014). Surgical resection remains the cornerstone of treatment of localized NF-PNETs, and curative intent is generally achievable when the tumor is confined to the pancreas. Surgical options may be distal pancreatectomy or Whipple procedure, depending on the size and site of the tumors. If NF-PNETs are of advanced stage, management by medical treatment is crucial using measures such as peptide receptor radionuclide therapy or targeted molecular therapies as indicated. The multidisciplinary approach to management emphasizes the overriding value of individualized measures that consider tumor characteristics and patient status.

With continuing research, further insight into the molecular etiology of NF-PNETs will continue to refine treatment strategies and improve patient outcomes. Lastly, future research and summations are crucial to refining our understanding and management of this challenging group of tumors (Bartsch et al., 2023) (Figure 12.14).

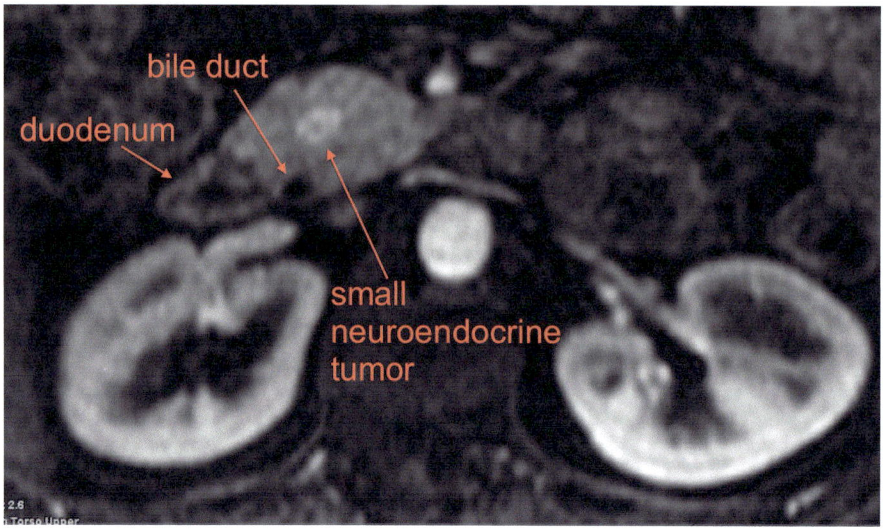

Figure 12.14. Pancreatic lesion.

Source: https://external-content.duckduckgo.com/iu/?u=https%3A%2F%2Fbodymri.stanford.edu%2Fwp-content%2Fuploads%2F2023%2F05%2FDedicatedPancreas-Example-DCE-neuroendocrine-1.png&f=1&nofb=1&ipt=cd8c1e74cb894ce73034b7ade03f4060c4680da435c847c48f90a995d097599e.

12.5.1. Clinical Presentation and Diagnosis

For PNETs, clinical presentation varies widely between functioning and non-functioning tumors. Functioning PNETs, such as insulinomas, gastrinomas, and VIPomas, are characterized by hypersecretion of insulin, gastrin, and vasoactive intestinal peptide, respectively. These hormone secretions generate distinctive clinical manifestations; for instance, patients with insulinomas have attacks of hypoglycemia, which are accompanied by palpitations, sweating, and confusion. Alternatively, non-functioning tumors may not be linked with hormone-related symptoms unless advanced, typically causing abdominal pain or obstructive jaundice. Having an insight into these manifestations is extremely crucial for early diagnosis and management as the development of symptomatic endocrine hyperfunction may provide valuable clues towards the underlying pathology of the tumor. PNETs are diagnosed by a multi-modality approach that involves biochemical, imaging, and histopathological investigations. Biochemical markers are of paramount significance in the diagnosis of viable tumors, where levels of the hormones are measured to determine the hypersecretion. Gastrin, for example, rises in gastrinomas, thereby aiding their detection. Imaging procedures such as CT, MRI, and EUS are pivotal in the localization of the tumors and determination of size and metastatic capability. Furthermore, the confirmed diagnosis often relies on histopathologic examinations, which are accompanied by immunohistochemical examinations for differentiation between various neuroendocrine tumors. Accurate understanding of these diagnostic modalities ensures proper classification and management of PNETs, which finally influences patient outcome in survival and quality of life (Andrysiak-Mamos et al., 2014). The development of updated clinical guidelines attempts to enhance the diagnostic and treatment management of PNETs. Current recommendations emphasize the necessity of a multi-disciplinary, combined strategy whereby specialists enhance diagnostic efficacy and individualize plans of treatment based on patients' requirements. The application of biochemical assays, high-tech imaging modalities, and immunohistochemistry is underscored to serve as an effective therapeutic pipeline. Surgery, particularly for localized functioning and non-functioning tumors, remains a pillar of care. Concurrently, integrated therapies like biotherapy, peptide receptor radionuclide therapy, and molecular-targeted therapies are covered to allow ongoing care of advanced disease patients. This well-planned system not only maximizes clinical practice for diagnosis and management of PNETs but also provides a platform for ongoing research and treatment modality refinement (Kos-Kudła et al., 2017).

12.5.2. Risk of Malignancy and Metastasis

The malignancy and metastatic potential in PNETs clearly vary with tumor type and biology. Cushing's syndrome, insulinoma, gastrinoma, and somatostatinoma are examples of functioning PNETs with readily apparent endocrine syndromes to complicate and delay appropriate treatment. The tumor grade according to histopathologic characteristics and immunohistochemical findings is an important factor determining the likelihood of malignant transformation. High-grade tumors are more prone to having aggressive characteristics, including early metastatic dissemination to regional and distant lymph nodes and organs, and thus the aggressive surveillance regimens both for functioning and non-functioning tumors. These characteristics have clinical implications when managing the patient, with the early detection of metastatic disease being able to greatly improve outcomes and guide treatment (Bartsch et al., 2023). Metastasis remains the main challenge in clinical management, as it has a strong influence on prognosis and therapeutic management of patients with PNETs. It is revealed that up to 60% of the patients have metastatic disease, predominantly those with non-functioning tumors, which are typically asymptomatic until advanced stages. Imaging modalities, e.g., CT and MRI, play an important role in the detection of metastasis and assessment of tumor burden. The revised diagnostic guidelines emphasize the necessity of a multidisciplinary assessment and treatment of PNET patients, particularly in view of the fact that resection is the only hope for a cure (Andrysiak-Mamos et al., 2014). However, with metastatic disease, systemic therapies in the form of somatostatin analogs, chemotherapy, and targeted therapy become central to the therapeutic armamentarium, indicate the complexity of the management of such neoplasms. In addition, PNET management includes precautionary stratification of patients on the basis of individual risk for malignancy and metastatic potential. Hereditary predispositions based on mutations in the MEN1 gene as well as other inherited syndromes can predispose patients to more aggressive disease patterns and thus mandate the initiation of active surveillance and early intervention. Incorporation of biochemical monitoring to monitor hormonal activity with imaging by radiology permits intervention at an optimal time, which can be maximally salvaged. Thus, the understanding of tumor biology, clinical presentation, and metastatic potential is all the more significant in optimizing patient outcomes. With evolving treatment modalities, ongoing research and adherence to established guidelines will remain to be of critical significance in evolving techniques in treating PNETs and mitigating the risk of malignancy and metastasis (Andrysiak-Mamos et al., 2014; Bartsch et al., 2023).

12.5.3. Treatment Options: Observation Versus Intervention

The treatment approaches for PNETs are a spectrum from active surveillance to aggressive treatment, and the choice of approach depends predominantly upon tumor characteristics and the patient's clinical status. If tumors are asymptomatic and are demonstrated to be indolent in nature, observation may be considered as an ideal option. Studies have shown that in certain non-functioning PNETs, particularly in those with no evidence of metastasis, the tumor growth might advance at a slow rate, hence in favor of a watchful waiting policy.

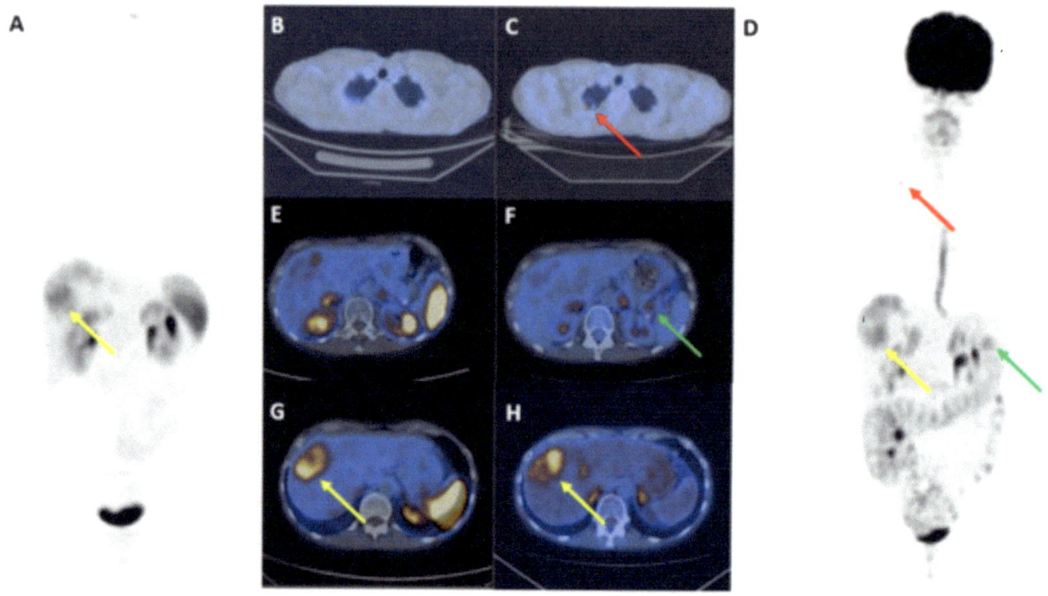

Figure 12.15. Treatment flowchart of pancreatic neuroendocrine neoplasms.

Source: Calabrò, Diletta, Giulia Argalia, and Valentina Ambrosini. 2020. "Role of PET/CT and Therapy Management of Pancreatic Neuroendocrine Tumors" *Diagnostics* 10, no. 12: 1059. https://doi.org/10.3390/diagnostics10121059

However, in functioning tumors such as insulinomas and gastrinomas, whose clinical impact is caused by physiological disruption as a result of hypersecretion of hormones, early surgery is often indicated to effect relief from symptoms and prevent complications of the hypersecretion syndromes. Therefore, careful evaluation of tumor behavior and patient presentation is critical to directing the treatment decision-making process, balancing the risk of over-treatment against potential for benefit by intervention. In evaluating the transition from observation to intervention, the extent and nature of tumor involvement is critical in directing management approaches. Where PNETs show signs of disease progression or metastatic disease, surgery is an integral component of treatment modalities. Surgical removal is still the standard for localized tumors, with potential curative results. In particular, removal of the primary tumor, as has been supported in studies, proves to result in better survival when compared to observation alone. Nonetheless, surgical decision is frequently clouded by the behavior of the tumors, like aggressive growth or more widespread metastasis, thus requiring a multidisciplinary evaluation to establish the best course of treatment. For patients who present with advanced disease, there are many non-surgical modalities, including targeted therapy and chemotherapy, that play a significant role as adjunctive treatments to minimize disease progression and symptom palliation. Finally, the treatment dilemma in PNETs is not one of observation versus treatment but rather one of patient considerations, tumor biology, and expected outcomes. Active surveillance may be suitable in non-vigorous tumor patients, as demonstrated in populations such as those with MEN-1, where conservative management has been shown to be effective without harm in the short term. Complications such as surgical resection or systemic treatment are however required for patients with vigorous disease patterns, not just maintaining the tumors under control but also with a significant impact on overall mortality. Given the character of PNETs and their varied presentations, ongoing patient counseling about the risk and benefit of each approach remains essential to offer informed choice and optimize results with the management of these tumors (Kulke et al., 2011; Hilli et al., 2016) (Figure 12.15).

12.6. Medical Management of Pancreatic Neuroendocrine Tumors (PNETs)

Clinical management of PNETs demands an equal understanding of both functioning and non-functioning tumors, as well as their relative clinical importance. Functioning tumors like insulinomas and gastrinomas need specialized pharmacologic therapy to control hormone secretion and symptom palliation. Insulinoma, for instance, can lead to devastating hypoglycemia, necessitating maneuvers such as oral ingestion of glucose or diazoxide to avert episodes. Treatment of gastrinomas also typically involves PPIs for the management of elevated gastric acid production, improving patients' quality of life. Also important is hereditary syndrome screening, such as MEN1, which is necessary in guiding medical management plans since early detection will lead to preemptive surveillance and potentially curative therapy, emphasizing the need for collaborative care models in treating PNET. Non-functional PNETs are typically a diagnostic challenge, given that they are asymptomatic in early stages. Nevertheless, their management is on no less a priority since they may be symptomatic by virtue of mass effect or metastatic disease. Medical management consists primarily of follow-up of the disease using imaging modalities and biomarkers with assessment of surgical potential. Somatostatin analogues, particularly octreotide, have become the prime option in treating non-functioning PNETs as they play a role in symptomatic relief and can perhaps slow tumor progression, thereby assuming their therapeutic benefit in clinical practice. Integration of novel therapies in the form of targeted therapies and PRRT is being explored in ongoing trials, which will hopefully give a fillip to the medical management of advanced non-functioning PNETs and make a positive impact on patient outcomes in the long term.

The shift in emphasis of molecular profiling in neuroendocrine tumors underscores the significance of precise diagnostics in tailoring medical treatment of PNETs. Histopathologic classification directs the selection of therapeutic modalities in conformity with tumors biological behavior and patient-specific factors, according to present guidelines. WHO grading system also guides oncologists to stratify PNETs by grade and stage, which is important for therapeutic decision-making and prognostic assessment, especially in advanced disease. Diagnostic modalities such as serum biomarkers and receptor imaging assist in detection of aggressive disease, also supporting early interventions. The multidisciplinary treatment of PNET is very important, incorporating genetics, pathology, and medical oncology to offer a complete treatment plan addressing the disease's complexity while enhancing patients' quality of life and survival rates (Marini et al., 2017; Cuccurullo et al., 2021) (Figure 12.16).

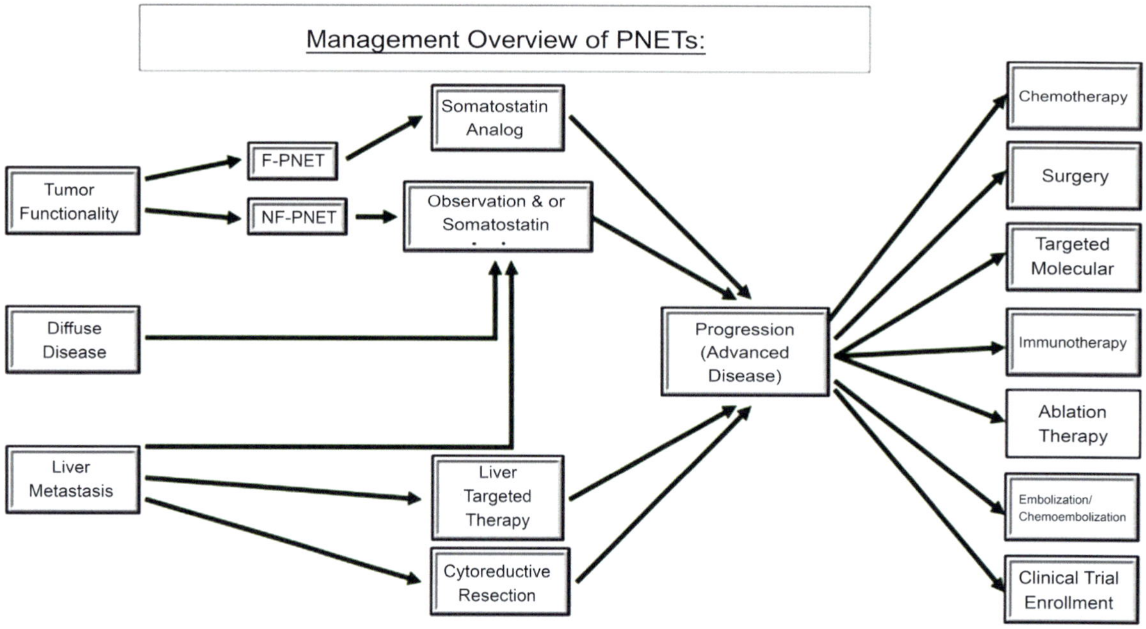

Figure 12.16. Management of pancreatic neuroendocrine tumors (PNETs).

Source: https://media.springernature.com/lw685/springer-static/image/chp%3A10.1007%2F978-3-030-37482-2_39-1/MediaObjects/487143_0_En_39-1_Fig1_HTML.png.

12.6.1. Role of Somatostatin Analogs

The role of somatostatin analogs in the management of PNETs is significant, particularly for functioning tumors that lead to the secretion of excessive hormones, resulting in disabling clinical symptoms. Somatostatin is a peptide hormone secreted from the hypothalamus and pancreas with a natural capacity to inhibit secretion of a number of hormones. The introduction of synthetic somatostatin analogs—octreotide and lanreotide—has revolutionized the treatment scenario in insulinomas, gastrinomas, and VIPomas. These drugs act by binding the somatostatin receptors of the tumor cells and thus suppressing hormone release and therefore the hypersecretory symptoms. Secondly, the somatostatin analogs have proved to exert antiproliferative activity and reduce the rate of advancement and increase of the tumors in patients with advanced disease, thus providing opportunities for treatment of challenging cases (Adamiec et al., 2024). The therapeutic application of the somatostatin analogs extends beyond symptom management to influence total treatment outcomes in PNET patients. Clinical experience has shown that long-acting somatostatin analogs are also able to deliver improved quality of life for hormone-related symptoms, particularly gastrinomas, where uncontrolled gastrin is the cause for severe gastrointestinal pain. Further, in chosen subsets of PNETs, the somatostatin analogs have been demonstrated to be associated with a reduction in tumor size, hence making it possible to have better surgical resectability in chosen instances. The agents not only complement surgery but also naturalize the requirement for long-term management modalities in individuals in whom surgery is not possible due to late presentation or disseminated disease (Kraszkiewicz et al., 2024).

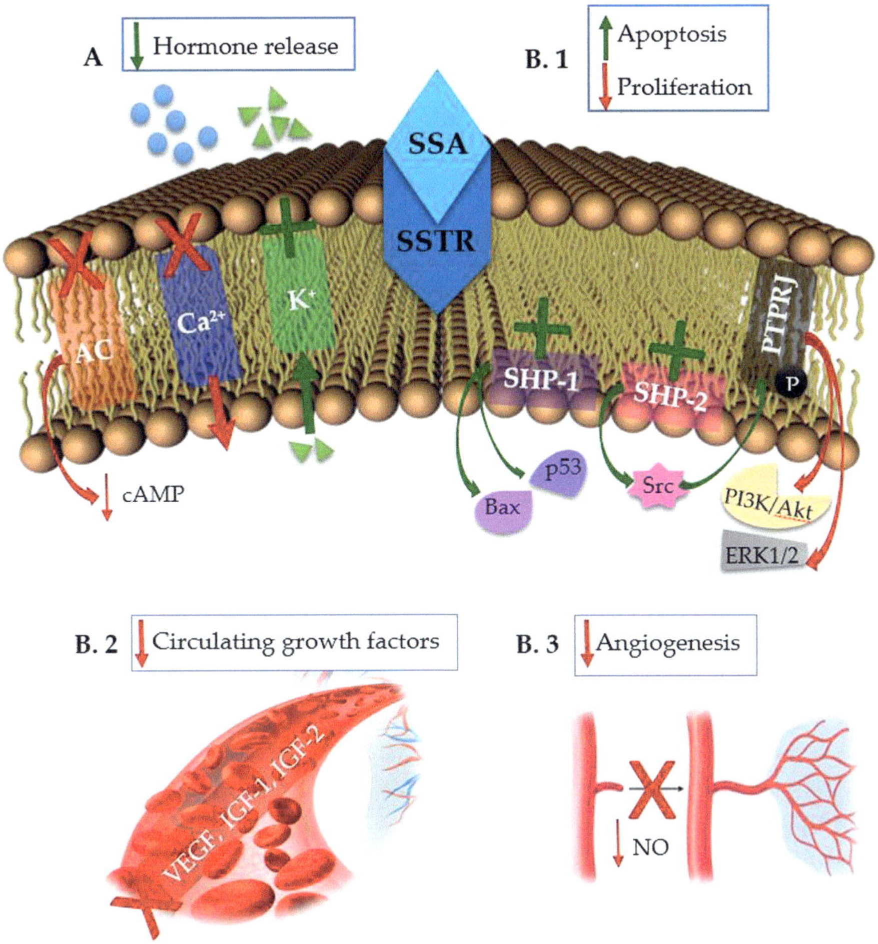

Figure 12.17. Somatostatin analogs in clinical practice.

Source: Gomes-Porras M, Cárdenas-Salas J, Álvarez-Escolá C. Somatostatin Analogs in Clinical Practice: A Review. *International Journal of Molecular Sciences*. 2020; 21(5):1682. https://doi.org/10.3390/ijms21051682

Consequently, the use of somatostatin analogs in treatment regimens is of multifactorial benefit, and they are critical in managing symptoms and disease progression. Despite their vast utility, the use of somatostatin analogs is not completely effective in all forms of PNET. Heterogeneity of somatostatin receptor expression among different tumor subtypes suggests that while some patients may experience substantial symptom relief and tumor control, others may not respond much to these therapies. Therefore, it is crucial for clinicians to modify treatment strategies accordingly, utilizing newer imaging techniques to identify receptor expression and selecting patients most likely to derive benefit from somatostatin analogs. In addition, ongoing research on new compounds and combination regimens provides potential for enhancement of the efficacy of somatostatin analogs, particularly in those PNETs that have developed resistance. With the advancement of a deeper understanding of the molecular basis of these tumors, the somatostatin analogs will remain a component of the armamentarium against PNETs, bridging the gap between symptom management and better prognostic outcomes (Figure 12.17).

12.6.2. Chemotherapy and Targeted Therapies

Management of PNETs is a complicated procedure that encompasses chemotherapy and targeted therapy as essential components of management. Chemotherapy is primarily a systemic method of combating the development of malignant cells in advanced PNET patients who are not candidates for surgical resection. Traditional chemotherapy regimens such as fluorouracil with streptozocin or doxorubicin have proved effective in some cases, especially for advanced forms of the disease. Nevertheless, response is usually restricted to a degree, and therefore more effective therapeutic interventions are required. Targeted therapy development has been a significant milestone in PNET treatment since they can target molecular pathways that are significant in tumor growth. Personalized medicine is essential in tumor and patient-specific stratification of therapy. Targeted agents like everolimus and sunitinib have encouraging outcomes through pathway inhibition that is significant to tumor growth and survival. Everolimus, an inhibitor of mTOR, has been promising in extending progression-free survival in unresectable, functioning, or non-functioning PNET patients, as demonstrated clinically. Similarly, sunitinib, a multikinase receptor tyrosine kinase inhibitor, has been beneficial in the treatment of patients with unresectable tumors by showing overall response rates improvement. Among the interesting features of these therapies is the relatively benign side effect profile relative to conventional chemotherapy, which can produce marked adverse effects, making it difficult to manage the patient. Incorporation of these target therapies into therapeutic protocols will require close collaboration among multijdisciplinary teams in order to maximize patient selection and therapeutic efficacy and toxicity monitoring. The role of chemotherapy and targeted therapy is particularly relevant in the context of operative PNETs, i.e., insulinomas, gastrinomas, and VIPomas, that may produce individualized hormones leading to debilitating symptoms. Management of these tumors is typically with a combination of operation and medical management as symptom control is critical to maximize quality of life. For instance, chemotherapy may be available in unresectable and advanced disease in gastrinoma patients, whereas targeted therapy can decrease symptoms through the inhibition of secretion at tumor level. Multidisciplinary management becomes a necessity, as pointed out by updated guidelines that advocate for individualized diagnostic and therapeutic approaches according to the individual needs of the patient (Andrysiak-Mamos et al., 2014; Kos-Kudła et al., 2017). To address both hormonal activity and tumor burden with a spectrum of modalities is a paradigm shift in the effective management of PNETs.

12.6.3. Palliative Care Considerations

Management of PNETs necessitates a prolonged strategy that includes consideration of palliative care, particularly since the tumors can generate significant morbidity and altered quality of life. Patients with PNETs are likely to present with disabling signs such as pain, gastrointestinal dysfunction, and psychological distress due to the disease. Palliative care is focused on the relief of symptoms regardless of whether the disease is at any phase or the treatment is intended to be curative. Through the use of an interdisciplinary team comprising oncologists, pain specialists, nutritionists, and mental health clinicians, health care practitioners can design a specific plan that meets the complex needs of the patient. Integration of palliative care in combination with standard medical treatments has been shown to greatly improve the quality of life of patients, enabling them to enjoy activities during their cancer treatment process. The primary palliative therapies for the treatment of patients with PNET may include pharmacological management of pain, i.e., by using opioids or adjuvant analgesics. Psychosocial management is also required in handling the emotional and psychological impact of cancer. The integration of counseling and support groups, along with the particular emotional problems of PNET patients, can act as a coping strategy for the patients as well as their families. Moreover, it is also necessary to maintain open communication between patients and healthcare providers that enables them to address advanced directives and goals of care. Such an anticipatory discussion enables the care to conform to the patients' wishes, particularly in managing expectations and preparation for end-of-life concerns once curative treatments become ineffective. Also, the role of palliative care in addition to medical management comes to the forefront while traversing the treatment scenario of different types of PNETs. Tumors that are resectable, such as insulinomas and gastrinomas, present challenges with their hormone-secreting functions, bringing forth symptoms necessitating immediate intervention. Treatment may have surgical interventions, as indicated above, but when surgery is not feasible, palliation comes into play. Palliative management for these conditions may involve the use of somatostatin analogs in an effort to alleviate hormone-generated symptoms, as well as widespread psychiatric care. As research continues into the molecular nature of PNETs and their variabilities concerning treatment options, particular emphasis on palliative care could enhance the therapeutic experience and aid in achieving a better quality of life, particularly for those with advanced or complex disease. With the changing dynamics of pNET management, it is all the more necessary to integrate curative and palliative objectives harmoniously (Heidsma, 2021; Balasundaram, 2024).

A CLOSER LOOK

FUTURE TREATMENT OF PANCREATIC NEUROENDOCRINE TUMORS (PNETS)

The development of treatment modalities for PNETs is critically dependent on continued research to elucidate tumor biology and individual patient responses. Future research is increasingly directed towards the genetic mutations and molecular pathways of PNETs, which may further define current classification systems and result in individualized therapeutic approaches. For instance, understanding the role of mutations in the MEN1 gene and other important oncogenes could prepare clinicians to predict the aggressiveness of such tumors and modify clinical interventions appropriately. Furthermore, incorporation of high-throughput sequencing technologies in the diagnostic toolkit of PNETs can potentially not only promote precision medicine but also unveil novel tumor-specific targets that can be harnessed for drug development and synoptic therapy. These developments are key to transitioning from a one-size-fits-all treatment paradigm to a more individualized care model in the treatment of PNETs. Besides genetic research, new pharmacological agents may also improve patient outcomes with PNETs.

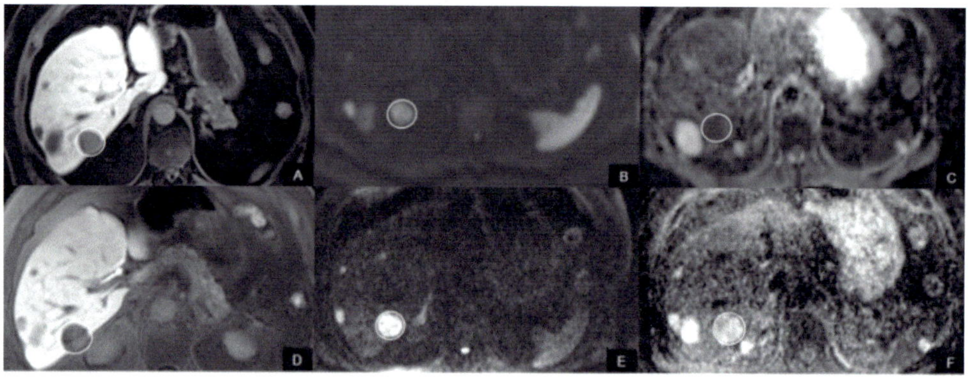

Source: https://external-content.duckduckgo.com/iu/?u=https%3A%2F%2Fpub.mdpi-res.com%2Fbiomedicines%2Fbiomedicines-10-02618%2Farticle_deploy%2Fhtml%2Fimages%2Fbiomedicines-10-02618-g004.png%3F1666089176&f=1&nofb=1&ipt=f110f1a0d5f9e52f3e55103df59b016f10514445103c823f8088bf9d9cc83238.

Present trials are evaluating multi-targeted agents that can inhibit multiple signaling pathways involved in tumor development and survival. The possibility of pairing known therapies, i.e., somatostatin analogues, with newer drugs acting on the vascular endothelial growth factor (VEGF), might introduce synergistic results, preventing the limitations of single-agent monotherapy. Immunotherapy is also becoming increasingly acceptable in PNET patients. Developments in the tumor microenvironment and immune checkpoint areas have opened the door to the use of checkpoint inhibitors to enhance the immune system against neuroendocrine tumors. A deeper understanding of the immune landscape would enable increased stratification of patients in clinical trials and thus maximize outcome and survival rates in patients with both functioning and non-functioning PNETs. Lastly, surgical intervention in PNETs will also be improved by improvements in minimally invasive surgery and new imaging modalities. With continued improvements in laparoscopic and robotic-assisted surgical methods, these should be able to reduce morbidity and shorten recovery for patients who have PNET resection. Improvement also in imaging technology, such as functional MRI and PET scans with newer tracers, may permit more accurate staging and better surgical planning. Such imaging modalities may allow for even minute or metastatic lesion detection, responsible for determining the surgical appropriateness. With ongoing research, integration of these advancements in technology with an understanding of PNET biology would likely implement a shift in paradigm for the surgical management strategies, yielding improved outcomes and enhanced quality of life for affected patients (Matyašovská, 2024) (Figure 12.18).

SUMMARY

Briefly, research on PNETs has illustrated the complexity of both functioning and non-functioning types, particularly regarding their clinical management. Functioning tumors, such as insulinomas and gastrinomas, are difficult to treat individually because they have hormone-driven symptoms, which can be a potential factor in the quality of life of patients. Surgical resection tends to remain the primary treatment, especially for localized lesions. Notwithstanding this, advancements in medical treatment, including targeted therapy and personalized therapy, complement surgical intervention to enhance PNETs. Through an increasing knowledge of the nuances of these tumors, medical professionals are able to craft treatment regimes specific to patients' individualized needs and enhance curative efficacy, thereby achieving enhanced overall prognoses. The understanding of PNETs evolves, particularly with the integration of molecular profiling techniques that enable diagnosis and personalized therapy. As reflected by ongoing studies, microRNA and mRNA dysregulation offer promising avenues towards elucidating the molecular pathogenesis of PNETs in a way that enables enhanced stratification of patients based on tumor characteristics. This stratification is significant for the prediction of treatment outcome and response, pointing to the importance of a multidimensional perspective that incorporates both molecular and clinical data. These findings may develop more effective biomarkers and treatments, ultimately influencing the clinical environment for PNET patients. The capacity of treatment plans to adapt with ongoing advances points to the dynamic nature of oncology and the emphasis on patient-centered care. Future research is important in further dissecting the complexity inherent in PNETs and refining existing treatment protocols. The following is reported in the evolving guidelines on the management of these tumors; the utilization of national protocols for conservatively managing low-risk PNETs reflects an extent of commitment to the improvement of patient outcomes while preventing unnecessary intervention. Prioritizing knowledge gap-filling research, especially in metastasis risk and best-practice surveillance methods, can provide the foundation for treatment paradigm innovations by researchers. Facilitating interdisciplinary collaborations between oncologists, researchers, and clinical biochemists can also propel PNETs' understanding . The potential for integration of state-of-the-art therapies and biomarker-based strategies will, with certainty, lead to improved management strategies, promising patients suffering from these otherwise under-emphasized yet highly impactful neoplasms (Donegan et al., 2017).

PNETs are a heterogeneous group of neoplasms derived from the islet cells of the pancreas. They are divided into functioning and non-functioning types of which functioning tumors secrete hormones that may lead to specific clinical syndromes such as insulinoma, gastrinoma, and VIPoma. Functioning tumors can have typical symptoms after hormone secretion, such as insulinoma, can lead to hypoglycemia, while gastrinoma results in Zollinger-Ellison syndrome. On the other hand, non-functioning tumors do not produce hormones and can be asymptomatic until it is advanced or present with mass effects. It is important to understand this classification so that management as well as diagnosis can be effectively done, since the clinical behavior and therapeutic modalities can be significantly different depending on whether the tumor is hormone-producing or not. Treatment of PNETs involves a multidisciplinary approach, with medical and surgical treatment combined to suit the function and behavior of the tumors. Surgery is the therapy of choice for localized disease and is curative, but operative decision-making depends on tumor size, location, and metastasis. For disseminated or metastatic disease, systemic treatment can incorporate targeted therapy, biotherapy, and peptide receptor radionuclide therapy. The current developments in the diagnostic methods, such as imaging methods and biochemical markers, have enhanced our ability to accurately diagnose and follow-up PNPs. As put forward in recent recommendations, histopathological verification through immunohistochemical techniques is still crucial in determining proper management plans for patients with PNEN (Kos-Kudła et al., 2017). Furthermore, clinical behavior of gastroenteropancreatic neuroendocrine tumors (GEP-NETs) highlights the intricacy associated with such tumors, whereby variations in symptoms and prognosis can be justified based on the unique biological behavior of every tumor type. The growing prevalence of GEP-NETs globally necessitates ongoing research to elucidate the pathogenesis and progression of such tumors. Studies on the role of angiogenesis, neuropeptides, and matrix metalloproteinases have shed light on other potential therapeutic targets. Although today markers for GEP-NETs exist, they are not sensitive and specific enough in their capacity to predict tumor growth and thus additional studies are indicated to elucidate correct biomarkers for improved management (Kuiper, 2011). In-depth understanding of PNETs finally leads to maximal patient care through intelligent interventions and new therapies.

KEY TERMS FROM THIS CHAPTER

- Neuroendocrine cells
- Functional tumors
- Insulinoma
- Glucagonoma
- Somatostatinoma
- Hypoglycemia
- Islet cells
- Non-functional tumors
- Gastrinoma
- VIPoma
- Hormonal secretion
- Zollinger–Ellison syndrome

References

1. Adamiec, D. K., Gonciarz, M. J., Dąbrowska, A., Zaliwska, D., Kienanh Do , M., Strojny, A. A., ... Czach, M. (2024). Pancreatic neuroendocrine tumors: classification, diagnosis and treatment – A review of the most frequent neuroendocrine tumors. *Quality in Sport*, *19*, 53611. https://doi.org/10.12775/QS.2024.19.53611 (accessed on 26 May 2025).
2. Donegan, D., Singh Ospina, N., Rodriguez-Gutierrez, R., Al-Hilli, Z., Thompson, G. B., Clarke, B. L., & Young, W. F., Jr (2017). Long-term outcomes in patients with multiple endocrine neoplasia type 1 and pancreaticoduodenal neuroendocrine tumours. *Clinical endocrinology*, *86*(2), 199–206. https://doi.org/10.1111/cen.13264 (accessed on 26 May 2025).
3. Andrysiak-Mamos, E., Bednarczuk, T., Blicharz-Dorniak, J., Bolanowski, M., et al. (2014). *Nowotwory Neuroendokrynne Trzustki–Zasady Postępowania (Rekomendowane Przez Polską Sieć Guzów Neuroendokrynnych)*. https://core.ac.uk/download/268441641.pdf (accessed on 26 May 2025).
4. Balasundaram, P. (2024). *Improved Detection of Pancreatic Neuroendocrine Tumors Through the Development of a Biomarker Panel* [Doctoral dissertation]. https://core.ac.uk/download/618291180.pdf (accessed on 26 May 2025).
5. Kos-Kudła, B., Rosiek, V., Borowska, M., Bałdys-Waligórska, A., Bednarczuk, T., Blicharz-Dorniak, J., Bolanowski, M., Boratyn-Nowicka, A., Cichocki, A., Ćwikła, J. B., Falconi, M., Foltyn, W., Handkiewicz-Junak, F., Hubalewska-Dydejczyk, A., Jarząb, B., Jarząb, M., Junik, R., Kajdaniuk, D., Kamiński, G., Kolasińska-Ćwikła, A., ... Zgliczyński, W. (2017). Pancreatic neuroendocrine neoplasms - management guidelines (recommended by the Polish Network of Neuroendocrine Tumours). *Endokrynologia Polska*, *68*(2), 169–197. https://doi.org/10.5603/EP.2017.2016(accessed on 26 May 2025).
6. Kulke, M. H., Bendell, J., Kvols, L., Picus, J., Pommier, R., & Yao, J. (2011). Evolving diagnostic and treatment strategies for pancreatic neuroendocrine tumors. *Journal of hematology & oncology*, *4*, 29. https://doi.org/10.1186/1756-8722-4-29
7. Marini, F., Giusti, F., Tonelli, F., & Brandi, M. L. (2017). Management impact: effects on quality of life and prognosis in MEN1. *Endocrine-related cancer*, *24*(10), T227–T242. https://doi.org/10.1530/ERC-17-0203 (accessed on 26 May 2025).
8. Brighi, N. (2022). *The Role of MGMT Promoter Methylation as a Predictive Factor for Temozolomide-Based Treatment in Neuroendocrine Neoplasms: A Prospective Observational Study* [Doctoral dissertation]. https://core.ac.uk/download/511394018.pdf (accessed on 26 May 2025).
9. Cardona, K., Dillhoff, M., Fields, R. C., Idrees, K., et al. (2019). The impact of failure to achieve symptom control after resection of functional neuroendocrine tumors: An 8-institution study from the US Neuroendocrine Tumor Study Group. *Journal of Surgical Oncology*. https://deepblue.lib.umich.edu/bitstream/handle/2027.42/147162/jso25306_am.pdf?sequence=1&isAllowed=y (accessed on 26 May 2025).
10. Andersen, K. Ø., Detlefsen, S., Brusgaard, K., & Christesen, H. T. (2024). Well-differentiated G1 and G2 pancreatic neuroendocrine tumors: a meta-analysis of published expanded DNA sequencing data. *Frontiers in endocrinology*, *15*, 1351624. https://doi.org/10.3389/fendo.2024.1351624

11. Cuccurullo, V., Iacomino, A., & Marino, A. (2021). *Neuroendocrine Tumors: From Anatomopathological to Clinical Presentation*. https://core.ac.uk/download/534976287.pdf (accessed on 26 May 2025).

12. Evans, D. B., Pisters, P. W. T., & Abruzzese, J. L. (2002). *Pancreatic Cancer*. Springer Science & Business Media. http://books.google.com/books?id=Fd8h89YGdX8C (accessed on 26 May 2025).

13. Gill, P. (2017). *Studies in Patients with Surgically Resected Pancreatic Neuroendocrine Tumors–Micron Expression and Clinical Correlation* [Doctoral dissertation]. https://core.ac.uk/download/212692797.pdf (accessed on 26 May 2025).

14. Heidsma, C. M. (2021). *Risk-Stratification and Management of Pancreatic Neuroendocrine Tumors* [Doctoral dissertation]. https://core.ac.uk/download/489785454.pdf (accessed on 26 May 2025).

15. Kraszkiewicz, A., Strojny, A. A., Dąbrowska, A., Adamiec, D. K., Zaliwska, D., Czach, M., Gonciarz, M. J., et al. (2024). *Pancreatic Neuroendocrine Tumors: Classification, Diagnosis and Treatment–A Review of The Most Frequent Neuroendocrine Tumors*. https://core.ac.uk/download/628504732.pdf (accessed on 26 May 2025).

16. Kuiper, P. (2011). *GEP-NET: Rare Tumor Connections. Pathophysiological Aspects of Gastroenteropancreatic Neuroendocrine Tumors* [Doctoral dissertation]. https://scholarlypublications.universiteitleiden.nl/handle/1887/17584

17. Matyašovská, N. (2024). *Molekulární Profilování K Odhalení Nových Signatur U Nádorových Onemocnění* [Doctoral dissertation]. https://core.ac.uk/download/651302032.pdf (accessed on 26 May 2025).

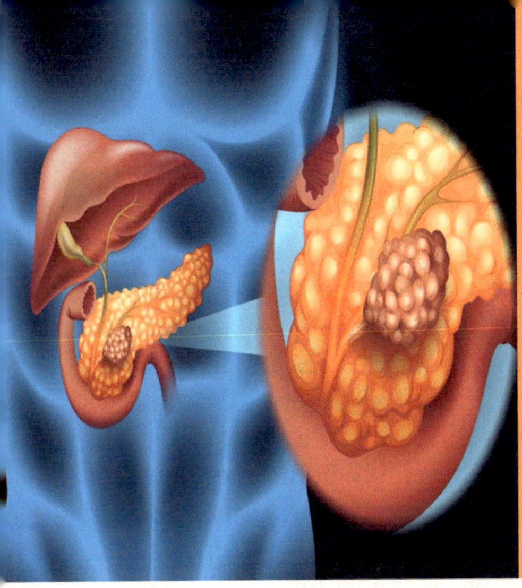

Chapter 13

METASTATIC AND RARE TUMORS OF THE PANCREAS

Contents

Introduction

The pancreas plays a significant role in both endocrine and digestive physiology, but is also a site for an enormous spectrum of tumors, some being rare and metastatic in nature. They encompass lymphomas and secondary tumors such as renal cell carcinoma metastasis. They reflect the intricacy of pancreatic pathology and the imperative necessity of precise diagnostic and therapeutic interventions. Lymphoma, a hematologic malignancy that either originates or metastasizes to the pancreas, presents some unique therapeutic challenges due to its varied biological behavior compared to pancreatic adenocarcinoma. The presence of such tumors, although infrequent, emphasizes the importance of awareness among clinicians to recognize and treat the affected patients promptly. With the changing face of pancreatic neoplasms, the growing significance of stromal and acinar cell tumors also serves as a turning point. Stromal tumors, fewer in percentage of pancreatic tumors, exhibit histopathological differences and varied clinical behaviors. Unlike the more frequent pancreatic ductal adenocarcinoma, stromal tumors may have a more indolent clinical course despite their presentation often in advanced stages of the disease. Acinar cell tumors further complicate the clinical scenario with their bidirectional acinar and ductal differentiation. The nuances of these rare tumors must be understood to customize treatment strategies because standard treatment protocols may prove inadequate for managing these heterogenous cancers (Cannon et al., 2020). When managing these heterogenous pancreatic tumor types, it is necessary to keep in mind contemporary treatment modalities involving both surgery and multimodal therapy. Surgical resection remains the pillar for potentially curative treatment in localized lesions, whereas systemic therapies can offer palliation or survival extension for advanced lesions. Immunotherapies and targeted therapies are increasingly being incorporated into regimens, particularly in the setting of poorly differentiated or advanced tumors. Development of an integrative model of treatment, based on robust diagnostics—molecular analysis and genetic studies, is going to enhance the survival of metastatic and rare pancreatic tumors. The biology behind such complexity dictates further research to perfect the method of treatment and devise a better prognosis for these patients as a whole (Figure 13.1).

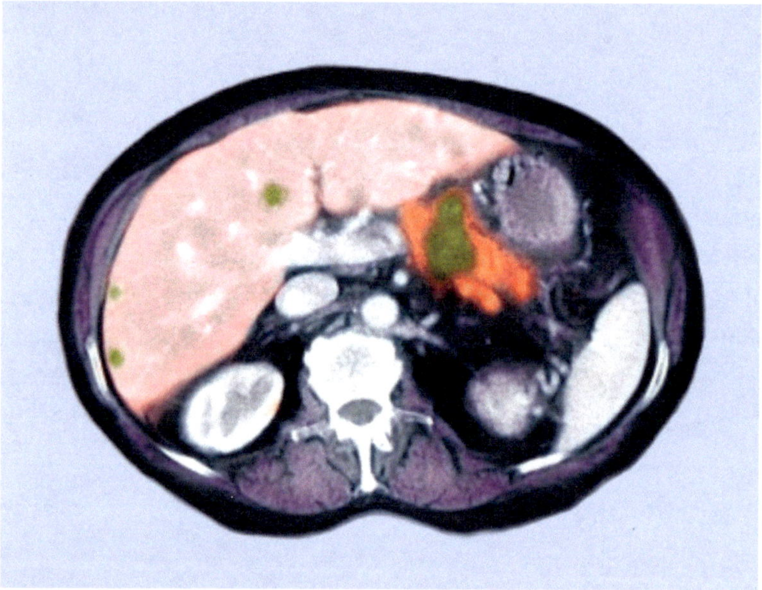

Figure 13.1. Metastatic pancreatic cancer.

Source: https://external-content.duckduckgo.com/iu/?u=https%3A%2F%2Fimages.fineartamerica.com%2Fimages-medium-large%2F2-metastatic-pancreatic-cancer-ct-scan-du-cane-medical-imaging-ltd.jpg&f=1&nofb=1&ipt=7c38bb741665ad86bbfbc903442e793a963c0861a3c83377c41e65ddd73a56fe.

Overview of Pancreatic Tumors

The pancreas, a significant organ positioned in the rear of the stomach, helps in digestion and metabolism by releasing digestive enzymes and hormones such as insulin. Among the various conditions of the pancreas, tumors are a serious concern and affect both exocrine and endocrine forms in the majority of instances. The most frequent pancreatic neoplasm is pancreatic ductal adenocarcinoma (PDAC), characterized by its malignancy and sinister prognosis, particularly in late stages. PDAC arises from the epithelial lining of the pancreatic ducts and has a tendency to present late, and thus, the five-year survival rate is miserably low. By taking into account the intricate character of pancreatic tumors in terms of histological subtypes and related difficulties, a clearer vision of their clinical implications and the need for effective treatment methods becomes apparent, which underlines the significance of ongoing research in this area. Metastatic pancreatic tumors, particularly those originating from the origin in other primary sites, complicate the clinical scenario even further. Lymphoma and renal cell carcinoma are two good examples where malignancies from other sites metastasize to the pancreas and contribute to the tumor burden. The metastatic processes are composed of complex interactions between metastatic tumor cells and the pancreas microenvironment that may change metastatic lesion biology and behavior. Importantly, TME is a predictor of treatment outcomes and survival for patients. Research into whether the TME may be modulated to maximize treatment efficacy is gaining momentum, reflected in ongoing research that explores the immune environment of pancreatic cancer. Increased understanding of such interactions may usher in new treatment paradigms with a better chance of overcoming the inherent resistance of pancreatic tumors (Coffelt, & de Visser, 2015).

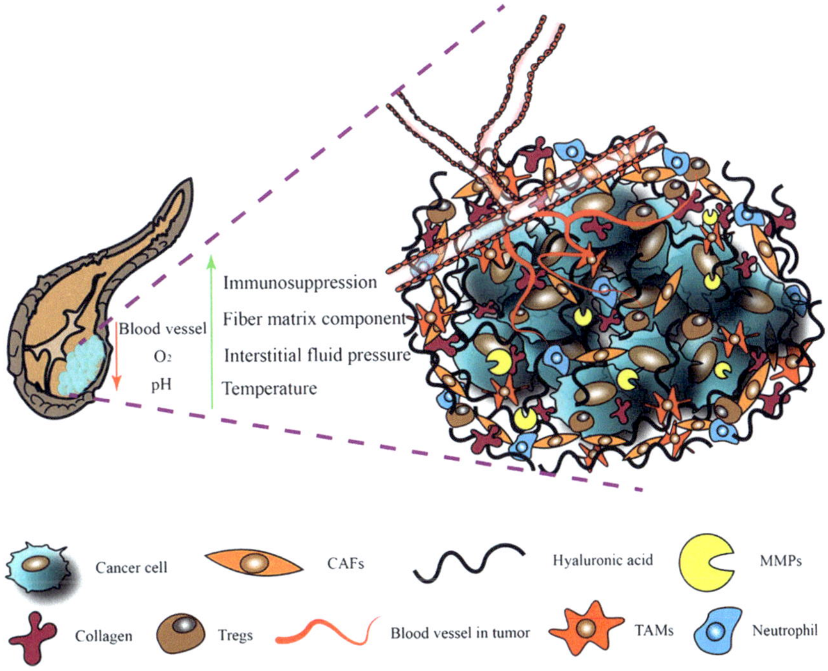

Figure 13.2. The tumor microenvironment (TME) in pancreatic cancer.

Source: https://www.researchgate.net/publication/356440392/figure/fig1/AS:1093173409513477@1637644259315/The-tumor-microenvironment-TME-in-pancreatic-cancer-The-expanded-extracellular-matrix.png.

In the field of pancreatic tumors, these uncommon varieties such as stromal and acinar cell tumors further broaden the scope of this crucial body of work. Stromal tumors, or what are also referred to as desmoplastic neoplasms, typically arise from the supportive tissue of the pancreas and may present with characteristic clinical features different from those of their more common counterparts. Acinar cell carcinoma, though less frequent, is another rare tumor that has its origin in the acinar cells responsible for secreting enzymes. The clinical presentation of such tumors is typically lacking in the usual markers of more frequent types and needs specialized diagnostic tests to diagnose them accurately. With continuous study delving deeper into the biological behavior and treatment response of such infrequent tumors, there is ever-growing recognition of the unique challenge presented by them that requires certain therapeutic approaches, like possibly targeting therapies and immunotherapy protocols, which may possibly be effective against such refractory tumors, in combination with findings of studies on the association between inhibition of AXL and cancer treatment, as described in Haaland et al. (2017) (Figure 13.2).

Importance of Studying Metastatic and Rare Tumors

The study of metastatic and uncommon tumors is of utmost significance in expanding the understanding of cancer biology, particularly concerning their unique pathophysiological mechanisms. Metastatic tumors, originating from primary tumors and spreading to secondary sites, such as the pancreas, are diagnostically and therapeutically difficult to identify clinically due to their heterogeneity. For example, pancreatic metastasis can occur from various tissues, thus making it difficult to establish a treatment protocol and predict prognosis. With the investigation of these tumors, biomarkers and pathways involved in tumor development and metastasis can be detected by researchers and clinicians, leading to more targeted therapies. Such need is emphasized by investigations that show the complexity of histological diagnosis and treatment modalities for various tumors. Continuing research is a critical necessity to improve survival and patient results with metastatic cancer, again pointing to the imperative of targeted investigation in this context. Furthermore, investigation into rare tumors, which are either exclusively present in special populations or have few treatment options, is also critical. These tumors have a tendency to be characterized by special molecular characteristics, which can greatly differ from those of common malignancies. For instance, information on the immunohistochemical profiles of such tumors, such as their use of biomarkers like ZBTB16 in germ cell tumors, will enhance diagnostic specificity and facilitate individualized treatment approaches.

This is significant because misdiagnosis leads to inappropriate treatment protocols and adverse patient outcomes. Identification of rare tumors, as well as research into their biology, uncovers individualized therapeutic avenues that otherwise would never be investigated. Thus, investment in research endeavors dealing with rare tumors has the potential to advance the overall understanding of cancer heterogeneity and improve clinical practice for every cancer (Aron et al., 2017). Moreover, there is greater awareness of the necessity to bring in a multidisciplinary study of metastatic and rare tumors. Multidisciplinary studies by oncologists, pathologists, radiologists, and researchers can enhance knowledge about tumor behavior and management strategies. For example, incorporation of advanced imaging modalities such as PET/CT in the evaluation of pancreatic cancer aids in enhanced characterization and staging, ultimately leading to better outcomes. As the face of cancer treatment evolves, particularly with the advent of personalized medicine, the findings from the studies on rare and metastatic tumors will be pivotal in fueling the creation of new treatment approaches. Hence, prioritizing research in these subjects not only strengthens our understanding of cancer but also energizes the innovation of efficacious treatment modalities to confront such challenging aspects of oncological practice.

13.1. Understanding Pancreatic Anatomy and Function

Understanding of pancreatic physiology and anatomy is basic to comprehending the intricacy of metastatic and rare pancreatic tumors. The pancreas is a significant organ situated retroperitoneally; hence its accessibility for investigation processes is limited. It is made up of two primary tissues: the exocrine tissue, which secretes digestive enzymes, and the endocrine tissue, which regulates blood glucose levels by releasing hormones, namely insulin and glucagon. This bipotentiality is the foundation of the organ's critical role in digestion and metabolic regulation. Consequently, any interference with the pancreatic architecture, such as metastasis of other malignant processes or development of rare tumors (e.g., acinar cell carcinoma or pancreatic stromal tumors), can have deleterious effects on digestive and hormonal health.

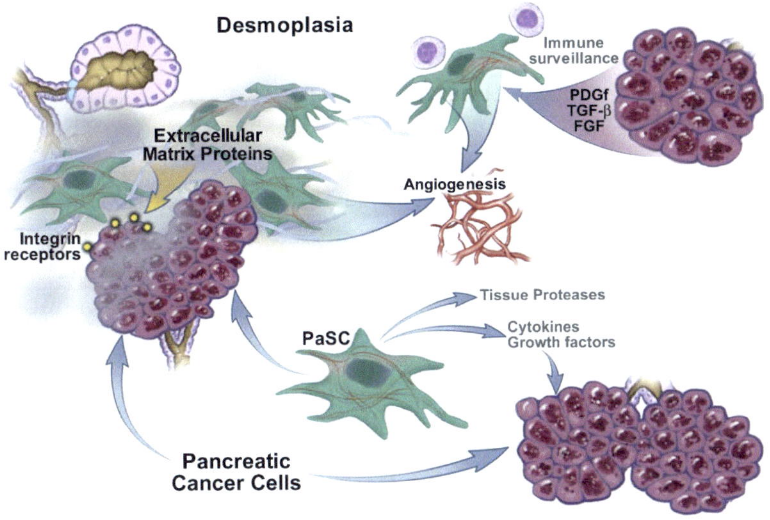

Figure 13.3. Desmoplasia of pancreatic ductal adenocarcinoma (PDAC).

Source: https://external-content.duckduckgo.com/iu/?u=https%3A%2F%2Fwww.cghjournal.org%2Fcms%2Fattachment%2F5423a225-cbc7-43c9-b253-dbc659b6a015%2Fgr1_lrg.jpg&f=1&nofb=1&ipt=e6d26f484f6225642271eeec9090c3d87d6e6b3d73ae7099457518b378b61a63.

An understanding of these anatomical and physiological attributes is necessary for the design of effective diagnostic and therapeutic regimens. Its vascular supply and supporting structures also mirror the anatomical intricacy of the pancreas, which contribute significantly to tumor behavior and responsiveness to therapy. The pancreas is richly supplied by the celiac trunk's branches, specifically the gastroduodenal and splenic arteries, which provide it with essential nutrients and oxygen. Moreover, it is anatomically related to significant organs such as the duodenum and spleen, so operating on pancreatic tumors becomes challenging. The metastatic lesions, for instance, renal cell carcinoma, also require meticulous examination because they have the propensity to block pancreatic ducts or vessels, resulting in further issues such as pancreatitis or systemic effects (Curran et al., 2015). Appreciation of how these anatomical connections affect both the function of the pancreas and the development of tumors is important for clinical practitioners treating pancreatic cancers. In addition, the pathophysiology of pancreatic cancer is frequently representative of the complex interaction among genetic, environmental, and immunological influences on both the development and growth of tumors. Genetic mutations in genes such as KRAS, TP53, and CDKN2A are most frequently implicated in pancreatic cancer, particularly Pancreatic Ductal Adenocarcinoma (PDAC) and the rarer forms, e.g., pancreatic lymphoma. The complexity of this form demands an integrative model of therapy with both traditional treatments and emerging options such as immunotherapy and targeted therapies to break tumor-specific pathways. By enhancing our understanding of pancreatic anatomy and function, clinicians can gain a greater appreciation of the mechanisms that dictate tumor behavior and modulate treatment approaches to patients with metastatic and rare tumors of the pancreas. Only through this complete understanding can patient outcomes be optimized and the field of pancreatic oncology advance (Figure 13.3).

13.1.1. Structure of the Pancreas

The pancreas, which is an abdominal cavity organ, plays a central role in both the exocrine and endocrine systems. Anatomically, it is divided into four areas: head, neck, body, and tail. The head rests in the duodenal curve and serves to secrete digestive enzymes secreted into the small intestine. They act as catalysts for digesting the macronutrients, such as proteins, fats, and carbohydrates. The neck is a transition area between the body and head, and the body and tail extend towards the spleen. The pancreas has a complex structure with groups of cells referred to as islets of Langerhans dispersed throughout the acinar cells. The islets have a direct role in the secretion of insulin and glucagon and thus are important for the metabolism of glucose and homeostasis. In addition to its distinctive anatomical compartments, the pancreas also has a distinctive microenvironment in support of its bicomponent function. Interstitial tissue harbors a dense vascular bed required for the delivery of hormones and nutrients, as well as for facilitating the exchange of gases in pancreatic tissue. Additionally, the presence of pancreatic stellate cells is relevant since such cells are responsible for the structural integrity of the organ and play a critical role in responding to injury and fibrosis. Interestingly, under pathological conditions like cancer, these stellate cells can be activated, and this can result in a fibrotic reaction that compromises the normal function of the pancreas. Tumorous invasion of various kinds of cells, including immune cells and myofibroblasts, complicates the pancreas's already intricate anatomy further, thereby significantly contributing to the tumor microenvironment and cancer growth that is essential for research into metastatic and rare tumors arising in this organ. An understanding of the pancreas anatomy is imperative to researching the character of particular tumor types that are able to arise within it, particularly in relation to metastasis. The unique structure of the pancreas dictates the path of metastasis; for instance, renal cell carcinoma and lymphoma can metastasize to the pancreas via hematogenous routes, complicating treatment plans. Pancreatic tissue-derived tumors, like acinar cell and stroma tumors, also demonstrate the central importance of pancreatic structure in disease mechanisms. Moreover, the intrinsic pancreas architecture is of extraordinary importance in therapeutic strategies, including how therapies could be delivered in order to be able to target specifically tumor microenvironments or the vasculature feeding tumor development (Gupta, 2017. Hence, a detailed understanding of the structural complexity of the pancreas is essential in developing effective interventions for metastatic and rare tumors (Figure 13.4).

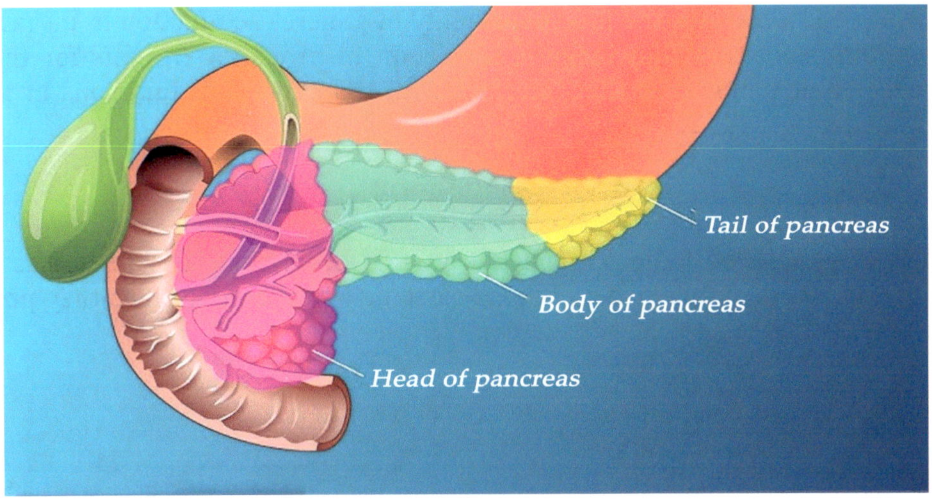

Figure 13.4. Structure of the pancreas.

Source: https://i.ytimg.com/vi/NZ4zcrTzUjA/hq720.jpg?sqp=-oaymwEhCK4FEIIDSFryq4qpAxMIARUAAAAAGAElAADIQj0AgKJD&rs=AOn4CLA-2lY0KqAtSIEXYaQ351iRtNcveA.

13.1.2. Role of the Pancreas in Digestion and Metabolism

The pancreas plays a twofold role in the human body, both as an endocrine and as an exocrine organ. As an exocrine organ, the pancreas releases digestive enzymes such as amylase, lipase, and proteases into the small intestine to facilitate carbohydrate, fat, and protein digestion. This enzymatic role plays a crucial role in proper nutrient utilization and metabolism. The pancreas also secretes bicarbonate to neutralize gastric acid that flows into the duodenum, creating an ideal pH for digestive enzymes to function effectively. In conditions like tumors of the pancreas, including rare acinar cell tumors, this digestive process can be completely impaired, leading to malabsorption and additional nutritional insufficiencies, eventually compromising overall health and metabolism. As an endocrine organ, the pancreas releases important hormones, such as insulin and glucagon, required for glucose metabolism regulation. Insulin lowers blood glucose through the promotion of cellular uptake and storage of glucose, while glucagon acts to increase blood glucose levels during fasting or stress. This hormonal balance is essential in the maintenance of homeostasis of energy metabolism. Metastatic diseases of the pancreas, such as metastasis of renal cell carcinoma, can impair this endocrine function further, also making a patient more prone to dysregulated blood glucose and, in extreme cases, diabetes mellitus. Scientific research has found that tumors in the pancreas can redefine hormonal profiles so that the ensuing metabolic situation is more complex for the patient and needs specialized treatment modalities to manage both malignancy and its metabolic effects. In addition to its vital roles in digestion and metabolism, the pancreas is also frequently involved in most pathologies, including endocrine tumors and neuroendocrine tumors. The latter tumors may manifest as hypersecretion of hormones, thus leading to secondary metabolic derangements. Gastrinomas, for instance, may lead to hypersecretion of gastric acid, which contributes to gastrointestinal morbidity. The advances in imaging techniques, such as 18F-DOPA PET and 11C-5-HTP PET, have enhanced the diagnosis of pancreatic neuroendocrine tumors, which are difficult to diagnose since they can have very minimal symptoms. Proper identification is important as early intervention will not only improve the survival rate but also metabolic control in the patients, which demonstrates the indispensability of pancreatic function in disease and health management. Additionally, this knowledge is important in providing insights for the generation of therapies targeted at tumor cells that interfere with the pancreas's functions in digestion and metabolism (Koopmans et al., 2015).

13.1.3. Implications of Pancreatic Tumors on Overall Health

The appearance of pancreatic tumors, particularly rare forms such as lymphomas and stromal tumors, renders the health status of the patients extremely challenging since they possess unique biological features and inevitable diagnostic complexities.

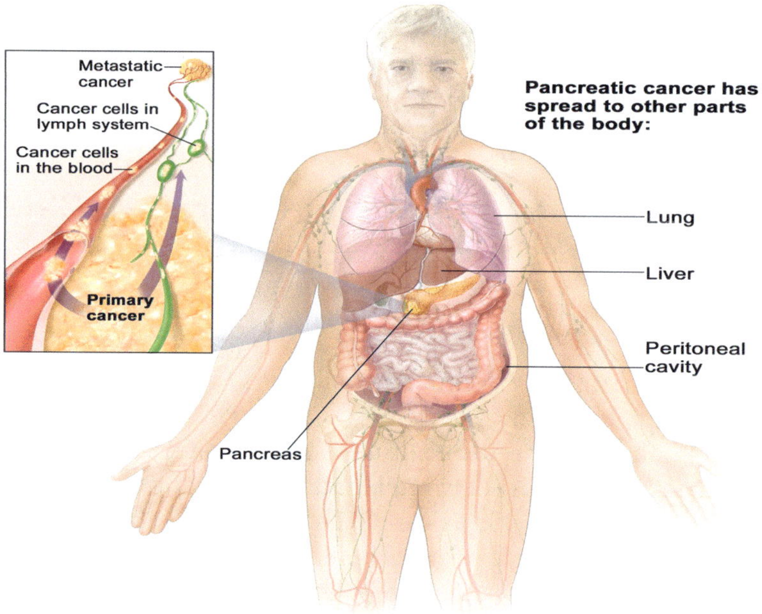

Figure 13.5. Pancreatic tumors on overall health.

Source: https://nci-media.cancer.gov/pdq/media/images/687943.jpg.

The tumors tend to express nonspecific symptoms, such that their diagnosis is delayed after they have already advanced. Hence, the late diagnosis is to blame for worse prognoses and fewer treatment options, which not only have the potential to impact survival rates but also the quality of life in the affected patients. Even tumors like acinar cell carcinomas disrupt the normal functioning of the pancreas, leading to malabsorption, nutritional deficiencies, and other systemic issues (Casey et al., 2015). Therefore, an extensive understanding of the importance of these tumors is important both to the healthcare practitioners and patients in the treatment process and general health. Involvement of the tumor microenvironment in pancreatic cancer yet again illustrates the complexity associated with these tumors. The microenvironment consists of heterogeneous cell types and signaling molecules and can influence tumor development, metastasis, and responsiveness to treatments. For instance, dysregulation of the primary signaling pathways RAS/MAP kinase and RAS/PI3K/AKT are pan-cancer in pancreatic cancer and are pivotal in the maintenance of cell proliferation and survival (Regad, 2015). The interaction of tumor cells with their environment can also lead to evasion of the immune system and resistance to treatment by targeting the tumor itself. An understanding of these interactions will be needed to offer newer treatment approaches that not only target the tumor but also reprogram the microenvironment to inhibit progression and maximize patient overall health gains. Additionally, systemic activity by pancreatic tumors extends beyond site-specific symptoms to impact global health through many mechanisms, such as systemic inflammation and dysregulated metabolic states. Patients usually experience extreme weight loss, weakness, and metabolic derangement secondary to the nutritional requirement and interference with normal pancreatic function of the tumor. These alterations can lead to cachexia, a syndrome of weight and muscle loss that seriously reduces a patient's quality of life and complicates treatment regimens. The psychological effect of dealing with a pancreatic tumor, especially unusual types with indeterminate prognostic factors, cannot be overstressed. As the patient begins their treatment journey, the physical as well as psychological implications of these tumors emphasize the need for a multidisciplinary care strategy that covers the various aspects of health impacted by pancreatic tumors (Casey et al., 2015) (Figure 13.5).

13.2. Lymphoma as a Pancreatic Tumor

As a rare but significant cause of pancreatic disease, lymphoma presents unique clinical challenges. As pancreatic adenocarcinoma dominates the forum on pancreatic neoplasms, lymphoma can present as a primary or secondary presentation and thus be difficult to diagnose. If lymphoma presents primarily in the pancreas, it can present with symptoms of more common pancreatic neoplasms such as pain, weight loss, and obstructive jaundice. The ability to differentiate lymphoma from adenocarcinoma is crucial but difficult since imaging techniques yield results that overlap and need sophisticated histological and immunohistochemical examinations to diagnose accurately. The multiplicity of lymphomas developed from different cell types such as B- or T-cells complicates this further, compelling physicians to make their diagnostic process more sophisticated and include lymphoma as a significant differential when evaluating pancreatic masses. Historically, the prognosis of patients with pancreatic lymphoma, and more so those who have primary pancreatic lymphoma (PPL), has been favorable relative to other forms of pancreatic neoplasms. So favorable is such an outcome, in large measure due to the efficacy of systemic chemotherapy, which is frequently tolerable and has shown to be highly responsive. Paradigms for treatment these days have been increasingly tailored, with use of molecular profiling to generate customized therapy regimens. These advancements are particularly important for the scenario of cancer of unknown primary (CUP), when the tissue of origin is elusive and has important implications for treatment planning (Ambrosini et al., 2021). The evolution of treatment strategies underscores the necessity of ongoing research as an understanding of the molecular profile of lymphoma can guide the development of new therapies that potentially lead to improved patient outcomes. Moreover, the overlap of the pancreas and lymphomas requires rethinking traditional assumptions regarding tumor classification and therapy. In response to emerging data, such as genetic data on BRCA2 mutations in regard to cancer mechanisms (Mathias et al., 2016), there is a greater requirement for interdisciplinarity in the management of pancreatic cancers. Oncologists, pathologists, and radiologists will be required to coordinate very closely to address questions of lymphoma presentations within the pancreas. Besides, exploration of the expression profile of non-coding RNAs in CUPs is suggesting that a targeted molecular therapy may one day become individualized treatment regimens for metastatic lymphoma patients with pancreatic involvement. With evolving therapeutic paradigms, an integrative and new approach will increasingly play a critical role in optimizing outcomes for this unique subset of pancreatic tumors (Figure 13.6).

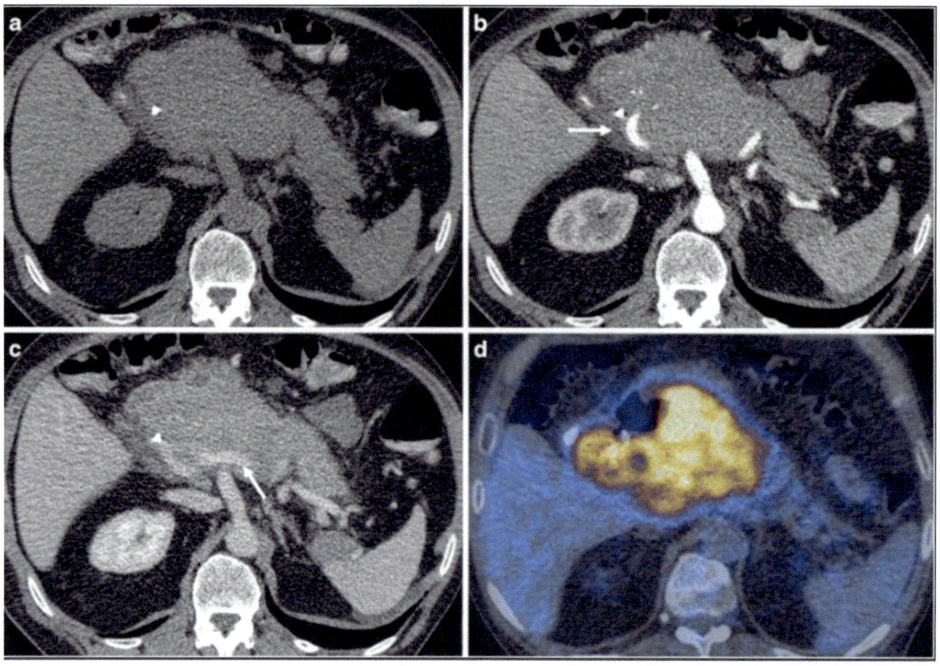

Figure 13.6. Computer tomography (CT) imaging of primary pancreatic lymphoma.

Source: https://media.springernature.com/lw1200/springer-static/image/art%3A10.1007%2Fs13244-017-0585-y/MediaObjects/13244_2017_585_Fig3_HTML.gif.

13.2.1. Definition and Types of Pancreatic Lymphoma

Pancreatic lymphoma is a rare form of malignancy that presents unique diagnostic as well as therapeutic dilemmas. In contrast to the more common primary pancreatic carcinomas, pancreatic lymphoma arises essentially from lymphoid tissue, with the pancreas either presenting as a primary tumor or presenting secondarily due to systemic lymphoproliferative disorders. The two most significant forms of pancreatic lymphoma are the diffuse large B-cell lymphoma (DLBCL) and the mantle cell lymphoma. These aggregations portend differential prognoses and responsiveness to therapy, thus complicating the management of patients with this disease. Due to its rarity, pancreatic lymphoma is likely to be missed or diagnosed late, its presenting signs being abdominal pain, weight loss, and jaundice, which are also similar to those of more frequent pancreatic diseases, thereby emphasizing the need for more awareness among health providers. The heterogeneity of pancreatic lymphoma complicates its treatment scenario further. Differently from solid neoplasms, lymphomas, including those of pancreatic origin, tend to appear as intra-tumor heterogeneity, which promotes tumor evolution as well as resistance to treatment. This characteristic is the primary therapeutic challenge, and an understanding of the underlying biological behavior of the lymphoma is of crucial value in designing an efficient therapy. Current advancements in the role of the tumor microenvironment have unraveled how it contributes to phenotypic heterogeneity seen in lymphomas and how it influences overall treatment and patient survival outcomes. These have further emphasized the importance of personalization of therapy, particularly the situation with pancreatic anatomical constraints brought about by risks of making adjacent tissues highly toxic (McGranahan & Swanton, 2017). In addition, differentiating primary pancreatic lymphoma from metastatic illness is important to manage the patient successfully. Distant metastases of aggressive lymphomas may cause CUP situations, where the tissue of origin cannot be identified, thus making the treatment course challenging (Ambrosini et al., 2021). Because of the infrequency of pancreatic lymphoma, it often may be a secondary site of systemic lymphoma, either by direct leukemic invasion or by generalized illness. Accurate diagnosis and recognition of pancreatic lymphoma are paramount to therapeutic management; therefore, new diagnostic techniques, including sophisticated imaging and molecular phenotyping, need to address the complexities of this illness. This investigation of these techniques can enhance knowledge regarding pancreatic lymphomas and lead to improved therapeutic outcomes.

13.2.2. Symptoms and Diagnostic Challenges

Expression of symptoms in metastatic and rare tumors of the pancreas is a serious diagnostic problem, primarily due to the anatomical and functional nuances of the organ. Indistinct and non-specific symptoms such as abdominal pain, weight loss, and jaundice are frequent in patients and easily can be attributed to a variety of gastrointestinal illnesses. This sharing of symptoms makes it harder for early detection and diagnosis, and hence treatment is delayed and may be poorer. Furthermore, the heterogeneity of such tumors, as noted in intratumor variation studies, introduces additional complication in establishing a final diagnosis since different components of the tumor may present with different features and inclinations (McGranahan & Swanton, 2017). The resulting diagnostic uncertainty often demands advanced imaging modalities and histopathologic examinations to adequately differentiate between intimately coexisting pathological conditions. Furthermore, the diagnostic process is also complicated by the fact that standard imaging modalities cannot possibly unveil the intricate nature of these tumors. As a result, clinicians are increasingly turning to techniques such as PET/CT to enhance the sensitivity and specificity of tumor detection in cases of rare pancreatic lesions. PET/CT is not yet widely available, however, and interpretation does require some expertise that may simply not be available in all clinical settings. This discrepancy may lead to variation in diagnosis and treatment algorithms between institutions. Further, the dynamic interaction between the immune system and the tumor microenvironment can impair the efficacy of imaging, threatening misinterpretation of tumor response to therapy. Integration of present advanced imaging technology with pathologic examinations still remains key to overcoming these challenges. Finally, treatment of metastatic and rare pancreatic tumors is often hindered by the lack of proven treatment regimens not considering the unique biology of the cancers. For instance, standard chemotherapy protocols may be unable to address the typical molecular characteristics and adaptive phenotypes exhibited by different types of tumors, including lymphoma and renal cell carcinoma metastasis. Strategies for the best approach to overcoming tumor heterogeneity, such as introducing precision medicine approaches, are still in their embryonic stages (McGranahan & Swanton, 2017). With more research needed to better understand the complexity of pancreatic tumors, treatment protocols must be tailored for each patient to improve prognosis. Emphasizing the importance of an interdisciplinary approach involving skilled diagnostic methods and personalized therapies can successfully advance the treatment of these intractable cancers (Figure 13.7).

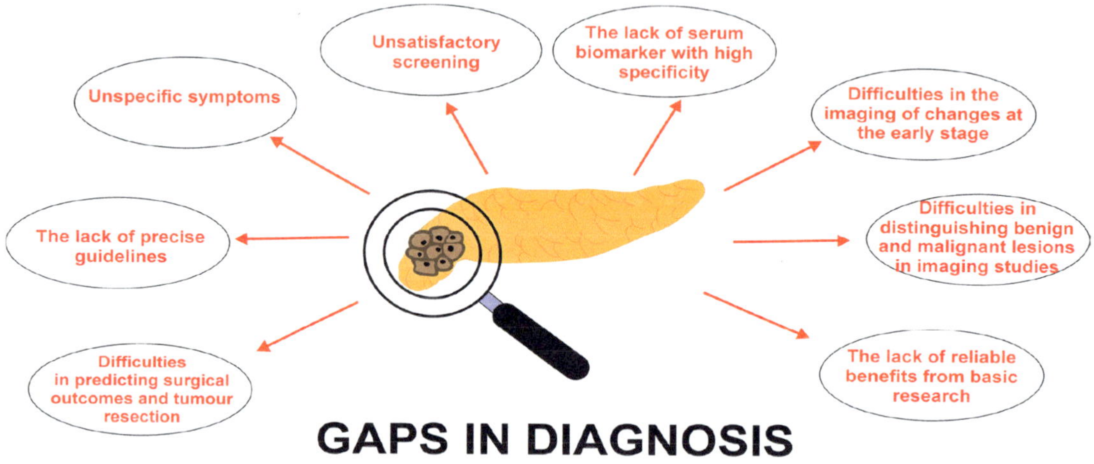

Figure 13.7. Gaps and opportunities in the diagnosis and treatment of pancreatic cancer.

Source: Caban M, Małecka-Wojciesko E. Gaps and Opportunities in the Diagnosis and Treatment of Pancreatic Cancer. *Cancers*. 2023; 15(23):5577. https://doi.org/10.3390/cancers15235577

13.2.3. Treatment Options and Prognosis

The treatment situation for pancreatic metastatic and rare tumors is complex and often challenging due to the inherent biological characteristics of these tumors, particularly PDAC. The response to conventional treatments, such as chemotherapy, is poor also in locally advanced or metastatic disease. This lack of efficacy can be attributed to the peculiar tumor microenvironment, which tends to complicate drug penetration and activity. Current evidence highlights that being aware of the tumor microenvironment may be pivotal to the development of novel, more potent regimens. For instance, a study of immune-related factors and inflammatory infiltrates suggests that patients with a positive immune context show a better response to immunotherapy, which suggests that this may be a promising first-line therapeutic modality combined with chemotherapy in the treatment of advanced pancreatic cancer. Aside from PDAC, the treatment and outcome for other uncommon pancreatic tumors, such as pancreatic lymphoma and metastasis of renal cell carcinoma, are rather different. For pancreatic lymphoma, less common but separate, the general rule of treatment is more chemotherapy and less resection surgery, particularly for advanced cases. The high response rate to specific chemotherapy regimens can greatly improve patient outcome. Conversely, metastatic renal cell carcinoma to the pancreas may call for a different approach, including the targeted therapies that are now valuable tools in the oncologic arsenal. Success with such treatments is often contingent on the molecular characterization of the metastatic tumors, and thus personalized medicine becomes essential to determining the best course for patients suffering from such rare cancers (Pfister et al., 2021). Moreover, acinar cell tumors and stroma-rich pancreas tumors have individual specific factors for treatment and prognosis. Acinar cell carcinoma, say, may have certain characteristics that make different treatment models essential where surgery may prove to be a valuable intervention in early disease due to the possibility of cure. Stroma-rich tumors, by contrast, are likely to complicate the treatment owing to their very fibrous composition, which is likely to hamper drug delivery. This raises the issue of ongoing research and clinical trials for the development of novel therapeutic drugs capable of targeting the stroma of a tumor effectively. Understanding the dynamics of these various types of tumors will be crucial to improving the overall patient prognosis and developing personalized treatment regimens that enhance the quality of life for such patients undergoing treatment for such chilling diagnoses.

13.3. Renal Cell Carcinoma (RCC) Metastasis to the Pancreas

The metastasis process of RCC to the pancreas, though uncommon, influences patient prognosis and treatment. Because RCC primarily arises in the kidney, it commonly metastasizes to the lungs, liver, and bones, with pancreatic metastasis occurring less frequently.

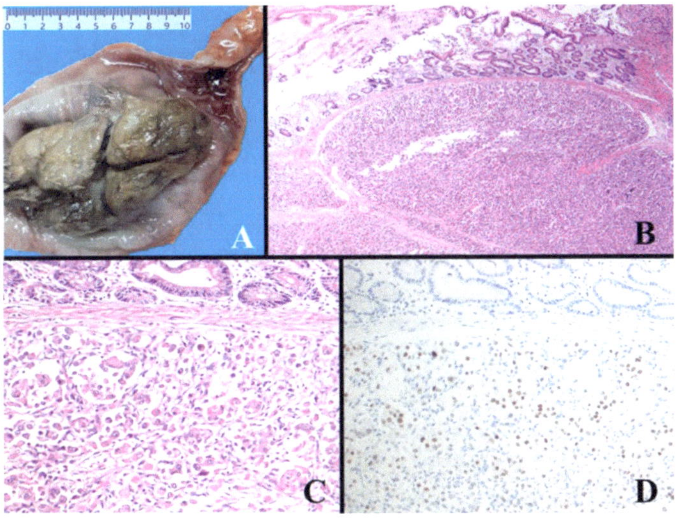

Figure 13.8. Metastatic renal cell carcinoma to pancreas and gastrointestinal tract.

Source: https://media.springernature.com/lw685/springer-static/image/art%3A10.1186%2Fs12894-021-00854-z/MediaObjects/12894_2021_854_Fig1_HTML.jpg.

This atypical metastatic pathway can complicate diagnosis because pancreatic lesions can commonly be mimicked by primary neoplasm of the pancreas, such as pancreatic ductal adenocarcinoma. Understanding the metastatic pattern and route of RCC is significant since pancreatic involvement may predominantly alter treatment prospects and overall prognosis. Radiological imaging with modalities like computed tomography (CT) and magnetic resonance imaging (MRI) plays a vital role in distinguishing primary from metastatic disease, thus dictating treatment prospects based on individual patient scenarios. The presentation of pancreatic metastases in RCC is most often nonspecific, typically presented with weight loss or abdominal pain, thereby necessitating a high index of suspicion among clinicians. Interestingly, prognosis in patients with pancreatic metastasis from RCC is most often poor, owing to the adverse prognostic factors of renal and pancreatic cancers. The presence of metastasis indicates advanced cancer, worsening the overall survival rate. Treatment approaches today also often include systemic therapy as targeted agents and immunotherapy, which has been shown to be efficacious for the management of RCC. However, pancreatic metastases treatment also considers local treatments such as resection in select situations, depending on the extent of the disease and the performance status of the patients (Sohal et al., 2021). Investigation also uncovers the mechanisms behind the metastatic capability of RCC to the pancreas and further deepens our insight into tumor biology. Molecular changes research and tumor microenvironment research may hopefully uncover therapeutic targets, leading to novel approaches to treating this disease. In addition, the genomics of RCC suggest that specific mutations would predispose the tumors to secondary spread to unusual sites, including the pancreas. This evolving understanding highlights the importance of a multi-specialty approach including oncologists, radiologists, and pathologists in patient management with presumptive pancreatic metastases of RCC. Additionally, the ongoing progress in personalized medicine by way of molecular analysis can further enhance management plans, improving patient outcomes over these aggressive malignancies (Figure 13.8).

13.3.1. Mechanisms of Metastasis from Renal Cell Carcinoma (RCC)

RCC is also characterized by a unique ability to metastasize, which includes a complex range of mechanisms facilitating tumor spread from the point of origin to the distant organs. It begins with local invasion of the adjacent tissues, during which renal cancer cells reorganize the tumor microenvironment and exploit multiple pathways to escape from the primary tumor. These processes have a tendency to activate the epithelial-to-mesenchymal transition (EMT) where the cancer cells lose their epithelial characteristics and gain migratory properties, hence enhancing their invasive potential. Additionally, the function of angiogenesis is crucial; RCC causes new blood vessel development by upregulation of vascular endothelial growth factor (VEGF), which not only sustains the growth of tumors but also offers a channel for cancer cells to access the bloodstream and spread to other organs. RCC metastatic dissemination is not only controlled by intrinsic cellular mechanisms but also by interaction with the hosts immune response. Tumors will often employ mechanisms to evade immune surveillance; RCC, for instance, can secrete programmed death-ligand 1 (PD-L1), allowing it to inhibit T-cell activation and establish an immunosuppressive environment. In addition, RCC can hijack the local immune microenvironment, recruiting regulatory T cells and myeloid-derived suppressor cells that further repress anti-tumor immunity. Immune evasion significantly enhances the likelihood of metastasis, enabling renal cancer cells to survive and proliferate in remote organs, like the pancreas. An understanding of these immune interactions offers promising therapeutic strategies, especially with immune checkpoint inhibitors that may foil the tumors immunosuppressive tactics. It has been emphasized in recent studies that major pathways such as the mammalian target of rapamycin (mTOR) pathway play a key role in RCC development and metastasis. The mTOR pathway is core to the growth and metabolism of cells, and its dysfunction is prevalent in RCC. mTOR signaling not only promotes cell growth but also metastasis by various means, including EMT and control of the tumor environment. Direct mTOR inhibition has not been successful in the clinic, but more recent evidence suggests that combination therapies would be effective by bypassing resistance mechanisms. This is in line with growing realization that a more sophisticated treatment approach, drawing on understanding from such as pathways as mTOR and immune modulation, will yield better clinical outcomes in metastatic RCC patients and serve to improve protocols of management of associated conditions, including metastasis to the pancreas (Munoz et al., 2014; Conciatori et al., 2018) (Figure 13.9).

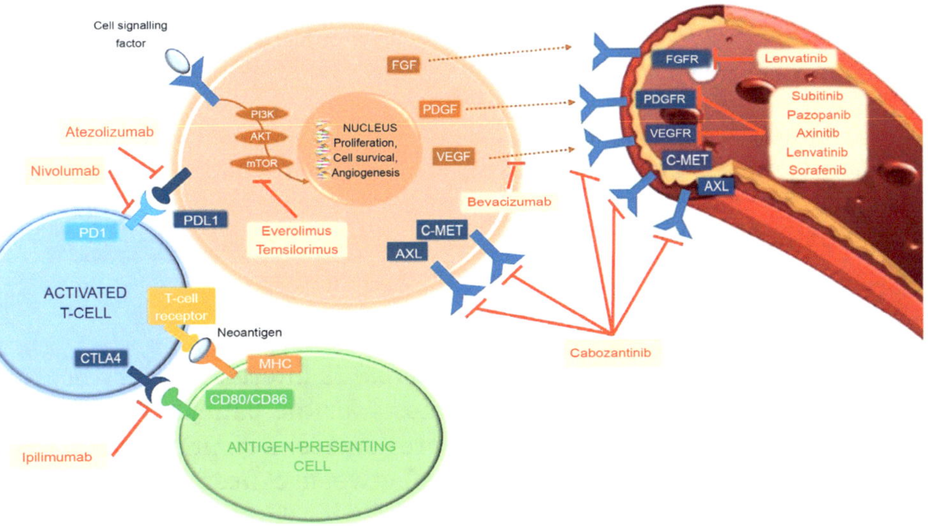

Figure 13.9. Mechanisms of metastasis from renal cell carcinoma.

Source: Roberto M, Botticelli A, Panebianco M, Aschelter AM, Gelibter A, Ciccarese C, Minelli M, Nuti M, Santini D, Laghi A, Tomao S and Marchetti P (2021) Metastatic Renal Cell Carcinoma Management: From Molecular Mechanism to Clinical Practice. Front. Oncol. 11:657639. doi: 10.3389/fonc.2021.657639

13.3.2. Clinical Presentation and Diagnostic Imaging

The presentation of pancreatic metastatic and rare tumors is often nonspecific and can contribute to the diagnostic complexity. The patients typically present with abdominal pain, weight loss, jaundice, and change in bowel habit, which can be common with more common pancreatic disorders, such as pancreatitis or pancreatic adenocarcinoma. In metastasis of lymphoma and renal cell carcinoma, there are systemic symptoms, including fever and night sweats. The variability in symptoms mandates careful clinical assessment to separate the potential pathologies. A thorough history and physical examination are key, as they guide the use of imaging tests and laboratory tests to establish the underlying cause. Given the higher incidence of atypical tumors, clinicians must have a high suspicion for the diseases when unusual pancreatic presentation is encountered. Diagnostic imaging is the key to making a diagnosis of pancreatic tumors and assessing the degree of spread. CT is usually the first imaging technique employed due to its ready availability and ability to define pancreatic anatomy and pathology. In particular, CT will identify mass lesions, lymphadenopathy, and other signs of metastatic disease, e.g., renal cell carcinoma metastasis. Furthermore, MRI and positron emission tomography (PET) scans are more commonly utilized for their ability to provide extensive information on the biology of tumors. These modalities offer improved contrast of the soft tissues and functional imaging, respectively, and as such, are of great utility in evaluating pancreatic lymphoma and stromal tumors. Accurate staging and optimal therapeutic planning rest on good utilization of these imaging modalities that, in turn, guide patient management results. Technological evolution in imaging technology has remained on the rise and has enhanced diagnostic accuracy for pancreatic tumors, and image interpretation has become more sophisticated. Integration of traditional methods of imaging with innovative technologies such as functional MRI and PET/CT allows a better understanding of the tumor microenvironment. For instance, the PET/CT ability to differentiate between benign and malignant lesions has been highlighted since it is possible to detect malignancy-associated metabolic activity. Moreover, advanced radiological examinations can help in the detection of network webs of lymphatic spread characteristic of lymphoma, with significant prognostic consequences. The incorporation of novel imaging techniques, as mentioned in studies on disease of the abdomen and pelvis, emphasizes the need for radiologists and clinicians to remain abreast of novel developments in the specialty to deliver optimal treatment to the patient.

13.3.3. Management Strategies and Outcomes

Treatment of metastatic and rare tumors of the pancreas is interdisciplinary because the diseases present a special challenge in treatment and prognosis for the patient. Tumor microenvironment complexity is crucial in tumor behavior and drug resistance. Definition and clarity of the tumor microenvironment (TME), that is, an interaction between cancer, stromal, and inflammatory cells, is critical to construct viable management modalities. Through identifying the mechanisms by which the TME supports tumorigenesis, therapy can be more effectively modulated so that not just the tumor cells, but also the supportive cellular components of the TME, are targeted. Introduction into therapeutic modalities those able to break these interactions could improve treatment effectiveness, hence patient prognosis. Thus, therapeutic approaches must encompass direct cytotoxicity in addition to indirect action on the tumor-promoting microenvironment in an attempt to attain maximum therapeutic gains in patients with pancreatic tumors like lymphoma and renal cell carcinoma metastasis (Kumar, 2023). Recent breakthroughs on targeted therapy and the development of somatostatin analogs are promising areas in the treatment of pancreatic tumors. Somatostatin (SST) plays a crucial role in inhibiting tumor growth through receptor-mediated pathways with direct antiproliferative effects and indirect control of tumor microenvironmental growth factors. The presence of five different somatostatin receptor subtypes (SSTR1-5) allows for target-specific modulation of tumor characteristics. Following the identification of new SST analogs and receptor-specific agonists, their implications in changing the course of treatment strategy in rare pancreatic tumors keep unfolding. In individuals suffering from some tumors, these agents can reliably impede tumor growth and improve survival rates. Accordingly, addition of SST-based therapies to the field of individualized management regimens has potential to enhance outcomes in rare pancreatic neoplasms (Kumar, 2023). Along with this, exploration of biologic markers within the tumor itself offers a window for maximizing management regimens in metastatic pancreatic tumors. One of these markers is tumor necrosis factor receptor-associated factor 6 (TRAF6), which participates in some of the most critical processes that control tumor growth and metastasis. Through inhibiting TRAF6 and the associated signaling pathways, a stronger therapeutic approach can be designed, able to halt or even reverse tumor progression. The discovery of markers enabling targeted treatments can also make the intervention possible at an earlier stage and direct treatment decisions specific to the patient's disease state. This management plan that is based on research emphasizes the importance of ongoing research into the tumor biology since it can eventually link the recent scientific discoveries into clinical practice and thus improve outcomes for metastatic and rare pancreatic tumors (Li et al., 2023) (Figure 13.10).

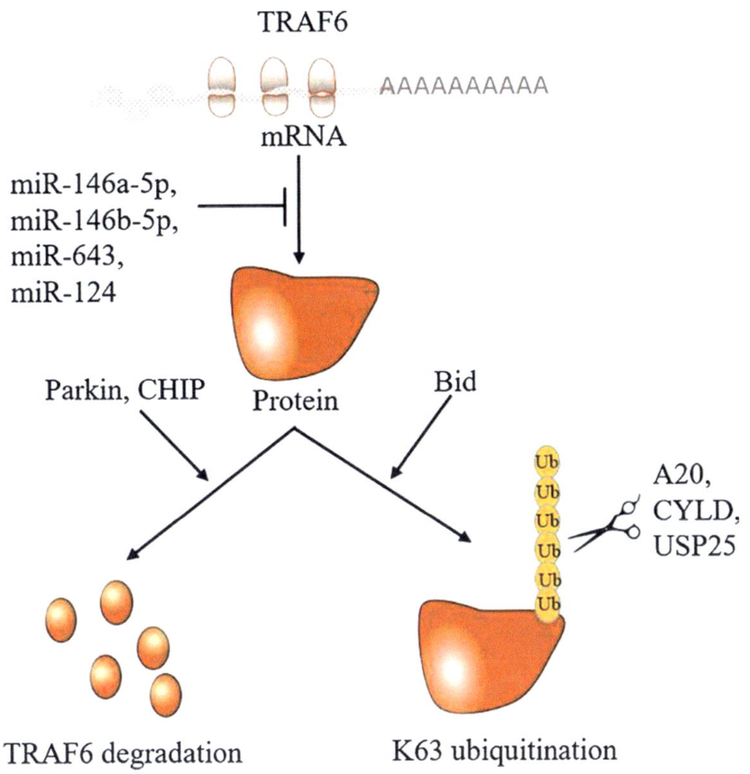

Figure 13.10. The relationship between tumor necrosis factor receptor-associated factor 6 (TRAF6) and tumors.

Source: https://media.springernature.com/lw685/springer-static/image/art%3A10.1186%2Fs12935-020-01517-z/MediaObjects/12935_2020_1517_Fig4_HTML.png.

13.4. Stromal Tumors of the Pancreas

Pancreatic stromal tumors, both PNETs and pancreatic fibromas, represent an interesting category of pancreatic neoplasms. Unlike more frequent pancreatic adenocarcinoma, the tumors originate from the pancreas's stroma and neuroendocrine cells and present with distinct biological behaviors and clinical features. PNETs may be functioning and, through hormone secretion, lead to syndromes such as insulinoma or gastrinoma, influencing both diagnosis and treatment. Conversely, pancreatic fibromas most often present as silent masses, and it is challenging to diagnose at an early age. Stromal tumors constitute a small subgroup of neoplasms of the pancreas and present an ordeal to clinicians to stay vigilant and well-informed about what they are and their implications for therapeutic maneuvers, such as surgery and therapeutics that can differ dramatically from those applied in exocrine tumors. Pathophysiological features of stromal tumors define their uniqueness from more common pancreatic cancers that have a tendency to trigger multiple signal pathways, for example, the RAS/MAP kinase and RAS/PI3K/AKT pathways. Receptor Tyrosine Kinases (RTKs) and the associated signal cascades are implicated in the proliferation and survival of most tumors, including pancreatic adenocarcinoma. In stromal tumors, the underlying defects and genetic alterations may be other, as studies have identified different genetic patterns in pancreatic neuroendocrine tumors compared to adenocarcinomas. Hence, targeted therapy to inhibit deranged RTK signaling might not be universally translatable, and interventions will have to be specifically identified depending on the unique characteristics of tumor biology in stroma and its response to therapeutic intervention, as outlined in more recent literature (Regad, 2015). Treatment of pancreatic stromal tumors is an area of high priority in ongoing investigation and clinical research. Surgical resection remains the standard therapy for locally confined tumors, as it holds the highest hope of long-term survival. For cases in which surgery cannot be performed, however, other therapeutic approaches come into play. The role of conventional anticancer drugs, including chemotherapy and radiotherapy, is limited; however, recent research reveals that immunotherapeutic regimens hold good options, especially when taking into consideration immune responses being generated by cytotoxic therapies (Coffelt & de Visser, 2015). Elucidation of the interactions between tumor microenvironment and host immune system is of prime importance in the development of successful regimens. With advancement in research, deeper insights into the immunological basis of pancreatic stromal tumors can be made, and novel treatment modalities addressing both tumor biology and immune landscape are needed to enhance clinical outcomes and provide better therapeutic alternatives for impacted patients (Figure 13.11).

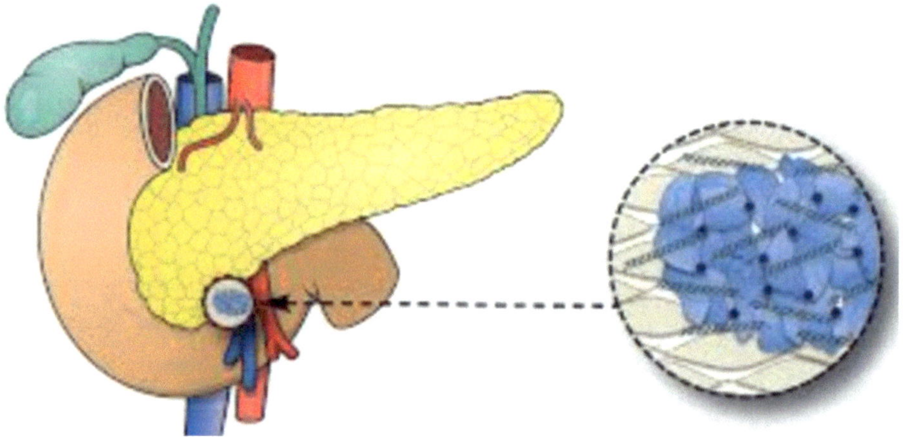

Figure 13.11. Pancreatic stroma.

Source: https://encrypted-tbn0.gstatic.com/images?q=tbn:ANd9GcT9JmwTNqWFw7gvlJtP9IfvhsWRMiPAU4CGQw&s.

13.4.1. Types of Pancreatic Stromal Tumors

Pancreatic stromal tumors are rare neoplasms that consist of the pancreas's connective tissue and represent a collection of heterogeneous tumor entities with uniform histological and biological characteristics. The two primary categories are PNETs, which are characterized by their origin from the neuroendocrine cells, and pancreatic acinar cell tumors (PACTs), which originate from acinar cells secreting the enzymes. Specifically, the PNETs are either functioning or non-functioning tumors based on the endocrine activity, and this plays an important role in patient presentation and treatment. The tumors might also be of variable aggressiveness, with certain PNETs being associated with syndromes like Multiple Endocrine Neoplasia (MEN), with a multifaceted interplay between genetic predisposition and clinical presentation. Therefore, understanding the different types of pancreatic stromal tumors is crucial for effective management methods and prognosis. One of the pancreatic stromal tumors is acinar cell carcinoma (ACC), which is distinguished by its unique pathology and clinical relevance. The tumor, though less common, is known to be extremely aggressive and has a poor prognosis, with presentation normally at advanced levels. ACCs typically have a firm architecture of the tumor with typical acinar differentiation, pathologically confirmed by the demonstration of zymogen granules and enzyme secretion such as lipase. Because these tumors are exceedingly common in young patients compared to more common pancreatic ductal adenocarcinomas, they pose some diagnostic and management challenges. Immunohistochemical analysis and new molecular techniques are important to detect ACC accurately and differentiate it from other pancreatic tumors. Mechanistic studies, including the contribution of the tumor microenvironment, may provide insight into the targeted treatment of patients with this recalcitrant malignancy (McGranahan & Swanton, 2017). Furthermore, there is a crosstalk between pancreatic stromal tumors and the tumor microenvironment that significantly influences tumor behavior and treatment responsiveness. The importance of such factors as the endothelin axis in pancreatic cancer has become highlighted, and it suggests a sophisticated relationship between the stromal components and tumor cells. Endothelins and their receptors are important in the development of tumors by controlling processes such as angiogenesis, fibrosis, and inflammation. Therapeutic approaches against the endothelin axis in such situations could offer new targets for intervention, especially in more aggressive pancreatic stromal tumors. Evidence indicates that modulating such interactions may be a potentially valuable strategy towards enhancing the efficacy of conventional chemotherapeutic agents by altering the fibro-inflammatory tumor microenvironment (Gupta, 2017). Understanding such dynamics is essential in devising integrated treatment approaches towards the improvement of patients suffering from pancreatic stromal tumors.

13.4.2. Pathophysiology and Risk Factors

The intricate pathobiology that accompanies metastatic and rare pancreatic tumors, e.g., renal cell carcinoma metastasis and lymphoma, is underscored by a number of molecular mechanisms and crosstalks of the tumor microenvironment. A determinant factor that controls the aggressiveness of pancreatic cancers is the stimulation of some growth factor signaling pathways, including the endothelin axis. There is evidence to suggest that endothelins, particularly ET-1, play a role in disease progression via stimulation of proliferation and angiogenesis and crosstalk between tumor and stroma. It has been demonstrated through research that expression of ET receptors, like ETAR and ETBR, on stromal and cancer cells is accountable for a tumorigenic environment that could ultimately find expression in an unfavorable prognosis for the patient as evidenced by the correlation between ETBR positivity and poor clinical outcome in pancreatic cancer patients (Gupta et al., 2017). Chemokines and their receptors are also pivotal to the pathophysiology of pancreatic cancers. For instance, the chemokine receptor CXCR4 is known to play a role in tumor cell invasion, migration, and survival, particularly metastatic dissemination. High expression of CXCR4 in metastatic pancreatic cell lines supports that it mediates chemotaxis toward its ligand, CXCL12, and thereby enhances processes such as transendothelial migration and remodeling of the tumor microenvironment. Furthermore, the activity of CXCR4 has also been identified as activating matrix metalloproteinases, which degrade the extracellular matrix and allow the spreading of tumors (Marchesi et al., 2006). These findings highlight the involvement of chemokine signaling in the aggressiveness of pancreatic cancer and suggest that therapy of the pathway could have therapeutic potential. The pathophysiologic landscape of pancreatic neoplasms is also complicated by a number of risk factors, including genetic predispositions, environmental exposures, and previous comorbidities. Predominantly, familial syndromes like Familial Pancreatic Cancer and conditions like diabetes mellitus predispose the individual to develop pancreatic cancers. Chronic inflammation such as that in pancreatitis is also a central mechanism of carcinogenesis through eliciting widespread fibrosis and the release of pro-inflammatory cytokines capable of changing cellular phenotype. Moreover, lifestyle problems such as smoking and obesity have also been implicated in elevated pancreatic cancer risk, pointing towards the etiology of its multifactorial origin. Awareness of these risk factors alongside their pathophysiologic consequences will be crucial in developing targeted prevention and intervention strategies in the management of metastatic and rare pancreatic tumors (Figure 13.12).

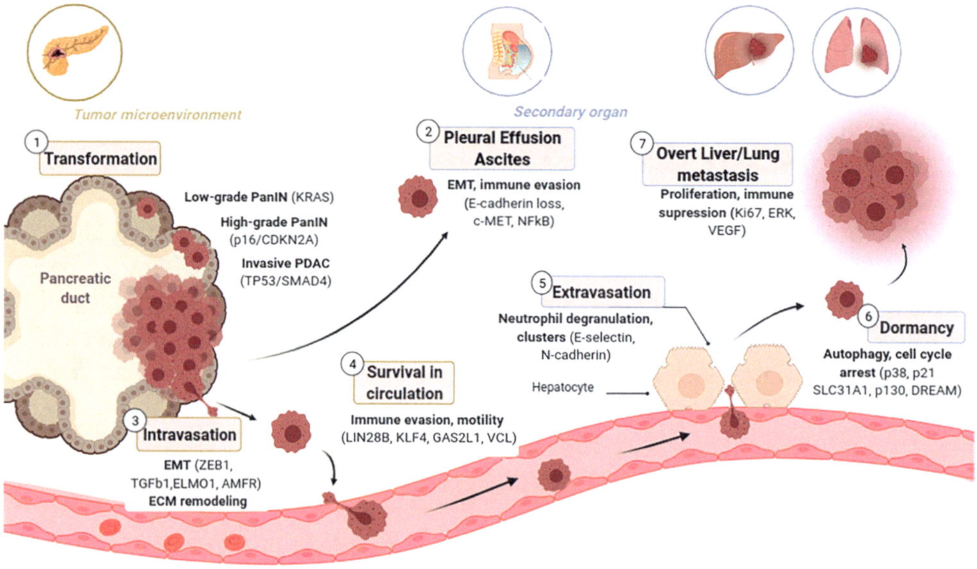

Figure 13.12. Pre-clinical models of metastasis in pancreatic cancer.

Source: Miquel M, Zhang S and Pilarsky C (2021) Pre-clinical Models of Metastasis in Pancreatic Cancer. Front. Cell Dev. Biol. 9:748631. doi: 10.3389/fcell.2021.748631

13.4.3. Treatment Modalities and Survival Rates

The treatment modalities for metastatic pancreatic cancers are extremely variable and based on the nature of the tumor as well as the extent of the tumor's growth. Chemotherapy is the treatment of choice for pancreatic lymphomas, with the administration of regimens such as CHOP (cyclophosphamide, doxorubicin, vincristine, and prednisone). This has been shown to prolong survival markedly in patients whose lymphoma is localized or is treatable. By contrast, metastatic renal cell carcinoma typically requires an interdisciplinary strategy involving targeted therapies and immunotherapy, which have become associated with prolongation of survival in advanced disease. The therapeutic modality divergence reflects the importance of tumor characterization because survival outcomes are not only based on the specific therapeutic maneuvers themselves but also on their timely delivery within clinical decision-making contexts. In addition to chemotherapy and immunotherapy, new modalities are assuming importance in the management of rare pancreatic neoplasms like stromal and acinar cell tumors. Surgical management remains a mainstay for local neoplasms; however, the infrequency of such presentations typically makes the treatment modality difficult. Such new modalities like radiotherapy and regional therapy are being explored as adjuvant treatments, with encouraging results. For instance, stereotactic body radiotherapy (SBRT) holds potential in the control of localized disease and overall survival. The integration of imaging modalities such as PET/CT facilitates enhanced tumor mapping, aiding in treatment response assessment and allowing for personalized medical approaches. Such emerging imaging is central to the optimization of outcomes in both rare and metastatic pancreatic cancer. Survival rates using these treatment approaches can be very varied based on numerous factors, including the patients' overall health, presentation stage, and the specific type of tumor. It has been discovered that early presentation followed by effective treatment regimens can significantly enhance the survival probabilities of pancreatic tumor patients. Current research highlights that for some intrapancreatic lymphomas, there can be a 50% complete response to chemotherapy, leading to survivorship benefits. Further, outcomes from treatment can be generally enhanced using multidisciplinary management teams where the experts combine efforts to develop custom-made treatment plans for each patient. These materials like those indicated in literature are highly resourceful when establishing the complexities of abdominal imaging and treatment techniques, all adding up to more advanced methodologies intended to enhance survival rates among patients with metastatic and uncommon pancreatic tumors.

13.5. Acinar Cell Carcinoma (ACC)

ACC, though rare, is an appreciable subset of pancreatic neoplasms, characterized by its distinctive histologic appearance and natural history. Unlike other more common pancreatic ductal adenocarcinoma, ACC occurs from acinar cells of the pancreas, the cellular element responsible for the production of enzymes. ACC is usually diagnosed late since its symptoms are vague and mimic other gastrointestinal pathologies. Thus, the patients come to the clinic with advanced disease most of the time, with disseminative metastasis to peritoneum and liver. The clinicopathological heterogeneity of ACC also makes treatment planning an intricate process, requiring multidimensional understanding of its unique biology compared to other neoplasms of the pancreas. Thus, optimal treatment remains an ongoing subject of research and inquiry in the dynamic landscape of oncology. Treatment of acinar cell carcinoma is extremely problematic due to the lack of chemotherapy protocols specifically approved for this subtype. Retro regimens with agents such as gemcitabine and 5-fluorouracil have been partially effective, and this again demonstrates the requirement of personalized treatments. New case reports have proposed emerging combinations, such as liposomal irinotecan plus S-1, with promising results in individual cases. This foresees a likely shift towards personalized therapy in the treatment of ACC, with various clinical trials ongoing to further refine the treatment protocols and improve the patient outcomes. Further, molecular targeting medications may also provide directions for enhancing the therapeutic index in this rare form of tumor. Thus, future researches and clinical trials are needed to further standardize and optimize treatment in patients suffering from acinar cell carcinoma. Survival rates for patients with advanced acinar cell carcinoma remain suboptimal, particularly with metastatic disease. Unlike those who come in with other forms of pancreatic cancer, ACC patients' outcomes can be unpredictable, with some research showing a relatively higher survival rate than that of patients with pancreatic ductal adenocarcinoma. Studies have revealed that pancreatic metastasis due to renal cell carcinoma can be associated with improved overall survival, suggesting the potential influence of tumor biology on outcomes (Crosby et al., 2025). Moreover, the rarity of ACC necessitates cross-institutional studies to generate large databases, which can lead to a better grasp of disease course. The development of better treatment modalities and the investigation of combination therapies can potentially improve the prognosis for patients with this uncommon pancreatic cancer, eventually propagating the survival rates through concerted efforts (Figure 13.13).

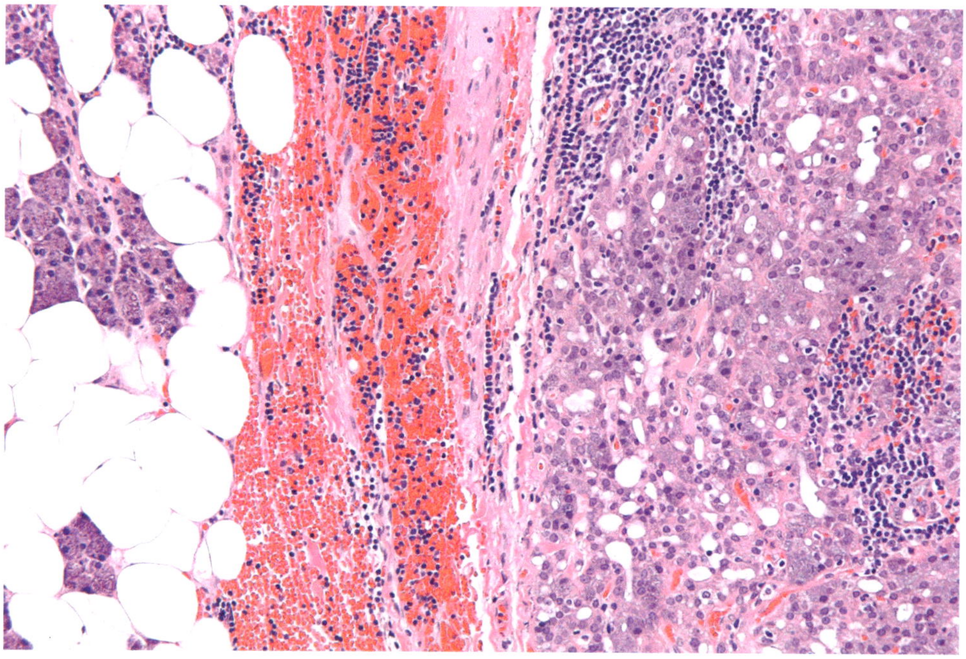

Figure 13.13. Acinic cell carcinoma.

Source: https://upload.wikimedia.org/wikipedia/commons/6/6b/Acinic_cell_carcinoma_-_high_mag.jpg.

13.5.1. Characteristics and Incidence of Acinar Cell Carcinoma (ACC)

ACC is a rare form of pancreatic tumor characterized by differentiating acinar cells, which are responsible for secreting digestive enzymes. The tumor occurs in approximately 1%–2% of all exocrine pancreatic malignancies. It is particularly rare compared to the more common pancreatic cancers, such as pancreatic ductal adenocarcinoma, which accounts for most of all cases. ACC tends to happen in older people, predominantly in people aged in their 60s and 70s, and is a particular diagnostic challenge as the often nonspecific and vague symptoms can mimic more typical conditions. Furthermore, the relatively low incidence of ACC complicates the development of effective treatment modalities and thus is a focus area of active research in oncology as evidenced by ongoing epidemiological studies targeting the demographics and characteristics of pancreatic tumors (AIRTUM Working Group, 2016). The clinical presentation of ACC is a tendency towards a better prognosis compared to other forms of pancreatic cancer, but rarity and unpredictability of behavior may make it challenging to treat. Symptoms could be abdominal pain, weight loss, and obstructive jaundice signs, possibly appearing late in the disease process. Histologically, ACC is marked by the presence of zymogen granules, and the tumor cells have a tendency to display acinar morphology. It may be associated with genetic syndromes such as familial pancreatitis or hereditary breast and ovarian cancer syndrome, and thus genetic counseling would be crucial in these families. Treatment modalities for ACC remain limited and largely surgical resection, with radiation therapy and chemotherapy providing variable efficacy in this malignancy. It is crucial to define the unique features and genetic factors that make up ACC in order to tailor treatment strategies (Haaland et al., 2017). The incidence of acinar cell carcinoma, while much lower than for other cancers of the pancreas, has serious public health and cancer treatment consequences globally. The annual incidence is fewer than one per 100,000 individuals, thus, by official definition, a rare cancer, founded on data gathered from a wide range of population-based cancer registries. Research has shown that the incidence of ACC has been found to vary geographically, with some areas reporting higher incidences, a trend possibly determined by variations in environmental risk factors, dietary patterns, and genetic susceptibility. In addition to this, survival rates analysis shows that while some patients achieve long-term survival post-diagnosis, a significant proportion of them still have poor prognoses, necessitating the need for greater awareness and clinic study of not only the clinical presentation of the cancers but also of the optimal management pathways (AIRTUM Working Group, 2016).

13.5.2. Diagnostic Criteria and Staging

The radiologic features of metastatic and rare tumors of the pancreas are mostly founded on a broad understanding of imaging modalities and clinical presentation. When assessing pancreatic lymphoma, for instance, imaging modalities such as CT and PET are highly beneficial in delineating the extent of disease spread. CT scanning is crucial in the assessment of pancreatic lesions and associated lymphadenopathy, while PET scans offer greater visualization of metabolically active areas. These diagnostic tools guide clinicians regarding confirmation of the diagnosis and treatment planning strategies, supporting the criticality of precise imaging protocols to stage the tumor accurately, particularly in the case of aggressive lymphoma. Such imaging technology has added tremendous value to a reflective strategy in diagnosing and managing pancreatic malignancies, ultimately with a view to optimizing patient outcomes in such complex situations. Understanding the staging of pancreatic cancers, including renal cell carcinoma metastasis and stromal cancers, is essential in the individualization of treatment approaches. The American Joint Committee on Cancer (AJCC) provides classification schemes that categorize tumors based on the tumor-node-metastasis (TNM) staging system. This approach enables practitioners to assess tumor size, lymphatic invasion, and metastasis presence, hence informing decision-making about treatments. Accurate staging not only yields information for prognosis but also guides therapeutic interventions, and these importantly differ across the various tumor types encountered in pancreatic oncology. Moreover, advancements in imaging technology have led to additional staging precision, allowing for additional distinction between localized and metastatic disease, something important in making decisions regarding treatment (AIRTUM Working Group, 2016). Besides imaging studies, histopathological examination is pivotal in making the diagnosis and staging of rare pancreatic tumors. Tissue sampling by endoscopic ultrasound-guided fine-needle aspiration (EUS-FNA) or surgery biopsy provides information about the cellular origin of the tumors, and differentiating between various types of tumors such as acinar cell carcinoma and pancreatic neuroendocrine tumors. This is important because histological subtypes will respond differently to treatment modalities. Integration of histopathology with imaging and clinical data allows for an integrated staging approach. Coordination between radiologists, pathologists, and oncologists is thus necessary to ensure accurate diagnosis and appropriate care of patients with pancreatic metastatic and rare tumors (Figure 13.14).

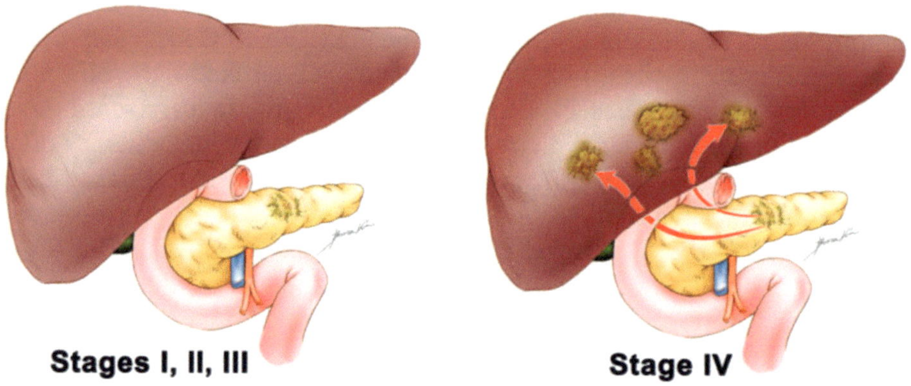

Figure 13.14. Stage and grade - Pancreatic cancer.

Source: https://pathology.jhu.edu/build/assets/pancreas/_image800/pancreas-stage.jpg.

13.5.3. Therapeutic Approaches and Clinical Trials

The therapeutic scenario of metastatic and pancreatic rare tumors has seen a vast transformation with the advent of personalized medicine. The traditional treatment methods, such as chemotherapy and radiotherapy, have been mostly ineffective in tackling pancreatic neoplasms, which are highly resistant and heterogeneous. This has prompted the quest for targeted therapies and immunotherapies directed at specific molecular pathways behind the tumor growth. The success of these new approaches, however, is contingent upon careful molecular profiling to establish the patient-specific genetic aberrations present in neoplasms. Not only would such profiling enable identification of possible targets for targeted therapies but also enhance the validity of existing clinical trials, extending thus the therapeutic armamentarium for the management of complex pancreatic neoplasms including but not limited to lymphoma and renal cell carcinoma metastasis. An important step forward toward enhanced treatment paradigms is the design and conduct of clinical trials in which biomarkers are deliberately integrated into therapy on an individualized basis. Because pancreatic cancers are so heterogeneously described, clinical trials based on biomarkers have never been more needed. The identification of molecular drivers, e.g., those of the PI3K and MAPK pathways, has underlined the potential of targeted therapies against such pathways. By testing in parallel the efficacy of combination therapies that capitalize on these pathways, researchers aim to improve patients' clinical responses from pancreatic tumors. Hence, the novel frameworks that explain intra-tumoral heterogeneity can significantly supplement the design of clinical trials, resulting in better therapeutic options and offering hope for patients commonly burdened with a poor prognosis, as seen in the hallmark results unveiled in Conway et al. (2019). The tumor microenvironment also plays a significant role in determining therapy responses. Interplay between cancer cells and invading stromal elements accounts for tumor behavior heterogeneity and drug resistance. New therapeutic approaches are engineered to modulate this microenvironment to maximize existing therapies and improve outcomes in patients. The development of immune-based therapies, coupled with a profound understanding of the evolution of cancer, provides an opportunity for the redefinition of treatment paradigms. For instance, leveraging the adaptability of micro-environment-immune system and also limiting mechanisms of resistance mediated by tumors can lead to more effective results. Thus, an emphasis on integrating such multi-component approaches into clinical trials, as reflected by McGranahan & Swanton (2017), places the spotlight on the requirement for innovative trial designs that will identify both intratumor heterogeneity and dynamic tumor evolution, thus informing future metastatic and rare pancreatic cancer treatment directions.

13.6. Treatment Approaches for Metastatic and Rare Pancreatic Tumors

Treatment of metastatic and uncommon pancreatic cancers is challenging clinically due to their heterogeneity and the nature of tumor evolution. They exhibit extreme intratumor heterogeneity, such that it becomes challenging to devise a treatment strategy and influence patient outcomes as a whole. It leads to varying response to treatment, wherein more than one mode of treatment usually is needed to attain maximum benefit. Current studies recognize the role of macro-evolutionary mechanisms like chromosomal alterations in tumor growth and metastasis in such cancers. The treatment, thus, will also need to target not only the death of the tumor cells but disruption of the adaptive mechanisms within the tumor microenvironment that culminate in drug resistance. For this, new strategies combining novel immunotherapy with conventional therapies are required as they can optimally utilize the interaction between cancer biology and immune elements (McGranahan & Swanton, 2017). Chemotherapy remains a cornerstone in metastatic pancreatic tumor therapy, particularly when surgery is unresectable. Regimens such as FOLFIRINOX or gemcitabine combined with nab-paclitaxel are employed prophylactically due to their well-established efficacy for this cancer's management. However, such routine measures' effectiveness is frequently dampened by utmost side effects and incremental returns to overall survival, leading quality of life for the patient to be an issue. The introduction of targeted treatments offers a sound remedy to such constraints. Of special interest is the receptor tyrosine kinase AXL as a key player in cancer development, being overexpressed in most cancer types, including pancreatic cancers. Research on the pharmacological targeting of AXL, such as with the anticoagulant warfarin, is promising through metastatic dissemination inhibition and improved patient outcomes and so indicates the need for further research into such targeted therapies within the clinic (Haaland et al., 2017). Furthermore, the formation of personalized medicine is central to the therapeutic strategy in metastatic and orphan pancreatic cancer. The new model emphasizes the importance of tailoring treatment methods based on patient and tumor profiles. Genomic profiling technology facilitates the identification of targetable mutations and alterations for therapy decisions and optimal achievement of treatment benefit. Through a customized approach, clinicians are well positioned to manage the complexities of tumor biology, such as variability in drug sensitivity and mechanisms of resistance inherent in these cancers. Such advances also provide momentum for the design of new clinical trials aimed at assessing novel combination therapies designed to maximize therapeutic gain. Overall, with the growing elucidation of molecular complexities of pancreatic neoplasms by research, the integration of targeted therapy, personalized medicine, and integrative treatment regimens will be essential for metastatic and rare pancreatic tumor optimization (Figure 13.15).

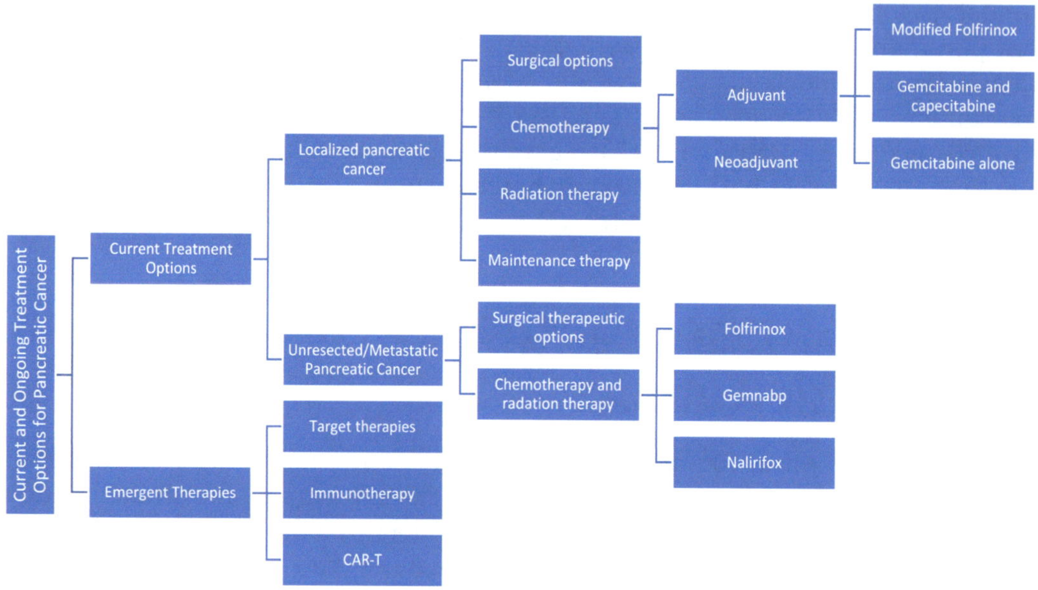

Figure 13.15. Metastatic pancreatic cancer: Current treatment options for patients.

Source: Hayat U, Croce PS, Saadeh A, Desai K, Appiah J, Khan S, Khan YI, Kumar K, Hanif A. Current and Emerging Treatment Options for Pancreatic Cancer: A Comprehensive Review. *Journal of Clinical Medicine*. 2025; 14(4):1129. https://doi.org/10.3390/jcm14041129

13.6.1. Surgical Interventions and Their Effectiveness

Surgical interventions have become a focus in the management of metastatic and rare tumors of the pancreas. Surgical resection in situations such as pancreatic lymphoma and renal cell carcinoma metastasis can significantly enhance patient outcomes, mostly through the alleviation of obstructive jaundice and pain symptoms. Technological advances in imaging, which were highlighted in current literature, allow for more precise tumor targeting, hence increased diagnostic and therapeutic yields. The union of endoscopic practices and minimally invasive surgical approaches further transformed the treatment regimen of pancreatic cancer, providing patients with improved quality of life following surgery and reduced recovery times. These developments underscore the effectiveness of operative interventions as a component of a multimodal therapeutic regime, making them priceless in the treatment of pancreatic abnormalities (AIRTUM Working Group, 2016). Even though potentially advantageous, the effectiveness of operative interventions is offset by the unique biological features of rare tumors. These are pancreatic stromal and acinar cell tumors, both having specific pathophysiological mechanisms that may make operative interventions complicated. These tumors are reported to arise in their late stage, so their resection is challenging and their treatment approaches should be tailored on a thorough knowledge of their molecular biology. For instance, gene expression profiling, as outlined in recent oncological studies, suggests that some molecular signatures may predict which way these tumors will react to treatment and even guide preoperative intervention and postoperative management (Iacobelli et al., 2012). Therefore, while surgery remains the mainstay of therapy, its success relies heavily on proper diagnosis and personalized treatments according to molecular data. Lastly, while surgical treatment for pancreatic cancer is promising in terms of patient management, tumor heterogeneity mandates judicious use of such therapies. Multidisciplinary care teams, including surgical oncologists, medical oncologists, and radiologists, are required to optimize treatment. The addition of a preoperative assessment with advanced-technology imaging modalities and genetic analysis can lead to more informed surgical planning, therefore maximizing treatment effect for metastatic and rare tumors. As the knowledge of these cancers continues to progress, the ongoing coupling of surgical methods with newly developing biomarkers will remain pivotal in fine-tuning therapy regimens, ultimately with the goal of enhancing survival and improving quality of life in afflicted patients (Iacobelli et al., 2012).

13.6.2. Chemotherapy and Targeted Therapies

Treatment of metastatic and uncommon pancreatic tumors, in this case PDAC, typically involves a combination of chemotherapy and targeted therapies. Since PDAC is a virulent and late-stage diagnosed tumor, standard chemotherapy regimens such as gemcitabine alone or in combination with nab-paclitaxel have become the standard.

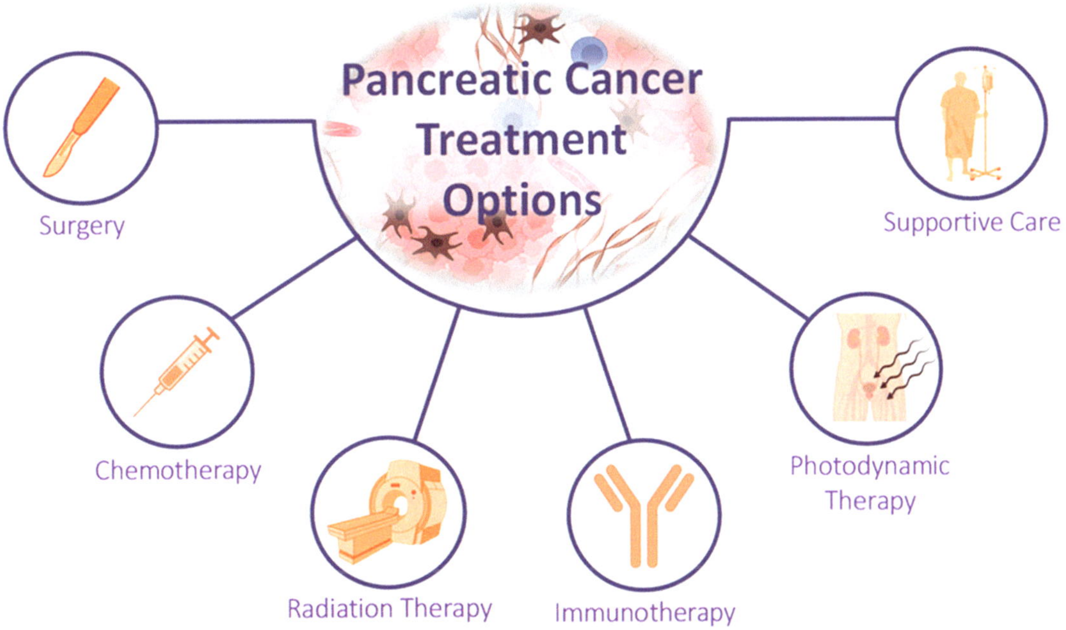

Figure 13.16. Chemotherapy and targeted therapies for pancreatic tumors.

Source: https://www.researchgate.net/publication/380014435/figure/fig2/AS:11431281239083083@1714151399720/Treatment-Options-for-Pancreatic-Cancer.tif.

However, these therapies provide only a partial survival benefit, justifying the need to enhance it using precision medicine. Chemotherapy is predominantly applied for the reduction of the tumor size and control of symptoms but generally encounters limitations due to the heterogeneity of pancreatic tumors, which also possesses an extremely high degree of resistance to conventional therapy. This underscores the requirement for therapies that will better specifically target the person genetic alterations in each tumor, providing a rationale for the increased focus on molecular stratification and personalized treatment regimens in the therapy of PDAC and other pancreatic neoplasms. Targeted therapies are revolutionizing the care of pancreatic cancers by acting against particular molecular pathways implicated in tumor growth and survival. There have been recognized main pathways such as the mitogen-activated protein kinase (MAPK) and phosphoinositide 3-kinase (PI3K) pathways to be pivotal in the pathogenesis of PDAC. Targeted agents modulating these pathways are being more aggressively pursued, particularly in combination with other treatments. For instance, the identification of mTOR, a key component downstream of the Kras mutation, which affects tumor growth and metabolism, has triggered clinical trials using mTOR inhibitors. Studies have indicated that the inhibition of mTOR through medication such as AZD6244 aimed at the MAPK pathway presents synergistic effects in cancer cell lines, with the significance of combined therapy for improving patient outcomes in pancreatic cancers brought to the fore (Jenq, 2012). Also, the complex tumor microenvironment and the prevalence of molecular abnormalities in pancreatic cancer call for a multidimensional treatment plan encompassing novel agents along with conventional modalities. Biomarker-based clinical trials are increasingly becoming the norm, as they will allow therapy to be selected on the basis of certain genetic profiles. This transition to target medicine is critical because the majority of PDACs have Kras gene mutations, and targeting downstream effects may limit tumor progression. Therapists can maximize treatment strategies through evidence from large-scale genomics to target drugs with high potential for inducing dramatic responses based on tumor type. These specifically targeted therapies can potentially transform pancreatic cancer management, finally aiming at optimizing survival and quality of life in affected patients while addressing the inherent molecular heterogeneity typical of these cancers (Conway et al., 2019) (Figure 13.16).

13.6.3. Emerging Treatments and Research Directions

The last few decades have seen metastatic and rare pancreatic tumors treated with a new wave of novel treatment modalities. Among these, one that has generated significant interest is the targeting of the endothelin axis (ET-axis), which has been a focus point due to its multifaceted participation in cancer biology. Studies indicate endothelin-1 as a molecule that affects tumor microenvironment dynamics, particularly in pancreatic cancer (PC), and that it promotes fibrosis as well as inhibits effective therapies. For instance, inhibition of ET receptors using antagonists such as Bosentan has been promising in suppressing tumor growth and enhancing the efficacy of treatment by modifying the tumor environment, thereby offering a novel therapeutic avenue for aggressive pancreatic cancer (Gupta, 2017). With science gradually unlocking the complexities of the ET-axis, it also creates windows of opportunity for combination therapies that involve these findings with traditional therapeutic approaches. There is also the quest for immunotherapies as emerging possibilities for treating rare pancreatic tumors. Building on the promise of the immune system, treatment modalities such as checkpoint inhibitors and adoptive cell transfer are being studied in clinical trials. These methods are intended to reverse the immunosuppressive nature of the tumor microenvironment common with pancreatic tumors, i.e., by focusing on tumor-associated antigens uniquely expressed in restricted kinds of tumors like lymphoma and renal cell carcinoma metastasis. Through new approaches, researchers anticipate enhanced visibility of the tumor along with robust immune reactions and ultimately improved patient results. Significantly, ongoing efforts at biomarker identification are necessary for patient stratification and maximization of these therapies, so that immunotherapeutic strategies can be individualized to tumor signatures (Kaushik, 2019). In parallel with this, the development of personalized medicine is also revolutionizing treatment modalities for metastatic pancreatic cancer. Precision oncology, which is dependent on the application of tumor genomic profiling to guide the selection of therapy, is proving to be effective in rare tumor subtypes like acinar and stromal tumors. This approach allows clinicians to detect functional mutations and select targeted therapy that is in line with the individual patient's specific genetic makeup. For instance, the use of next-generation sequencing techniques has revealed specific mutations in the KRAS pathway that can be addressed with novel therapies and thereby enhance outcomes. Besides, the integration of bioinformatics and data analytics is providing new opportunities for better insight into tumor heterogeneity and resistance mechanisms. As such, research waves move ahead, they promise hope for personalized treatment, improved prognosis, and improved quality of life for these aggressive cancer patients (Gupta, 2017).

A CLOSER LOOK

METASTATIC SQUAMOUS CELL CARCINOMA TO THE PANCREAS

Metastatic squamous cell carcinoma (SCC) to the pancreas is an exceedingly rare clinical occurrence because the pancreas is an uncommon site of metastasis and primary squamous cell carcinoma of the pancreas is extremely uncommon because pancreatic tissue lacks indigenous squamous epithelium. Most pancreatic SCCs are secondary, resulting from a primary tumor elsewhere in the body, most commonly the lung, esophagus, head and neck, or cervix. Metastatic tumors can present as a single or multiple masses within the pancreas and can frequently be mistaken clinically as well as on imaging for primary pancreatic adenocarcinoma. They tend to present with nonspecific symptoms such as abdominal pain, weight loss, jaundice, or intestinal obstruction, making their diagnosis without a history of known primary SCC elsewhere challenging. Imaging techniques such as CT and MRI can give evidence of a pancreatic mass, but histopathological confirmation using immunohistochemical staining is most often needed for a firm diagnosis, which will differentiate metastatic SCC from primary pancreatic neoplasms. Markers such as p40, p63, and cytokeratin 5/6 are supportive of a squamous phenotype, and correlation with the patient's clinical history is required for determination of the primary site. The prognosis of metastatic SCC to the pancreas is usually poor and suggests extensive disease. Treatment is non-existent and is generally palliative only, in the form of systemic chemotherapy or biologic agents based on the primary site of origin. Surgery is not generally recommended unless for control of symptoms or if the metastasis is limited and the primary tumor is controllable. Since it is an infrequent occurrence, each case has to be specifically evaluated by a multidisciplinary panel, and diagnosis must be established to avoid mistaking it as primary pancreatic cancer, whose management would be different (Yilmaz, 2023) (Figure 13.17).

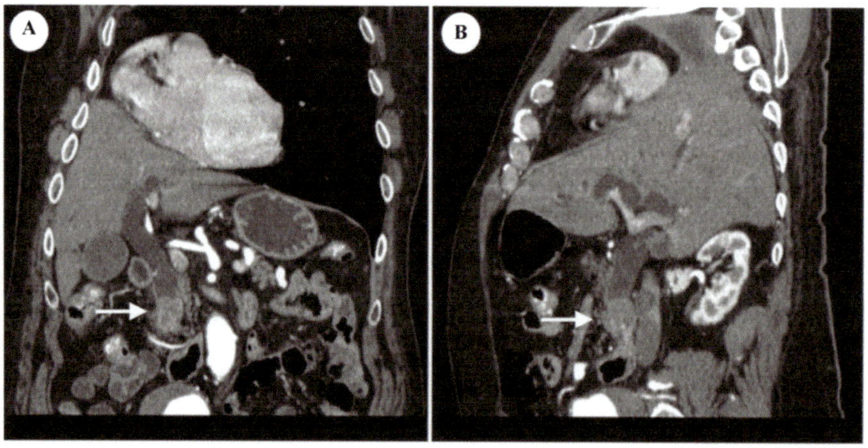

Source: https://external-content.duckduckgo.com/iu/?u=https%3A%2F%2Fwww.spandidos-publications.com%2Farticle_images%2Fmco%2F10%2F1%2Fmco-10-01-0144-g00.jpg&f=1&nofb=1&ipt=cf462805c7f7c61200ac90d5f07e9ddbee6b34439c3331d2c53a43c6aa83c252.

SUMMARY

The research of rare and metastatic pancreatic tumors points to the pressing need for more knowledge, diagnosis, and treatment in oncology practice. The biology of pancreatic tumors, leading indicators among them being lymphoma and renal cell carcinoma metastases, poses very serious problems that call for comprehensive research activity. Analysis of the TME imposes strict interactions among cancer cells and other cellular elements. For instance, the endothelin axis has been a prominent character, influencing not just tumor growth but also its microenvironmental characteristics. Understanding these interactions is essential to create targeted therapies that might disrupt tumor development and enhance patient prognosis, as seen in studies on ET signaling pathways (Gupta, 2017). In addition, the role of cytokines in PDAC illustrates the complexity of tumor interactions with the immune system. The identification of overexpressed cytokines CXCL9 and CXCL10 in PDAC even more strongly indicates their probable impact on disease progression and patient prognosis. With evidence of correlations of these cytokines with poor survival, clinicians need to consider immunological factors when designing treatment regimens (Cannon et al., 2020). This school of thought not only shifts the paradigm to one of individualized treatment but also emphasizes the need for a multi-factorial approach while addressing pancreatic cancers that are resistant to conventional therapies. The findings presented in this essay emphasize the need to continue to investigate therapeutic approaches that consider the different types of tumors and the biology pertaining to each. Specifically, novel treatment strategies acting on specific pathways, such as the endothelin axis and other cytokine receptors, may hold promise in the enhancement of treatment in patients with pancreatic cancer. In the continued advancement in oncology practice, further investigation of the molecular underpinnings of metastatic tumors and uncommon tumors will be essential in more sharply delineating current therapy and potentially unveiling new treatments. This dynamic effort relies on the synergy of researchers, clinicians, and patients in concert with each other because together, they all seek enhanced survival rates and quality of life in patients afflicted with these conditions.

Metastatic and rare pancreatic tumors have yielded important information on their pathophysiology and the approaches to treatment. Among these tumors, pancreatic lymphomas with their nonspecific presentation are difficult to diagnose. Histological diversity of these tumors necessitates a detailed understanding of the behavior of these tumors and their reactions to the treatments. Intratumor heterogeneity has been outlined more recently as one of the factors in the morphologic complexity of lymphomas. By tumor evolution, this heterogeneity is also further complicating treatment, pointing towards an imperative necessity for individualized approaches to therapy, taking into account the distinctive characteristics of each tumor subtype (McGranahan & Swanton, 2017). The newer imaging techniques, especially PET/CT, have also significantly improved diagnostic yield, enabling easier differentiation between lymphoma and other masses in the pancreas, thus making it easier to implement appropriate interventions at an early stage. Further, the degree of metastatic disease, particularly from renal cell carcinoma, underlines the virulent character of certain pancreatic tumors. Renal cell carcinoma often metastasizes to the pancreas, and awareness of the presentation and evolution of these tumors can help to optimize treatment plans. Communication between the metastatic cells and the microenvironment of the pancreas can encourage marked phenotypic change, influencing metastatic potential and therapeutic resistance. Notably, tumor stroma coexisting with tumors enhances the tumors' resistance to conventional therapies, thereby necessitating new strategies that may target tumor and supportive stroma in unexplored ways. The emerging body of evidence supporting such interactions calls for more robust research platforms to explore drug combinations that can disrupt such pathways and improve patient outcomes effectively (McGranahan & Swanton, 2017). In the study of stromal and acinar cell tumors, we are also interested in the peculiar challenges that they present in clinical management. Such rare tumors do not typically possess robust histopathological characteristics; hence, presentation and pre-treatment planning are complex. Effective management entails multi-disciplinary management and is dependent on exposure to recent developments in imaging and molecular typing. Realization of dynamic tumor evolution in response to genetic and epigenetic drivers only increases the call for adaptive therapy. By channeling the insights that have been derived from tumor microenvironment research, we can improve targeted therapies, ushering us into greater therapeutic gains. Embracing such key findings not only explains the complexities that underlie the different types of pancreatic tumors but also advocates for the value of ongoing research and creativity in treatment models.

KEY TERMS FROM THIS CHAPTER

- Metastasis
- Melanoma
- Breast carcinoma
- Sarcoma
- Acinar cell carcinoma
- Pancreatoblastoma
- Renal cell carcinoma (RCC)
- Lung carcinoma
- Colorectal carcinoma
- Lymphoma
- Solid pseudopapillary neoplasm (SPN)
- Undifferentiated carcinoma

References

1. Coffelt, S. B., and de Visser, K. E. (2015) Immune-mediated mechanisms influencing the efficacy of anticancer therapies. Trends in Immunology, 36(4), pp. 198-216. (doi:10.1016/j.it.2015.02.006)
2. Adamo, M. S., Adorni, A., Alessi, D., Aletta, F., et al. (2016). *Italian Cancer Figures–Report 2015: The Burden of Rare Cancers in Italy=I Tumori in Italia–Rapporto 2015: I Tumori Rari in Italia*. https://core.ac.uk/download/pdf/162429352.pdf AIRTUM Working Group, Busco, S., Buzzoni, C., Mallone, S., Trama, A., Castaing, M., Bella, F., Amodio, R., Bizzoco, S., Cassetti, T., Cirilli, C., Cusimano, R., De Angelis, R., Fusco, M., Gatta, G., Gennaro, V., Giacomin, A., Giorgi Rossi, P., Mangone, L., Mannino, S., ... Dal Maso, L. (2016). Italian cancer figures--Report 2015: The burden of rare cancers in Italy. *Epidemiologia e prevenzione*, *40*(1 Suppl 2), 1–120. https://doi.org/10.19191/EP16.1S2.P001.035 (accessed on 26 May 2025).
3. Pfister, S. M., Reyes-Múgica, M., Chan, J. K. C., Hasle, H., Lazar, A. J., Rossi, S., Ferrari, A., Jarzembowski, J. A., Pritchard-Jones, K., Hill, D. A., Jacques, T. S., Wesseling, P., López Terrada, D. H., von Deimling, A., Kratz, C. P., Cree, I. A., & Alaggio, R. (2022). A Summary of the Inaugural WHO Classification of Pediatric Tumors: Transitioning from the Optical into the Molecular Era. *Cancer discovery*, *12*(2), 331–355. https://doi.org/10.1158/2159-8290.CD-21-1094 (accessed on 26 May 2025).
4. Ambrosini, E., Ferracin, M., Klec, C., Laprovitera, N., et al. (2021). Cancer of unknown primary: Challenges and progress in clinical management. https://core.ac.uk/download/554143116.pdf (accessed on 26 May 2025).
5. Casey, S. C., Amedei, A., Aquilano, K., Azmi, A. S., Benencia, F., Bhakta, D., Bilsland, A. E., Boosani, C. S., Chen, S., Ciriolo, M. R., Crawford, S., Fujii, H., Georgakilas, A. G., Guha, G., Halicka, D., Helferich, W. G., Heneberg, P., Honoki, K., Keith, W. N., Kerkar, S. P., ... Felsher, D. W. (2015). Cancer prevention and therapy through the modulation of the tumor microenvironment. *Seminars in cancer biology*, *35 Suppl*(Suppl), S199–S223. https://doi.org/10.1016/j.semcancer.2015.02.007(accessed on 26 May 2025).
6. Aron, M., Idrees, M. T., Priemer, D. S., Wei, S., et al. (2017). ZBTB16 is a sensitive and specific marker in detection of metastatic and extragonadal yolk sac tumor. https://core.ac.uk/download/84832024.pdf (accessed on 26 May 2025).
7. Conciatori, F., Ciuffreda, L., Bazzichetto, C., Falcone, I., Pilotto, S., Bria, E., Cognetti, F., & Milella, M. (2018). mTOR Cross-Talk in Cancer and Potential for Combination Therapy. *Cancers*, *10*(1), 23. https://doi.org/10.3390/cancers10010023 (accessed on 26 May 2025).
8. Koopmans, K.P., Dierckx, R.A., Elsinga, P.H., Links, T.P., Kema, I.P., Fiebrich, H.-B., Walekamp, A.M.E., de Vries, E.G.E. and Brouwers, A.H. (2015). Other Radiopharmaceuticals for Imaging GEP-NET. In Somatostatin Analogues (eds A. Hubalewska-Dydejczyk, A. Signore, M. de Jong, R.A. Dierckx, J. Buscombe and C. Van de Wiele). https://doi.org/10.1002/9781119031659.ch7(accessed on 26 May 2025).
9. Cannon, A. C. (2020). *The Role of the CXCR3 Signaling Axes in Pancreatic Ductal Adenocarcinoma* [Doctoral dissertation]. https://core.ac.uk/download/327938243.pdf (accessed on 26 May 2025).

10. Conway, J. R., Herrmann, D., Evans, T. J., Morton, J. P., & Timpson, P. (2019). Combating pancreatic cancer with PI3K pathway inhibitors in the era of personalised medicine. *Gut, 68*(4), 742–758. https://doi.org/10.1136/gutjnl-2018-316822 (accessed on 26 May 2025).
11. Crosby, B., Frazer, R., McGrane, J., Challapalli, A., Charnley, N., Jiang, X. Y., Malik, J., et al. (2025). First line treatment of pancreatic metastases in metastatic renal cell carcinoma: Insights from the UK Renal Oncology Collaborative (UK ROC)—Tyrosine kinase inhibitors time to shine? *Journal of Clinical Oncology*. https://www.semanticscholar.org/paper/9110dfe85192fb9945a2bbf9793b6a20c69cb49a (accessed on 26 May 2025).
12. Curran, M., Fox, B., & Redmond, W. L. (2015). Editorial: Advances in combination tumor immunotherapy. *Frontiers in Oncology, 5*. https://www.semanticscholar.org/paper/5e997a247773022102d42d5a223e91c67c0a0ff1 (accessed on 26 May 2025).
13. Gupta, Suprit, "Role of Endothelin Axis in Pancreatic Tumor Microenvironment" (2017). *Theses & Dissertations*. 203. https://digitalcommons.unmc.edu/etd/203(accessed on 26 May 2025).
14. Haaland, G. S. (2017). *Investigations of the Cancer Therapeutic and Protective Effects of Warfarin-Mediated Inhibition of The Receptor Tyrosine Kinase AXL* [Doctoral dissertation]. https://core.ac.uk/download/479092661.pdf (accessed on 26 May 2025).
15. Jenq, H. (2012). *Identifying Genes That Are Required for The Maintenance of Pancreatic Ductal Adenocarcinoma* [Doctoral dissertation]. https://core.ac.uk/download/10129746.pdf (accessed on 26 May 2025).
16. Kaushik, G. (2019). *Developing Targeted Therapy Against Pancreatic Cancer* [Doctoral dissertation]. https://core.ac.uk/download/268253012.pdf (accessed on 26 May 2025).
17. Kumar, U. (2023). Somatostatin and somatostatin receptors in tumor biology. *International Journal of Molecular Sciences, 25*(1), 436. https://doi.org/10.3390/ijms25010436.
18. Munoz, J., Wheler, J. J., & Kurzrock, R. (2015). Androgen receptors beyond prostate cancer: an old marker as a new target. *Oncotarget, 6*(2), 592–603. https://doi.org/10.18632/oncotarget.2831
19. Li, T., Lei, Z., Wei, L., Yang, K., Shen, J., & Hu, L. (2023). Tumor necrosis factor receptor-associated factor 6 and human cancer: A systematic review of mechanistic insights, functional roles, and therapeutic potential. *Journal of Cancer, 15*, 560–576. https://doi.org/10.7150/jca.90059.
20. Marchesi, F. (2006). *Chemokines and Their Receptors in The Metastatic Behaviour of Human Pancreatic Ductal Adenocarcinoma* [Doctoral dissertation]. https://core.ac.uk/download/227755341.pdf (accessed on 26 May 2025).
21. Mathias, A. C., Synnott, A. J., Small, D. L., von Hoff, D., Couch, F. J., Colon-Otero, G., Hall, J. C., et al. (2016). Novel patient-derived xenograft mouse model for pancreatic acinar cell carcinoma demonstrates single agent activity of oxaliplatin. https://core.ac.uk/download/pdf/81888742.pdf (accessed on 26 May 2025).
22. McGranahan, N., & Swanton, C. (2017). Clonal Heterogeneity and Tumor Evolution: Past, Present, and the Future. *Cell, 168*(4), 613–628. https://doi.org/10.1016/j.cell.2017.01.018(accessed on 26 May 2025).

23. Regad T. (2015). Targeting RTK Signaling Pathways in Cancer. *Cancers*, *7*(3), 1758–1784. https://doi.org/10.3390/cancers7030860(accessed on 26 May 2025).

24. Sohal, D., Sun, W., & Haller, D. (2021). Pancreatic, gastric, and other gastrointestinal cancers. *DeckerMed Family Medicine*. https://www.semanticscholar.org/paper/fae1f44408f95974f2af160050bfde74de02ba8a (accessed on 26 May 2025).

25. Teng, Ling-Chiao[1,*]; Shih, Yu-Hsuan[2,3]. A Liposomal Irinotecan and S-1 Combination is Shown to be Efficacious in the Treatment of Metastatic Pancreatic Acinar Cell Carcinoma: A Case Report. Journal of Cancer Research and Practice 11(3):p 118-121, Jul–Sep 2024. | DOI: 10.4103/ejcrp.eJCRP-D-24-00009 (accessed on 26 May 2025).

26. Yilmaz, Y. (2023). *Roles of ADAM8 and PRMTs in Tumor-Stroma-Interactions in Pancreatic Ductal Adenocarcinoma* [Doctoral dissertation]. https://core.ac.uk/download/586348240.pdf (accessed on 26 May 2025).

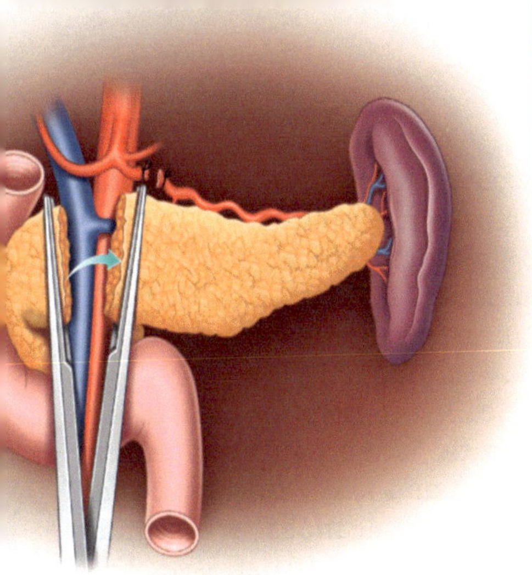

Chapter 14

TRAUMA TO THE PANCREAS

Contents

Introduction

The pancreas performs many physiological roles, including digestion and glucose metabolism. The organ is nevertheless extremely vulnerable to trauma, resulting from both blunt and penetrating injuries. Such trauma is capable of leading to massive clinical morbidity, ranging from hemorrhage, infection, to even organ failure. The increasing number of pancreatic injuries renders a complete knowledge of their etiology, presentation, and management compulsory. A critical analysis of the literature points out significant gaps in knowledge and therapeutic handling of these injuries, as the majority of literature has not made systematic assessment available for their evaluation. This highlights the importance of further refining present surgical methods and improving patient outcomes by targeted research aiming to solve the complexities of pancreatic trauma. Grading and classification of pancreatic injury are crucial in the planning of the operation and outcome estimation. Several grading systems have been proposed, but usage and efficacy are patchy. For instance, various systems might grade injuries based on the severity of parenchymal injury or the involvement of major vascular structures. Furthermore, the lack of standardized protocols creates significant problems for clinical decision-making. Krige et al. (2017) emphasizes the need to surmount these limitations by research focussed on proper data collection and analysis that can be utilized for upgrading clinical assessment and management plans. Adoption of a standardized grading system not only aids in grading injury severity but is also a foundation for creating personalized treatment protocols. Additionally, complications occurring post-trauma because of pancreatic injuries can potentially lead to long-term diseases for the individuals involved. These complications, potentially from pancreatic fistula, deranged insulin production, and pain syndromes, often complicate the recovery process and lower quality of life. Understanding the biochemical and physiological pathways in these complications is essential to provide optimal surgical care and postoperative management. Ball et al. (2010) stresses the need for a multidisciplinary approach to intervention with strict follow-up and patient support in recovery from pancreatic injury. With the development of the area, linking clinical experience with ongoing research will be the imperative in enhancing patient outcomes for those experiencing the deleterious effects of pancreatic injuries (Figure 14.1).

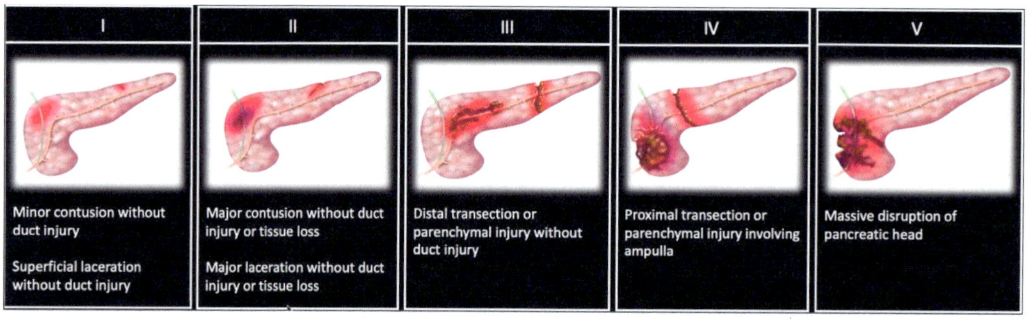

Figure 14.1. Trauma to pancreas.

Source: https://pancreas.thecommonvein.net/wp-content/uploads/2021/10/pancreas-trauma-grade.jpg.

Definition of Pancreatic Trauma

Pancreatic trauma is a continuum of pancreatic injuries caused primarily by blunt or penetrating forces. Blunt trauma, also very common in road traffic accidents or falls, is due to forceful deceleration and can cause laceration or contusion of the organ. Penetrating trauma caused by gunshot or stab injuries can lead to immediate disruption of pancreatic tissue with resulting more severe injury. The uniqueness of pancreatic injuries is their potential to evolve complications such as hemorrhage or development of a pancreatic fistula, making patient management drastically more complicated. Understanding these definitions is of utmost importance as it lays the platform for assessment of the severity of the injury, which is crucial in guiding the management and the surgical interventions in affected patients. A careful assessment of pancreatic trauma requires the application of a formal grading system, facilitating the determination of the therapeutic approach. Grading typically ranges from classifying injuries as minor, such as superficial lacerations, to major disruption involving extensive pancreatic destruction or compromise of vessels. This grading is significant in guiding the surgeons decision-making since dealing with a grade I laceration would be different from dealing with a grade III one requiring surgery. Further, evaluation of the mechanism of injury and its clinical presentation also allows for important individualized therapeutic interventions. In clinical practice, studies aim to clarify such grading protocols and their relevance in outcomes of surgery so that patients are provided with suitable amounts of care along with a reduced risk of post-traumatic complications (Krige, 2017). Both the trauma surgeons and the rest of the medical team working together are most important in dealing with pancreatic trauma. Trauma surgery as a subspecialty involves operative and non-operative management, with highly coordinated intervention in the emergency setting to resuscitate and assess abdominal trauma patients. Multidisciplinary care is needed due to the pancreas's anatomical position and its significant functional role, making decision-making more difficult. Effective surgical intervention is resection in severely injured segments of the pancreas, while less invasive methods, such as observation and medical management, are suitable in less severe cases. Lastly, proper definition and full comprehension of pancreatic trauma enable physicians to improve surgical outcomes and better control post-traumatic complications, bringing about further development in the field of trauma surgery and improving patient care.

Importance of Understanding Pancreatic Injuries

Pancreatic injuries must be comprehensively understood, particularly due to their severity and potential for serious complications. The pancreas, as a vital organ with both endocrine and exocrine functions, presents unique challenges when injured. Blunt or penetrating pancreatic injury can disrupt these functions and lead to acute pancreatitis, a disease that can become very severe. The clinicians must have a high index of suspicion because pancreatic injuries are often overlooked due to the retroperitoneal location of the organs and their nonspecific clinical presentations. Detection and management of pancreatic trauma at an early phase are paramount for reducing morbidity and mortality rates of such injuries. Heightened sensitivity among physicians about the complexity of pancreatic trauma forms the cornerstone for initiating early interventions to minimize the risk of major complications, as emphasized in recent studies on the treatment of acute pancreatitis and grading scores of pancreatic trauma (Stecca et al., 2023). The use of imaging modalities cannot be overstressed in the management of pancreatic trauma. High-technology imaging modalities such as CT scans play a pivotal role not just in the diagnosis but also in the follow-up of pancreatic pathology. Both modalities provide high-resolution data regarding the degree of tissue damage, enabling clinicians to make the appropriate choice as regards surgical intervention or conservative management. Accurate visualization of pancreatic trauma is of crucial importance, as misinterpretation would lead to faulty management strategies that could further aggravate the patient's condition. Understanding the strengths and limitations of various imaging modalities, such as CTA and MRA, is critical in maximizing diagnostic returns and ensuring patient outcomes. As expounded in contemporary studies, a detailed understanding of the imaging framework facilitates practitioners in resolving the complexities involved in the evaluation of pancreatic injuries (Ghouri et al., 2019). Also, addressing the potential complications stemming from pancreatic injuries corroborates the need for detailed management protocols. Complications of post-traumatic origin, such as pancreatic necrosis, pseudocysts, and chronic pancreatitis, can negatively impact a patient's quality of life unless they are addressed appropriately. Clinicians must be able to identify early warning signs of these complications so that they can implement prompt intervention ranging from increased monitoring to surgery. Moreover, the pathophysiologic mechanisms of pancreatic injury and healing direct not only acute but also long-term patient outcomes. By an understanding of the three-dimensional aspect of pancreatic trauma, however, clinicians can develop holistic management plans with both acute and long-term follow-up, ultimately improving survival and decreasing chronic morbidity (Stecca et al., 2023) (Figure 14.2).

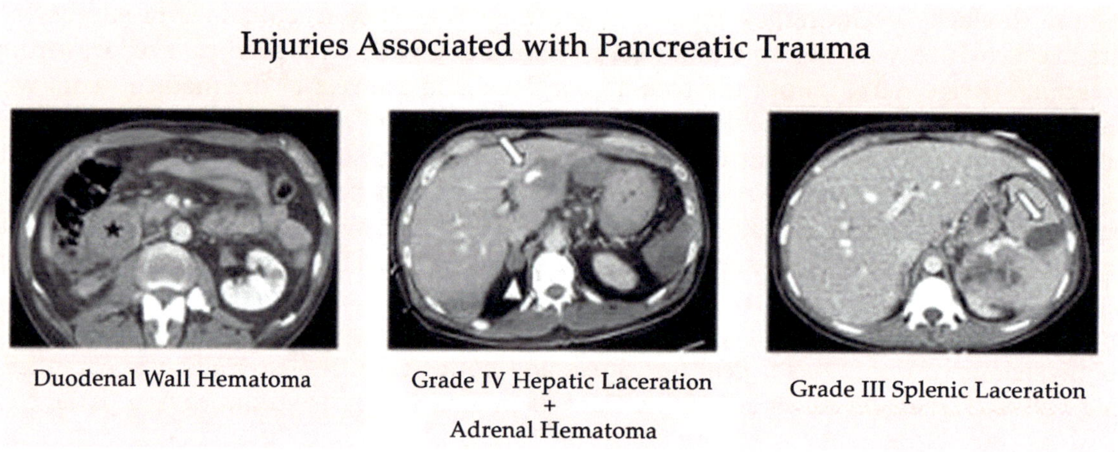

Figure 14.2. Trauma pancreatic injuries.

Source: https://pubs.rsna.org/cms/10.1148/rg.2021200077/asset/images/medium/rg.2021200077.va.gif.

14.1. Anatomy and Function of the Pancreas

The pancreas is a vital organ located in the retroperitoneal space with a dual role in digestion and endocrine function. The pancreas is anatomically separated into four sections: the head, neck, body, and tail. Each of these sections has unique anatomy and function and the broadest portion is the head in the hook of the duodenum. Functionally, the pancreas is a digestive exocrine gland secreting digestive enzymes, amylase, lipase, and proteases, into the duodenum to permit digestion of carbohydrates, fats, and proteins. It is also an endocrine gland secreting essential hormones such as insulin and glucagon in order to control blood glucose levels. Knowledge of this intricate anatomy and multi-convoluted function is essential when evaluating the impact of trauma on pancreatic function and health. Pancreatic trauma is indicated by both blunt and penetrating trauma and is subject to extensive clinical evaluation and management strategies. Blunt abdominal trauma, the most frequent cause of which is motor vehicle accidents or falls, has the capacity to result in pancreas contusion or laceration. Penetrating trauma—most commonly from stab wounds or gunshot injuries—tends to cause more direct and complex pancreatic tissue injury. Because of the proximity of the pancreas to critical structures like the duodenum, biliary tract, and great vessels, any trauma significantly complicate surgical intervention. The contemporary literature emphasized the merit of a graded grading system to assess the severity of the pancreatic injury, which determines surgical interventions from conservative management to advanced reconstruction techniques. The grading allows personalized therapeutic strategy that can enhance patient prognosis while diminishing those with pancreatic trauma. Surgical management of pancreatic injury must be considered in terms of the unique challenges posed by the organs anatomical position and its contacts with the neighboring structures. Depending on the grading of the injury, management can vary considerably. Low-grade injuries can be managed by simple repair mechanisms, while high-grade injuries can be managed by more advanced procedures such as distal pancreatectomy or pancreatoduodenectomy. In those who present with concurrent duodenal injuries, synchronized surgical procedures are warranted, according to Mohanasundaram et al. (2019). Surprisingly, complications after surgery such as pancreatic fistulas or abscesses can form and need ongoing management efforts, as in recent literature regarding complications following pancreatic injury (Krige, 2017). Hence, an accurate knowledge of pancreatic anatomy and physiology is essential for surgeons who take care of the traumatic injuries to this complex organ.

14.1.1. Location and Structure of the Pancreas

The pancreas, being the vital organ of the digestive and endocrine systems, lies retroperitoneally, extending outwards horizontally upon the posterior abdominal wall. From vertebrae levels L1 to L2, between the right duodenum and the left spleen, it lies. Its division is divided into four major regions: head, neck, body, and tail.

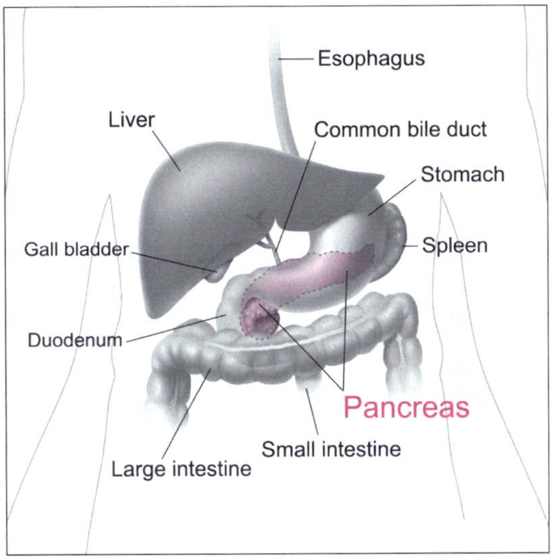

Figure 14.3. Location and structure of the pancreas.

Source: By Don Bliss (Illustrator) - This image was released by the National Cancer Institute, an agency part of the National Institutes of Health, with the ID 4363 (image) (next)., Public Domain, https://commons.wikimedia.org/w/index.php?curid=24052171

The head is over the curve of the duodenum, and the neck is a thin tube to the body, which is the largest part of the organ. The tail is in the direction of the spleen and typically located close to branches of the splenic artery and vein. Understanding the anatomical relationships of the pancreas is important, particularly within the framework of mechanisms of trauma related to penetrating as well as blunt trauma, which can severely compromise its function and complicate surgical treatment. Pancreatic trauma can manifest in the form of lacerations, transections, and hematomas, all of which present varying difficulties based on the location and extent of injury. The pancreas is particularly vulnerable due to its anatomical position, as trauma is most often in the context of abdominal trauma to adjacent organs. For instance, in duodenal trauma, trauma to the pancreas can occur because the pancreas is near the duodenum; they are often both involved in trauma because of the interconnectedness of abdominal trauma. Surgical intervention for pancreatic trauma is quite varied and is based on the severity and type of injury, highlighting the importance of knowing in depth the anatomy of the pancreas and the implications of its location in resolving post-traumatic pathology, such as pancreatitis or pancreatic juice leakage (Mohanasundaram et al., 2019). Complications following pancreatic injuries following trauma are primarily due to the complexity of the vascular and ductal anatomy of the organs. Pancreatic duct discontinuity can lead to extravasation of the digestive enzymes and hence generate local inflammation and abscess. Additionally, injury to nearby blood vessels can complicate the picture, with consequent major hemorrhage or ischemia. During surgery, repair of the duct or removal of damaged tissue is commonly necessary, and precise knowledge of pancreas anatomy is thus essential for optimal results. Further, the high frequency of related injuries, particularly in the context of blunt trauma, demands intensive assessment and management strategies that not only consider the pancreas but also contiguous organs, including the duodenum and bile ducts (Brohi et al., 2020). Therefore, the priority on early diagnosis and intervention is crucial in optimizing patient outcomes following pancreatic trauma (Figure 14.3).

14.1.2. Role of the Pancreas in Digestion and Metabolism

The pancreas also plays a central part in digestion and metabolism as a vital nexus that enables food to be digested and absorbed. The pancreas is an exocrine and endocrine gland that releases digestive enzymes and hormones that contribute directly to the metabolic functions of the body. The exocrine portion of the pancreas discharges enzymes such as amylase, lipase, and proteases into the duodenum that play a crucial role in carbohydrates, fats, and protein digestion, respectively. Proper maintenance of the pancreas is required for there to be proper nutrient uptake; derangement through trauma can significantly hamper these crucial processes, resulting in systemic metabolic disturbances and insufficiency of nutrients. This is increasingly critical to realize when quantifying the implications of injury since destruction of the pancreas may lead to both acute and chronic derangement of gastrointestinal function and metabolic function, complicating recovery from trauma to the patient. In a situation of trauma, both blunt and penetrating injury to the pancreas may be severely injurious to both digestive efficacy and metabolic homeostasis. These traumas can disrupt pancreatic function to some extent, leading to such complications as pancreatitis, diabetes, or syndromes of malabsorption.

Penetrating wounds are usually in need of immediate surgery because failure to repair the damage can lead to such complications as hemorrhage or bursting of the digestive enzymes into the peritoneal cavity and chemical peritonitis. Blunt trauma, conversely, may present with less immediate symptoms which mask the critical internal damage that may compromise the function of the pancreas in the long term. Grading and evaluation of the latter are significant, providing a guideline for surgical management to prevent pancreas-related complications due to its indispensible role in digestion and metabolism (Devarajani et al., 2010). Post-operative management of pancreatic injuries also identifies close monitoring for metabolic and endocrine function following surgery as crucial. Clinical outcome hinges on early diagnosis and treatment since, if left delayed, complications like sepsis or hypoglycemia may aggravate. Patients may develop varied post-operative complications due to the dual role of the pancreas, e.g., improper secretion of enzymes or deranged glucose metabolism, both of which require special treatment. Accordingly, awareness of the function of pancreas in digestion and metabolism is critical to establish effective surgical plans and post-operative management strategies. This overall practice needs to be combined with personalized nutritional support to overcome the deficit as a result of the failing of the pancreas, highlighting the role of pancreas in maintaining overall metabolic status following trauma (Juillard et al., 2010).

14.1.3. Vascular Supply and Innervation of the Pancreas

The blood supply to the pancreas is of utmost importance, particularly in the context of traumatic injury. The pancreas is supplied by branches arising from the celiac trunk in the form of the pancreatico-duodenal arteries and the splenic artery. These arteries provide a rich supply to the pancreas, which is vital for both its endocrine and exocrine functions. In blunt or penetrating trauma, the integrity of these vessels can be lost and result in disastrous complications in the form of hemorrhage or ischemia.

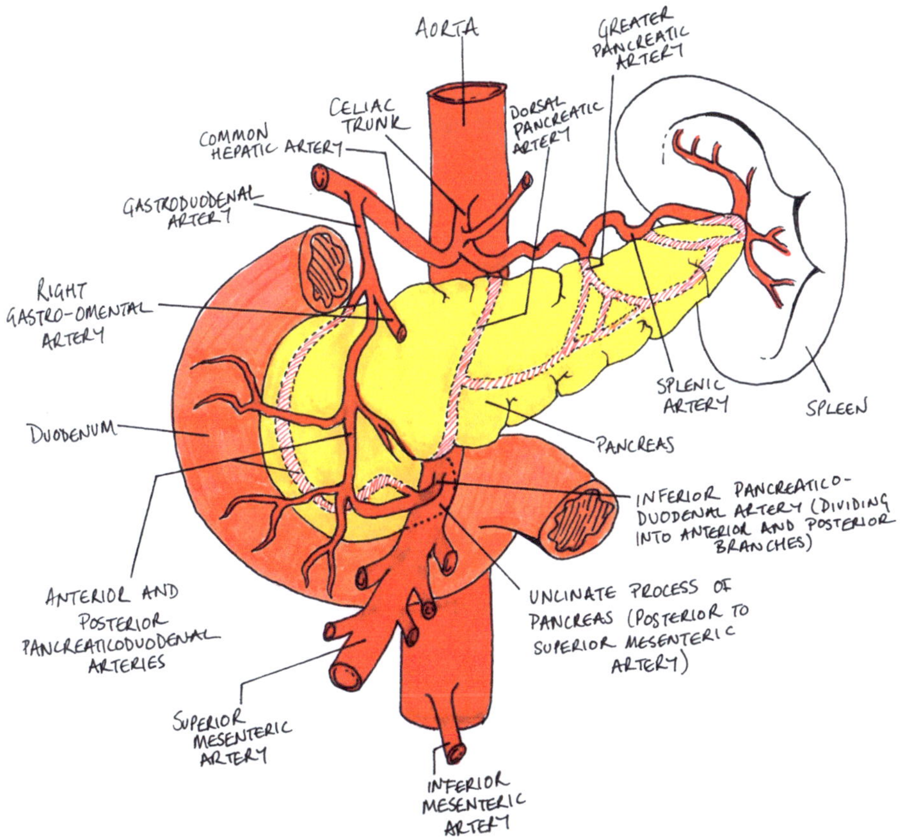

Figure 14.4. Pancreas vascular anatomy.

Source: https://i.pinimg.com/originals/51/5c/96/515c9602d4594e15fc758f1e9a4e6730.jpg.

Pancreatic parenchymal injuries typically involve surrounding structures and hence necessitate careful assessment of the vascular supply during surgery. Surgical management methods depend greatly on preserving the vascular supply to prevent necrosis, particularly in instances of resection or repair for an injury (Mohanasundaram et al., 2019). Additionally, innervation of the pancreas plays a role in determining its function and response to injury. The pancreas is innervated by both enteric and autonomic nervous system with inputs from the celiac plexus. This complex network of nerves controls the release of digestive enzymes and hormones like insulin and glucagon to maintain glucose homeostasis. Trauma impairs pancreatic function and produces metabolic derangements due to nerve damage. Post-operative complications such as pancreatic fistulae or delayed gastric emptying may result if innervation is impaired during surgery. Understanding this innervation is crucial to surgeons in planning surgical procedures, as maintaining nerve function will aid in the recovery process and improve patient outcome following injury (Rethinavelu et al., 2016). In general, vascular supply and innervation of the pancreas are directly related to its overall health and recovery following traumatic injury. The interaction of these systems with blunt or penetrating trauma necessitates a complex understanding from the surgeons to address the nuances involved in pancreatic injuries. Effective assessment and management of these anatomical structures can significantly reduce the risk of complications and improve the patient's prognosis. As discussed in case reports, precise surgical techniques are required to restore function without interfering with the nearby vasculature and neural tracts (Rethinavelu et al., 2016; Mohanasundaram et al., 2019). Thus, comprehension of the sensitive balance of these factors forms the foundation for successful surgical results and post-trauma recovery (Figure 14.4).

14.2. Types of Pancreatic Injuries

The pancreas can be subjected to a variety of different types of injury, and they are largely categorized into blunt or penetrating. Blunt pancreatic injury is frequently associated with high-energy deceleration, such as motor vehicle accidents or falls. These can lead to contusion, laceration, or transection depending on the force of the trauma and direction of trauma. These injuries may not become clinically evident promptly and hence it is difficult to diagnose and treat. Penetrating trauma, whether from gunshot wounds or stab injuries, will be more likely to cause focal injury to the pancreas. The severity and nature of the injury will dictate the approach in management, echoing the intensity required in assessment within the trauma environment. Most importantly, advancements in trauma evaluation have identified the role of imaging modalities, which can enable a wider understanding of the extent of pancreatic injuries and assist in the delineation of effective surgical treatment strategies, thereby improving patient outcomes. Pancreatic grading is important in guiding surgical management and determining the possibility of complications. The American Association for the Surgery of Trauma (AAST) has established a grading system that classifies pancreatic injury from I (milder contusions) to IV (obliteration of major transections). The grades yield prognostic factors and guide treatment plans, since various grades denote varied levels of tissue damage and resultant risks of complications such as pancreatitis or pancreatic fistula. For instance, grades I and II generally can be treated non-surgically, while grades III and more typically need surgery due to the danger of significant ductal damage or devascularization of pancreatic tissue. Recent studies emphasize the importance of the use of granular data in grading pancreatic injuries, as some studies indicate that enhancement of grading systems can lead to more precision-oriented management strategies for reducing late complications in trauma patients (Krige, 2017). Surgical intervention for pancreatic injuries requires thorough understanding of the nature, severity, and complication of the injury. For less severe injury, there is an option for non-operative management, especially if the injury is grade I or II since these are commonly recoverable with supportive care. For more severe injury, most especially those grade III or IV, operative intervention is generally necessary, and this can involve resection or drainage procedures to address damage and prevent issues like abscess formation or frank hemorrhage. It is the role of trauma surgeons that is central to stabilizing patients, evaluating injuries, and taking evidence-based action for interventions. Further, ongoing studies on surgical management and complications emphasize the need for integrated strategies that not only address the acute trauma but also provide long-term recovery and quality of life for the patients (Figure 14.5).

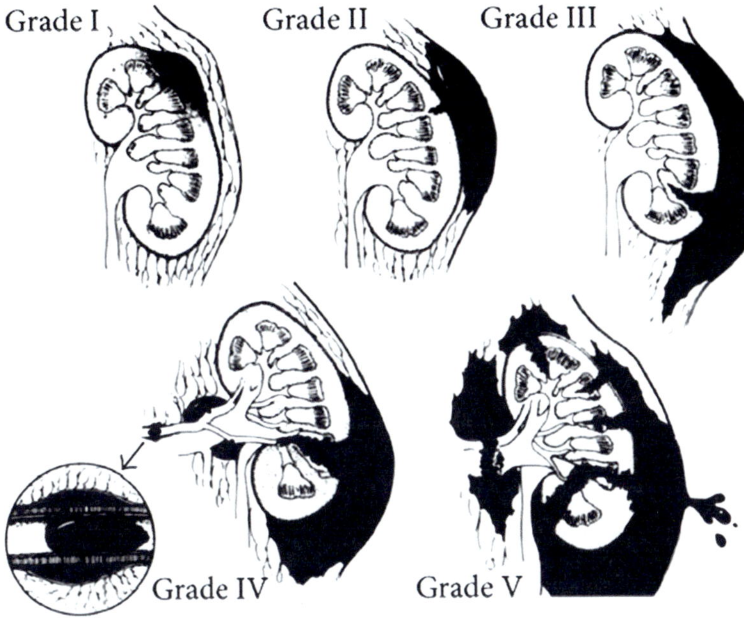

Figure 14.5. American Association for the Surgery of Trauma (AAST) organ injury.

Source: https://www.researchgate.net/publication/237200832/figure/fig7/AS:1089016678088715@1636653217276/American-Association-for-the-Surgery-of-Trauma-AAST-Organ-Injury-Severity-Score-for-the.jpg.

14.2.1. Blunt Pancreatic Injuries

Blunt pancreatic injuries are a significant challenge in abdominal trauma, typically secondary to high-energy injuries such as motor vehicle collisions or falls. Being a retroperitoneal organ, the pancreas is most susceptible to injury given its anatomical position, and this can lead to a spectrum of injuries ranging from minor contusions to complete ductal disruption. The management of such injuries depends on the full understanding of their grading, which is essential in determining appropriate surgical or conservative treatment. Proper assessment is required because misdiagnosis will lead to severe complications such as infections and necrosis of the pancreas, hence the need for having standardized criteria during the assessment of these injuries (Krige, 2017). Technological advancements in imaging, especially computed tomography (CT), have greatly enhanced the diagnostic accuracy regarding blunt pancreatic trauma. A study evaluating the utility of initial and follow-up CT scans showed excellent sensitivity in the detection of pancreatic injury, with initial scans detecting injury in 81% of patients (Alhilli et al., 2008). This advancement underscores the need to incorporate serial imaging modalities to track the evolution of injuries, as initial scans may be subject to false negatives. These advances also allow for improved decision-making between surgical and non-surgical management based on the extent and nature of injury identified through imaging. Early recognition of associated complications, such as ductal injury or bleeding, is an important factor in determining patient outcomes in trauma. Further, effective surgical treatment of blunt pancreatic injury follows a meticulous grading system that characterizes the spectrum of pancreatic injury. This grading system assists in helping surgeons decide on interventions ranging from observation to resection or reconstruction of the pancreatic tissue. Comparative research among patient outcomes has emphasized the importance of individualized surgery according to the grade of injury, with higher-grade injuries generally needing more invasive surgical interventions to prevent potentially life-threatening post-traumatic complications. The application of a multidisciplinary approach to the treatment of blunt pancreatic trauma, as highlighted by Krige (2017), offers integrative care that heals not just the acute trauma but also considers long-term healing, reducing complications of this challenging form of trauma (Figure 14.6).

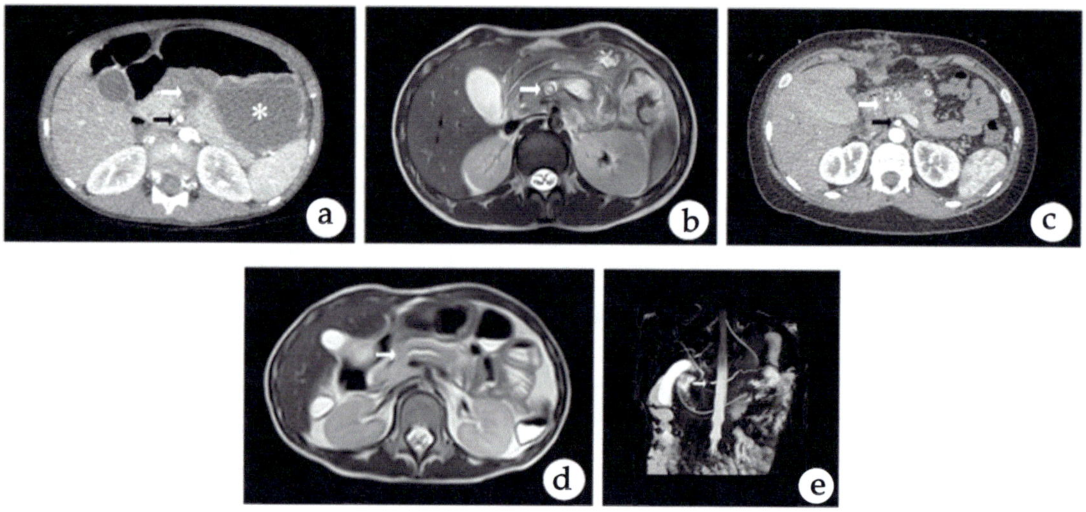

Figure 14.6. Nonresection management of the pancreas for grade III and IV blunt pancreatic injuries in children.

Source: https://media.springernature.com/lw685/springer-static/image/art%3A10.1186%2Fs12887-021-02535-0/MediaObjects/12887_2021_2535_Fig1_HTML.png.

14.2.2. Penetrating Pancreatic Injuries

Penetrating pancreatic injury, even though less common than blunt trauma, is a rather severe issue in surgical treatment due to its complex character and severe complications. These injuries mostly occur with stab or gunshot injuries and necessitate good knowledge of their mechanism and their impact on patient therapy. Proper diagnosis and grading of the injury are crucial, since treatment maneuvers may be significantly different depending on the severity of pancreatic injury, along with the presence or absence of concomitant vascular or visceral injuries. The grading system that was formulated by the American Association for the Surgery of Trauma permits a systematic approach to predicting the severity of pancreatic injuries, allowing clinicians to select the most appropriate intervention, from nonoperative care to operative intervention and repair.

The prevalence of pancreatic injuries, particularly in trauma, emphasizes the need for meticulous evaluation and aggressive management. A retrospective study conducted at Aga Khan University Hospital demonstrated that pancreatic injuries accounted for merely 1.5% of abdominal trauma in adults, with a very high complication rate of 80% in patients who were operated on for these injuries (Memon et al., 2013). This is evidence of the complicated nature of pancreatic trauma, with the interaction between factors such as the timing of presentation and severity of concomitant injuries determining patient outcomes to a large extent. The 23.3% mortality rate among this population only highlights the criticality of surgical intervention at the appropriate time. Given that the severity of penetrating injuries necessitates individualized management protocols, surgeons must exercise caution in assessing and treating every patient. Further studies on the management of penetrating pancreatic injuries need to be attentive to new operative procedures and techniques that work towards reducing the risk of complications. Research aimed at addressing the deficits in the assessment and investigation of these injuries paints a picture of an absence of robust data and sound surgical practices, ones that Krige et al. (2017) sought to address through detailed research. By analyzing detailed data of a large population treated in dedicated trauma centers, it is clear that the management of pancreatic injuries needs to be revised to take into consideration not just the immediate repair of damaged tissues but also the long-term outcome of patients. This paradigm shift necessitates standardization of surgical management protocols with a promise to enhance outcomes and decrease the burden of complications of penetrating pancreatic trauma (Figure 14.7).

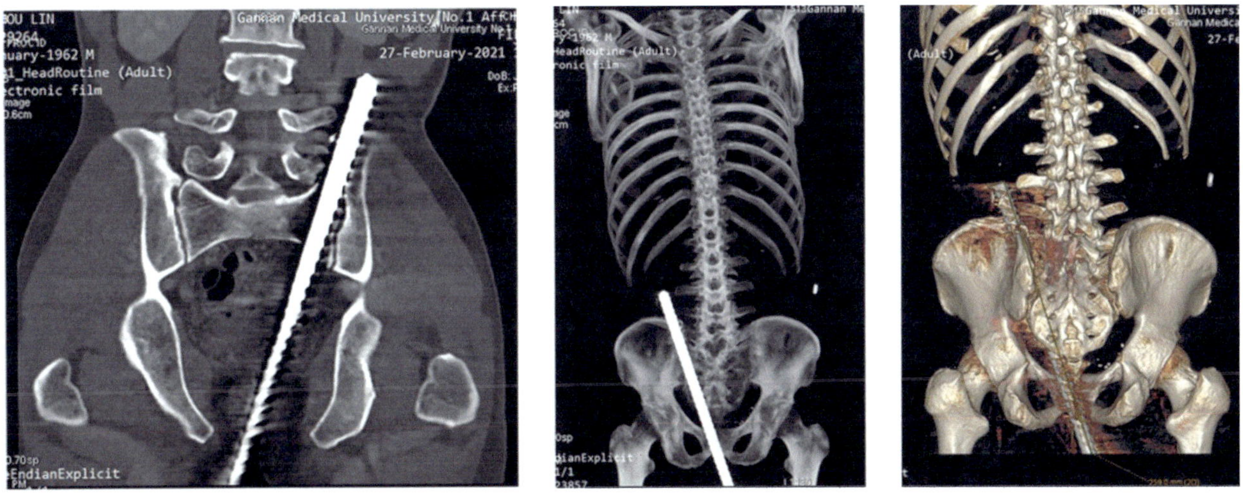

Figure 14.7. Rare penetrating abdominal injury caused by falling.

Source: Liu Y, Xu Q, Zhu H, Wang J, Zeng F and Lin J (2022) Rare penetrating abdominal injury caused by falling from height: Miraculously good prognosis. Front. Surg. 9:1018003. doi: 10.3389/fsurg.2022.1018003

14.2.3. Mechanisms of Injury and Their Implications

Understanding the pathophysiology of pancreatic injury is crucial for correct diagnosis and management. Pancreatic trauma can primarily be due to blunt or penetrating trauma. Blunt trauma, typically secondary to a motor vehicle collision or fall, can cause parenchymal laceration, contusion, or transection and significantly make surgery more difficult. Alternatively, penetrating injury, i.e., stab or gunshot wounds, may breach pancreatic tissue and its vascular supply directly. The site and severity of the injury dictate the risk for such complications as hemorrhage, necrosis, and infection. Analysis of the mechanisms helps to lay a foundation for discerning judicious grading of injury, following surgical treatment appropriate to the severity of trauma. Careful comprehension of these mechanisms of injury finally directs preoperative planning and postoperative care algorithms and thus maximizes patient outcomes while avoiding complications of pancreatic trauma. Pancreatic injuries bear long-term implications in the form of immediate physical injury; they also encompass significant clinical and management problems. Correct grading of pancreatic injuries is critical as it dictates the decision-making process regarding surgery. For instance, minor lacerations may be treated conservatively, while extensive injury can require complex surgical treatment in the way of distal pancreatectomy or pancreaticoduodenectomy. Additionally, assessment of concomitant injury, particularly those that involve contiguous organs such as the colon or spleen, is critical due to the impact on prognosis in the patient. Furthermore, late complications in the form of post-traumatic pancreatitis and abscess formation can also occur, and closer monitoring, followed by further treatment, may be indicated. Thus, understanding these implications is crucial for trauma surgeons and healthcare providers in responding to the intricate issues of pancreatic injuries and reorienting their management strategies to match evolving needs in patients. Management of the mechanisms of injury with subsequent implications demands a solid basis for surgical intervention in trauma. Current evidence indicates that careful evaluation of pancreatic trauma, facilitated by a comprehensive knowledge of its pathophysiology, maximizes the treatment outcome (Krige, 2017). Both operative and non-operative treatments together, as highlighted in the trauma surgery literature, remain of paramount significance. Trauma surgeons are strategically placed along the care pathway of stabilization, early management, to complex procedures, based on the unique patient presentation. Standardized protocols allow for equal treatment, accommodating the heterogeneity of pancreatic injuries. The multi-faceted system also has the long-term objective of optimizing recovery and preventing long-term sequelae of pancreatic trauma, thereby establishing the supreme value of adequate assessment of the injury and individualized therapy in the setting of trauma care.

14.3. Grading of Pancreatic Injuries

Grading of pancreatic injury plays an important role in the determination of proper surgical management and prediction of the outcome of patients. The grading is typically done based on the severity of the trauma, from a minor contusion to severe laceration and transection. AAST has developed a standardized grading system. In the system, the injuries are classified into five grades, each corresponding to the different degree of damage to pancreatic tissue and vasculature. This grading system must be comprehensible and adhered to by clinicians because it helps them conditionally treat the patient, either to adopt conservative treatment or a surgery for the purpose of repair, which increases efficiency in patient care. Dependence on such a grading system is proportionate to the ongoing quest for maximization of treatment regimens and outcomes of the patient being treated for pancreatic trauma (Krige, 2017). Also, imaging tests are at the forefront of efficient grading of the pancreatic injury. Techniques such as CT have become the benchmark of the initial evaluation of pancreatic trauma because of their capacity for non-invasive but comprehensive understanding of the injury. A research demonstrated that the early use of CT can reveal some features such as organ fractures, swelling, and collection of fluids, which are components of injury grading (Alhilli et al., 2008). Misdiagnosis might occur, particularly for initial CT scanning, necessitating repeated imaging for confirmation in cases where the cause is unknown. Thus, while imaging plays a significant role in grading, it should not be employed for independent clinical decision-making; rather, a broad spectrum of evaluation including clinical assessment and laboratory tests is required.

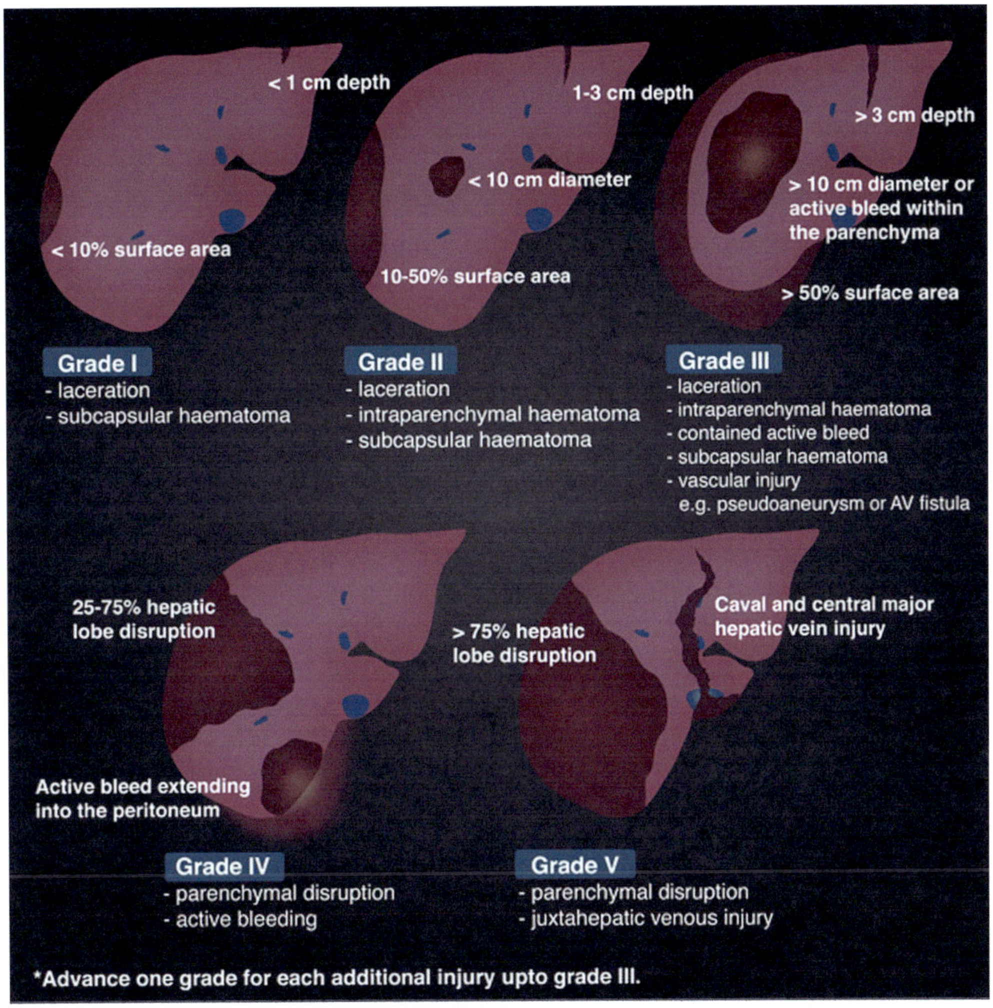

Figure 14.8. American Association for the Surgery of Trauma (AAST) has developed a standardized grading system that facilitates this process.

Source: https://prod-images-static.radiopaedia.org/images/44955209/9b54ec4db08e75b767da356bf6ba77_big_gallery.jpeg.

This multi-disciplinary approach is most important in facilitating maximum intervention based on subjective injury grade. By embracing newer advances in surgical interventions and post-traumatic care, management of pancreatic injuries has achieved considerable progress. Surgical treatments can range from simple drainage to a large resection, and the choice would largely be based on the grade of injury. For instance, lower grades of injury could be well managed with conservations treatment, while high-grade injuries typically require surgery to deal with widespread ductal disruption in addition to vascular compromise. The importance of proper grading extends beyond the immediate management and also influences the ultimate outcome of the patient as well as the potential for complications, such as the formation of pancreatic fistula (Krige, 2017). With the development of improving surgical technique and recovery practices, the importance of proper grading systems further remains a key in bridging the gap between the severity of the injury and the best treatment pathways and ultimately the destiny of trauma surgery (Figure 14.8).

14.3.1. Overview Of Grading Systems (e.g., American Association for the Surgery of Trauma (AAST))

The grading systems used in the classification of pancreatic injuries are significant in guiding treatment and also predicting outcomes of patients following trauma. The AAST has established a popular grading system that categorizes pancreatic injuries according to severity. The grading is from Grade I, which represents minor contusions or lacerations, to Grade IV and V, which are severe injuries with major vascular structures and complete pancreas transections, respectively. Such systemic grading facilitates a more uniform process for the management of trauma and allows clinicians to communicate effectively in terms of the extent of injury. The grading system also plays an important role in prospective studies for evaluating the efficacy of therapy, which aids in advancing surgical protocols and management methods in trauma care. As increasing evidence of the evolution of knowledge in pancreatic trauma is observed, the trend now shifts towards non-operative management (NOM) with increasing influence from developments in imaging modalities and interventional strategies. The incorporation of thorough grading systems, in combination with advances in technology such as enhanced CT, has facilitated acute decision-making with a tendency for conservative treatment in stable patients. NOM holds the potential for significant reduction in surgical morbidity while maintaining effective hemostatic control by interventional measures such as embolization. These developments necessitate continuous refinement of grading systems. They must be attuned to fresh data and methods so that the classification of injuries and how they are treated can keep up with what is being practiced currently and improve patient outcomes for trauma patients (Wallis et al., 2010). Ultimately, the ongoing development of grading systems for pancreatic injury transcends classification; it's a system that dictates clinical protocols and operative techniques. A comprehensive understanding of the extent of injury, as specified by accepted grading criteria, allows multidisciplinary teams to implement individualized treatment protocols in accordance with the specific needs of patients. Furthermore, a thorough study of published literature on pancreatic trauma illustrates areas to be investigated and researched. For instance, research comparing surgical methods according to AAST grading can clarify the dynamics of the treatment of complex pancreatic traumas. By addressing these fields, researchers can contribute effectively to evidence-based practices that enhance surgical outcomes and patient safety in the event of penetrating and blunt pancreatic trauma (Krige, 2017).

14.3.2. Criteria for Grading Blunt Injuries

The grading of blunt pancreatic trauma is significant in determining the treatment modality and surgical strategy. AAST grading gives a systematic approach, grading the injury from grade I to grade V based on its severity. Grade I is a laceration or contusion with no ductal injury, and grade II is moderate laceration with potential minor duct involvement. Increased grades reflect greater injuries, such as total disruption of the pancreatic duct and related vascular injury. By evaluating these criteria in an organized fashion, surgeons are able to anticipate patient outcome and complications, enabling individualized treatment strategies.

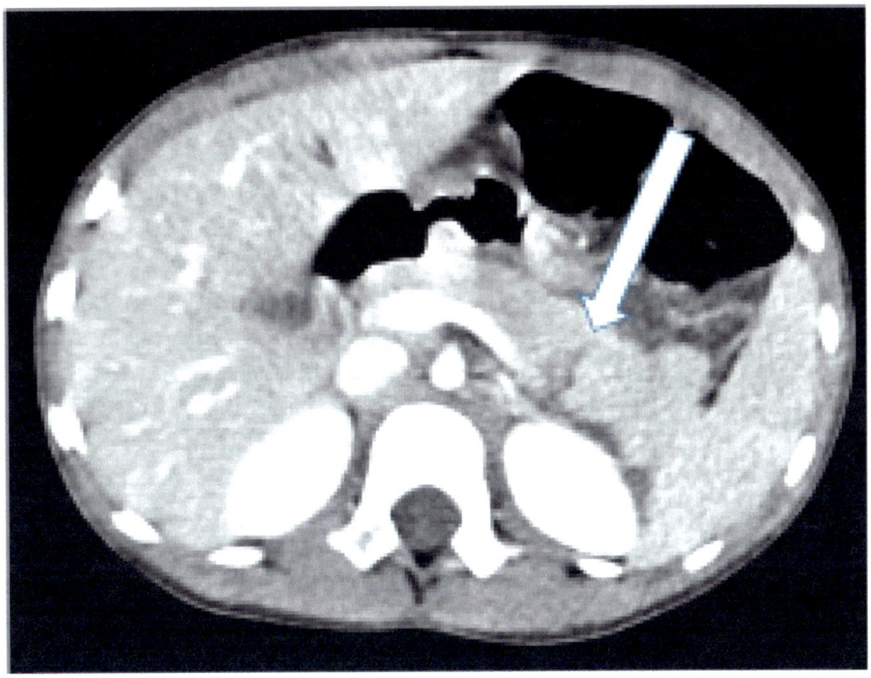

Figure 14.9. Management of blunt pancreatic trauma.

Source: Sukhotnik I, Cohen N. Management of Blunt Pancreatic Trauma in Children: A Persistent Controversy—Case Report and Comprehensive Literature Review. *Children*. 2024; 11(1):135. https://doi.org/10.3390/children11010135

The importance of maintaining a robust grading system is highlighted by existing research to reflect the necessity of such systems in addressing the multitude of the application in the treatment of pancreatic trauma, as suggested by various clinical studies in examining injury patterns and outcomes of care in trauma settings (Krige, 2017). In blunt pancreas injuries, it has been reported that a large proportion of the cases are associated with other intra-abdominal injuries, complicating diagnosis and management. Studies among children patients in North Queensland indicated that blunt trauma is the causative factor for the majority of pancreatic injuries, with repeated traumas from motor vehicle incidents and other causes of blunt trauma common among the present patients. This aids in the justification for having a stepwise and logical grading system, as injuries often do not present alone. The grading system helps not only with short-term clinical decision-making but also with long-term management plans, including surveillance for possible complications like pancreatic pseudocyst formation and postoperative pancreatic fistula (Everson et al., 2023). Therefore, clinicians need to become familiar with the correlations between grading of pancreatic injury and blunt trauma to optimize patient outcomes and customize surgical interventions. Besides informing direct clinical practice, the implications of AAST grading also have research and development implications for standardized treatment protocols. More effective data collection and analysis methods, including those addressed in pancreatic trauma research, point out existing knowledge gaps regarding outcomes across differences in injury grades. The detailed differentiation of patient groups within trauma centers allows for a more nuanced appreciation of the correlation between specific grades of injury and complications and the requirement for surgery. Thus, being part of systematic clinical research not only validates grading requirements but also aids in developing evidence-based protocols addressing the unique challenges posed by blunt pancreatic injury. Speaking to these shifting attitudes within the clinical setting is key as surgical management practices are constantly evolving, ultimately toward improved patient care (Krige, 2017) (Figure 14.9).

14.3.3. Criteria for Grading Penetrating Injuries

Grading of pancreatic penetrating injuries is a critical component in surgical planning and management. There are numerous systems of grading, but all offer an assessment of the severity of tissue damage, damage to the vessels, and associated concomitant complications. The majority of grading systems place the injury on a severity scale, ranging from minor injury requiring conservative treatment to severe injury requiring complex operation. This stratification is not only required to guide clinical decision-making but also dictates the surgical plan and desired outcome. The grading criteria can also encompass the mechanism of injury and the patient's overall stability, further enhancing the precision of the assessment. This systematic approach is essential, considering that effective management is all about proper grading, where surgeons prioritize interventions that aptly respond to the degree of injury sustained by the pancreas in trauma. Considering the complexity involved in pancreatic trauma, current literature has underscored the need for a standardized approach to grading penetrating trauma. The use of large cohort studies has revealed significant discrepancies in treatment outcomes based on the grading systems employed. For instance, research is that an integrated grading schema will improve clinical outcomes through facilitating the ability to achieve consistency in treatment protocols and surgical approaches. This is well exhibited in trauma centers with extensive experience in managing such cases, as identified by the work of Krige (2017). Ideally, a grading system that takes into account both radiological and clinical findings can make more precise prognostic estimates, thereby ultimately assisting in selecting the treatment modalities based on the severity of injury. Continuous efforts towards formulating and polishing these grading criteria are therefore essential to enhance the quality of care provided to patients with penetrating pancreatic injuries. In addition, the implications of effective grading do not only apply to immediate surgery interventions but extend to controlling long-term complications of pancreatic trauma. Being aware of what grading criteria are will allow clinicians to foresee potential sequelae such as necrosis of the pancreas, abscess, or even organ failure. An effective grading system not only facilitates intervention in a timely fashion but also enables practitioners to implement follow-up measures according to individual patient needs. Cooperation is ongoing to create consensus guidelines for specialists, as presented in Park et al. (2021). With continued harmonization of data from various specialties, including surgical oncology and transplant surgery, better knowledge of pancreatic injuries can be established, which will ultimately lead to improved patient outcomes. Therefore, addressing the grading criteria for penetrating injuries is not an exercise in academic pedantry; it is an integral component of improving trauma care and surgical practice.

14.4. Surgical Management of Pancreatic Trauma

In the treatment of pancreatic injury during trauma, care must be taken to properly grade the injury as treatment protocols are greatly reliant on the grading system. AAST grading system groups injury into categories based on the involvement of ducts, vascular compromise, and laceration extent. This grading is important in determining the need for surgical intervention, from conservative management in low-grade injury to more extensive surgical procedures in high-grade injuries. Surgeons must consider whether operative intervention is even necessary, given that the majority of pancreatic injuries are managed without operation, especially with limited hematoma and duct injury. In addition, the choice of surgical procedure—resection, drainage, or repair—needs to agree with the character of the injury and patients' general status, emphasizing personalized care for maximizing recovery and outcomes (Krige, 2017).

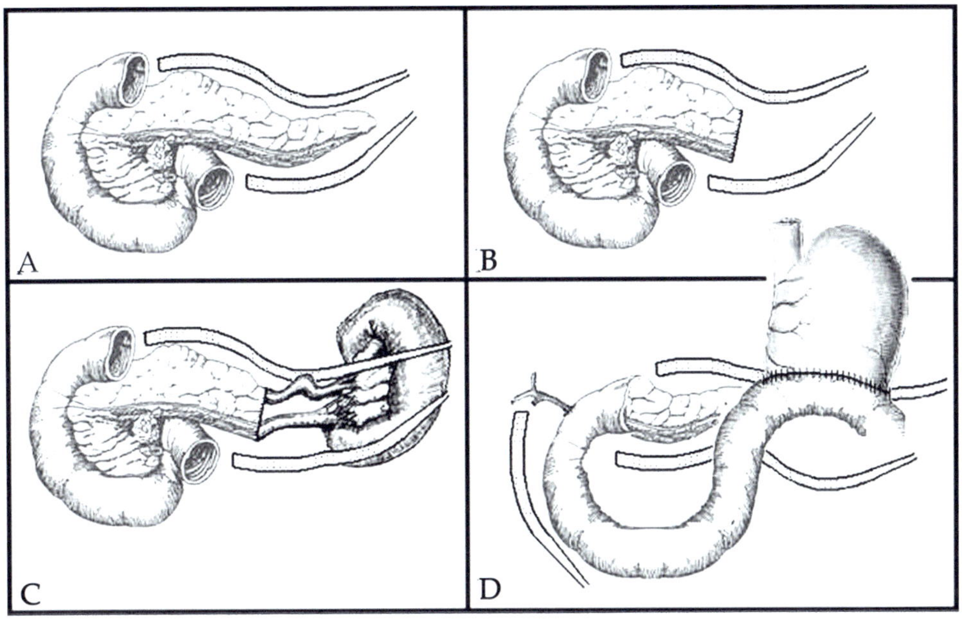

Figure 14.10. Commonly used surgical techniques in the setting of pancreatic trauma. (A) Simple drainage—sufficient in a significant number of cases. (B) Distal pancreatectomy with splenectomy and wide drainage. (C) Distal pancreatectomy with splenic preservation and wide drainage. (D) Whipple procedure with wide surgical drainage.

Source: https://www.researchgate.net/figure/Commonly-used-surgical-techniques-in-the-setting-of-pancreatic-trauma-A-Simple_fig1_23679082.

Clinical decision-making for surgical management of pancreatic injury also needs to incorporate advanced imaging modalities to facilitate clinical management. Early and follow-up CT scans play a very important part in assessing the severity of pancreatic injury and any comorbid conditions that will impact surgery. The literature is such that strict assessment of CT scans, with the laboratory tests and examination by surgery, is vital in planning management. Particularly, the use of endoscopic retrograde cholangiopancreatography (ERCP) or magnetic resonance cholangiopancreatography (MRCP) can additionally clarify, particularly in suspected primary pancreatic duct injuries. Surgeons are permitted to maximize their procedures using sequential, systematic assessment of pancreatic status by this multimodal imaging technique, resulting in improved surgical outcomes (Alhilli et al., 2008). Complications following pancreatic surgery can significantly affect the recovery of the patient as well as the overall prognosis. Complications covered by these include infections and abscesses all the way through to those related to handling of pancreatic leaks and endocrine deficiency. Surgical teams need to establish robust follow-up mechanisms for screening for these potential issues, with an emphasis on early detection and control. Further, as therapeutic modalities improve, the application of minimal access surgical techniques may provide advantages in reducing recovery time and complications. Continuing research is important in setting evidence-based practices for the management of difficult pancreatic injuries that have been highlighted in ongoing investigations of important aspects of surgical techniques and outcomes in traumatic patients (Krige, 2017). By optimization of surgical techniques and post-operative care, healthcare professionals are able to significantly enhance the outcome of patients with traumatic injury of the pancreas (Figure 14.10).

14.4.1. Indications for Surgical Intervention

The management of pancreatic injury requires a strong appreciation of the indications for surgery. Surgical treatment becomes major in patients with penetrating injuries in whom vascular compromise may be present. For patients who present with abdominal pain, hemodynamic instability, or peritonitis, prompt surgical assessment is necessary. The emergency is illustrated by the potential for rapid deterioration associated with pancreatic trauma since they are at risk for severe complications such as hemorrhage or infection. Therefore, on clinical assessment of significant injury, especially in hemodynamically unstable patients, immediate intervention is often necessary to avoid further organ injury or systemic infection, initiating a critical time frame in trauma patient care. The decision-making process for surgical intervention must also consider the therapeutic advancement in NOM approaches. As the strong trend towards NOM for stable hemodynamics patients has emerged, defining the cut-offs for selecting surgical intervention becomes crucial.

As in current literature, interventions such as embolization have been on the rise in popularity in order to achieve hemostasis with preserved organ function without the adverse effects inherent to surgery. They emphasize the usefulness of imaging technologies, particularly developments in CT, allowing for precise evaluations of the severity of injury and integrity of organs. Through a deliberate attempt to consider each patient's unique case, medical professionals are able to maximize outcomes by determining whether or not surgical intervention is truly necessary (Wallis et al., 2010). In the treatment algorithm of pancreatic trauma, the fine-grading system plays an important role in establishing indications for surgery. The grading of pancreatic injury, based on tissue damage severity, ductal injury, and associated vascular injury, dictates clinical management. It is rather the more complex injuries, particularly grade III and higher, that are likely to necessitate surgery to address potential complications effectively. Evidence indicates that pancreatic trauma, which involves massive disruption of the pancreatic duct or the presence of devascularized tissue must be treated operatively to avoid severe complications like pancreatic necrosis or the development of an abscess. As evidenced by existing research, these findings attest to the necessity for greater specificity in surgical decision-making, ultimately striving to balance risk versus benefit of intervention against the backdrop of patient anatomy and degree of injury (Krige, 2017).

14.4.2. Surgical Techniques for Managing Pancreatic Injuries

The management of pancreatic injuries from either blunt or penetrating trauma necessitates a thorough command of various surgical techniques to properly treat the complexities of such injury. Previously, operations have focused on those that either resect injured pancreatic tissue or allow drainage of necrotic tissue. For instance, in the case of the classical Whipple procedure, it is employed for individuals with a large extent of injury requiring the resection of part of the pancreas with the adjacent structures. On the other hand, in milder presentations, more conservative approaches such as debridement and drainage but not resection can be performed. This hybrid approach acknowledges heterogeneity of pancreatic damage and addresses surgical management based on the specific grade of damage and patient condition, in accordance with contemporary practice guidelines that favor patient-specific care and conservative management wherever feasible (Krige, 2017). In the perioperative setting, intervention timing is of paramount importance to the success of patients with pancreatic injury. Early intervention is usually preferable, particularly with penetrating trauma when instantaneous damage control takes precedence. Resuscitation and stabilization have to be weighed by trauma surgeons against the intricacies of pancreatic anatomy, where operative access is dependent on careful planning around surrounding structures. Techniques such as laparotomy or laparoscopy are frequently used, allowing for an internal exploration and treatment of the injury. Additionally, non-operative management adoption in the form of percutaneous drainage and observation has increasingly taken center stage, particularly for stable presentations and lower-grade injuries. This shift in paradigm underscores the importance of ongoing evaluation and selective use of surgery based on patient presentation. Complications following surgery remain a critical problem for the management of pancreatic injury by surgery. The friable nature of pancreatic tissue makes it prone to procedural mishaps such as pancreatic fistula, abscess, and even delayed gastric emptying. Prevention of these is through careful surgical technique, drains, and careful monitoring of the patient's post-procedure clinical status. Improvements in surgical technology in the guise of newer imaging techniques and minimal access surgery have aided in better outcomes. Secondly, meta-analysis of numerous clinical trials has also brought forth important aspects of how to care for such complications (Krige, 2017). Lastly, individualization of the operation procedure based on the specific patient requirement, along with anticipation of post-surgery complications, still tops recovery as well as long-term outcome in patients of pancreatic trauma.

14.4.3. Post-Operative Care and Monitoring

Care and monitoring in the postoperative period are major components following surgical management for pancreatic trauma, emphasizing the highest need for careful management and observation to avoid complications. All patients who have received trauma to the pancreas by blunt or penetrating trauma are at risk for developing numerous postoperative complications, such as leaks from the pancreas, abscesses, and infection. The pancreatic anatomy with intricate blood supply and duodenal and biliary system relationship demands vigilant postoperative care. It is essential to closely monitor vital parameters, laboratory investigations such as amylase and lipase levels, and imaging studies to detect any sign of complications at an early stage. As pointed out in most studies, early diagnosis and intervention can greatly minimize morbidity and mortality rates, so extensive monitoring is most important for the best recovery results in such patients (Juillard et al., 2010). In addition, post-operative management encompasses not only physical but also psychological support for complete recovery. The patients undergoing surgical treatment for pancreatic injuries are prone to extreme pain and emotional stress and so need efficient pain control measures and psychological counseling. The nursing staff plays an essential role in teaching the patient about pain management techniques and how to report any atypical signs and symptoms, such as increased pain or changes in gastrointestinal function. Coordination of care among the healthcare providers guarantees that care is integrated in the management of the complicated and often multifaceted needs of these patients. Along with this, as recovery goes on, nutrition becomes a necessary priority; post-operative nutrition needs to be taken care of carefully, beginning with enteral nutrition once tolerated, to contribute towards healing and prevent gastrointestinal complications (Juillard et al., 2010). Last but not least, the importance of rehabilitation and follow-up cannot be overestimated in the post-operative management of pancreatic trauma. Surgeons must develop a personalized follow-up plan to evaluate for late complications such as pancreatic insufficiency or the development of diabetes, both of which have a considerable impact on the quality of life of the patients. Integration of dietitians and endocrinologists can improve healing by providing meticulous attention to nutritional and metabolic requirements. Regular follow-up visits are a must to evaluate the functional status of the patients, apply lifestyle changes, and monitor complications that can arise as a result of the trauma and surgery. This whole process of post-operative care not only improves outcomes but also empowers patients to regain control of their path to recovery (Coccolini et al., 2019) (Figure 14.11).

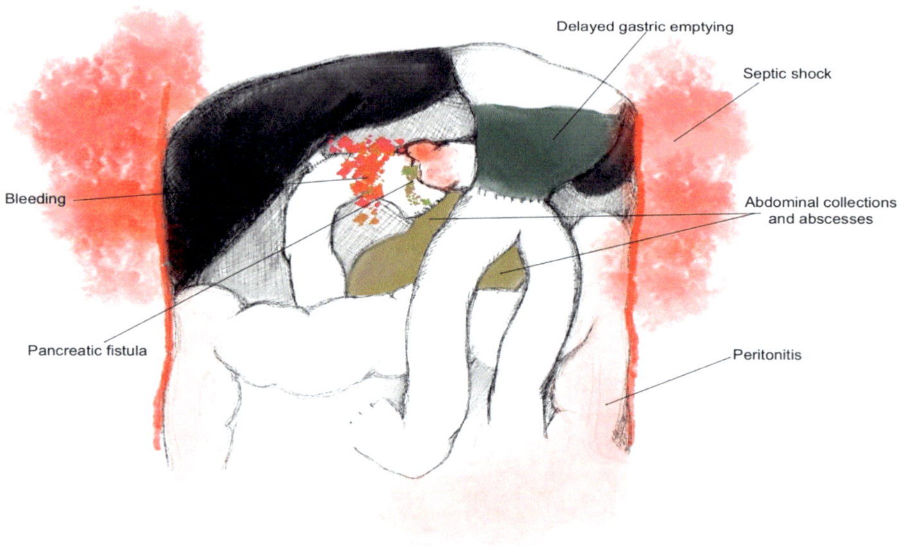

Figure 14.11. Post-operative care and monitoring of surgical intervention for pancreatic injuries.

Source: Gajda M, Grudzińska E, Szmigiel P, Czopek P, Rusinowski C, Putowski Z, Mrowiec S. Risk Factors of Postoperative Acute Pancreatitis and Its Impact on the Postoperative Course after Pancreaticoduodenectomy—10 Years of Single-Center Experience. *Life*. 2023; 13(12):2344. https://doi.org/10.3390/life13122344

14.5. Non-Surgical Management Strategies

Non-surgical management modalities of pancreatic injury have gained increased popularity because they facilitate effective healing with less risk incurred as opposed to surgical options. One of the secrets of these modalities is accurate grading of the injury, which determines whether one adopts conservative management or surgery. Some of the non-surgical procedures include monitoring, resuscitation with fluids, and nutritional support.

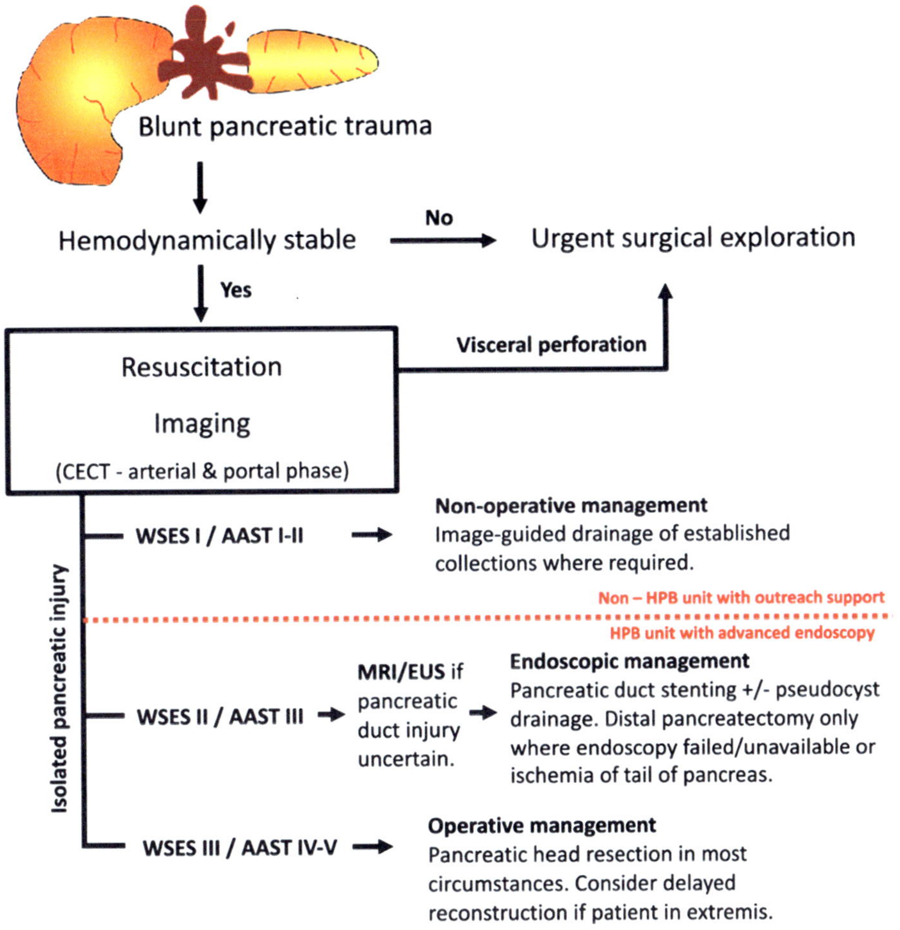

Figure 14.12. Non-surgical management strategies for pancreatic trauma.

Source: https://www.researchgate.net/publication/371773533/figure/fig3/AS:11431281172817408@1688659638890/Management-flow-chart-for-blunt-pancreatic-trauma-Proposed-flow-chart-for-the.png.

These methods are meant to enhance healing and prevent complications arising from pancreatic trauma, particularly in minor or moderate trauma patients. Such interventions can lower morbidity associated with invasive interventions, pointing to the importance of tailor-made and cautious management of pancreatic trauma. Research shows that application of non-surgical management is capable of delivering positive outcomes in carefully selected cases, which points toward patient-specific treatment in trauma care (Krige, 2017). The role of imaging in non-surgical management cannot be emphasized enough, as it aids in estimating the extent of pancreatic injury and guiding clinical decisions. With methodologies like CT scans, clinicians are able to completely visualize the pancreas and identify associated complications such as pancreatic fluid collections or necrosis. In the presence of a suspected pancreatic duct injury, imaging methodologies can be used to stratify treatment protocols. In particular, non-surgical therapeutic regimens may include percutaneous drainage of pancreatic pseudo cysts and somatostatin analog use, allowing pancreatic secretions to decrease, thus healing. By monitoring patients closely and employing these adjunctive treatments, healthcare professionals are able to maximize the rate of recovery while minimizing surgeries to an absolute minimum (Memon et al., 2013). Although ideal treatment is non-surgical, there should always be awareness of its limitations and also the possible complications. Aggressive monitoring and supportive therapy are indispensable while keeping in mind that not all patients may react favorably to conservative strategies. Complications such as infection or persistent hemorrhage in certain cases may necessitate surgical intervention, even after initial management with non-operative methods. To this end, a multidisciplinary team with trauma surgeons, radiologists, and intensivists becomes important for managing complex pancreatic injury. Thorough assessment of each patient's individual presentation and course with non-surgical intervention will ultimately determine treatment, enabling the best possible outcome (Krige, 2017) (Figure 14.12).

14.5.1. Indications for Non-Operative Management

Non-operative therapy is an appropriate choice for certain patients in the context of pancreatic trauma with specific patterns of injury and clinical presentation. The approach is strongly indicated in stable hemodynamic patients, absence of peritonitis, and grade I and grade II injuries based on the AAST classification. The benefit of non-operative treatment is that it decreases surgical complications and maintains pancreatic function wherever possible. Conservative management strategies such as observation, nutritional care, and pain management can be successful while avoiding complications of surgical treatment. Clinicians should remain watchful for developing complications, with delayed presentation potentially advancing morbidity with pancreatic trauma, leading to the necessity of an adequate initial evaluation. The management of pancreatic injury now includes more endoscopic and percutaneous procedures, which significantly enhance the available non-operative care. Endoscopic procedures can help in managing ductal injuries and preventing the spread of complications, thus allowing patients to avoid immediate surgery, as per the guidelines of the World Society of Emergency Surgery (WSES). Percutaneous drainage techniques can also be utilized very effectively for any resulting abscesses or collections of fluid, further confirming the non-operative course. By utilizing these minimally invasive techniques, physicians are better able to enhance recovery capacity and reduce the need for more invasive surgical interventions, often commonly associated with increased morbidity. The capability of treating certain injuries non-operatively is evidence of a shift toward more individualized care strategies in trauma management. While the benefits of non-operative management are obvious, it is equally important to realize the limitations and potential risks of such an approach. Some injury patterns, such as those with severe extrahepatic biliary and duodeno-pancreatic injuries, are typically not amenable to non-operative management due to the associated high morbidity and mortality. The presence of hemodynamic instability or signs of peritonitis could determine the need for urgent surgical intervention, highlighting the importance of meticulous examination in initial management. As explained, the possibility of late diagnosis and treatment can complicate courses, reaffirming the importance of watchfulness and follow-up. Overall, while non-operative management is a great choice for some patients with pancreatic injury, thorough assessment of the severity of the injury and stability of the patient is required for optimal outcomes in accordance with modern management guidelines (Coccolini et al., 2019; Hecker et al., 2019).

14.5.2. Role of Imaging in Non-Surgical Management

Imaging is an important modality in the non-operative management of pancreatic trauma, allowing for early diagnosis, grading of the severity of injury, and planning. Recent advances in imaging modalities such as CT have revolutionized the evaluation of blunt and penetrating pancreatic injuries. CT scan provides exquisite visualization of the pancreas and associated structures that allows for accurate grading of injury based on established criteria.

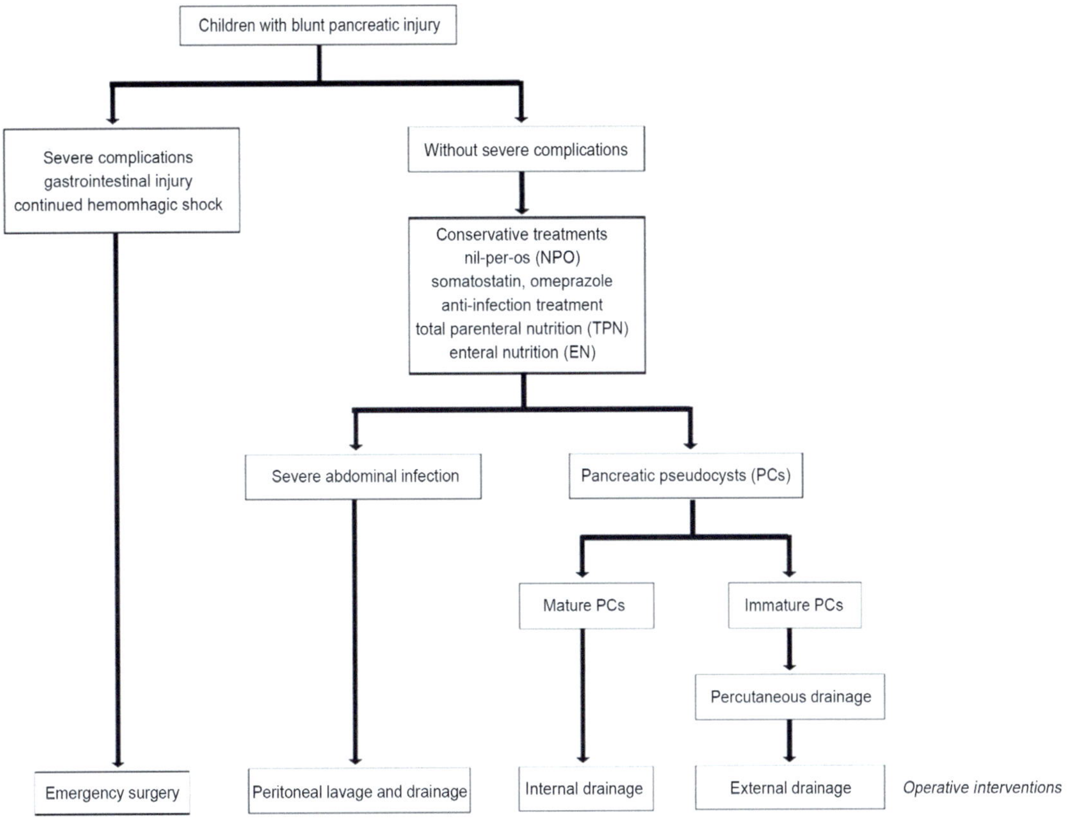

Figure 14.13. Role in the non-surgical management of pancreatic trauma.

Source: Zhang, D., Yan, J., Siyin, S.T. *et al.* Nonresection management of the pancreas for grade III and IV blunt pancreatic injuries in children: a single center's experience. *BMC Pediatr* **21**, 75 (2021). https://doi.org/10.1186/s12887-021-02535-0

This imaging is critical in determining whether a non-operative approach is feasible, especially where hemodynamic stability is maintained. Non-surgical management becomes more prominent through the potential of preventing complications of invasive treatment, alongside advancing early detection of subtle injuries, which could evolve over time (Hecker et al., 2019). This reliance on imaging serves the purpose of enabling clinicians to make evidence-based decisions regarding the care of patients with pancreatic trauma, ultimately improving outcomes. The role of imaging is also supplemented by the fact that it enables follow-up of post-traumatic complications after non-operative management of pancreatic injury. Following the initial assessment and management, patients require follow-up imaging for the detection of complications such as fluid collection, abscess, or delayed hemorrhage. These complications can develop insidiously and manifest overtly only when they need treatment. Complications can be recognized early and managed appropriately, either conservatively or by endoscopic means, using modalities like ultrasound or follow-up CT scans. Even for late-presenting sequelae patients, it has been linked with significantly reduced morbidity and mortality (Coccolini et al., 2019). Thus, regular imaging monitoring supports the plan of non-surgical management, ultimately contributing to better patient outcomes in pancreatic injury. Apart from its diagnostic and monitoring roles, imaging also guides therapeutic procedures within non-surgical management. Techniques such as endoscopic drainage or percutaneous catheter placement solely rely on imaging to ensure accurate guidance, minimizing risks associated with such interventions. As a case point, when patients are seen with pancreatic pseudocysts or fluid collections, imaging can aid in determining the optimal size and location of catheter placement for successful drainage and reduced risk of potential complications. The imaging-interventional radiology interaction is a paradigm shift towards minimally invasive treatment methods, especially in patients who are not suitable candidates for surgical treatment (Hecker et al., 2019). With advancing technology, imaging continues to be a key part of the non-operative management of pancreatic trauma, emphasizing its pivotal function in enhancing patient care in an area that is susceptible to complexity (Figure 14.13).

14.5.3. Nutritional Support and Management of Complications

Nutritional care of the patient following pancreatic injury is crucial in recovery, particularly after surgery. After surgeries such as pancreas-sparing duodenectomy, early enteral nutrition post-surgery is required to reinitiate gastrointestinal function as well as support metabolic needs. For instance, studies report that enteral nutrition can be started within 20 hours of surgery, significantly reducing malnutrition-related complications and having a highly impactful effect on the rate of recovery. In trauma care, provision of sufficient nutritional support not only helps in the healing of wounds but also contributes toward reducing the rate of postoperative complications. Proper nutritional planning for patients with traumatic pancreas injuries is fundamental since it directly reflects their quality of life and overall outcome, which highlights the need to incorporate nutrition into postoperative protocol (Dudek et al., 2009). Complication management after pancreatic trauma involves not just surgical treatment but also optimal nutritional care. Complications such as pancreatitis, fistula, and sepsis can complicate the recovery course and might necessitate a shift in nutrition plans. Nutritional support can be switched from normal enteral feeds to specialized low-fat feeds with easily absorbed proteins in such patients. Such adjustment can aid in the control of symptoms as well as healing in a poor post-operative setting. Moreover, active monitoring of nutritional status during recuperation allows for physicians to provide interventions in a timely fashion against deficiency. Good standards of personalized nutrition care are thus the solution to the avoidance of long-term consequences on health since better nutritional care is synergistic with better surgical recovery and less prolonged hospitalization, illustrating the interconnected nature of nutrition and clinical recovery (Krige, 2017). In addition to managing acute nutritional needs, long-term follow-up is indicated for patients with pancreatic trauma. Regular nutritional assessment must be a component of post-trauma care to prevent chronic conditions such as weight loss and malnutrition that may arise from excessive diet restriction or surgical manipulation over time. Interventions and proper modifications in dietary planning can be implemented in time owing to frequent assessments. It should be noted that favorable long-term outcomes in patients who have undergone pancreas-sparing procedures highlight the benefit of being able to maintain a robust nutritional plan. The addition of multidisciplinary teams, including dietitians, can maximize the quality of care and promote the optimal recovery trajectory. By and large, aggressive nutritional management is established as a pillar in the successful treatment of complications following pancreatic trauma, emphasizing the importance of nutrition in medical recuperation (Dudek et al., 2009).

14.6. Post-Traumatic Complications

The consequence of pancreatic trauma, irrespective of whether it is caused by blunt or penetrating trauma, has the potential to generate a spectrum of post-traumatic complications that require careful management. These complications consist of pancreatic necrosis, pseudocyst formation, and ductal disruption, which follow as a result of the pancreas's central role in digestion and endocrine function.

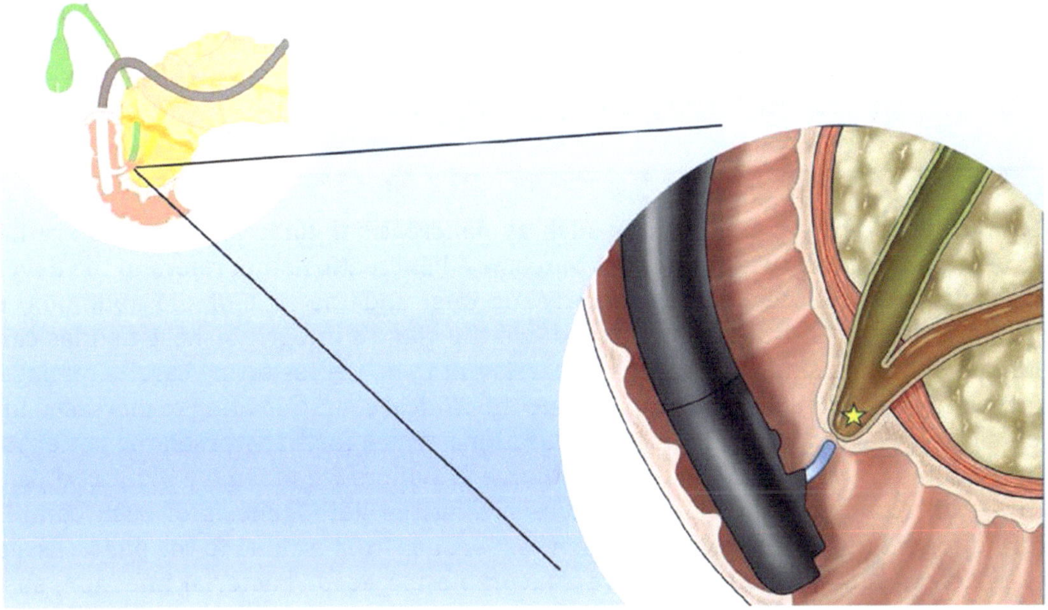

Figure 14.14. Post-endoscopic retrograde cholangiopancreatography pancreatitis.

Source: https://mednexus.org/cms/asset/fd8711e0-040c-4b86-9ce0-7d7bfc0d6f0d/jp9.0000000000000165.png.

Upon injury, physiological responses have the potential to generate severe impairments in pancreatic function, thus complicating the clinical scenario. Particularly, organ disruption and hematomas around the injured organs offer a rich soil for secondary infection and sepsis-related inflammatory syndrome. In a review of surgical versus conservative treatment of pancreatic trauma, post-traumatic evaluations from the study illustrated how the early identification and management could significantly curb long-term morbidity of such complications, illustrating the crux of postoperative follow-up and the need for individualized therapeutic treatment in a bid to improve patient outcomes (Krige, 2017). Modern imaging modalities have improved the management of post-traumatic complications of pancreatic trauma. The initial CT scans are crucial diagnostic tools to assess the severity of injury and identify complications like fluid collection or necrosis. These scan findings should, however, be correlated with follow-up imaging, e.g., MRCP or ERCP, for proper assessment. Research highlights that while the initial CT scans can produce false negatives or indeterminate results, their repetition will provide essential information about the ongoing pathological changes in the pancreas (Alhilli et al., 2008). Optimization of imaging protocols is also important for accurate diagnosis of trauma and planning appropriate surgery, further supporting the role of watchful imaging in preventing post-traumatic complications. Treatment of post-traumatic complications needs a multi-disciplinary approach, integrating surgical, medical, and radiological expertise. For necrosis or pancreatic pseudocysts, surgical management versus conservative care is based on clinical presentation and ongoing risk assessment. Serial imaging and laboratory evaluation are crucial because collections of fluid can represent complications necessitating intervention. A structured treatment plan for post-traumatic complications allows practitioners to handle the complexities that come with pancreatic trauma, significantly affecting patient recovery and quality of life. Continuous research into optimal modes of treatment and protocols, as noted in recent studies, is a sign of a desire to further advance in the context of pancreatic injuries, enhancing patient outcomes and treatment (Krige, 2017) (Figure 14.14).

14.6.1. Acute Complications (e.g., Pancreatic Fistula, and Abscess)

In pancreatic trauma, acute complications such as pancreatic fistulae and abscess are important concerns that may drastically change patient outcomes. Pancreatic fistula refers to the development of an irregular connection between the pancreatic duct and the rest of the abdomen, typically after surgical procedures or trauma, breaking down the gland's integrity. These fistulas can lead to substantial loss of fluid, malnourishment, and persistent pain, necessitating careful management to prevent additional morbidity. They also complicate the clinical course, leading to increased utilization of healthcare resources and longer in-hospital durations, which further worsen the patient's disease and recovery course (Al-Aref et al., 2024). Healthcare providers who manage blunt and penetrating injury to the pancreas must have knowledge regarding the pathogenesis of such complications. Abscess formation is another acute complication that ensues from trauma to the pancreas. Following injury, the pancreas gets infected and offers a favorable target for bacterial infection, so that pus accumulates in localized collections. Clinical presentation of pancreatic abscess is initially nonspecific, and it may present as fever and abdominal pain, such that diagnosis and treatment are delayed. This delay contributes to a cascading effect in patient healing, leading to increased surgeries and prolonged hospital stays (Krige, 2017). If it is not diagnosed and aggressively treated, abscesses can progress to systemic infection and sepsis, further advancing the risk of mortality. Therefore, a high degree of suspicion is warranted, most particularly in those high-risk patients who have experienced severe pancreatic trauma. Management of these acute complications must be tailored to the patient based on how extensive the injury and the overall clinical condition. For pancreatic fistulas, nonsurgical treatment, e.g., dietary modification and use of somatostatin analogs—may suffice at times. Severe complications, however, can necessitate surgical intervention to cover over the pancreatic duct and prevent additional complications. Similarly, pancreatic abscesses typically also require drainage, to be achieved either percutaneously or operatively, depending on their size and location. The operative management of such complications points to the delicate balance of maintaining pancreatic function and addressing potentially life-threatening processes (Al-Aref et al., 2024). Creating standardized protocols for their management, as espoused in the literature in recent years, holds the potential to improve the outcomes in severely injured patients, offering a means to reduce associated morbidity and optimize recovery.

14.6.2. Long-Term Complications (e.g., Diabetes, Chronic Pancreatitis)

The pancreas, while not always really talked about when trauma is being considered, is an important endocrine and exocrine system organ. Injury to the organ, either blunt or penetrating trauma, can lead to significant long-term complications such as diabetes mellitus and pancreatitis. Following trauma, damage to the pancreatic tissue can lead to defective insulin production, causing hyperglycemia and potentially leading to the formation of diabetes. Studies indicate that patients who are subjected to pancreatic injuries have a higher risk of developing insulin-dependent diabetes in the later stages of their life, particularly if the injury results in partial or complete pancreatectomy. Not only does it affect metabolic control, but also raises the patient's risk for comorbidities, further complicating the patient's state in the long term. The result of such a chronic condition necessitates ongoing medical attention and lifestyle changes to maintain glucose within normal levels. Chronic pancreatitis is also a potential complication that arises from damage to the pancreas. It typically occurs due to ongoing inflammation and fibrosis, processes that may be triggered by initial trauma or repeated pancreatic injuries. The long-term inflammation causes injury to the structure and function of the pancreas, resulting in permanent damage and often pain, malabsorption, and endocrine deficit. Patients with chronic pancreatitis may experience debilitating pain that significantly impacts their quality of life. Moreover, research has shown that patients with chronic pancreatitis are more likely to have pancreatic cancer, contributing to the long-term effects of traumatic insult to this organ. The long-term nature of such conditions highlights the importance of multidisciplinary management of patients, combining surgical treatment, pain relief, and nutrition. Management of long-term complications of pancreatic trauma requires unified effort on the part of clinicians to manage both short-term and long-term illness. Preventive management is needed to monitor and reverse the complications of diabetes and chronic pancreatitis. Recommendations to the affected individuals usually involve frequent follow-ups with specialists in endocrinology and gastroenterology to individualize treatment regimens that include dietary changes, pharmacological management, and lifestyle modifications. Education concerning identifying symptoms of complications is necessary to enable the patients to manage their health proactively. Such an exhaustive approach not only improves the quality of the patients' lives but also attempts to reduce the healthcare burden of the long-term pancreatic injuries, highlighting the importance of precise post-trauma management in surgical practice (Juillard et al., 2010; Park et al., 2021).

14.6.3. Strategies for Prevention and Management of Complications

Efficacious management of complications secondary to pancreatic trauma demands aggressive strategy in prevention and intervention. Initiation of patient assessment is paramount, with thorough imaging to establish the extent of injury and associated risk, guiding individualized treatment strategy. Standardized assessment processes enhance the ability for early detection of injuries, allowing timely interventions. Such structured evaluation is particularly relevant as pancreatic injury has varied presentations and a wise approach to management is the only requirement. The employment of evidence-based recommendations derived from large-scale studies, e.g., a big cohort analysis, will provide a similar response to similar patterns of injury, thus encouraging training and decision-making in acute care (Krige, 2017). Furthermore, immediate resuscitation and stabilization of the patient are paramount to decreasing complications and can affect overall recovery outcomes. Surgical intervention remains a pivotal intervention in traumatic pancreatic injury treatment, with techniques carefully selected based on grade of injury and patient status. In the case of significant hemorrhage or tissue necrosis, early operative exploration and debridement can go far in reducing infection and other complication risk. The operative or non-operative management should be decided based on the nature of the injury and the physiological condition of the patients, with trauma surgeons playing the central role in making such critical decisions. The integration of a multidisciplinary effort with radiologists and critical care providers will further improve patient outcomes through comprehensive treatment planning. Additionally, setting up post-operative care routines with focus on monitoring for complications such as necrosis of the pancreas or abscess can also simplify the recovery process. Implementation of trauma care education programs also holds a central role in prevention and treatment procedures. Professional education in new protocols for pancreatic injury and complication management can lead to improved clinical outcomes as well as decreased complications. Collaboration through periodic workshops and simulated trauma cases enhances learning and readiness for real-life emergencies, where rapid decision-making is vital. Emphasis on interprofessional collaboration, such as in Australia's South Metropolitan Health Service, encourages an integrated model of care in which communication channels between surgical teams, nurses, and allied health personnel are optimized. Finally, ongoing investigation to refine current limitations to knowledge about pancreatic trauma will guide future management, making the trauma surgery community responsive and capable of adapting to new evidence (Krige, 2017) (Figure 14.15).

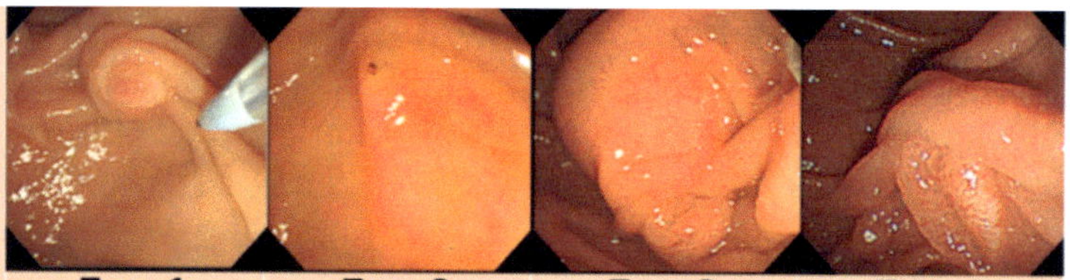

PAPILLA MORPHOLOGY	Type 1 (Regular)	Type 2 (Small)	Type 3 (Protruding)	Type 4 (Creased/Ridged)
Prevalence	56%	13%	23%	8%
Cannulation Failure	2% (REF)	12% (OR 7.9)*	11% (OR 7.3)*	6% (OR 3.9)
Difficult Cannulation	36%	52%*	48%*	43%
Pancreatitis	7%	20%*	2%	6%

Figure 14.15. Post-ERCP pancreatitis: Prevention, diagnosis, and management.

Source: Cahyadi O, Tehami N, de-Madaria E, Siau K. Post-ERCP Pancreatitis: Prevention, Diagnosis and Management. *Medicina*. 2022; 58(9):1261. https://doi.org/10.3390/medicina58091261

A CLOSER LOOK

PANCREATIC DAMAGE CONTROL

Pancreatic damage control is an emergency surgical and medical treatment employed in the treatment of severe pancreatic trauma or inflammation in unstable patients where immediate definitive repair can be avoided. The procedure is most commonly used for blunt or penetrating pancreatic injuries that are severe, severe acute necrotizing pancreatitis, or iatrogenic injury during abdominal procedures. The goal of control of pancreatic damage is to stabilize the patient at the physiological level and reduce ongoing contamination, bleeding, and enzymatic injury. Early surgical management focuses on hemorrhage control and containment of pancreatic enzymes and infected material from dissemination. External drainage of the pancreas, packing of points of bleeding, and temporary closure of the abdomen with a vacuum-assisted device or other techniques that allow re-exploration (Figure 14.16) can be performed.

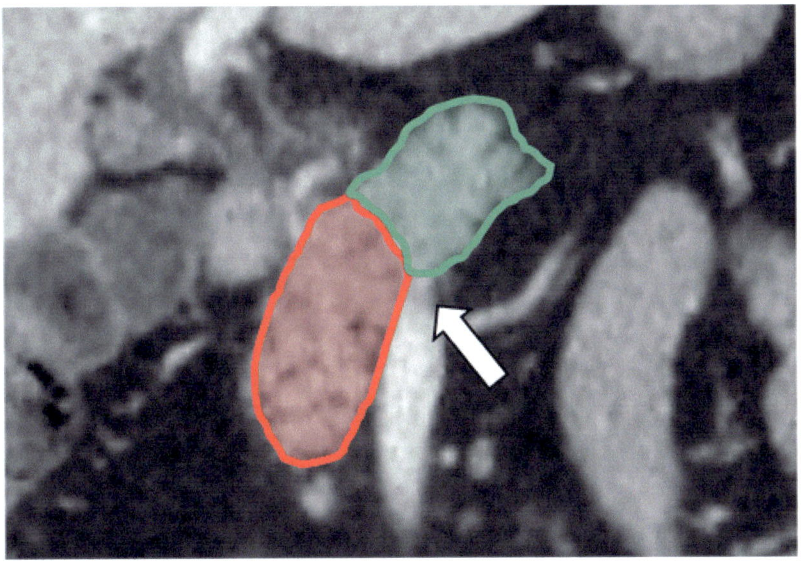

Source: https://external-content.duckduckgo.com/iu/?u=https%3A%2F%2Fpubs.rsna.org%2Fcms%2F10.1148%2Frg.2021200077%2Fasset%2Fimages%2Fmedium%2Frg.2021200077.fig7b.gif&f=1&nofb=1&ipt=ff7a5c1f5210de50234b9cfdb24c62ca947640dd2e036d1073259444e28b984b.

In trauma, particularly of the pancreatic duct, a major problem is pancreatic enzyme leakage, which can lead to autodigestion, abscess, and systemic inflammatory response. In the event of suspected injury to the duct but inability to properly assess it in the acute situation, drains are placed about the pancreas for the control of leakage and deferring definitive reconstruction until the patient is stabilized hemodynamically. In necrotizing pancreatitis, early surgical intervention is normally avoided with the exception of in the case of established infected necrosis, where a step-up approach is optimal, initiating with percutaneous or endoscopic drainage and progressing to necrosectomy as needed. Postoperatively, patients are managed in intensive care with aggressive fluid resuscitation, nutrition, usually by enteral feedings, and broad-spectrum antibiotics should infection be impending. Serial imaging and lab monitoring allows for assessment of need for further intervention. Definitive therapy, e.g., distal pancreatectomy or pancreaticojejunostomy, is delayed until inflammation has resolved and patient stability allows. Multidisciplinary management by surgeons, intensivists, gastroenterologists, and interventional radiologists is critical for optimal outcomes. Pancreatic damage control has enhanced critically ill patients' survival by prioritizing physiologic stabilization and staged intervention over early definitive surgery in complex pancreatic injuries.

SUMMARY

Pancreatic trauma treatment involves a differential consideration of both the mechanism of trauma and the general clinical status of the patient. The findings from the extensive literature support the importance of individualizing treatment modalities in the context of such variables as the nature and severity of injury, and the hemodynamic stability of the patient. The increasing trend towards NOM in stable patients has significant consequences for the surgical approach, necessitating a more conservative approach in some cases. This shift is an acknowledgment of the benefits of preserving pancreatic function and eliminating the morbidity of more complex surgical interventions, harmonizing with improvements in imaging modalities and interventional radiology, enabling these choices. Furthermore, the grading of pancreatic injuries with standardized grading systems is valuable for clinical decision-making and communication. Implementation of a uniform grading approach assists with improved understanding of the severity of injury, guiding operative management where necessary. As can be observed, the evolution of diagnostic imaging technology, such as CT, has significantly enhanced speed and precision in trauma assessment. These advancements are essential in developing appropriate management channels, as they allow for direct recognition of complications and the selection of appropriate treatment modalities (Krige, 2017). Additionally, an evidence-based discussion of surgical management approaches is essential, as such debate brings forth information on best practices that can drive patient outcomes for complicated pancreatic trauma cases. Lastly, ongoing research in overcoming the shortcomings put forth in current methodology is required for pancreatic trauma care to be improved constantly. Exploration of overlooked avenues and establishment of robust clinical evidence are imperative for the further enhancement of surgical methods and patient treatment. As indicated in recent studies, the value of learning from an extended patient cohort underlines the requirement of well-structured clinical guidelines responsive to emerging evidence (Krige, 2017). Only through such evidentiary standards is the surgical community capable of learning towards improved outcomes and reducing the post-traumatic morbidity of pancreatic trauma, so that patients can be given the most effective and safest treatment possible.

Traumatic pancreatic injuries, either penetrating or blunt, present extreme challenges for surgical management. Grading of pancreatic injury is to guide management because it puts the magnitude of the trauma into grades according to established criteria. These grades range from minor injury that may be managed conservatively to major injury that needs to be operated on. The anatomical intricacy of the pancreas, as well as its relationship with surrounding structures, complicates diagnosis and planning for treatment. Moreover, the lack of adequate robust clinical evidence does not allow for the consistent implementation of treatment protocols, making the adoption of consistent practice within trauma centers to facilitate improved patient outcomes (Krige, 2017). The process guarantees a decrease in inherent pancreatic trauma-related complications while optimizing the resuscitation and surgical handling process. With surgical treatment, operative and non-operative interventions both take a central role in the management of pancreatic injury. Literature suggests that trauma surgery remains patient-dependent and must find a balance between conservative and aggressive treatment based on the grading of the injury. Assessment of individual cases usually includes imaging studies that inform assessment of the extent of injury and make up part of the planning for the operation. Resuscitation, along with successful subsequent surgical intervention, is key in reducing morbidity for pancreatic trauma. Additionally, identifying complications after trauma to the pancreas—pancreatic fistulas, infection, and abscesses—glimpses long-term patient management, tremendous developments in surgical techniques can yield better outcomes. Overall, treating pancreatic injury encompasses a myriad of factors from initial assessment to long-term treatment. The interplay between injury grading, surgery, and subsequent complications underscores the critical role of multi-disciplinary collaboration in trauma care. Ongoing research has worked towards filling gaps in research and improving the model for diagnosing and managing pancreatic injuries optimally. Pooling data from large-volume trauma centers can further enable refinement of current management guidelines to ultimately advance improvements in patient care. These advances are seminal to the handling of the complexities of trauma to the pancreas such that prompt and later clinical needs are fulfilled effectively (Krige, 2017).

KEY TERMS FROM THIS CHAPTER

- Blunt pancreatic injuries
- Duodenum
- Formal grading system
- Ischemia
- Minor contusion
- Nutrition
- Pancreatic grading
- Blunt pancreatic injury
- Endocrine
- Grading systems
- Lacerations
- Non-operative management (NOM)
- Pancreatic fistula
- Pancreatic parenchymal injuries

References

1. Aarabi, S., Durand, R., Evans, L. L., Jensen, G., et al. (2021). *Torso Vascular Trauma*. https://core.ac.uk/download/617035627.pdf (accessed on 26 May 2025).
2. Coccolini, F., Kobayashi, L., Kluger, Y. *et al.* Duodeno-pancreatic and extrahepatic biliary tree trauma: WSES-AAST guidelines. *World J Emerg Surg* **14**, 56 (2019). https://doi.org/10.1186/s13017-019-0278-6 (accessed on 26 May 2025).
3. Zingg, T., Agri, F., Bourgeat, M., Yersin, B., Romain, B., Schmidt, S., Keller, N., & Demartines, N. (2018). Avoiding delayed diagnosis of significant blunt bowel and mesenteric injuries: Can a scoring tool make the difference? A 7-year retrospective cohort study. *Injury*, *49*(1), 33–41. https://doi.org/10.1016/j.injury.2017.09.004 (accessed on 26 May 2025).
4. Al-Aref, R., Choron, R. L., Kirsch, M., et al. (2024). *Pancreaticoduodenectomy in Trauma Patients with Grade IV–V Duodenal or Pancreatic Injuries: A Post Hoc Analysis of An EAST Multicenter Trial*. https://core.ac.uk/download/643771889.pdf (accessed on 26 May 2025).
5. Alhilli, S., Allam, H., Darweesh, A., Ismail, H., et al. (2008). Imaging of blunt pancreatic trauma: The value of initial and sequential CT examinations. Scientific Exhibit DOI-Link: https://dx.doi.org/10.1594/ecr2010/C-0181 (accessed on 26 May 2025).
6. Park, K. M., Rashidian, N., Mohamedaly, S., Brasel, K. J., Conroy, P., Glencer, A. C., He, J., Passeri, M. J., Katariya, N. N., Alseidi, A., & TrainHPB research group (2021). Unifying the Hepatopancreatobiliary Surgery Fellowship Curriculum via Delphi Consensus. *Journal of the American College of Surgeons*, *233*(3), 395–414. https://doi.org/10.1016/j.jamcollsurg.2021.06.004 (accessed on 26 May 2025).
7. Juillard, C., Etoundi Mballa, G. A., Bilounga Ndongo, C., Stevens, K. A., & Hyder, A. A. (2011). Patterns of injury and violence in Yaoundé Cameroon: an analysis of hospital data. *World journal of surgery*, *35*(1), 1–8. https://doi.org/10.1007/s00268-010-0825-5
8. Brohi, I. B., Kalhoro, N., Laghari, H. R., et al. (2020). Complication rates in managing hepatic trauma: A cross-sectional study stratifying their outcomes. https://core.ac.uk/download/543135762.pdf (accessed on 26 May 2025).
9. Everson, E., Buschel, H., Carroll, J., & Palamuthusingam, P. (2023). Paediatric pancreatic trauma in North Queensland: a 10-year retrospective review. *BMC pediatrics*, *23*(1), 88. https://doi.org/10.1186/s12887-023-03904-7 (accessed on 26 May 2025).
10. Devarajani. (2010). *Evaluation of Patients with Penetrating Injury to Abdominal Organs at K.A.P.V Government Medical College and Annal Gandhi Memorial Government Hospital, Trichy* [Master's thesis]. https://core.ac.uk/download/235667013.pdf (accessed on 26 May 2025).
11. Dudek, W., Hart, C. A., Lowery, K., Paluszkiewicz, R., et al. (2009). Pancreas sparing duodenectomy as an emergency procedure. https://core.ac.uk/download/pdf/8295296.pdf.
12. Ghouri, M., Gupta, N., Bhat, A. P., Thimmappa, N., Saboo, S. S., Khandelwal, A., & Nagpal, P. (2019). CT and MR imaging of the upper extremity vasculature: Pearls, pitfalls, and challenges. *Cardiovascular Diagnosis and Therapy, 9*(Suppl 1), S152–S173. https://doi.org/10.21037/cdt.2018.09.15.
13. Hecker, A., Kirkpatrick, A., Leppaniemi, A., Pikoulis, A., Mefire, A. C., De Simone, B., Sakakushev, B., et al. (2019). *Duodeno-Pancreatic and Extrahepatic Biliary Tree Trauma: WSES-AAST Guidelines*. https://core.ac.uk/download/288798568.pdf (accessed on 26 May 2025).

14. Wallis, A., Kelly, M. D., & Jones, L. (2010). Angiography and embolisation for solid abdominal organ injury in adults - a current perspective. *World journal of emergency surgery : WJES, 5*, 18. https://doi.org/10.1186/1749-7922-5-18

15. Ball, C. G., Dixon, E., Kirkpatrick, A. W., Sutherland, F. R., Laupland, K. B., & Feliciano, D. V. (2010). A decade of experience with injuries to the gallbladder. *Journal of trauma management & outcomes, 4*, 3. https://doi.org/10.1186/1752-2897-4-3

16. Krige, J. 2017. A prospective evaluation to define optimal surgical strategies in the management of complex pancreatic injuries based on the analysis of patients treated at a major South African academic institution. University of Cape Town.https://core.ac.uk/download/185391081.pdf.

17. Memon, A. A., Zafar, H., Raza, R., & Murtaza, G. (2013). Traumatic pancreatic injury--an elusive diagnosis: experience from a developing country urban trauma referral centre. *JPMA. The Journal of the Pakistan Medical Association, 63*(4), 440–444. (accessed on 26 May 2025).

18. Mohanasundaram, N. (2019). *Comprehensive Management of Duodenal Injuries and Its Outcome* [Master's thesis]. https://core.ac.uk/download/235671057.pdf (accessed on 26 May 2025).

19. Rethinavelu, C. (2016). *One-Year Prospective Study on Accuracy of Diagnostic Peritoneal Paracentesis in Acute Abdominal Condition Requiring Emergency Surgical Intervention* [Master's thesis]. https://core.ac.uk/download/235659061.pdf (accessed on 26 May 2025).

20. Stecca, T., Nistri, C., Pauletti, B., Di Giacomo, A., Colaut, F., Ruperto, M., & Caratozzolo, E., et al. (2023). *Management of Acute and Chronic Pancreatitis*. In IntechOpen eBooks. https://doi.org/10.5772/intechopen.109115.

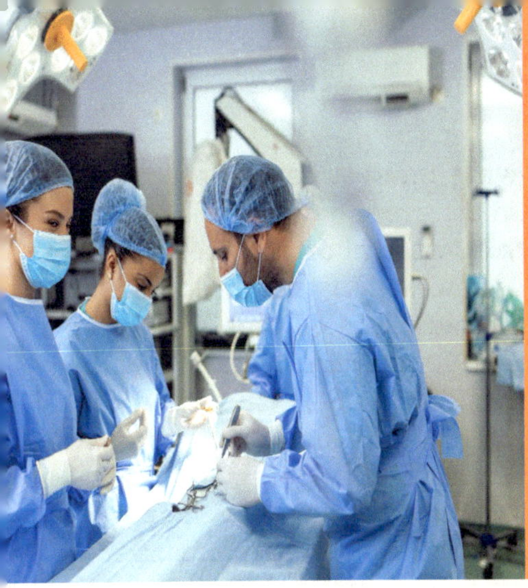

Chapter 15

SURGICAL INTERVENTIONS IN PANCREATIC DISEASES

Contents

Introduction

Surgical interventions for pancreatic conditions are an essential aspect of treating severe diseases such as pancreatic cancer, pancreatitis, and pancreatic trauma. The pancreas, being at the core of the digestive and endocrine systems, demands delicate surgical techniques to help effectively manage a range of conditions. Surgical interventions such as the Whipple procedure and distal pancreatectomy are essential in the removal of tumor tissue while minimizing traumatic impacts on pancreatic function. As indicated within literature, there is a pressing need to address gaps in data and surgical strategies, as it pertains to pancreatic injury as well as treatment (Krige, 2017). Through optimization of existing surgical methods, medical personnel are better equipped to individually tailor the outcomes of patients and provide patients with individualized care options that better reflect the diversity of each patient's disease. Furthermore, the necessity of establishing robust management guidelines is stressed by the high rates of complications for pancreatic procedures. The drainage therapy for pseudocysts and necrosis of the pancreas is of growing interest as inappropriate treatment can lead to significant morbidity. The variability of clinical presentations relating to pancreatitis, including the potential for gastrointestinal bleeding from visceral artery aneurysms, further clouds the operating picture. It is comprehension of these interactions that will enable diagnostic practice to be enhanced and the risks of surgery decreased. Detailed studies taking into account these complications suggest that early diagnosis and intervention are necessary, with improper handling resulting in lethal outcomes, demonstrating the initiative of the surgical team in preoperative planning and postoperative care (Johnson et al., 2006). In summary, pancreatic surgery is a dynamic branch of medical science and practice that necessitates ongoing evaluation of procedure efficacy and patient outcome. New technologies, such as minimally invasive therapies and newer imaging techniques, possess promising potential for enhancing the accuracy of surgery and reducing recovery time. Through ongoing review and reaction to changing evidence in the treatment of pancreatic disease, surgical techniques can more closely accommodate the complexities of individual patient conditions. Integration of improved data collection, advanced methodology of surgery, and comprehensive treatment regimens is essential in transversing challenges with the treatment of pancreatic diseases, effectively reshaping the landscape of surgical interventions in this life-sustaining area of medicine (Figure 15.1).

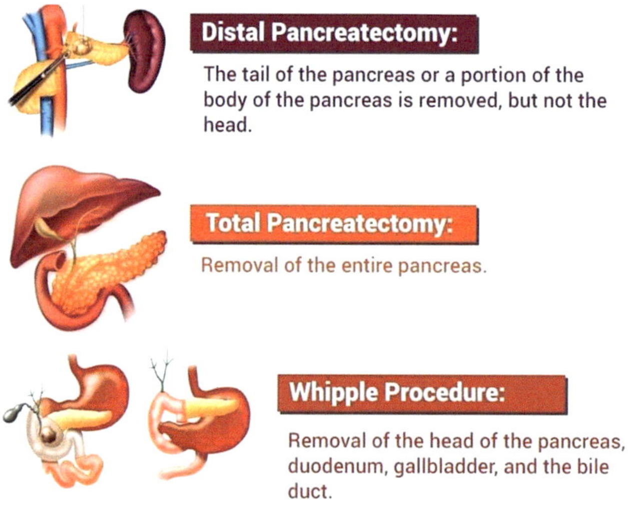

Figure 15.1. Surgical interventions in pancreatic diseases.

Source: https://www.drnikhilagrawal.com/assets/images/pancreatic-cancer-surgery.jpg.

Overview of Pancreatic Diseases

The pancreas is a vital organ with a fundamental contribution to endocrine and exocrine functions, playing a significant role in metabolic function and digestive well-being. Pancreatic disease encompasses a wide variety of conditions, ranging from acute and chronic pancreatitis to pancreatic cancer and pancreatic trauma. Acute pancreatitis can occur secondary to obstruction of the bile ducts or excessive alcohol ingestion and results in intense inflammation and potential systemic disease. On the other hand, chronic pancreatitis is characterized by irreversible morphological alterations, typically resulting in chronic pain and diminished endocrine and exocrine function, directly affecting a patient's quality of life. Prevalence of predisposing factors such as alcohol consumption also plays a significant role in making chronic pancreatitis an increasingly important issue in most populations, reflecting the complexity of the disease and the requirement for multidisciplinary approach to management. Pancreatic disease presents unique diagnostic and therapeutic difficulties, highlighting the need for intense clinical guidelines. Chronic pancreatitis is a classic difficulty regarding its heterogeneity and absence of absolute classificatory approach to therapeutic regimens. The South African guidelines highlight the importance of individual therapeutic methods, addressing variability in the etiological factors resulting in pancreatic y disturbances. This includes looking at the effectiveness of surgical and medical management, the need to continue research in the interplay of factors causating the disease. Purposeful focus on cooperative, interdisciplinary management can work significantly to improve patient outcomes in the management of such complicated disorders (Krige, 2017). Pancreatic trauma, often underestimated, is another major component of pancreatic diseases. Pancreatic injury management demands careful attention given the organ's delicate structure and complex vascular supply. Research has described existing limitations in understanding pancreatic trauma, which can lead to inappropriately untimely surgical results (Krige, 2017). Innovation in surgical techniques and the availability of standard protocol are central in meeting these limitations. The overall complexity of pancreatic conditions requires an integrated approach, combining robust data and technologies, to facilitate advancements in procedures such as the Whipple procedure and distal pancreatectomy with the aim of achieving optimal patient care and rehabilitation outcomes in the presence of such debilitating diseases (Figure 15.2).

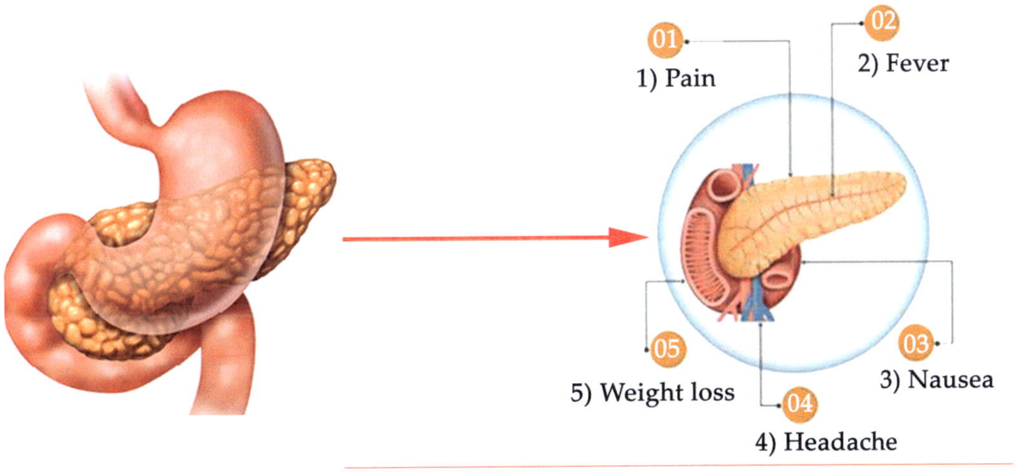

Figure 15.2. Pancreatic function in pancreatic diseases.

Source: https://liverandpancreasclinic.com/blog/wp-content/uploads/2018/09/What-Happens-To-Pancreatic-Function-In-Pancreatic-Diseases.jpg.

Importance of Surgical Interventions

Surgical management is of paramount importance in the management of pancreatic diseases due to the complex nature of the conditions affecting this organ, notably chronic pancreatitis, pancreatic malignancy, and trauma. The success of surgical interventions such as the Whipple procedure and distal pancreatectomy is of paramount importance in symptom relief and improving survival rates among patients with these debilitating conditions. The capacity to remove diseased or damaged pancreatic tissue is treating the cause of why a patient is ill. Moreover, surgical procedures can serve as final restoration measures once every avenue has been pursued. This capacity to relieve much, or even cure, is an advancement in surgical gastroenterology and oncology and evidently proves how surgical techniques can influence patient outcomes in usually hopeless circumstances. As highlighted by clinical studies, the cumulative nature of pancreatic diseases necessitates early and effective surgical procedures capable of addressing life-threatening complications (Krige, 2017). In addition to contributing towards better clinical outcomes, surgical interventions can provide life-saving support to patients suffering from chronic pancreatitis, a rapidly recognized complex and heterogeneous disease. Treatment of the disease is typically a multidisciplinary effort, as is evident with the recommendations for interventions that include surgical modalities in conjunction with medical management (Bornman et al., 2010). Surgical intervention, such as drainage of necrosis or pseudocysts, is pivotal to prevent further complications, such as infection or systemic sepsis. These interventions serve not only to manage the presence of ongoing complications but also play a key role in the restoration of pancreatic function where indicated. As learning continues to mature, it is evident that surgical options are not so much adjuncts as critical components in the global management of chronic pancreatitis, functioning as insurance measures against the mounting health emergencies that the disease can exact. Moreover, the post-operative situation of pancreatic procedures places considerable emphasis on the surveillance of possible complications and vigilant follow-up. Though surgical procedures have short-term benefits, they may lead to a series of post-operative challenges like delayed gastric emptying, endocrine deficiency, and pain. The complexity associated with these outcomes makes evidence for individualized patient care that intervenes in both the physical and psychological aspects of recovery highly pertinent. By being aware of the risks and benefits of surgical procedures, health professionals are better positioned to instruct their patients, guiding them through the experience. The exploration of new ways of performing surgery, best management practices, and ongoing research all indicate an investment in ensuring maximum patient outcomes for patients with pancreatic diseases. Surgical procedures, therefore, continue to be the focal point of therapeutic practice, contributing importantly to relief from the burdens of these complicated health conditions (Bornman et al., 2010).

15.1. Anatomy and Function of the Pancreas

Pancreas, which is a stomach organ, plays a dual vital role in the body's digestive system and metabolism. Both as an exocrine and endocrine gland, it produces vital hormones such as insulin and glucagon that regulate blood glucose levels, and digestive enzymes necessary for carbohydrate, protein, and fat digestion. The endocrine component is found in clusters of cells called islets of Langerhans, which release hormones directly into the bloodstream. The exocrine system, constituting the majority of pancreatic tissue, releases enzymes via a ductal system into the duodenum to permit digestion. Understanding this anatomy and function is crucial for evaluating surgical treatments, such as the Whipple procedure to resect parts of the pancreas to control malignancies and often has significant impact on both the exocrine and endocrine functions of the gland. Chronic inflammation and neoplastic proliferation of disease in the pancreas can erode the function of the pancreas. Illnesses such as chronic pancreatitis cause irreversible damage to pancreatic tissue and tend to end up in incapacitating chronic pain and loss of both exocrine and endocrine function. The pathogenesis of chronic pancreatitis is characteristically related to chronic alcoholism, particularly in middle-aged males, and is a significant indication for surgical treatment when medical management fails. Operative procedures such as the Frey procedure aim to reduce pain and improve pancreatic function by removing the diseased tissue while maintaining the drainage of digestive enzymes. The relationship between pancreatic anatomy and surgical techniques lies at the heart of optimizing patient outcomes, where procedure choice often relies on the specific disease process and anatomical configuration of the diseased pancreas. The intricate pancreatic anatomy is transposed to the extensive postoperative management of complications, particularly following procedures like the Whipple operation and distal pancreatectomy. Perhaps the most dreaded postoperative complication is the development of postoperative pancreatic fistula (POPF), which refers to the leakage of pancreatic enzymes from the operative site. Studies have indicated that POPF risk can range between 15%–26%, which affects overall patients' morbidity following pancreatic surgery. Factors such as pancreatic softness and duct size can be pivotal in the prediction and management of these complications, underlining the significance of thorough intraoperative assessment. For instance, the employment of standardized intraoperative pancreatic risk assessments (IPRA) will enhance clinical decision-making by offering stratification of postoperative complication risk and thereby presenting surgeons valuable information to avoid adverse outcomes as well as improve the quality of life of patients who are subjected to such complex surgery procedures (Ansorge, 2013; Sivakumar, 2015) (Figure 15.3).

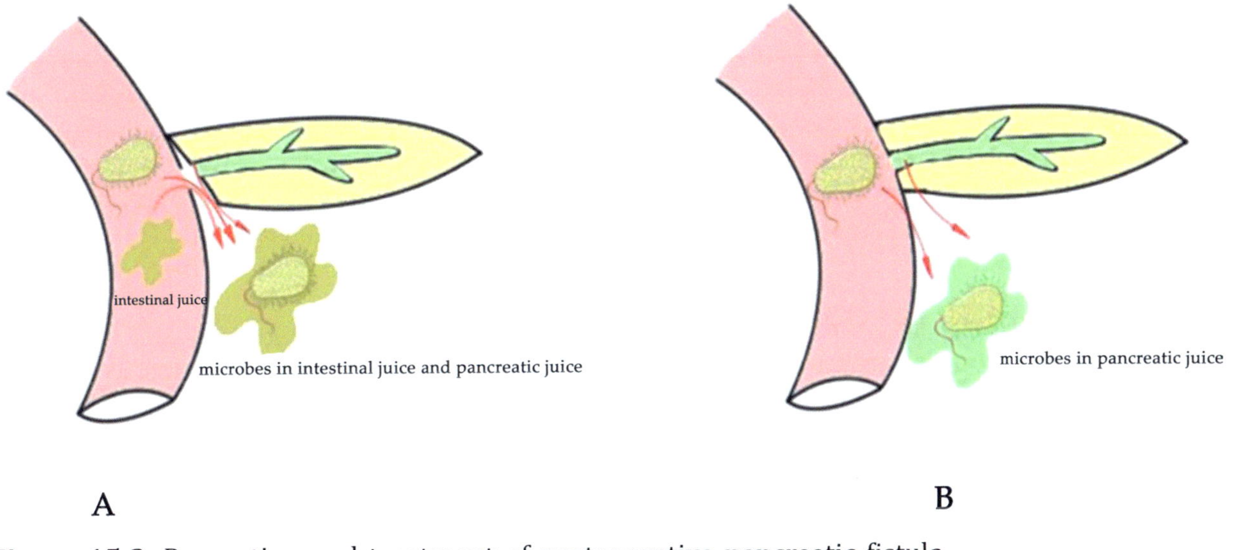

Figure 15.3. Prevention and treatment of postoperative pancreatic fistula.

Source: Xiang C, Chen Y, Liu X, Zheng Z, Zhang H, Tan C. Prevention and Treatment of Grade C Postoperative Pancreatic Fistula. *Journal of Clinical Medicine.* 2022; 11(24):7516. https://doi.org/10.3390/jcm11247516

15.1.1. Structure of the Pancreas

The pancreas, located in the retroperitoneal cavity, is an important organ that performs both endocrine and exocrine functions. Its anatomy consists of a series of various regions: head, body, and tail, all of which contribute to its overall functionality. The head of the pancreas lies within the duodenum curve, and it houses structures such as the pancreatic duct that transports digestive enzymes to the small intestine. The body and tail, lying towards the spleen, have a group of cells known as islets of Langerhans, responsible for the secretion of hormones like insulin and glucagon. Knowledge of the anatomy and functional correlation of these regions is crucial in surgeons' handling operations like the Whipple procedure or distal pancreatectomy because changes in pancreatic anatomy can lead to severe postoperative complications and affect the overall cure. The pancreas also contains acinar cells that are primarily involved in exocrine functions by secreting digestive enzymes. The enzymes, including lipases, amylases, and proteases, play significant roles in fat digestion, carbohydrate digestion, and protein digestion, respectively. The pancreas also secretes a bicarbonate-rich fluid that neutralizes the gastric acid in the duodenum and hence creates an optimal pH for enzyme function. The ductal system of the pancreas runs parallel to the biliary system anatomically, an expression of a functional synergy between the pancreas, liver, and gallbladder. Pancreatic pathology operations necessitate a close understanding of this intricate ductal anatomy since obliterations or disruptions in the ducts can initiate disastrous complications. Some conditions, such as pancreaticoduodenal adenocarcinoma or chronic pancreatitis, are typically responsible for requiring surgery to address complications arising from ductal disease, as in the setting of multiple interventions, including drainage procedures for necrosis and pseudocysts (Bornman et al., 2010). Furthermore, anatomical variations in the pancreas can significantly impact surgery. For example, the presence of anatomical abnormalities like encasement of vessels or ectopic branching of the splenic artery can make procedures such as the Whipple or distal pancreatectomy challenging. All of these operations necessitate careful pre-operative imaging studies to precisely delineate the anatomy of the pancreas and plan for it accordingly. The risk of complications like bleeding from visceral artery aneurysms points towards a high index of suspicion and vigilant technique on the part of surgeons during surgery, particularly in diseases of the pancreas. Familiarity with the architectural intricacies of the pancreas also aids in the prevention and anticipation of post-operative complications and the overall enhancement of patient outcomes in the treatment of pancreatic pathology (Johnson et al., 2006).

15.1.2. Role of the Pancreas in Digestion

The pancreas plays an important role in digestion through its two-pronged function as both an endocrine and exocrine gland. During digestion, the exocrine aspect secretes diverse enzymes such as amylase, lipase, and proteases, which play crucial roles during carbohydrate, fat, and protein digestion, respectively. The enzymes are secreted in an inactive form and discharge into the duodenum via the pancreatic duct. Their activation only after arrival at the intestinal environment to prevent autolytic destruction of the pancreatic tissue. Aside from this, the pancreas also secretes bicarbonate to neutralize gastric acid, which creates an ideal pH for enzyme activity. Therefore, any compromise in pancreatic function can potentially severely disrupt digestion, placing supreme importance on this organ in the backdrop of gastrointestinal health and on surgical interventions designed to cure pancreatic disease, which often arises as a consequence of such malfunction. Chronic pancreatitis (CP) is a case in point regarding the deleterious effects of pancreatic malfunction on digestion. Pathognomonic of persistent inflammation and chronic pancreatic damage, CP leads to a decline in exocrine and endocrine function. With worsening exocrine function, patients can have malabsorption of nutrients, presenting with weight loss, diarrhea, and malabsorption of nutrients. Alcoholism is the most frequent etiology of CP in the majority of the world, including the Western world, and it enhances pancreatic inflammation and consequent tissue scarring. Moreover, the management of patients with CP typically requires surgical procedures, which in certain instances can be the Whipple procedure or distal pancreatectomy, as explained in the surgical treatments outlined within this essay. An appreciation of the role of the pancreas in digestion does act to highlight the paramount importance of effective surgical treatment in patients with such disease, especially when other nonsurgical interventions are ineffective (Bornman et al., 2010). The interface between surgical practice and the function of the pancreas is most critical; the pancreas must be considered not just a region of disease but an essential actor within the digestive function. Procedures such as drainage procedures for pancreatic pseudocysts and management of pancreatic necrosis illustrate the need to re-establish pancreatic function for digestive processes to be effective. Following surgical management, patients are likely to experience complications that can largely influence digestive efficiency, requiring vigilant post-operative observation and treatment. The healing process may include changes in diet, enzyme replacement therapy, and regular follow-up to evaluate digestive function. The intricate mechanisms of digestion and pancreatic activity underscore the need for a thorough understanding of the pancreas function to provide an apparatus of the surgical intervention taken to ease allied complications and restore the overall status of the gastrointestinal tract (Johnson et al., 2006) (Figure 15.4).

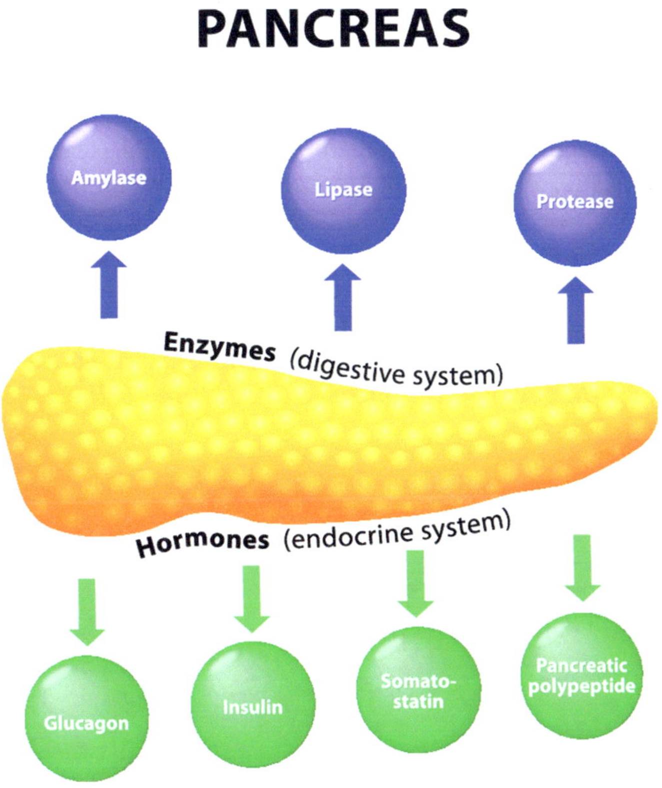

Figure 15.4. Role of the pancreas in digestion.

Source: https://external-content.duckduckgo.com/iu/?u=https%3A%2F%2Fctocrx.com%2Fwp-content%2Fuploads%2F2019%2F10%2FiStock-536892277.png&f=1&nofb=1&ipt=5ffa0391d3b084eb6c11230576ae88766bbbc09c15419131f0c78f86f6d724fa.

15.1.3. Hormonal Functions of the Pancreas

The pancreas plays a critical role in the endocrine system by exercising control over metabolic processes through its hormonal activities. It secretes crucial hormones, including insulin, glucagon, and somatostatin, primarily from the islets of Langerhans. Insulin released from beta cells enhances glucose uptake by tissues, lowering blood sugar levels. On the other hand, glucagon released from alpha cells stimulates glucose release from hepatic stores when blood sugars are low. The balance of these hormones is responsible for glucose homeostasis and hence any imbalance will lead to diabetic melitus as an abnormal condition. Such endocrine imbalance can complicate the clinical course of pancreatic disease and influence operative planning, so it is vital to know about the endocrine function of the pancreas in the context of surgery. Surgery of the pancreas, including the Whipple procedure and distal pancreatectomy, creates unique challenges for the endocrine balance of the organ. For instance, resection of segments of the pancreas can lead to reduced production of insulin, which may precipitate endocrine deficiency after surgery and diabetes. Yu (2020) highlights the importance of hormonal function evaluation in surgical planning and decision-making when the patient presents with tumors that result in hormonal dysregulation prior to surgery. Surgeons will thus have a need to prospectively screen for risk of developing diabetes post-surgery and plan for potential management solutions, which will include insulin therapy and dietary modification. The intricacies of the production and regulation of pancreatic hormones emphasize the importance of multidisciplinary management of patients, particularly where dietetic, surgical, and pharmacologic measures overlap. Postsurgical complications of surgery following pancreatic operation also directly affect the organs' capacity for hormone synthesis. Patients undergoing pseudocyst or necrosis drainage can have alterations in hormonal status resulting from damage to the remaining pancreatic tissue. Such physiological changes may manifest in the form of pancreatic insufficiency and malabsorption along with deranged glucose metabolism. Notably, Beger et al. (2018) opines that residual pancreatic function complications must be closely monitored since they can predispose patients to long-term endocrine dysfunction. The work of the surgeon does not just stop at surgery; vigilant monitoring of hormones and metabolic status is just as crucial in facilitating patient recovery. Knowing these hormonal actions is critical to optimizing postoperative care and enhancing patient outcomes after surgical procedures (Figure 15.5).

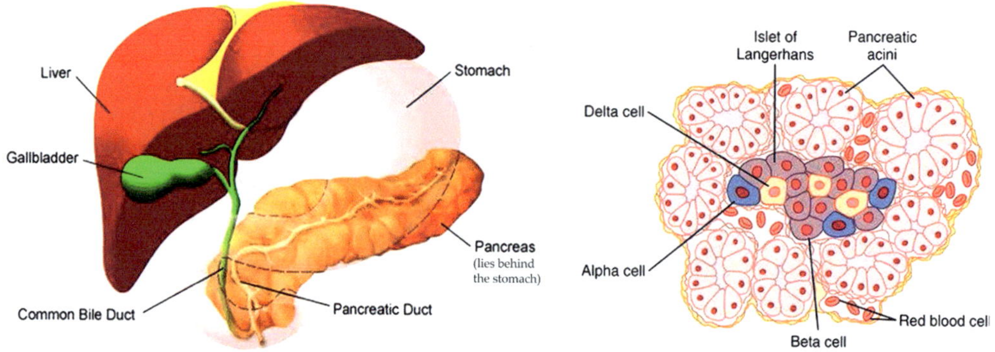

Figure 15.5. The pancreas: Structure, function, and hormonal secretions.

Source: https://external-content.duckduckgo.com/iu/?u=https%3A%2F%2Fclassnotes123.com%2Fwp-content%2Fuploads%2F2023%2F06%2Fstructure-of-pancreas.jpg&f=1&nofb=1&ipt=5def08299daf00c0f37c441403b167617ee4b15a3b4f975b10909f183107d6eb.

15.2. Indications for Surgical Intervention

Therapy by surgery for pancreatic disease is often based on a balance between disease severity and the potential advantage of surgery. The Whipple Procedure, for instance, is reserved primarily for pancreatic cancer patients with resectable pancreatic cancer, particularly if the tumor is located in the head of the pancreas. This prolonged process not only aims to remove the tumor but also addresses any involved localized tissues, particularly important for the achievement of negative margins and reducing recurrence rates. Other indications may also involve chronic pancreatitis complicated by those in which risks of irreversible conditions are greater than the risks of surgery. Surprisingly, empirical evidence points toward a stark disparity in knowledge on surgical modalities for pancreatic trauma, as evidenced by studies with emphasis on robust analysis of operative care for optimization of interventions to meet needs efficaciously (Krige, 2017). Another surprising feature of surgical management is indications for distal pancreatectomy, particularly when the tumor is in the body or tail of the pancreas. This procedure can be applied to both malignancies and benign disease, as a means of eliminating symptomatology associated with more massive masses, e.g., obstructive jaundice or pain. As part of the entire management of chronic pancreatitis, surgical therapy, including distal pancreatectomy, can diminish debilitating pain that is usually not responsive to medical treatment. These procedures are vital in maximizing patient quality of life and functionality. A study highlights the importance of understanding the multifactorial factors of pain in chronic pancreatitis, as both medical and surgical management can play a crucial role in influencing the patient outcomes in this multifactorial disease process (Salim et al., 1997). Moreover, drainage of pseudocysts and necrosis is also a important surgical intervention when medical management fails or in case of symptomatic complication. Surgical indications also include enlarging size, infection, or pain associated with these disorders. Surgical approaches, either by laparoscopic or open techniques, permit relief of symptoms and avoidance of more serious complications like pancreatic necrosis or perforation. These procedures not only address the acute clinical issues but are also part of the overall plan of management for patients with chronic pancreatitis, including a multiaxial system of care. The integration of empirical data and clinical experience in addressing these surgical indications remains critical to refining treatment protocols and enhancing patient outcomes in pancreatic disease management (Krige, 2017).

15.2.1. Types of Pancreatic Diseases Requiring Surgery

The scope of pancreatic pathology which needs surgery is driven by a variety of different pathological processes, including malignancies, pancreatitis, both acute and chronic, and complications of pancreatitis. Among these, pancreatic cancer is especially a definite indication for surgery due to its delayed presentation and poor prognosis. Whipple's procedure, or pancreaticoduodenectomy, is most frequently utilized to resect resectable pancreatic carcinoma in the head of the pancreas. This huge operation involves the resection of the pancreatic head along with portions of the small intestine, bile duct, and gallbladder, with the aim of achieving tumor resection with preservation of gastrointestinal function and avoidance of metastasis. Awareness of indications for such operations is most crucial since timely action can have a significantly differing impact on patient prognosis, attesting to the reason for continuous research in pancreatic surgery, as underscored by Krige et al. (2017). Also, pseudocysts and necrosis, which occur as a direct sequel to acute pancreatitis, are optimally treated clinically. Pseudocysts or fluid collections can develop as a result of the inflammatory response of the pancreas and can manifest as pain, obstructive symptoms, or complications of infection. Obstruction or other secondary complications of these cysts require drainage operationally. Minimally invasive interventions, such as endoscopic or percutaneous drainage, have worked in others, while more invasive interventions are warranted. Treatment for these complications is also indicative of the measured choice-making in surgical interventions for pancreatic disease, reflecting the evolving understanding of treatment protocols as investigated in ongoing research projects (El-Badry et al., 2022). Chronic pancreatitis, with its progression into a multitude of complications, also induces scenarios in which surgery is indicated. Surgery, including distal pancreatectomy, is indicated when patients have incapacitating pain or develop into complications such as cyst formation or malignancy. These operations entail tail resection of the pancreas and can be curative of symptoms and complications. Above all, choosing surgical treatment is based on a thorough evaluation of the patient and complications involved. The literature indicates the need to balance surgical benefit against potential risks, once more reiterating the value placed on ongoing investigation into optimizing patient outcome and surgical procedure in the case of pancreatic disease, as demonstrated through findings gained from Krige et al. (2017), El-Badry et al (2022) (Figure 15.6).

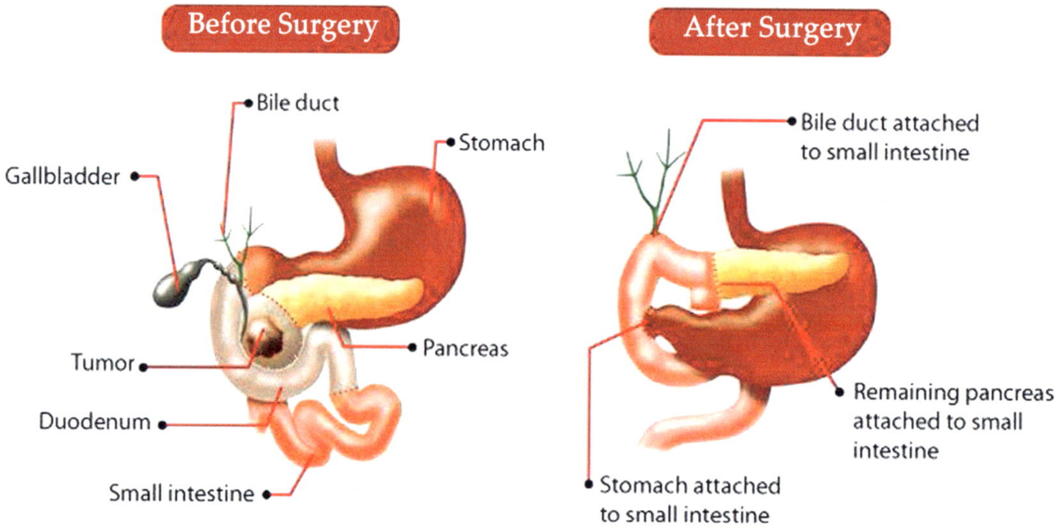

Figure 15.6. Pancreas surgery.

Source: https://external-content.duckduckgo.com/iu/?u=https%3A%2F%2Flivertransplantindia.net%2Fwp-content%2Fuploads%2F2021%2F05%2FWhipple-procedure-.jpg&f=1&nofb=1&ipt=c6880870fc68dc6943418fb66d6fdefa595439f5fd9b3d33843fae03824b7005.

15.2.2. Criteria for Surgical Candidacy

Surgical fitness evaluation for procedure against pancreatic pathology, such as Whipple surgery or distal pancreatectomy, is a strict analysis of a variety of clinical factors. Primarily, general health status of the patients is considered along with physiological reserve and presence of comorbidities that may affect the procedure of surgery. In the case of chronic pancreatitis patients, as researched in the study conducted in Thanjavur Medical College Hospital, nutritional assessment and endocrine or exocrine deficiency should be taken into account. All of these considerations are in favor of the need for a multidisciplinary method to select possible candidates for surgical intervention, particularly in the case of patients who are at risk for complications associated with the disease or postoperative recovery course (Anand, 2018). The second aspect of great relevance to evaluate when determining surgical candidacy is the extent and nature of pancreatic disease itself. For example, interventions such as drainage for pseudocysts and necrosis are largely contingent upon location, size, and nature of these diseases as well as symptomatology. Whether or not the disease is resectable or whether lesser interventions would be best is something that needs to be considered by surgeons. In addition, imaging studies take center stage in this determination, influencing decision in the area of surgical intervention feasibility. Remarkably, recent surgical hepatology literature has shown new procedures and principles, thereby expanding surgery eligibility and enhancing patient outcomes in cases of acute necrotizing pancreatitis or other complicated presentations (Akhaladze et al., 2014). Finally, the psychosocial support framework and psychological preparation of potential surgical candidates should not be discounted. Robust support is instrumental for recuperation after treatment and adherence to post-surgical regimens, including lifestyle management and follow-up. Psychological evaluation can provide some insight into the patient's preparedness for surgery at a psychological level, which is no less significant given the life-altering nature of such treatments. Thus, selection for surgical candidacy of pancreatic disease must include a holistic approach with every element of consideration varying from clinical factors to psychosocial factors and ultimately with the best possible surgical outcomes. Under this multi-dimensional approach, clinicians ensure proper analysis of candidates, hence increasing the chances of successful interventions and decreasing likely complications.

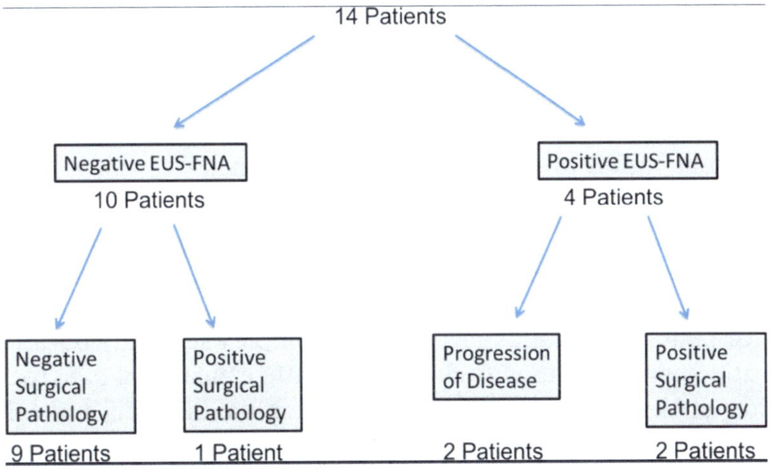

Figure 15.7. The utility of EUS-FNA to determine surgical candidacy.

Source: https://www.jogs.org/cms/10.1007/s11605-019-04415-6/asset/1ea81a7a-6cd7-4900-a5fd-5c11d0915d46/main.assets/Fig3_HTML_lrg.jpg.

15.2.3. Risks Associated with Non-Surgical Management

The management of pancreatic disease is frequently such that the non-surgical options are subjected to close consideration, particularly for diseases like chronic pancreatitis and pseudocysts of the pancreas. While in certain patients, conservative treatment may be beneficial, the risks are significant. Pain management, for example, often relies on analgesics, which are likely to promote dependency resulting in addiction, particularly when opioid drugs are employed. Furthermore, patients may develop disabling maldigestive symptoms of severe weight loss and gnawing abdominal pain. These symptoms not only compromise quality of life, but they are also often associated with inappropriate or delayed treatment, as evidenced by studies demonstrating that nearly 50% of patients who have chronic pancreatitis will eventually require surgical intervention following prolonged non-operative management (Sivasankar et al., 2006). This procrastination can contribute to increased morbidity and complicate the operative situation when interventions become critical. Non-surgical treatment harbors another critical risk, which is the likelihood of development of the disease and the complication. Chronic pancreatitis has been found to result from long-term conservative treatment with increased damage to pancreatic tissue, which, in turn, leads to exocrine and endocrine failure. Such complications manifest as diabetes and nutritional deficiencies, making patient management even more complicated. Moreover, patients also present with infection or acute exacerbation events that ultimately necessitate more aggressive treatment as the disease progresses. Recent literature suggests that without surgery, long-term outcomes for patients who present with chronic pancreatitis are still poor and highlight the extreme risks involved with continued non-surgical care (Krige, 2017). An intensive evaluation of the risk-benefit profile is thus indispensable. In addition, non-operative management does not generally cure the inherent pathophysiological process, i.e., inflammation or blockade. Such a deficiency may lead to psychosocial morbidity and reduced emotional function due to chronic pain and associated lifestyle limitation. Non-surgical treatments can also do indirectly to encourage a perpetuation of deleterious habits, such as alcohol consumption, which has been linked with adverse consequences and increased pain (Sivasankar et al., 2006). The synergistic impact of these psychological and lifestyle factors has the power to further deteriorate the overall well-being of a patient. Hence, medical practitioners must counterweigh the necessity of surgery with the often fluctuating benefits of conservative management. In summary, while non-surgical management may at first glance seem adequate in the case of some pancreatic diseases, the risks involved highlight the importance of strict monitoring and early surgical contemplation to optimize patient outcome.

15.3. The Whipple Procedure

Whipple procedure, or pancreaticoduodenectomy, is a complex surgical operation primarily for the treatment of pancreatic head conditions such as pancreatic cancer and pancreatitis. The operation involves the resection of the pancreatic head, duodenum, gallbladder, and bile duct, making for a complex surgical method. Its success also depends largely on early detection, as the outlook of pancreatic disease, particularly cancer, drastically worsens in later stages. The Whipple Procedure is rated a gold standard in surgical oncology, giving patients hope for high survival rates and symptom alleviation. But due to the intricacies of the anatomy involved and the general health status of the patients, success rates are unpredictable. Further, the results rely on the capabilities of the facilities and experience, and therefore specialized surgical centers must be able to conduct complex pancreatic surgery safely. In the subject of surgeries that are meant to cure pancreatic disease, the Whipple Procedure suggests not only an approach to treatment but also holds an intrinsic risk in developing complications after the operation. A few examples of popular complications developed during the procedure include pancreatic fistula, delayed gastric emptying, and infection, among others. These complications possess the ability to significantly alter the recovery course of a patient, extending hospital stays and necessitating additional interventions. For optimal recovery, Enhanced Recovery After Surgery (ERAS) strategies for patients undergoing pancreatic surgeries have been initiated in most institutions. These strategies provide intensive preoperative education, postoperative care, and early mobilization to avoid complications and make the recovery process smoother. The ERAS program organization has been shown to decrease the length of hospital stay and improve overall patient outcome, which is a paradigm shift in the provision of surgical care for the Whipple Procedure and other pancreatic resection operations. The performance of the Whipple Procedure is usually determined by a meticulous assessment of the patients' characteristics as well as the severity of their disease and thus is a multidisciplinary practice. Operating groups typically conduct long preoperative consultations to evaluate the probability of benefits and risks based on patient-specific profiles. Research indicates that the quality of evidence on postoperative complications and long-term survival following surgical operations remains highly heterogeneous and merits more research in clinical trials. Postoperative mile markers, quality of life, and other factors are targets for studies yielding richer insight into patient recovery trajectories. Future studies are needed to study these dynamics in more detail, more specifically fine-tuning surgical techniques and overall efficacy of the Whipple Procedure, and others for conditions affecting the pancreas, such as distal pancreatectomy and drainage procedures for pseudocysts and necroses, and improving the quality of care that can be provided to affected patients (Figure 15.8).

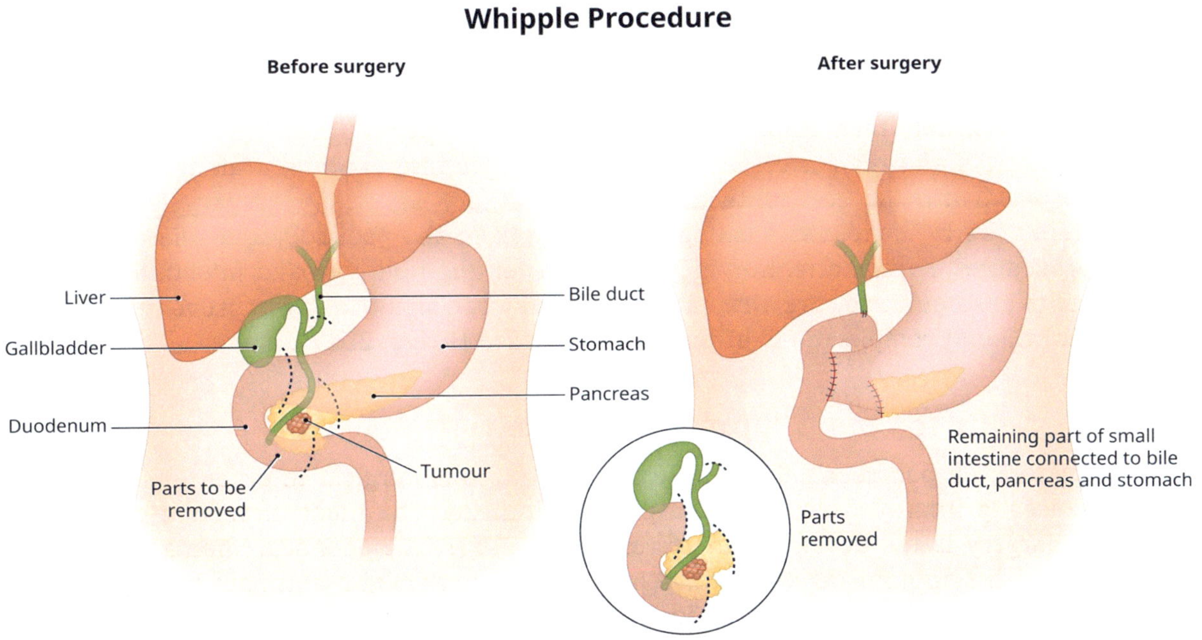

Figure 15.8. Whipple procedure.

Source: https://cdn-assets-eu.frontify.com/s3/frontify-enterprise-files-eu/eyJwYXRoIjoiaWhoLWhlYWx0aGNhcmUtYmVyaGFkXC9maWxlXC9DeFhyQ3BjaW9nSGp1eUFDd0dhTC5qcGcifQ:ihh-healthcare-berhad:_z_kV8q_Tf7Wfe4SsBV2rU5GQcIiQ8hskFIQQkDW7ZM?width=%7Bwidth%7D.

15.3.1. Description and Steps of the Procedure

Whipple procedure or pancreaticoduodenectomy is a highly complex operation employed primarily for the resection of tumor in the head of the pancreas. The procedure begins with the complex surgical exploration and mobilization of the pancreas, duodenum, and bile duct. The operating specialist then dissectively separates these structures while paying special attention to vascular integrity. Once the diseased tissue is removed, the remaining pancreas, stomach, and intestines are reconnected with a series of important anastomoses. Each connection is carefully constructed so that complications such as leaks or strictures, which can arise post-operatively, can be prevented. As a result of its invasive nature, the Whipple procedure necessitates multidisciplinary patient management with surgical skills combined with pre-and post-operative care to maximize recovery results and minimize complications (Krige, 2017). In comparison to the Whipple procedure, a distal pancreatectomy is the surgical removal of the body and tail of the pancreas, typically performed when malignancies or severe chronic illnesses are isolated in these regions. The surgical procedure starts by incising an adequate access path through the abdominal wall, followed by dissection to fully separate the pancreas. The spleen may also be removed at this point, especially when the disease has extended to the vasculature of the spleen. The surgeon ensures that the surrounding structures such as the stomach and adrenal glands are well protected throughout the operation. Post-resection, the residual pancreas is reconstructed, most commonly by a pancreatico-jejunostomy or by other drainage procedures. Having knowledge of the specific steps of a distal pancreatectomy is crucial since it dictates the patient's recovery pattern and overall quality of life following surgery (Rajkumar et al., 2014). Drainage procedures for pancreatic pseudocysts and necrosis are mandatory procedures for managing complications of acute and chronic pancreatitis. The process typically begins with imaging tests to gain a good understanding of pseudocysts size and location. The surgeon may then employ either endoscopic or percutaneous methods, depending on the nature of cysts and their access. Through endoscopic intervention, drainage is facilitated by inserting a stent into the gastrointestinal system. Otherwise, where surgery is required, a cystoenterostomy can be done, establishing a pathway from the pseudocyst to the intestine. In all of these procedures, special attention is given to preventing fluid loss and infection, which are critical aspects of postoperative care. Drains done carefully can significantly improve the prognosis and prevent continuing complications of pancreatic disease (Krige, 2017).

15.3.2. Indications for the Whipple Procedure

Whipple procedure, or pancreaticoduodenectomy, is a serious surgical intervention for various pancreas diseases, primarily cancers of the pancreatic head. The most important sign of this very complex surgery is the development of resectable pancreatic adenocarcinoma that may be combined with such symptoms as obstructive jaundice, loss of weight, and pain in the abdomen. This procedure not only resects the affected pancreatic tissue but also involves resection of the surrounding tissues, including the duodenum, gallbladder, and portion of the bile duct. This extensive resection is justified when diagnostic imaging has confirmed that the tumor is confined to the head of the pancreas without vascular encasement or distant metastases, thus offering the promise of curative resection. The critical review of these factors is most important in establishing candidacy for a patient to undergo the Whipple procedure. Furthermore, chronic pancreatitis can blossom into an environment in which surgical intervention is needed due to biliary obstruction or disabling pain. The Whipple procedure can be invoked where conservative measures have been futile and patients are experiencing significant lifestyle handicap. One of the treatment options, it aims to alleviate symptoms of chronic pancreatitis through resection of the pancreatic head and related structures for drainage of the obstructed ducts. However, keeping in view the danger and complexity of pancreatic surgery—like postoperative morbidity in the guise of gastrointestinal fistulas and sepsis—the selection of patients and preoperative workup are critical. Thus, the Whipple operation may serve as a two-in-one: both meeting oncological needs and alleviating chronic pain in suitably selected patients. Another indication for the Whipple operation is benign neoplasms or diseases such as neuroendocrine tumors when they arise in the head of the pancreas. Although less common, these tumors can become symptomatic and complicated with symptoms and complications of malignancy and can necessitate surgical removal for diagnosis and treatment. When strictures or obstructions of the bile duct system develop secondary to mass effect from these lesions, the Whipple procedure provides the best solution for restoring bile drainage. In addition, as pancreatic operations can lead to vascular complications that require a multidisciplinary treatment, the Whipple operation is in line with broader optimal care for pancreatic diseases. The preservation of vascular integrity should be addressed, especially when post-operative complication from such diseases as splanchnic pseudoaneurysms (Barge & Lopera, 2012) would be at risk. Hence, the Whipple procedure is a landmark in the surgical treatment of pancreatic pathologies where an appropriate understanding of potential complications plays a vital role (Figure 15.9).

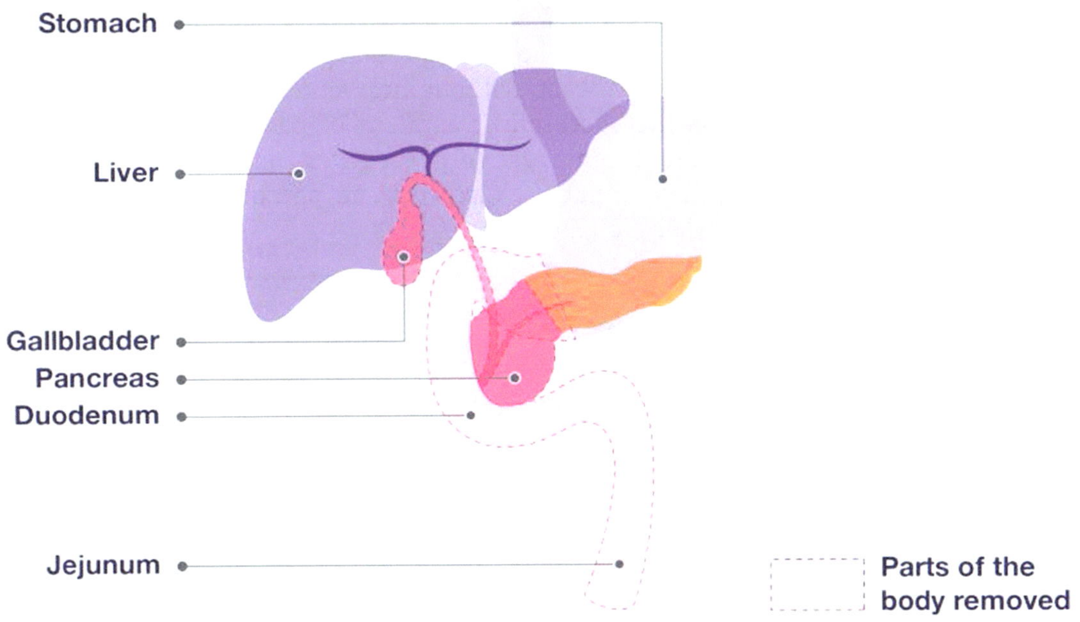

Figure 15.9. Indications for the Whipple procedure.

Source: https://pancreaticcanceraction.org/wp-content/uploads/2012/10/PCA_SurgicalDiagram_Whipples-Procedure_BEF-788x446.jpg.

15.3.3. Expected Outcomes and Survival Rates

The survival rate and prognosis of surgery in pancreatic disease vary significantly based on the type of procedure performed. For instance, the Whipple operation, involving the excision of the head of the pancreas, has been associated with varying survival rates based on the tumor stage and the health status of the individual prior to surgery. Survival is greater than 20% at five years for patients who receive the treatment for pancreatic adenocarcinoma, especially when detected at a younger age. General health, age, as well as comorbidities, all play vital roles in choosing prognosis for patients. Successful surgery, thus, is closely linked to pre-operative conditions and the biological behavior of the tumor, hence requiring a customized strategy for planning treatment and counseling the patient regarding expected outcomes and potential risks (Krige, 2017). Distal pancreatectomy is another common surgical intervention for pancreatic disease, namely for benign tumors and some malignant tumors occurring in the body and tail of the pancreas. The results of the process can cause marked benefit, including symptom alleviation and tumor removal, with survival rates being inclined to depend on the histological grade of the tumors and also on the medical condition of patients. Studies have indicated that five-year survival in patients for the process could be between 30%–65% depending mainly on the nature of pancreatic pathology. As with the Whipple procedure, the specific nature of the pancreatic pathology, patient population, and surgical experience are critical considerations in the probability of success in the patient after a distal pancreatectomy, highlighting the necessity for strict post-operative care and observation (Johnson et al., 2006). Drainage of pseudocysts and necrosis also has good expected outcomes when done appropriately. These processes, like endoscopic or percutaneous drainage, are to correct complications of inflammation of the pancreas, primarily fluid accumulation. These drainage processes are ideally low in morbidity risk and can suitably relieve symptoms without creating additional complications. Morbidity in patients who undergo such procedures is also high since they involve addressing non-cancerous conditions that, without intervention, can become complications of lethal nature. Generally speaking, the successful treatment of pancreatic disease by surgical means, either radical resection or more conservative procedures, underscores the importance of certain approaches based on individual patient histories and pathology to ultimately achieve maximization of survival and quality of life (Krige, 2017).

15.4. Distal Pancreatectomy

Distal pancreatectomy is a procedure in which the distal part of the pancreas is removed, often in cases of localized tumors, cysts, or chronic pancreatitis. The procedure has often been termed a treatment for a variety of pancreatic diseases, including pancreatic adenocarcinoma, neuroendocrine tumors, and chronic pancreatitis. By amputating the tail and sometimes the body of the pancreas, the surgeons aim to relieve symptoms, prevent complications, and check disease spread. As with all surgery, evaluation of the general condition of the patients and comorbidities is very much needed to determine distal pancreatectomy candidacy, which now is being performed in a minimally invasive procedure. These developments see to it that there is reduced pain postoperation and reduced periods of recovery, hence making the procedure more attractive to patients as well as surgeons. Healing from pancreatic conditions may be challenging and needs one to be conscious of the consequences and potential complications. Among the consequences of operation is leakage from the pancreas, whereby digestive enzymes leak out of the remaining pancreatic tissue due to pancreatic duct obstruction. These complications have the potential to lead to severe morbidity if not managed, usually through additional interventions or prolonged hospitalization. In terms of long-term outcome, patients can also suffer from endocrine dysfunction necessitating careful follow-up for postoperative diabetes mellitus. Complete explanation and follow-up are very much integral components of successful distal pancreatectomy management because they have great impacts on the overall well-being and quality of life of the patient following surgery. The decision to use a distal pancreatectomy must be a careful weighing of its risks versus benefits. As with the management of chronic pancreatitis, where surgery is considered when medical management fails, the decision to use this operation must also take into account the patient's specific condition, lifestyle, and anticipated postoperative needs. Attempts at enhancing surgical outcomes may be incorporation of better recovery protocols, which are based on lowering complications and shortening recovery time. In pancreatic interventions, condensing evidence-based practice into direct implications has bearing on postoperative recovery and satisfaction with care. Continuing research into surgical procedures and postoperative care is needed to advance the science, closing gaps in previous areas of knowledge as observed in studies on pancreatic trauma and treatment options (Krige, 2017; Anand et al., 2018) (Figure 15.10).

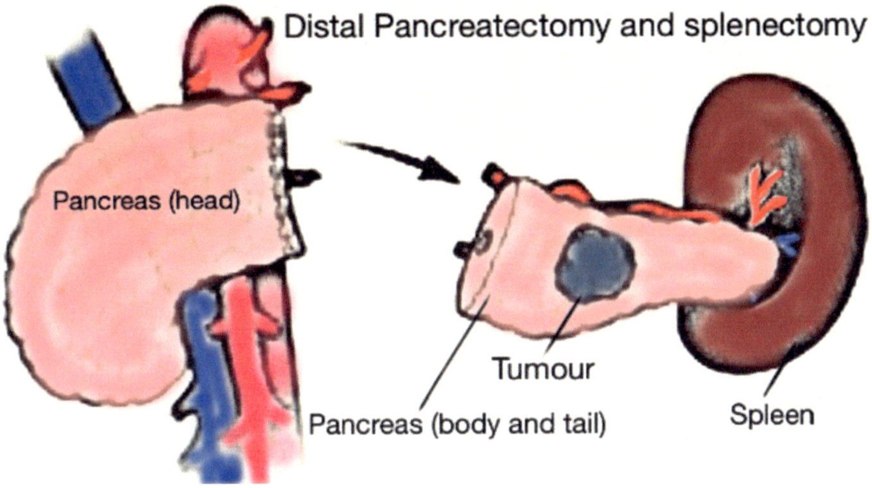

Figure 15.10. Distal pancreatectomy.

Source: https://external-content.duckduckgo.com/iu/?u=https%3A%2F%2Fwww.saboorkhan.co.uk%2Fwp-content%2Fuploads%2F2019%2F05%2FDistal-Pancreatectomy-and-Splenectomy.jpg&f=1&nofb=1&ipt=728292f32eb6280060bd06d4a798bc797d06607b54589565efdb0281702aaf12.

15.4.1. Definition and Surgical Technique

Surgeries for pancreatic disease involve a range of techniques intended to address various clinical issues posed by pancreatic dysfunction and trauma. The one unifying aspect of these surgeries is that they are tailored with the express goal of normalizing pancreatic function or addressing consequences of conditions like chronic pancreatitis, pancreatic cancer, or traumatic trauma. The Whipple operation, or pancreaticoduodenectomy, is also significant; it involves resection of the head of the pancreas, duodenum, a portion of the bile duct, and sometimes part of the stomach. This intricate operation is required for the treatment of malignancy of the pancreatic head and possibly curative for certain neoplasms confined to the region. Surgical techniques are continually evolving, such as minimally invasive techniques that try to keep recovery times as short as possible and increase surgical outcomes, showing an ongoing interest in maximizing patient care and safety in pancreatic surgery. Technique details are crucial to the success of pancreatic disorder treatments. For instance, the distal pancreatectomy, in which the body and tail of the pancreas are removed, is commonly employed in the case of tumors of these locations. The procedure requires utmost caution when dealing with the vascular structures around it, as poor dissection will result in widespread complications. Conversely, drainage procedures for pancreatic necrosis and pseudocysts are of significant concern in the complication management of chronic pancreatitis or trauma (Krige, 2017). The procedures are either surgical or percutaneous, depending on the size and symptoms of the cysts, and are used to alleviate pain without causing more complications. The proper application of these skills illustrates the overlap of clinical acumen and technical skill in producing the optimal patient outcomes. Postoperative complications of surgery are a fact of pancreatic surgical operations that depend on the type of surgery and preoperative condition of the patient. Delayed gastric emptying, fistula, and infection are some of the common complications. They can very much impact recovery as well as quality of life and need to be monitored as well as treated closely. Understanding the mechanisms of chronic pancreatitis pain is also crucial in the development of effective surgical methods for pain reduction during and after surgery (Salim et al., 1997). Strong preoperative assessment incorporated with using standardized protocols for managing pancreatic trauma is essential in the improvement of surgical outcomes and minimizing complications. Along with the development of surgical techniques, a focus on early as well as delayed postoperative management remains vital in enhancing overall efficacy of treatment of pancreatic diseases.

15.4.2. Indications for Distal Pancreatectomy

The indications for distal pancreatectomy mainly depend on the treatment of pancreatic tumors, chronic pancreatitis, and benign lesions. The surgery is generally indicated when patients present with neoplasms of the body or tail of the pancreas, such as pancreatic adenocarcinomas, neuroendocrine tumors, and cystic lesions like serous and mucinous cystadenomas. Also, long-standing pancreatitis with serious symptoms and complications, such as incapacitating pain or infection, may need distal pancreatectomy. In these instances, the purpose of the distal pancreatectomy is to alleviate pain with maximal control of the underlying disease for an improvement in the patient's quality of life. The extensive approach employed to create indications emphasizes the significance of extensive diagnostic workup, such as imaging studies and endoscopic examinations, in order to properly choose candidates for surgery for optimal beneficial results. Moreover, management of complications from chronic pancreatitis is a major indication for distal pancreatectomy. Patients are usually plagued by serious abdominal pain, maldigestion, and significant weight loss, which are detrimental to their overall well-being and lifestyle, as highlighted in the case of surgical management of chronic pancreatitis (Sivasankar et al., 2006). In the event that conservative measures fail to treat these effectively, surgery can be taken into consideration.

Distal pancreatectomy not only cures the pain cause by removing pathologically altered pancreatic tissue but also decreases the risk of subsequent complications, such as pancreatic necrosis or abscess. Surgical treatment, therefore, is a vital component of the long-term management strategy for those being bogged down by the complexity of chronic pancreatitis. Furthermore, the evolvability of pancreatic exocrine and endocrine deficiency often supports the indication of distal pancreatectomy in selected patient populations. With advancing chronic pancreatitis, patients may face the debilitating consequences of insulin-dependent diabetes mellitus due to loss of pancreatic tissue (Krige, 2017). Surgical interventions are indicated in situations where patients experience extreme weight loss as well as impaired digestion because removal of the affected segments can reinstate a more functional pancreatic environment. Operative outcomes, particularly those concerning endocrine function and overall metabolic status, play very important roles in directing surgical management. Thus, distal pancreatectomy not only addresses immediate symptoms but aims to reestablish a near-normalcy in metabolism, providing a solution to all for the complex issue presented in pancreatic disease management (Figure 15.11).

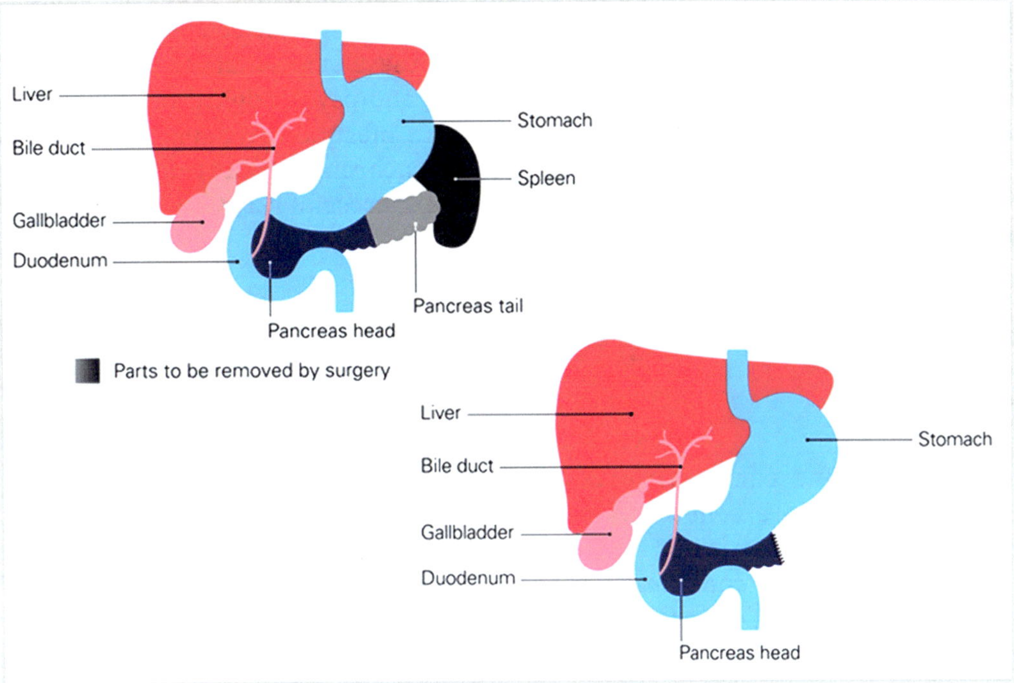

Figure 15.11. Indications for distal pancreatectomy.

Source: https://letswinpc.org/wp-content/uploads/2022/05/distal-pancreatectomy.gif.

15.4.3. Post-Operative Recovery and Care

Post-operative care and management are basic requirements in the delivery of successful surgeries for pancreatic conditions such as the Whipple procedure and distal pancreatectomy. These are complex surgical interventions that may lead to numerous post-operative complications, which can negatively affect patient recovery. Critical monitoring in the initial post-operative period is required for identification of common post-operative complications such as infections, bleeding, or pancreatic leaks. A planned care approach including pain management, dietary support, and gradual return to normal activities is essential to enhance recovery. Additionally, execution of evidence-based guidelines on strong data, as highlighted in Krige et al. (2017), can lead to improved outcomes by addressing patients' unique needs to recover following major pancreatic resections. Effective post-operative care is not only limited to monitoring in the immediate post-operative but also encompasses long-term planning for recovery. Patients would generally require intensive follow-up in managing their pattern of recovery, especially in cases where the surgery impacts pancreatic function. Nutritional counseling becomes necessary because these patients would often experience problems with digestion and enzyme secretion post-surgery. Taking an enrolled approach with the introduction of dietary changes and enzyme supplements can effectively address such issues. Apart from that, understanding the physiological changes that occur following surgery helps healthcare providers to create intervention and support systems that enhance optimal recovery and enhance the patient's quality of life. Psychosocial interventions are also an integral aspect of recovery after surgery for patients undergoing surgery to treat pancreatic diseases. The psychological and emotional journey following major surgery can be very stressful, and this can influence recovery compliance with procedures and overall health. Providing psychological treatment, like counseling services and peer support groups, will assist in helping patients overcome these emotional obstacles. Incorporating a multidisciplinary model that incorporates both medical and psychological intervention creates an overall recovery process. To that effect, the emphasis on lifestyle management and rehabilitation alongside medical control adds to the importance of synchronizing post-operative care with the unique needs of the patient to eventually ensure a more successful recovery process for pancreatic surgery.

15.5. Drainage Procedures for Pseudocysts and Necrosis

Treatment of necrosis and pancreatic pseudocysts often involves drainage procedures as a key intervention. Pseudocysts are collections of fluid which may develop after pancreatitis and can cause significant complications if not treated. Symptom relief, preventing further tissue damage, and limiting the occurrence of complications in these structures are the primary goals of drainage procedures. Percutaneous and endoscopic methods have gained popularity due to their minimally invasive nature and satisfactory outcomes. Studies indicate that the evolution in imaging modalities has immensely improved preoperative assessment, thereby allowing for adequate selection of the best draining option (Krige, 2017). Moreover, the decision-making process on whether to intervene and when and how is vital as timing of treatment influences long-term outcomes. After the decision to drain has been made, several techniques can be employed, each of which is tailored to the pseudocyst or necrotic tissue at hand. Endoscopic drainage, guided by fluoroscopy or ultrasound, allows direct access to the fluid-filled cyst immediately. Perforation of the skin to insert a catheter into the cyst for constant drainage is another option. Such procedures not only aim to drain the fluid but also stimulate the development of a mature fistula that will allow for permanent healing of the pseudocyst. Depending on where the cyst is, how large it is, and how healthy the patient is, even the modality of drainage can be decided. The use of these procedures is a significant shift in the management of pancreatic pathology, which establishes the significance of custom-made treatment plans (Krige, 2017).

Beyond the success of drainage procedures, potential complications must also be evaluated and managed appropriately. Common complications include infection, reaccumulation of the fluid, and injury to adjacent structures. Thus, close monitoring and follow-up imaging must be done after these procedures to prevent failed procedures. Studies indicate that, although complications are relatively low, the complexities of pancreatic anatomy can pose some odd intra- and post-operative challenges (Bhoopathi et al., 2009). Additionally, a transition from minimally invasive to more open surgical approaches may be warranted when initial drainage fails to bring relief. As in the case of any surgical intervention, there is a need for a multidisciplinary approach involving surgeons, radiologists, and gastroenterologists to understand the intricacies of managing complications and enhancing patient outcomes maximally (Figure 15.12).

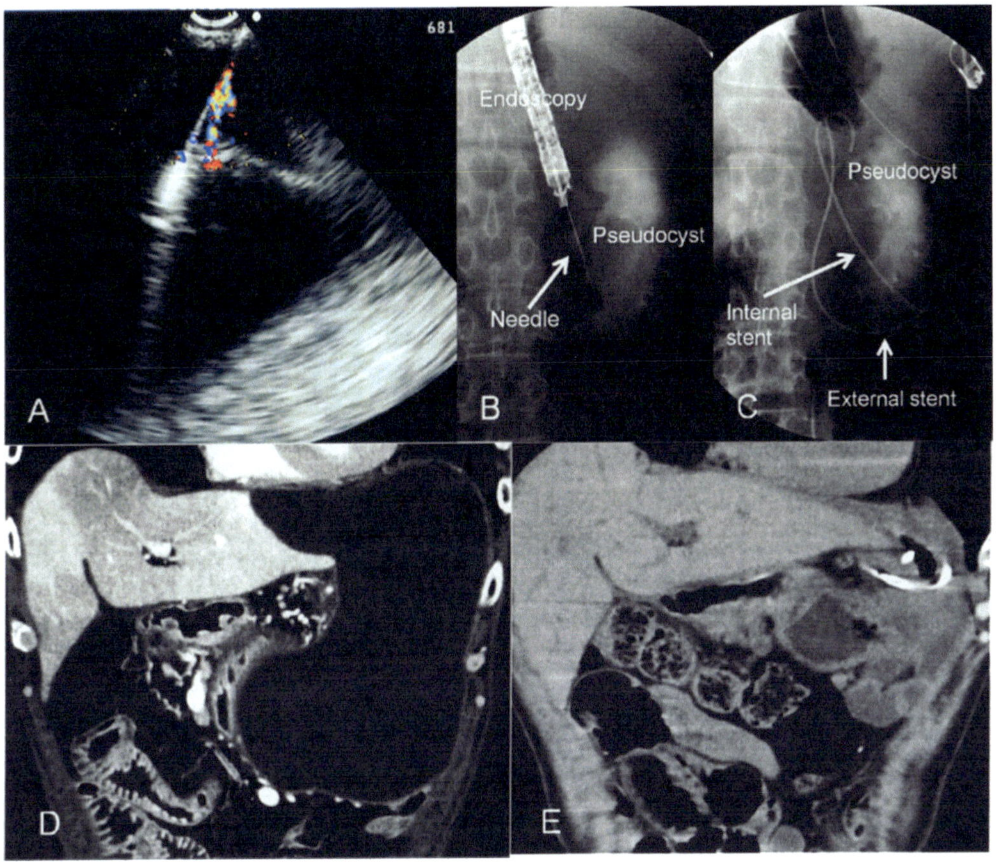

Figure 15.12. Endoscopic ultrasound (EUS)-drainage for pancreatic pseudocyst.

Source: https://www.researchgate.net/profile/Hiroshi-Imaizumi/publication/265532947/figure/fig1/AS:295805970862080@1447537047261/EUS-drainage-for-pancreatic-pseudocyst.png.

15.5.1. Types of Drainage Procedures

Drainage procedures are a critical component of the therapy for pancreatic disease, particularly in the care of complications such as pseudocysts and necrosis. Pseudocysts, which are fluid collections that can arise from pancreatic inflammation or injury, typically need to be treated when they produce pain, infection, or other problems. Percutaneous drainage therefore presents as an initial option in these circumstances, to the minimally invasive removal of unwanted fluid with marked symptom relief. Under imaging guidance, this is a procedure that is preferred for its ability to minimize complications resulting from more invasive surgery. Finally, percutaneous approaches are often able to be repeated if fluid recurs, and therefore provide a flexible means of maintenance (Krige, 2017). Apart from percutaneous drainage, surgical drainage constitutes an indispensable component of necrotizing pancreatitis treatment, an acute condition that can have severe morbidity. Surgical interventions, such as necrosectomy, are justified in the presence of extensive pancreatic tissue and surrounding structure necrosis. This involves the removal of necrotic tissue to prevent abscess formation and facilitate healing. Following this, the placement of drains in the bed of the pancreas is observed to allow constant drainage of left-over necrotic tissue and prevent fluid accumulation.

The incorporation of effective drainage techniques within the plan of surgical treatment is important towards reduction of post-operative complications, emphasizing the role of individualized drainage in complicated pancreatic conditions (Johnson et al., 2006). Besides, drainage procedures are not complication-free and do not involve an uncomplicated challenge, which underscores the need for especial care of clinical practice. While percutaneous and surgical procedures may significantly enhance patient outcome, they carry with them the risk of complications from infection, bleeding, and trauma to contiguous organs. A multidisciplinary approach is hence commonly required in a bid to optimize the results by engaging the surgical units, radiologists, and gastroenterologists. The cautious evaluation of each patient's unique case allows for an appropriate selection of drainage procedures to balance interventions properly between efficacy and safety. The ongoing evolution of imaging modalities and endoscopic techniques further sharpens the precision and success rates of these interventions, reaffirming the vital significance of their role in the entire management of pancreatic disease (Krige, 2017).

15.5.2. Indications for Drainage Interventions

In pancreatic disease, drainage interventions are of great value in the setting of complication of conditions such as acute pancreatitis or pancreatic pseudocysts. When fluid collections are created, they might present as symptomatic pseudocysts that generate abdominal pain, infection, or obstructive jaundice. Drainage interventions are needed to palliate symptoms and prevent further complications in these situations. The intervention choice is usually determined by the size of the pseudocyst, how long it has been present, and the patients' clinical condition. The interventions would be endoscopic drainage or percutaneous, both of which are established as successful for symptomatic pancreatic fluid collections. The real selection of intervention is determined by the location of fluid accumulation and the overall general health profile of the patient, underlining the significance of initial full evaluation prior to instituting drainage interventions. Endoscopic drainage methods have become leading interventions in recent years mostly due to their minimally invasive nature and favorable outcome. The indications for endoscopic interventions are mostly made up of symptomatic pseudocysts in whom intervention is warranted according to clinical presentation. Furthermore, infected pancreatic necrosis presentations may also need to be urgently drained to prevent the occurrence of systemic complications like sepsis. The conventional and modified endoscopic techniques are aimed at dealing with such cases effectively. Interestingly, the process of endoscopy is more than mere fluid drainage; it is a careful evaluation of the adjacent anatomy and potential underlying pathologies that can contribute to the overall patient presentation. The synergy between endoscopy and surgical interventions is a multidisciplinary process that is part of optimizing patient outcomes in complex pancreatic disease cases (Swartz & Obando, 2012; Vladimirov et al., 2015). Drainage in pancreatic necrosis treatment is not only therapeutic but also diagnostic. Because pancreatic necrosis has a tendency to form fluid collections that may contain infectious complications, early intervention is warranted. Indications for drainage therefore encompass symptomatic relief as well as the need to address infected necrotic tissue. These conditions are, in such cases, frequently particularly useful, enabling clinicians to puncture fluid for microbiological analysis and thus guide antibiotic therapy. Successful interventions also depend on imaging, e.g., ultrasound or CT scan, to assess fluid collection characteristics and ensure precision of placement. Lastly, through the use of drainage interventions with care, health professionals are able to transcend the multifaceted aspects of pancreatic disease without the risks associated with more invasive surgical techniques (Swartz & Obando, 2012; Vladimirov et al., 2015) (Figure 15.13).

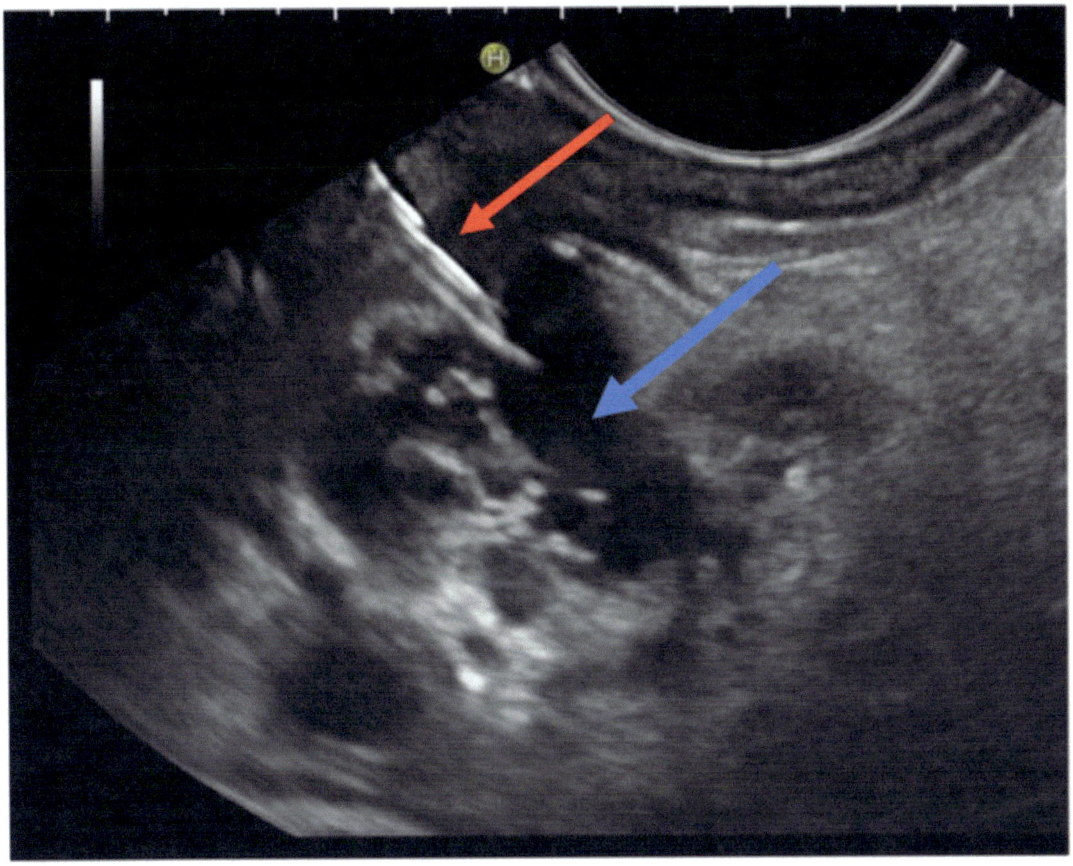

Figure 15.13. Endoscopic ultrasound (EUS)-guided pancreatic drainage for pancreatic strictures.

Source: Will U, Fueldner F, Buechner T, Meyer F. Endoscopic Ultrasonography-Guided Drainage of the Pancreatic Duct (EUS-PD)—Indications and Results with a Literature Review. *Journal of Clinical Medicine*. 2024; 13(24):7709. https://doi.org/10.3390/jcm13247709

15.5.3. Complications Associated with Drainage Procedures

The use of drainage methods in the management of pancreatic pseudocysts and necrosis is one of the essential aspects of treating pancreatic disease complications. They are not risk-free, however, even though they are often successful in alleviating symptoms and preventing worsening complications. The most common complications of these drainage methods are infection, fistula formation, and bleeding. These complications can occur due to the caustic nature of pancreatic secretions, which can result in the disruption of the surrounding tissue. Additionally, since drainage procedures often involve the manipulation of the delicate anatomy of the pancreas, there is always a risk of injury to adjacent organs, which complicates the recovery process and leads to additional morbidity (Ho et al., 2005). Besides the immediate problems secondary to the procedure itself, there are chronic sequelae that need to be taken into account. One particular worry is that of postoperative pancreatic fistula, leading to malnutrition and longer hospital stays as a result of secondary procedures. Such complications not only prolong the period of recovery but may also necessitate the placement of other drains or surgical re-entry to close the fistula and prevent further complications. Additionally, according to studies, the occurrence of such complications has been linked to severe derangement of the metabolic functions of the pancreas, with accompanying conditions like pancreatic exocrine insufficiency or diabetes mellitus (El-Badry et al., 2022). The necessity for intensive management and follow-up post-drainage thus becomes critical to optimize patient outcome. Complication management after drainage procedures will ultimately be a multidisciplinary effort to address the range of potential complications. Surgeons and clinicians will need to work together in order to implement preventive strategies, including intraoperative techniques reducing tissue trauma and proper selection of drainage based on individual patient factors. Also, proper follow-up care and patient education are necessary so that the patients would be able to recognize early complications. The overall goal is to enhance recovery and quality of life with minimal risk from drainage procedures. Working in the surgical setting with an emphasis on patient safety and ultimate health will benefit significantly those who are to receive these operations, since optimal practice management can lower the incidence of postoperative complications (Ho et al., 2005).

15.6. Post-Surgical Complications

Complications following operation are a critical aspect of interest in the field of pancreatic surgery such as the Whipple procedure and distal pancreatectomy. Complications can present as short-term or long-term effects, and they directly impact patient recovery and outcomes. Bleeding, infection, and development of pancreatic fistula are common post-operative complications, and the latter is particularly prevalent in procedures that involve manipulation of pancreatic tissue. Each of these complications has the ability to introduce additional morbidity and, in severe cases, mortality. Also, their management has a tendency to require supplementary interventions, making the patient's course still more complicated. Thus, familiarity with the risk factors surrounding these complications becomes relevant in the promotion of post-operative care and outcome for patients undergoing pancreatic surgery, validating the significance of careful surgical technique and postoperative monitoring. The complication rate is to a large extent dependent on the extent of the operation performed. The Whipple procedure, which is an extensive resection of pancreas, duodenum, and biliary tree, has been seen to carry a higher rate of complications than lesser procedures like distal pancreatectomy. Research indicates that the pathology, the skill of the surgeon, and the preoperative status of the patient contribute all to the risk of acquiring complications post-surgery. In particular, complications of delayed gastric emptying and infections have the potential to extend hospital stays and increase the cost of healthcare, highlighting the importance of meticulous planning and conduct of surgery. The importance of further investigation of the correlates of such complications cannot be overstated because it addresses critical gaps in knowledge regarding the intricacies of outcomes of surgery in the management of pancreatic disease (Krige, 2017). As a measure to minimize post-surgical adverse events, various interventions and protocols have been implemented in favor of favoring recovery and minimizing adverse occurrences post-surgery. Use of ERAS protocols that focus on multimodal analgesia, early mobilization, and optimal nutrition has proven fruitful in rewiring post-operative outcomes. There is a need for continuous monitoring and adjustment of these protocols based on evolving clinical evidence, especially due to the peculiarly challenging nature of pancreatic resections. Besides, the integration of advanced surgical techniques and technology, like minimally invasive surgery, may reduce the incidence of post-operative complications. Nevertheless, full understanding of factors related to the individual patient still remains significant in the process of personalizing intervention and designing better recovery experiences, highlighting the complexity of managing post-operative complications of pancreatic disease treatment (Bank et al., 2018) (Figure 15.14).

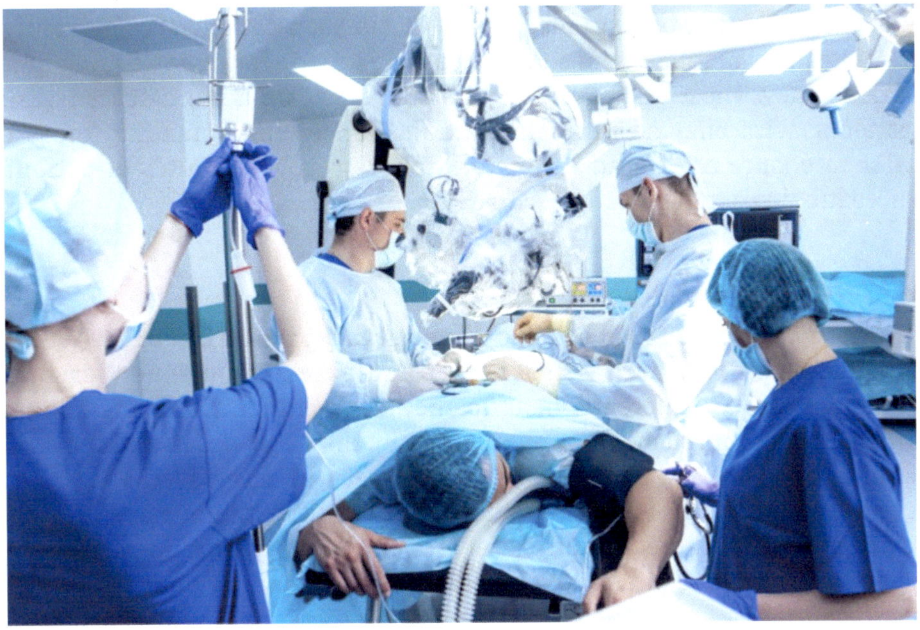

Figure 15.14. Post-surgical complications.

Source: https://yegthrive.ca/wp-content/uploads/2022/01/Post-Surgical-Complications-e1642695274295.jpeg.

15.6.1. Common Complications Following Pancreatic Surgery

Complications during pancreatic surgery are often a function of the intricate anatomy and critical functions of the organ. Procedures such as the Whipple procedure and distal pancreatectomy are essential in management of pancreatic disease but entail their own risks. Complications following these procedures are most commonly postoperative hemorrhage which can be caused by disruption of vascular structures during surgery. This bleeding may lead to significant morbidity if it is not detected and managed in a timely fashion. Secondly, leaks of the pancreas occur with increased frequency following resections, particularly following Whipples, where an anastomosis between the residual pancreas and the intestine is created. These leaks can lead to local infections or even to abscesses, which complicate the recovery process and necessitate multiple interventions (Krige, 2017). Infection is another prime risk factor in pancreatic operations, especially with conditions such as pseudocysts or necrosis of the pancreas. Postoperative infections can be of many causes, including wound infection, intra-abdominal abscess, or pneumonia. Because of the large number of vascular structures and organs that encompass the pancreas, any infection can quickly lead to systemic sepsis unless it is carefully controlled. Further, infectious complications have the tendency to prolong hospital stays, increase healthcare costs, and result in readmissions. The problem is infection management, hence making prophylactic antibiotics and strict postoperative care central to avoiding such complications and enhancing patient outcomes following pancreatic operations (Sivakumar, 2015). Finally, endocrine and exocrine deficiency are notable long-term consequences that can happen following pancreatic surgeries, significantly impacting patient quality of life. Intraoperative loss of pancreatic tissue can potentially result in diminished insulin production and, as such, new-onset diabetes mellitus. This derangement of metabolism needs to be monitored and controlled carefully, often with the use of insulin therapy in such patients. Concurrently, patients will suffer from gastrointestinal manifestations of decreased exocrine function, leading to malabsorption and nutritional deficiency. These issues need to be addressed on a multifaceted basis and include dietary changes along with enzyme supplementation. Hence, understanding these complications is crucial in order to ensure an overall care and improve recovery routes of patients undergoing surgery for pancreatic diseases (Sivakumar, 2015).

15.6.2. Management of Complications

Surgical complications of diseases such as pancreatic surgery in the form of the Whipple procedure and distal pancreatectomy have specific issues to be addressed and planned for. One of the major complications among these is pancreatic insufficiency, resulting in malabsorption and nutritional deficiencies. Postoperative course may be complicated by the deterioration of the ability to manage pain and metabolic disturbances, and such would need to be addressed with an individualized strategy to provide symptom relief and maintain quality of life. Studies have indicated that about 50% of chronic pancreatitis patients will ultimately require surgery, bringing them into the limelight of appropriate postoperative care in this context. Sustained vigilance of patients for signs of exocrine and endocrine deficiency enables health practitioners to implement diet modifications and enzyme replacement therapies to counteract insufficiencies arising from surgery, thereby enhancing patient outcomes as a whole (Sivasankar et al., 2006). Also, infection and delays such as delayed gastric emptying and infection are frequently observed after pancreatic surgery, which complicate recovery times and lengthen hospital stays. Infection can result from disruption of tissue or the pancreatic duct, which necessitates close observation and early implementation of antibiotics. Like any other complication, the development of delayed gastric emptying, one of the common postoperative complications, can preclude a patient from tolerating oral intake and lead to additional distress and risk of nutritional compromise. To adequately manage these complications, a multidisciplinary effort on the part of surgeons, dietitians, and pharmacologists is necessary. Using standardized monitoring regimes post-surgery can also aid in the timely detection of complications, which can permit interventions that can diminish their impact on patient prognosis (Krige, 2017). Psychological as well as emotional control is also vital in managing postoperative recovery complications of pancreatic surgery. The patients can endure a lot of distress, given the severity of the condition as well as the invasive nature of surgical therapy. The consequent modification in their lifestyle, dietary regimen, and potential loss of independence can lead to depression and anxiety. Incorporation of support systems, such as counseling and peer support, will promote mental health and improve coping mechanisms among patients experiencing chronic pain and lifestyle modifications post-surgery. The understanding that postoperative recovery tends to extend beyond recovery from somatic illness emphasizes the need for comprehensive care that encompasses the somatic and psychosocial aspects of the patient's rehabilitation (Sivasankar et al., 2006).

15.6.3. Long-Term Effects on Patient Health

The long-term effect on the health of the patient following surgical interventions for pancreatic disease is diverse and multifaceted. Among the surgical procedures, the Whipple procedure, or pancreatoduodenectomy, is notable due to the complexity of the procedure and its extensive effect on the digestive apparatus. Carbohydrate and fat metabolism can be permanently altered in patients as a consequence of the removal of significant portions of the pancreas and surrounding tissues. This can lead to greater dangers of malnutrition, diabetes mellitus, and changes in weight in the long term. Moreover, the need for lifelong monitoring and eventual supplementation becomes central, as the majority of these patients develop with exocrine and endocrine deficiencies, necessitating careful monitoring of their diet and insulin requirements.

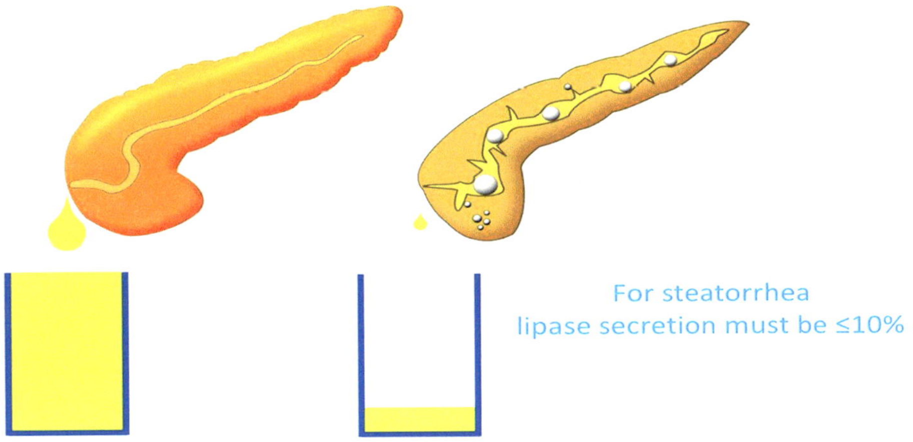

Figure 15.15. Steatorrhea for pancreatic diseases.

Source: https://external-content.duckduckgo.com/iu/?u=https%3A%2F%2Fpbs.twimg.com%2Fmedia%2FD-7bunTXsAAdti5.jpg&f=1&nofb=1&ipt=7cd0592e8886b2a30e3431d0dcbbb7e2f87cfe3c2b4bf5af3944c3954867eacb.

The gravitas of these physiological changes echoes throughout a patient's general state of well-being, highlighting the fundamental need for long-term follow-up and multi-disciplinary therapy following surgery. Other than the Whipple procedure, distal pancreatectomy also carries its own complications and effects on the health of a patient in the long term. Distal pancreatectomy involves the resection of the tail and even the body of the pancreas, which also results in the same metabolic effects. The patient would suffer from reduced insulin secretion, further elevating his or her chances of getting diabetes; this can also happen years after undergoing the surgery. The resultant overall endocrine dysfunction underscores the gravity of ongoing surveillance and potential dietary modification. Additionally, the impact on exocrine function can be observed as steatorrhea, which takes a significant quality of life impact on patients. The surgical treatment of pancreatic ailments therefore, must consider such long-term health implications, aiming to educate and ready patients for the way of life changes that will allow proper management of their diseases, as emphasized through a comprehensive study of pancreatic trauma and surgical treatment (Krige, 2017). Drainage of pseudocysts and necrosis carries significant long-term effects on the health of patients, particularly in the management of complications related to pancreatic fluid collections. While such procedures are at times less invasive compared to resections, they still carry risks for chronic diseases. The patient may have recurrent symptoms of abdominal pain and potential infection or pseudocyst recurrence, requiring ongoing medical treatment. Further, the risk of insufficiency of the pancreas is by no means trivial, impacting digestive function and leading to malabsorption syndromes. These considerations highlight the importance of customized patient education and vigorous management following drainage procedures. Systematic protocols-based evidence-based practices in long-term care, including dietary interventions and round-the-clock monitoring, are needed to optimize patients' quality of life and have them stay as fit as possible following surgical intervention, consistent with the need for systematic protocols in the management of pancreatic illness (Гончаров et al., 2023) (Figure 15.15).

A CLOSER LOOK

IMPACT OF SURGERY ON PANCREATIC DISEASE OUTCOMES

The therapy for pancreatic disease is crucial to the outcome of the patient, especially in the complexity and variability of surgery. The Whipple Procedure, widely used for pancreatic tumor treatment, illustrates the delicate balance between curative potential and severe postoperative complications. The more precise surgical methods become, the greater the impact on patient recovery and survival rate. This complex interplay highlights the necessity for surgeons to enforce rigorous data-based protocols, as highlighted by Krige (2017), whereby refinements to the limitations in pancreatic injury evaluations can have an impact on improved surgical strategies and results. Lastly, operating success is not solely dependent on technique but also on a deep acquaintance with each patient's individual physiological context.

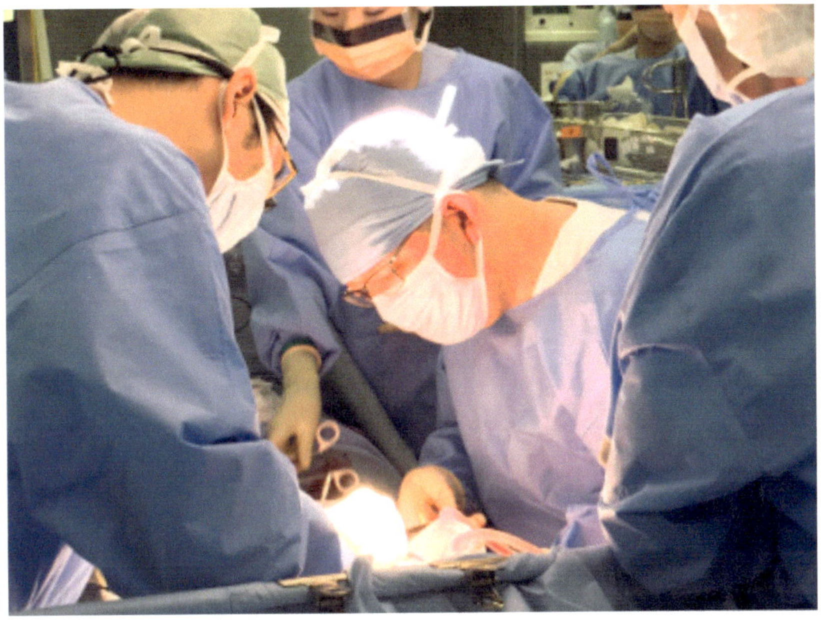

Source: https://external-content.duckduckgo.com/iu/?u=https%3A%2F%2Fwww.h.u-tokyo.ac.jp%2Fenglish%2Fcenters-services%2Fclinical-divisions%2Fhepatobiliary-and-pancreatic-surgery%2F_icsFiles%2Fafieldfile%2F2022%2F02%2F25%2FHPSurgery1.jpg&f=1&nofb=1&ipt=276360b68e74e6070dc29eeda25bc9fac239aebf3ce97ab6cdcf58599bf8ce1b.

Moreover, the complications of pancreatectomy pancreatic disease have a significant effect on patient quality of life and postoperative courses. Pancreatitis, sepsis, and gastrointestinal dysfunction following surgery are factors that come to illustrate the significance of precise preoperative assessment and postoperative care. Drainage of pseudocysts, for instance, should be undertaken with caution not to complicate secondary to associated pancreatic pathology. The data presented in recent literature indicates a greater focus on minimally invasive techniques, which can reduce recovery and complications. Thus, analyzing the long-term outcomes of various surgical interventions is critical to maximizing surgical approaches in the management of pancreatic disease. Overall, the success of operations in pancreatic disease is based on a vast number of factors that range from the specific surgical procedure employed to to patients' overall health status. As more collaborative research is conducted in the field, the advancement of postoperative care and surgical techniques represents a commitment towards bettering patient outcomes. The exploration of unresolved questions surrounding pancreatic injuries discloses a new paradigm in the management of patients that centers on data generation and evaluation, as emphasized in Krige (2017). And thus, as awareness of pancreatic disease intricacies expands, so does the likelihood that surgery not merely addresses immediate requirements but also improves the quality and longevity of survival among patients with such challenging diseases (Fisher, 2022) (Figure 15.16).

SUMMARY

A review of complications relating to surgical intervention in pancreatic conditions indicates that surgeries such as the Whipple procedure, distal pancreatectomy, and pseudocyst drainage procedures are significant advances in surgical treatment. These surgeries not only hold significance for the resection of malignant tissue but also for the decompression of pancreatitis complications. The heterogeneity of these surgical techniques encapsulates the intricacy of pancreatic diseases and underscores the importance of individualized surgical strategy. More efficacious data are required, as thought in more recent articles, to enhance better assessment of pancreatic injuries and better surgical techniques in a bid to enable better patient outcomes and reduce morbidity rates across various pancreatic diseases (Krigc, 2017). Apart from this, research on post-surgical complications is most significant. Side effects generally afflict patients after pancreas operations, which include bleeding, infection, and gastrointestinal malfunction. It is imperative to be aware of such complications to improve surgical operations and patient care. Research on such side effects must involve revolutionary imaging techniques and early intervention strategies, as highlighted by recent studies. These strategies can potentially prevent complications preoperatively and improve the success rates of the aforementioned surgeries overall. Effective complication control is not just dependent on proper post-operative care but also on active assessment of patient-specific risk factors for the aim of optimizing recovery and optimizing surgical results (Johnson et al., 2006). In conclusion, surgical management of pancreatic disorders is a key component of overall patient care. They emphasize the integration of surgical innovation and patient care, with emphasis placed on the need for a multi-faceted awareness of potential complications that can arise post-surgery. The use of newer imaging modalities can significantly help in early detection and management of complications, leading to better patient outcomes. With progressive field development, ongoing research is essential to help evolve best practices and improve surgical techniques. The emphasis should still be on improving surgical procedures that center on patient safety and overall well-being, which is a sign of devotion towards improving care in pancreatic disorders (Krige, 2017).

Surgical intervention of pancreatic pathologies comprises an array of surgeries, each tailored to a specific pathological status. The Whipple procedure or pancreaticoduodenectomy, is unique in its complexity and applies principally to the treatment of pancreatic cancer or tumor invasion into the head of the pancreas. Such a significant procedure involves resection of the duodenum, gallbladder, common bile duct, and a segment of the pancreas with intricate reconstruction. Distal pancreatectomy, however, is restricted to those lesions within the tail of the pancreas and represents a less invasive option with satisfactory results when resection of the tumor can be achieved. Other techniques, such as drainage procedures for pancreatic pseudocysts and necrosis, are aimed at complications of pancreatitis and illustrate the variety of surgical techniques employed in this area. Each method, either simple or complex, requires a careful selection of patients to ensure the best surgical outcomes and prevent morbidity. Postoperative complications are still an important issue in treating pancreatic diseases, which have a great effect on recovery and long-term outcome of the patient. Among the most common complications are pancreatic leaks and infections, which can develop due to the biological nature of the pancreas and its secretory function. Such complications are typically in need of further intervention in the form of drainage procedures and imaging studies in order to properly treat concomitant symptoms. Monitoring strategies for patients must be rigid, since early complication detection has a significant effect on outcomes.

Furthermore, evidence points toward the increasing prevalence of visceral artery aneurysm in the context of pancreatic surgery and the need for information regarding their likelihood to rupture and for adjunctive treatment modalities like trans-catheter embolization. The post-operative environment is complex and necessitates a multidisciplinary approach to enable proper care of the patient, underlining the significance of consistency in surgical practice in high-risk environments (Johnson et al., 2006). Advances in surgical intervention and postoperative care continue to characterize the discipline of pancreatic surgery, underlining evidence-based interventions that enhance patient outcomes. Detailed scrutiny of surgery data enhances understanding of specific risks and advantages associated with procedures like the Whipple and distal pancreatectomy, especially regarding trauma or pancreatitis treatment. According to existing studies, application of granular information collected from diverse patient groups has been highly beneficial in the development of standard care guidelines, emphasizing the call for urgency as well as accuracy in surgical practice (Krige, 2017). Advanced imaging techniques and diagnostic tests contribute to accurate assessments, thus directing surgical interventions and even reducing complications. In most instances, the coming together of scientific investigation and clinical practice tends to lead to improved management plans for pancreatic pathology, eventually dictating the importance of surgical intervention within this complex area.

KEY TERMS FROM THIS CHAPTER

- Biliary obstruction
- Comprehensive treatment
- Endocrine deficiency
- Enhanced Recovery After Surgery (ERAS)
- Fluid accumulation
- Gastric emptying
- Biliary system
- Distal pancreatectomy
- Endoscopic examinations
- Fat digestion
- Gallbladder
- Hormone synthesis

References

1. Barge, J. U., & Lopera, J. E. (2012). Vascular complications of pancreatitis: role of interventional therapy. *Korean journal of radiology, 13 Suppl 1*(Suppl 1), S45–S55. https://doi.org/10.3348/kjr.2012.13.S1.S45
2. Akhaladze, G. G., Akhmedov, S. M., Baymakhanov, B. B., Buriev, I. M., Vetshev, P. S., Vetshev, S. P., Gautier, S. V., et al. (2014). *Annals of Surgical Hepatology* (Vol. 19, No. 4). http://www.hepatoassociation.ru/journal (accessed on 26 May 2025).
3. El-Badry, A., Mahmoud, A., Ali, M. (2022). Enucleation Versus Standard Pancreatic Resection for Benign Lesions and Borderline Tumors: A Comparative Study. The Egyptian Journal of Hospital Medicine, 86(1), 486-492. doi: 10.21608/ejhm.2022.213801 (accessed on 26 May 2025).
4. Anand, V. (2018). *Chronic Pancreatitis and Its Management in Thanjavur Medical College Hospital*. https://core.ac.uk/download/pdf/235668720.pdf (accessed on 26 May 2025).
5. Ansorge, Christoph (2013). Pancreatic fistula following pancreaticoduodenectomy : risk assessment and early diagnosis. Karolinska Institutet. Thesis. https://hdl.handle.net/10616/41552 (accessed on 26 May 2025).
6. Bank, S., Louw, J. H., & Marks, I. N. (2018). *The Role of Surgery in The Management of Pancreatitis*. https://core.ac.uk/download/478314830.pdf (accessed on 26 May 2025).
7. Beger, H. G., Warshaw, A. L., Hruban, R. H., Büchler, M. W., Lerch, M. M., Neoptolemos, J. P., Shimosegawa, T., et al. (2018). *Index*. In *Pancreas*. https://doi.org/10.1002/9781119188421.index.
8. Bornman, P. C., Botha, J. F., Ramos, J. M., Smith, M. D., Van der Merwe, S., Watermeyer, G. A., & Ziady, C. C. (2010). Guideline for the diagnosis and treatment of chronic pancreatitis. *South African medical journal = Suid-Afrikaanse tydskrif vir geneeskunde, 100*(12 Pt 2), 845–860. https://doi.org/10.7196/samj.4530 (accessed on 26 May 2025).
9. Ho, C. K., Kleeff, J., Friess, H., & Büchler, M. W. (2005). Complications of pancreatic surgery. *HPB : the official journal of the International Hepato Pancreato Biliary Association, 7*(2), 99–108. https://doi.org/10.1080/13651820510028936
10. Gurusamy, K. S., Lusuku, C., Halkias, C., & Davidson, B. R. (2016). Duodenum-preserving pancreatic resection versus pancreaticoduodenectomy for chronic pancreatitis. *The Cochrane database of systematic reviews, 2*(2), CD011521. https://doi.org/10.1002/14651858.CD011521.pub2 (accessed on 26 May 2025).
11. Fisher, Natalie E., "Enriching the Perioperative Enhanced Recovery After Surgery (ERAS) Program for Patients Undergoing Whipple Procedure for Pancreatic Cancer" (2022). Doctor of Nursing Practice Final Manuscripts. 198. https://digital.sandiego.edu/dnp/198 (accessed on 26 May 2025).
12. Vladimirov, B., Getzov, P., & Ivanova, R. (2015). Endoscopic Treatment of Pancreatic Diseases. InTech. doi: 10.5772/60589 (accessed on 26 May 2025).
13. Johnson, M. (2006). *Management Options in Visceral Artery Pseudoaneurysms–A Critical Analysis at A Tertiary Care Referral Center*. https://core.ac.uk/download/235656426.pdf (accessed on 26 May 2025).

14. Krige, J. 2017. A prospective evaluation to define optimal surgical strategies in the management of complex pancreatic injuries based on the analysis of patients treated at a major South African academic institution. University of Cape Town.Swartz, David Keith, Obando, Jorge, Endoscopic Management of Peri-Pancreatic Collections, *Gastroenterology Research and Practice*, 2012, 906381, 7 pages, 2012. **https://doi.org/10.1155/2012/906381**

15. Rajkumar, R. (2014). *Analysis of Presentation, Management and Outcome of Chronic Calcific Pancreatitis in A Tertiary Care Center*. https://core.ac.uk/download/235656398.pdf (accessed on 26 May 2025).

16. Salim, A. S. (1997). *Perspectives in Pancreatic Pain*. https://core.ac.uk/download/pdf/8088439.pdf.

17. Saravana Bhoopathi, P. (2009). *Impact of Intraoperative Ultrasonogram (IOUS) in Drainage Surgery for Chronic Pancreatitis*. https://core.ac.uk/download/235655049.pdf (accessed on 26 May 2025).

18. Sivakumar, G. (2015). *Comparative Study of Drainage Procedures in The Management of Chronic Pancreatitis in Government Mohan Kumara Mangalam Medical College, Salem*. Dissertation submitted to THE TAMIL NADU DR. MGR. MEDICAL UNIVERSITY CHENNAI – 600 032 In partial fulfillment of the regulations For the awards of the degree of M.S. DEGREE BRANCH – I. https://core.ac.uk/download/235656756.pdf (accessed on 26 May 2025).

19. Sivasankar, A. (2006). *Outcome of Surgery for Chronic Calcific Pancreatitis*. https://core.ac.uk/download/235656428.pdf (accessed on 26 May 2025).

20. Yu, Z. (2020). Solid pseudopapillary neoplasm of the pancreas: Clinical-radiological-pathological characteristics of four pediatric cases. *Gastroenterology Pancreatology and Hepatobiliary Disorders*, *4*, 1–7. https://doi.org/10.31579/2641-5194/011.

21. Гончаров, А. С., Гончарова, Н. М., Нессонова, М. М., Тесленко, А. В., et al. (2023). Кістозні пухлини підшлункової залози: діагностика та хірургічне лікування [Cystic tumors of the pancreas: Diagnosis and surgical treatment]. https://core.ac.uk/download/570906284.pdf (accessed on 26 May 2025).

INDEX

C

F

G

H

I

K

L

M

N

Q

R

S